Laboratory Manual for Clinical Anatomy and Physiology for Veterinary Technicians

Laboratory Manual for Clinical Anatomy and Physiology for Veterinary Technicians

Fourth Edition

Thomas Colville, DVM, MSc

Attending Veterinarian
Red River Zoo
Fargo, North Dakota

Joanna M. Bassert, AB, VMD

Professor Emeritus
Program of Veterinary Technology
Manor College
Jenkintown, Pennsylvania

Prepared by:

Sherry Castle Boyer, BSDH, MS
Creative Director
Educational Development
Castle Media Consultants, LLC
Huntsville, Alabama

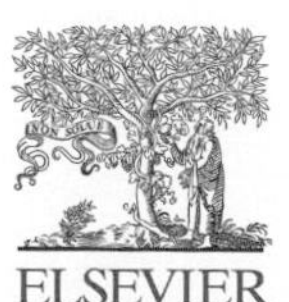

ELSEVIER

Elsevier
3251 Riverport Lane
St. Louis, Missouri 63043

LABORATORY MANUAL FOR CLINICAL ANATOMY AND PHYSIOLOGY
FOR VETERINARY TECHNICIANS, FOURTH EDITION

ISBN: 978-0-323-79342-1

Content Strategist: Melissa Rawe
Senior Content Development Specialist: Tina Kaemmerer
Publishing Services Manager: Deepthi Unni
Senior Project Manager: Thoufiq Mohammed
Design Direction: Amy Buxton

Printed in India

Last digit is the print number: 9 8 7 6 5 4 3 2 1

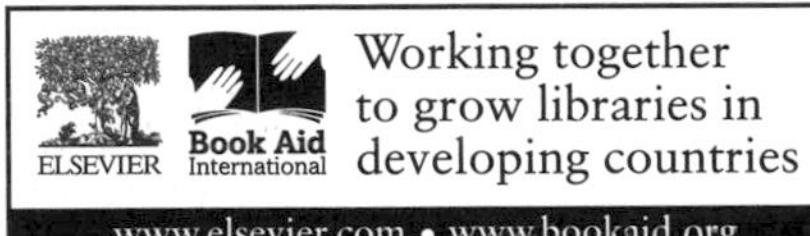

Preface

Holding, touching, and exploring the many organs and tissues that compose an animal's body can be an amazing experience. A remarkable organ such as the heart suddenly becomes real. The chambers, valves, and blood vessels discussed in lecture are there in your hands. As you probe the intricacies of this marvelous pump in the laboratory, a new level of understanding is acquired, one that can only be achieved through direct contact with the animal. The importance of hands-on learning in anatomy is what inspired the development of this laboratory manual. It has been specifically designed to accompany and complement the *Clinical Anatomy and Physiology for Veterinary Technicians*, Fourth Edition textbook, by helping readers to become conversant in the language of anatomy and physiology, to visualize important anatomic structures, and to understand key physiological concepts through an assortment of activities and exercises.

Key Features

- Overview at a Glance section in each chapter outlines the main proficiencies of each chapter and includes a list of all of the exercises in the chapter
- Concise summaries of important anatomy and physiology concepts
- Learning objectives for each chapter, including lists of structures to be identified
- An assortment of clinically oriented learning exercises to help readers become familiar with the language of anatomy and physiology as they identify structures and learn concepts
- Clear step-by-step dissection instructions for complex organs such as the heart
- Hundreds of full-color photographs and illustrations
- Suggestions for additional in-class learning activities
- Review questions and study exercises
- Detailed glossary

Evolve Online Resources

Student Resources

Student resources include Test Yourself Answers and Review Questions.

Instructor Resources

Instructor resources include a 1000-question test bank in ExamView format with rationales. Two image collections are included: one with all figures from the textbook, the second with all figures from the Laboratory Manual. A Power Point collection is arranged chapter by chapter with the textbook. The answers to the Laboratory Manual are available. Instructors also have access to all student resources. With the text, lab manual, and online student and instructor resources, we hope that the study of the animal body will come alive.

Contents

1 **Anatomical Terms, 1**
Anatomic Planes, 2
Directional Terms, 3
Left and Right, 3
Cranial, Caudal, and Rostral, 3
Dorsal and Ventral, 3
Medial and Lateral, 3
Deep and Superficial, 4
Proximal and Distal, 4
Limbs—Cranial, Caudal, Dorsal, Palmar, and Plantar Surfaces, 4
Common Regional Terms, 4
General Body Position Terms, 4
Dorsal, Sternal, and Lateral Recumbency, 4
Oblique Positions, 4
Dental Terms, 4
Dental Arch, Dental Arcade, Quadrant, 6
Incisor, Canine, Premolar, and Molar Teeth, 6
Crown and Root, 6
Mesial and Distal, 7
Buccal, Palatal, Labial, and Lingual Surfaces, 8
Coronal, Apical, and Gingival, 8
Incisal Edge and Occlusal Surface, 9
Interproximal Spaces and Surfaces, 9
Furcation, 9

Exercises, 9
Anatomic, Common, and Position Terms, 9
Dental Terms, 15
Critical and Clinical Thinking, 18

2 **Microscopy, 20**
Identification of Parts of the Microscope, 21
Oculars (Eyepieces), 21
Objective Lenses, 23
Degree of Magnification, 24
Parfocal, 24
Resolving Power (Resolution), 24
Working Distance, 24
Arm and Base, 24
Light Source, 24
Rheostat for Light Source, 24
Condenser, 24
Iris (Aperture) Diaphragm, 24
Coarse and Fine Adjustment, 25
Stage and Stage Brackets or Clips, 25
Care of the Microscope, 25
Putting the Microscope Away, 25

Exercises, 26
Parts of the Microscope, 26
Use of the Compound Microscope, 27
Critical and Clinical Thinking, 32

3 **Cell Anatomy, 34**
The Anatomy of the Cell, 35
Plasma Membrane, 35
Nucleus, 37
Cytoplasm: Cytosol, Cytoskeleton, and Organelles, 38
Stages of Cell Division, 42
Interphase, 42
The Stages of Mitosis, 43
Prophase, 43
Metaphase, 43
Anaphase, 44
Telophase, 44
Cytokinesis, 44
Cell Division in Sex Cells (Meiosis), 44

Exercises, 44
Cell Anatomy, 44
Cellular Microscopy, 46
Cell Division, 49
Fluid Therapy, 52
Critical and Clinical Thinking, 53

4 **Exploring Tissues, 54**
Identification of tissues, 55

Exercises, 55
Epithelial Tissue, 55
Connective Tissue, 58
Muscle Tissue, 59
Nervous Tissue, 60
Critical and Clinical Thinking, 60

5 **The Integumentary System, 70**
The Layers of the Integument, 71
Layers of the Epidermis, 71
Epidermis of the Nose and Paw Pads, 72
Ergots and Chestnuts, 74
Special Features of the Integument, 76

Identify the Structures Associated with the Dermis, 76
Structure of Hair, 78
Associated Structures, 80
Structure of Canine and Feline Claws, 80
Inspect the Retractable Nails of the Cadaver, 80
The Equine Foot, 80
The Skeleton, 82
The Corium, 82
The Hoof, 82
The Bovine Horn, 82

Exercises, 84
Layers of the Integument, 84
Special Features of the Integument, 86
Hair, 88
Assorted Structures, 90
Critical and Clinical Thinking, 93

6 The Skeletal System, 97
The Skeletal System, 99
Types of Bone, 99
Bone Shapes, 99
Long Bones, 99
Short Bones, 99
Flat Bones, 99
Irregular Bones, 101
Common Bone Features (Lumps, Bumps, Grooves, and Holes), 101
Articular Surfaces, 101
Condyles, 101
Head, 105
Facet, 105
Processes, 105
Holes and Depressed Areas, 105
The Skeleton, 112
Axial Skeleton, 112
Skull, 112
External Bones of the Cranium, 113
External Bones of the Face, 113
Internal Bones of the Face, 118
Hyoid Bone, 118
Spinal Column, 118
Ribs, 120
Sternum, 120
Appendicular Skeleton, 120
Thoracic Limb, 120
Pelvic Limb, 126
Joints, 130
Fibrous Joints, 130
Cartilaginous Joints, 130
Synovial Joints, 130

Suggested in-class activities, 132
Bone Shapes and Features, 132
Bone Shape and Feature Identification, 132
Bone Shape and Feature Hunt, 132
The Axial Skeleton, 132
Skull Bone Identification, 132
Live Animal Palpation, 132
Skull Bone Hunt, 133
Vertebral Process Identification, 133
Axial Assembly, 133
Radiographic Identification, 133
Live Animal Palpation, 133
The Appendicular Skeleton, 133
Appendicular Limb Assembly, 133
Radiographic Identification, 133
Live Animal Palpation, 133
Animals in Motion, 133
Appendicular Bone Hunt, 133

Exercises, 134
The Skeletal System, 134
The Skeleton, 137
Joints, 143
Critical and Clinical Thinking, 144

7 The Muscular System, 148
Laboratory I, 149
Extrinsic Muscles of the Thoracic Limb and Related Areas, 149
Items to Be Identified, 149
Muscles, 149
Terms, 149
Getting Started, 149
Dissection of the Musculature, 151
Extrinsic Muscles of the Thoracic Limb, 152
Superficial Pectoral Muscle, 152
Deep Pectoral Muscle, 153
Brachiocephalicus Muscle, 153
Omotransversarius Muscle, 155
Trapezius Muscle, 155
Rhomboideus Muscle, 155
Latissimus Dorsi Muscle, 155
Serratus Ventralis Muscle, 155
Question, 155
Muscles of the Neck and Head, 155
Sternocephalicus Muscle, 155
Platysma Muscle, 156
Muscles of Mastication, 157
Temporalis Muscle, 157
Masseter Muscle, 157
Digastricus Muscle, 157
Mylohyoideus Muscle, 158
Suggested In-Class Activity, 158
Live Animal, 158

Laboratory II, 159
Intrinsic Muscles of the Thoracic Limb, 159
Lateral Muscles of the Scapula and Shoulder, 161
Deltoideus Muscle, 161
Infraspinatus Muscle, 161
Supraspinatus Muscle, 162
Medial Muscles of the Shoulder, 162
Subscapularis Muscle, 162
Teres Major Muscle, 162

Cranial Muscles of the Foreleg, 162
Biceps Brachii Muscle, 162
Brachialis Muscle, 162
Caudal Muscles of the Foreleg, 162
Triceps Brachii Muscle, 162
Craniolateral Muscles of the Foreleg, 163
Brachioradialis Muscle, 163
Extensor Carpi Radialis Muscle, 165
Common Digital Extensor Muscle, 166
Lateral Digital Extensor Muscle, 167
Extensor Carpi Ulnaris (Formerly Ulnaris Lateralis), 167
Abductor Pollicis Longus Muscle, 167
Caudomedial Muscles of the Foreleg, 167
Flexor Carpi Radialis Muscle, 167
Flexor Carpi Ulnaris Muscle, 167
Superficial Digital Flexor Muscle, 167
Deep Digital Flexor Muscle, 167
Muscles of the Forefoot (Manus), 173
Suggested In-Class Activity, 173
Live Animal, 173

Laboratory III, 173
Muscles of the Pelvic Limb, 173
To Be Identified, 174
Muscles, 174
Structures, 175
Terms, 175
Dissection of the Musculature, 176
Lateral Muscles of the Hip, 176
Tensor Fasciae Latae, 176
Superficial Gluteal Muscle, 177
Middle Gluteal Muscle, 177
Deep Gluteal Muscle, 178
Caudal Muscles of the Thigh, 178
Biceps Femoris Muscle, 178
Semitendinosus Muscle, 179
Semimembranosus Muscle, 179
Medial Muscles of the Thigh, 181
Sartorius Muscle, 181
Gracilis Muscle, 181
Pectineus Muscle, 182
Adductor Muscle, 182
Cranial Muscles of the Thigh, 182
Quadriceps Femoris Muscle, 182
Craniolateral Muscles of the Hind Leg, 182
Cranial Tibial Muscle, 182
Long Digital Extensor Muscle, 182
Peroneus Longus Muscle, 182
Caudal Muscles of the Hind Leg, 182
Gastrocnemius Muscle, 182
Superficial Digital Flexor Muscle, 187
Deep Digital Flexor Muscle, 188
Popliteus Muscle, 189
Common Calcanean Tendon, 189
Muscles of the Rear Foot (PES), 189
Muscles of the Abdominal Wall, 189
External Abdominal Oblique, 190
Internal Abdominal Oblique, 190
Transversus Abdominis, 191
Rectus Abdominis, 191

Exercises, 192
Laboratory I: Extrinsic Muscles of the Thoracic Limb and Related Areas, 192
Laboratory II: Intrinsic Muscles of the Thoracic Limb, 194
Laboratory III: Muscles of the Pelvic Limb and Abdominal Wall, 199
Critical and Clinical Thinking, 203

8 The Nervous System, 204
The Brain, 205
External Structures of the Cerebrum, 207
External Structures of the Cerebellum, 207
Cranial Nerves, 209
Internal Structures of the Cerebrum and Cerebellum, 210
External Structures of the Diencephalon, 211
Internal Structures of the Diencephalon, 212
External Structures of the Brainstem, 213
Gray Matter and White Matter in the Brain, 214
The Spinal Cord, 215
The Meninges, 216
Peripheral Nerves of Clinical Importance, 217
Facial Nerve, 217
Vagus Nerve, 218
Brachial Plexus, Radial Nerve, Median Nerve, and Ulnar Nerve, 219
Cat Declaw Nerves, 220
Femoral Nerve, 220
Sciatic Nerve, 221

Exercises, 222
The Brain, 222
Peripheral Nerves of Clinical Importance, 225
Critical and Clinical Thinking, 228

9 Sense Organs, 232
Pain, 233
Taste, 233
Smell, 235
Hearing, 235
External Ear, 235
Middle Ear, 235
Inner Ear, 236
Equilibrium, 236
Vestibule, 236
Semicircular Canals, 237
Vision, 237
The Outer Fibrous Layer of the Eye, 237
The Middle Vascular Layer, 238
Iris, 238
Ciliary Body, 238
Lens, 238
Choroid, 238

The Inner Nervous Layer (Retina), 241
Optic Disc, 242
Optic Nerve, 242
Optic Chiasm, 242
Compartments of the Eye, 244
Eyelids and Conjunctiva, 244
Third Eyelid (Nictitating Membrane), 246
External Eye-Related Landmarks, 246
Extraocular Muscles, 246
Suggested In-Class Activities, 247
Dissection of a Sheep's Eye, 247
Materials Needed, 247
Gaze into Another's Eyes, 249
Materials Needed, 249
Clinical Significance, 249
Take a Trip Into the Depths of the Ear Canal, 249
Materials Needed, 249
Clinical Significance, 249
Witness the Amazing Nasolacrimal Ducts, 249
Materials Needed, 249
Clinical Significance, 249

Exercises, 250
Pain, 250
Hearing, 250
Vision, 251
Critical and Clinical Thinking, 256

10 The Endocrine System, 261
Control of Hormone Secretion, 262
Hypothalamus and Pituitary Gland, 262
In-class Activity, 262
Anatomy, 262
Hormone Physiology, 265
Hypothalamus, 265
Anterior Pituitary Gland, 265
Posterior Pituitary Gland, 265
Thyroid Gland, 265
In-class Activity, 265
Anatomy and Histology, 265
Hormone Physiology, 265
Clinical Applications, 265
Parathyroid Gland, 268
In-class Activity, 268
Anatomy and Histology, 268
Hormone Physiology, 268
Parathyroid Hormone, 268
Vitamin D, 268
Calcitonin, 268
Clinical Applications, 268
Equine Secondary Nutritional Hyperparathyroidism, 268
Adrenal Gland, 270
In-class Activity, 270
Anatomy and Histology, 270
Hormone Physiology, 270
Clinical Applications, 270
Hyperadrenocorticism in Domestic Animals, 270
Endocrine Pancreas, 270
In-class Activity, 270
Anatomy and Histology, 270
Hormone Physiology, 273
Clinical Applications, 273
The Gonads, 273
Other Endocrine Tissues, 273

Exercises, 273
Control of Hormone Secretion, 273
Hypothalamus and Pituitary Gland, 274
Thyroid Gland, 275
Parathyroid Gland, 278
Adrenal Gland, 279
Endocrine Pancreas, 281
Other Endocrine Tissues, 282

11 Blood, Lymph, and Lymph Nodes, 285
The CBC: A Veterinary Technician's Responsibilities, 286
The Blood Smear, 287
Hematology Stains, 287
Transfusions, 288
Blood Types or Groups, 290
Crossmatch Testing, 291
Immunoassays, 291

Exercises, 293
The CBC: A Veterinary Technician's Responsibilities, 293
The Blood Smear, 294
Hematology Stains, 295
Transfusions: Blood Types or Groups, 296
Transfusions: Crossmatch Testing, 297
Immunoassays, 297

12 The Cardiovascular System, 299
Basic Blood Flow Through the Cardiovascular System, 300
Helpful Heart Hints: Finding Your Way on the Outside of the Heart, 300
Helpful Heart Hints: Making Sense of the Inside of the Heart, 302
Important Blood Vessels of the Neck and Thoracic Cavity, 303
Important Blood Vessels of the Thoracic Limb, 308
Important Blood Vessels in the Abdominal Cavity, 309
Important Blood Vessels of the Pelvic Limb, 312
Suggested In-Class Activities, 315
Materials for Suggested In-Class Activities, 315
Trace the Flow of Blood Through the Heart, 315
Palpate Common Venipuncture Sites, 315
Auscultate (Listen to) the Heart, 315
Palpate Pulse Points, 315
Peek Inside the Living Chest, 315

Dissection of a Sheep Heart, 315
Materials Needed, 315
Procedure, 315
Trace the Flow of Blood Through the Heart, 317
Materials Needed, 317
Procedure, 317
Clinical Significance, 318
Palpate Common Venipuncture Sites, 318
Materials Needed, 318
Procedure, 318
Clinical Significance, 318
Auscultate (Listen to) the Heart, 318
Materials Needed, 318
Procedure, 318
Clinical Significance, 319
Palpate Pulse Points, 319
Materials Needed, 319
Procedure, 319
Clinical Significance, 319
Peek Inside the Living Chest, 319
Materials Needed, 319
Procedure, 319
Clinical Significance, 319

Exercises, 320
Basic Blood Flow Through the Cardiovascular System, 320
Critical and Clinical Thinking, 328

13 The Respiratory System, 334
Respiratory Revelations: Structures of the Upper Respiratory Tract in the Skull, 335
Respiratory Revelations: The Larynx, 338
Respiratory Revelations: The Trachea, 340
Respiratory Revelations: Structures of the Lower Respiratory Tract in the Thoracic Cavity, 342
Suggested In-class Activities, 347
Watch the Nares on Live Animals, 347
Materials Needed, 347
Procedure, 347
Clinical Significance, 347
Palpate the Neck of an Animal, 347
Materials Needed, 347
Procedure, 347
Clinical Significance, 347
Auscultate (Listen to) the Breath Sounds and Lungs, 347
Materials Needed, 347
Procedure, 347
Clinical Significance, 348
Peek Inside the Living Animal, 348
Materials Needed, 348
Procedure, 348
Clinical Significance, 348

Exercises, 349
The Skull and Neck, 349
The Larynx and Trachea, 350
Structures of the Lower Respiratory Tract in the Thoracic Cavity, 351
Critical and Clinical Thinking, 356

14 The Digestive System, 364
Salivary Glands, 366
The Oral Cavity, 367
Tooth Structure, 368
Types of Teeth, 368
In-class Activity, 369
The Esophagus and Stomach, 369
Dissection of the Esophagus and Stomach, 369
The Monogastric Stomach, 370
The Ruminant Stomach, 370
The Intestinal Tract, 373
Small Intestine, 373
Dissection of the Small Intestine, 374
Large Intestine, 375
Digestion-Related Organs, 379
Liver, 379
Pancreas, 379

Exercises, 379
The Oral Cavity, 379
Dental Formulas, 381
The Esophagus and Stomach, 382
The Intestinal Tract, 385
Digestion-Related Organs, 387
Review of Digestive Anatomy, 390
Review, 394
Critical and Clinical Thinking, 396

15 The Urinary System, 399
Blood Flow to and From the Kidneys, 400
Nephron Notables, 401
Urinary System Location, 401
Kidney, 402
External Kidney Features, 402
Internal Kidney Features, 403
Ureters, 405
Urinary Bladder, 406
Urethra, 407
The Urinary System on Radiographs, 408
Suggested In-Class Activities, 409
Palpate the Urinary Bladder of an Animal, 409
Materials Needed, 409
Clinical Significance, 409
Peek Inside the Living Animal, 409
Materials Needed, 409
Clinical Significance, 409

Exercises, 409
Blood Flow to and from the Kidneys, 409
Nephron Notables, 410
Urinary System Location, 411

Kidney—External, 414
Kidney—Internal, 415
Clinical and Critical Thinking, 416

16 The Reproductive System, 421
The Male Reproductive System, 422
The Scrotum, 422
The Testes, 422
Vaginal Tunics and Testis Capsule, 424
Epididymis, 424
Vas Deferens, 425
Spermatic Cord, 425
The Urethra, 427
The Accessory Reproductive Glands, 427
The Penis, 428
The Prepuce, 429
The Os Penis, 429
The Bulb of the Glans, 429
The Sigmoid Flexure, 431
The Female Reproductive System, 431
The Ovaries, 431
The Oviducts, 433
The Uterus, 433
Suspensory Ligaments, 434
The Cervix, 434
The Vagina, 436
The Vulva, 436
The Placenta, 437

Exercises, 440
Male Reproductive System, 440
Female Reproductive System, 444
Critical and Clinical Thinking, 445

17 Pregnancy, Development, and Lactation, 450
Pregnancy, 451
The Ovaries, 451
The Uterus, 451
The Placenta, 451
Development, 452
Lactation, 452
Mammary Glands, 452
Location, 452
Microscopic Anatomy, 452
Gross Anatomy, 452
Hormones, 452
Suggested In-Class Activities, 453
Dissection Questions, 453
Bibliography, 453

Exercises, 453
Pregnancy, 453
Development, 455
Lactation, 455
Clinical and Critical Thinking, 456

18 Avian Anatomy, 458
Feather Types and Structure, 459
Skeletal Anatomy, 460
Wing Anatomy, 460
Ocular Anatomy, 460
Beak Anatomy, 460
Digestive Anatomy, 460
Cardiac Anatomy, 461
Respiratory Anatomy, 461
Reproductive Anatomy, 461
In-class Necropsy Exercise, 461
Description of Exercise, 461
Procedure, 461

Exercises, 466
Feather Types and Structure, 466
Skeletal Anatomy, 469
Wing Anatomy, 471
Ocular Anatomy, 472
Beak Anatomy, 473
Digestive Anatomy, 474
Cardiac Anatomy, 475
Respiratory Anatomy, 475
Reproductive Anatomy, 476
Critical and Clinical Thinking, 477

Glossary, 480

Index, 488

Laboratory Manual for Clinical Anatomy and Physiology for Veterinary Technicians

1 Anatomical Terms[a]

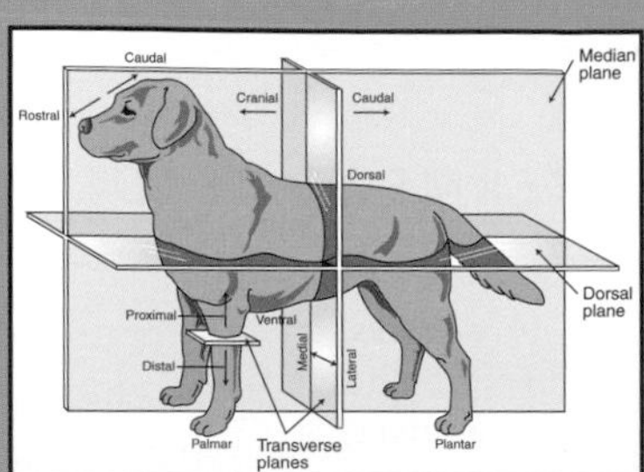

OVERVIEW AT A GLANCE

Anatomic Planes 2

Directional Terms 3

Limbs—Cranial, Caudal, Dorsal, Palmar, and Plantar Surfaces 4

Common Regional Terms 4

General Body Position Terms 4

Dental Terms 4

Exercises 9–18

Anatomic, Common, and Position Terms 9–15

1. *Write the Right Word 9*
2. *Definitions 10*
3. *Identification 11*
4. *Suggested In-Class Activities 15*

Dental Terms 15–16

5. *Write the Right Word—Definitions 15*
6. *Identification 16*

Critical and Clinical Thinking 18

7. *Clinical Thinking Challenge 18*
8. *Lab Partner Experience 18*

LEARNING OBJECTIVES

In this chapter, we will explore the descriptive language of anatomic terminology. We will cover anatomic planes, directional terms, common regional terms, general body position terms, and dental terms.

CLINICAL SIGNIFICANCE

Anatomic terminology is used daily in veterinary hospitals to facilitate communication among members of the veterinary staff. It also allows accurate information to be recorded in patients' medical records. For example, the location of a laceration or bone break, the correct position of an animal for a radiograph, or the site of a surgical incision can all be described using anatomic terminology. It is extremely important that anatomic terminology becomes part of your everyday vocabulary.

INTRODUCTION

Suppose you are an astronaut onboard the space shuttle shortly after launch, and you hear the commander tell the pilot that MECO was about to occur before SRB sep. Should you be concerned? To answer, you have to know what the terms "MECO" and "SRB sep" mean.[b] They seem as foreign to us as anatomic terminology probably seems to an astronaut or rocket scientist, yet both allow quick, accurate communication of important facts.

TERMS TO BE IDENTIFIED

Anatomic planes and directional terms
- Caudal
- Cranial
- Deep
- Distal
- Dorsal
- Dorsal plane
- Lateral
- Left
- Medial
- Median plane
- Palmar
- Plantar
- Proximal
- Right
- Rostral
- Sagittal plane
- Superficial
- Transverse plane
- Ventral

Common regional terms
- Barrel
- Brisket

[a]The authors and publisher wish to acknowledge Joann Colville and Amy Ellwein for previous contributions to this chapter.

[b]During a space shuttle launch, solid rocket booster separation (SRB sep) normally occurs about 2 minutes after launch. Shuttle main engine cut-off (MECO) does not take place until the vehicle has reached orbit nearly 8½ minutes after launch. MECO occurring before SRB sep would be a serious problem that would require an emergency landing.

TERMS TO BE IDENTIFIED—cont'd

Cannon (hoofed animals)
Fetlock (hoofed animals)
Flank
Hock
Knee (hoofed animals)
Muzzle
Pastern (hoofed animals)
Poll
Stifle
Tailhead
Withers
General body position terms
- Dorsal recumbency
- Lateral recumbency
- Oblique recumbency
- Sternal recumbency

Dental terms
- Apical
- Buccal
- Canine tooth
- Coronal
- Crown
- Dental arch
- Distal
- Furcation
- Incisal edge
- Incisor tooth
- Interproximal space
- Interproximal surface
- Labial
- Lingual
- Mesial
- Molar tooth
- Occlusal surface
- Palatal
- Premolar tooth
- Quadrant
- Root

Anatomic Planes

Anatomic planes describe imaginary slices through animal bodies (Fig. 1.1 and Box 1.1). We use them as reference points to describe positions or to indicate how a part of the body is being viewed. Each of the three basic planes is oriented at right angles to the other two. The three basic planes are the **dorsal plane,** which divides the body into dorsal (top) and ventral (bottom) parts; the **transverse plane,** which divides the body into cranial (front) and caudal (rear) parts; and the **sagittal plane,** which divides the body into left and right parts. A fourth plane, the **median plane,** is the

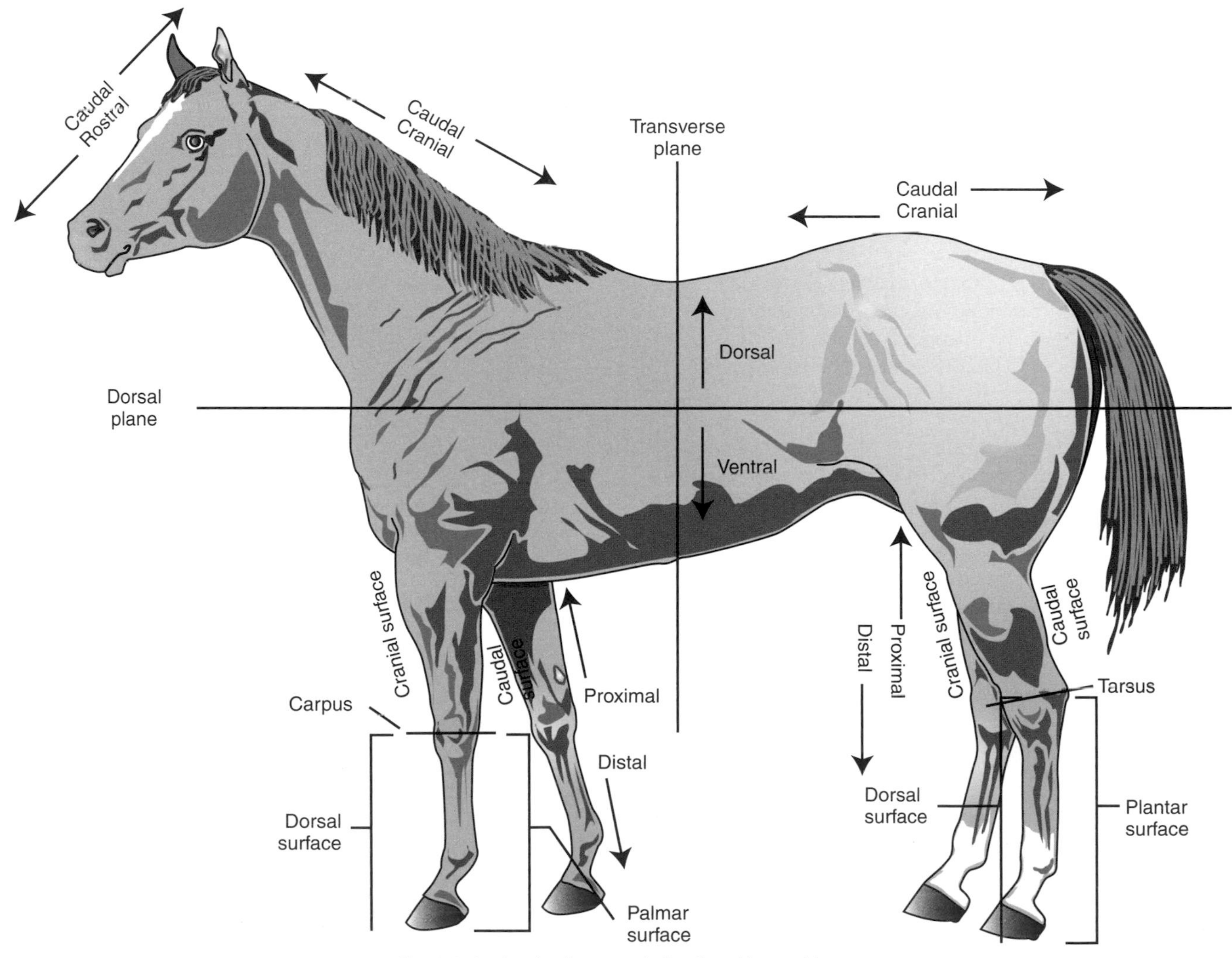

• **Fig. 1.1** Anatomic planes and directional terms. Horse.

• BOX 1.1 Anatomic Planes

Median plane Divides the body into equal left and right halves
Sagittal plane Divides the body into left and right parts that are not necessarily equal
Transverse plane Divides the body into cranial and caudal parts
Dorsal plane Divides the body into dorsal and ventral parts

sagittal plane that divides the body into equal left and right halves. It could accurately be called a midsagittal plane, but it is more commonly termed the median plane.

Directional Terms

Box 1.2 organizes directional terms into convenient pairs that mean the opposite of each other.

Left and Right

Left and **right** always refer to the animal's left and right, regardless of what direction we are viewing it from.

Cranial, Caudal, and Rostral

Cranial means toward the head (cranium), and **caudal** means toward the tail (cauda). The term "cranial" loses its meaning on the head itself, so we use the term **rostral** to mean toward the tip of the nose (rostrum). We only use the term rostral when describing directions or locations on the head.

Dorsal and Ventral

Dorsal means toward the backbone (top) surface of the body (Fig. 1.2), and **ventral** means toward the belly (bottom) surface of the body. When saddling a horse, the saddle is placed on the horse's dorsal surface, and the cinch goes down around its ventral surface to hold the saddle in place. (Note: If the cinch is not tight enough, the saddle and possibly the rider can end up on the horse's ventral surface. Ouch!)

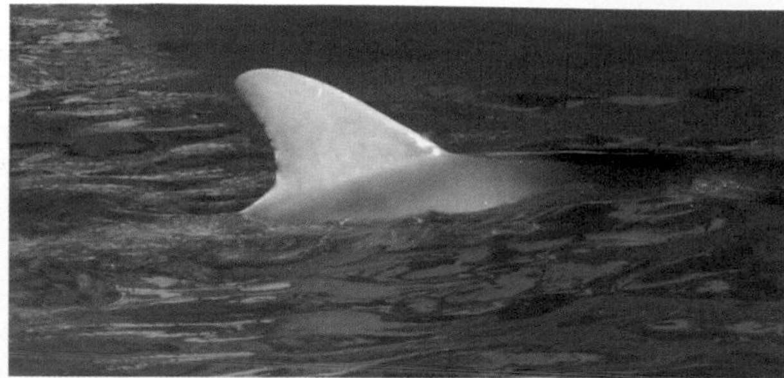

• Fig. 1.2 Dorsal fin of a porpoise.

• BOX 1.2 Directional Terms

Left The animal's left
Right The animal's right
Cranial Toward the head; also the "front" surface of a limb proximal to the carpus or tarsus
Caudal Toward the tail; also the "back" surface of a limb proximal to the carpus or tarsus
Rostral Toward the tip of the nose (used only on the head)
Dorsal Toward the top (backbone) surface of the body; also the top/front surface of a limb distal to the carpus or tarsus
Ventral Toward the bottom (belly) surface of the body
Medial Toward the median plane
Lateral Away from the median plane
Deep Toward the center of the body or a body part
Superficial Toward the surface of the body or a body part
Proximal Toward the body (used for appendages)
Distal Away from the body (used for appendages)
Palmar Ground/back surface of the front limb distal to the carpus
Plantar Ground/back surface of hindlimb distal to the tarsus

Medial and Lateral

Medial and lateral use the median plane as their reference point. **Medial** means toward the median plane, and **lateral** means away from it. The medial surface of a limb is the inside surface, and the lateral surface is the outside surface (Fig. 1.3).

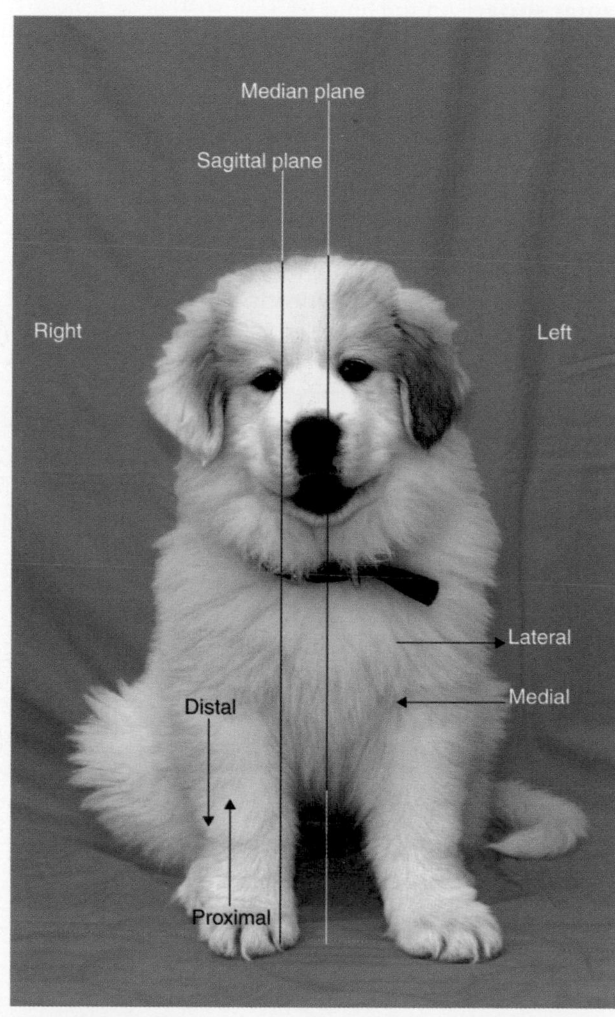

• Fig. 1.3 Anatomic planes and directional terms. Dog.

Deep and Superficial

Deep and superficial are pretty simple. **Deep** means toward the center of the body or a body part, and **superficial** means toward the surface.

Proximal and Distal

Proximal and distal are only used for appendages, such as the legs, the ears, or the tail. **Proximal** means toward the attachment of the appendage to the body, and **distal** means away from the attachment to the body (see Fig. 1.3).

Limbs—Cranial, Caudal, Dorsal, Palmar, and Plantar Surfaces

The terms for the front and back of the legs and feet get a little more complicated. Proximal to the **carpus** of the front leg and the **tarsus** of the rear leg, the "front" surface of the leg is called the **cranial surface,** and the "back" surface of the leg is the **caudal surface.** Distal to the carpus and tarsus, the area that includes the "front" of the leg and the top of the foot is called the **dorsal surface.** The area on the "back" of the limb, including the bottom of the foot, is called the **palmar surface** on the front leg and the **plantar surface** on the hind leg (Fig. 1.4).

Common Regional Terms

Common regional terms give us a shorthand way of communicating anatomic information. It is easier to refer to the "flank" than to write "the side of the abdomen between the last rib and the pelvis and hind leg." Box 1.3 gives the meanings of commonly used regional terms, including some unique to the horse and other hoofed animals (Fig. 1.5).

General Body Position Terms

General body positioning terms allow us to easily describe the position of a recumbent animal (one that is lying down) (Box 1.4). This can be useful for recording information in an animal's medical record and describing positions necessary for surgical, medical, and radiographic procedures.

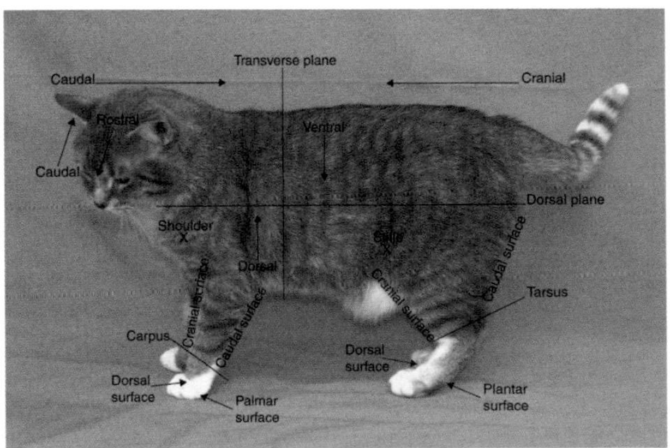

• **Fig. 1.4** Anatomic planes and directional terms. Cat.

• BOX 1.3 Common Regional Terms

Barrel Trunk of the body—formed by the rib cage and the abdomen
Flank Lateral surface of the abdomen between the last rib and the hind legs
Brisket Area at the base of the neck, between the front legs, that covers the cranial end of the sternum
Poll Top of the head between the bases of the ears
Muzzle Rostral part of the face formed mainly by the maxillary and nasal bones
Withers Area dorsal to the scapulas
Tailhead Dorsal part of the base of the tail
Hock Tarsus
Stifle Femorotibial/femoropatellar joint—equivalent to the human knee
Fetlock Joint between cannon bone (large metacarpal/metatarsal) and the proximal phalanx of hoofed animals
Knee Carpus of hoofed animals
Cannon Large metacarpal or metatarsal bone of hoofed animals
Pastern Area of the proximal phalanx of hoofed animals

Dorsal, Sternal, and Lateral Recumbency

The first word of general positioning terms tells us what body surface the animal is lying on—that is, which surface is downward. A **dorsal recumbent** animal is lying on its back (dorsal surface) with its belly facing upward (Fig. 1.6). An animal in **sternal recumbency** is the opposite. It is lying on its sternum (ventral surface) with its back facing upward (Fig. 1.7). **Lateral recumbency** describes an animal lying on its side. Adding the words "left" and "right" indicates which side the animal is lying on. An animal in the right lateral recumbency is lying with its right side down (Fig. 1.8).

Oblique Positions

Sometimes animals are positioned with their bodies tilted between true dorsal or sternal and true lateral recumbency. This is known as **oblique recumbency,** and its description requires a combination of the other position terms. For example, an animal in dorsal–left lateral oblique recumbency is lying on its back with its body tilted to the left between true dorsal recumbency and true left lateral recumbency. Oblique positions are sometimes used in radiography to prevent body structures from overlapping, as sometimes occurs in the "straight" positions.

Dental Terms

Dental terms help us describe positions and directions on individual teeth and for groups of teeth (Box 1.5). The tight, often curving arrangement of the teeth makes directional terms used for the rest of the body inadequate for describing positions and directions in dental records.

Poll
Forehead
Muzzle
Withers
Point of hip (ilium)
Barrel
Tailhead
Thigh
Shoulder
Flank
Brisket
Stifle
Elbow
Hock (tarsus)
Knee (carpus) hoofed animals
Cannon hoofed animals
Pastern hoofed animals
Fetlock hoofed animals

• **Fig. 1.5** Common regional terms. Horse.

• BOX 1.4 General Body Position Terms

Dorsal recumbency Lying on the back (dorsal body surface) with the ventral surface facing up

Lateral recumbency Lying on the side—left lateral recumbency means left side down, and right lateral recumbency means right side down

Sternal recumbency Lying on the sternum (ventral body surface) with the dorsal surface facing up

Oblique recumbency The body is tilted between dorsal or sternal recumbency and lateral recumbency; referred to by a combination of the other position terms

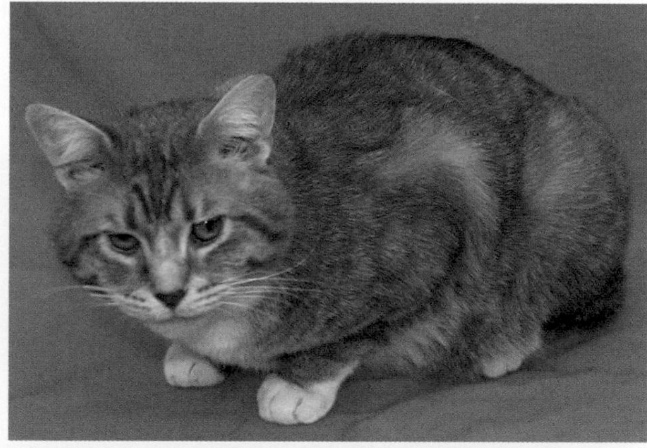

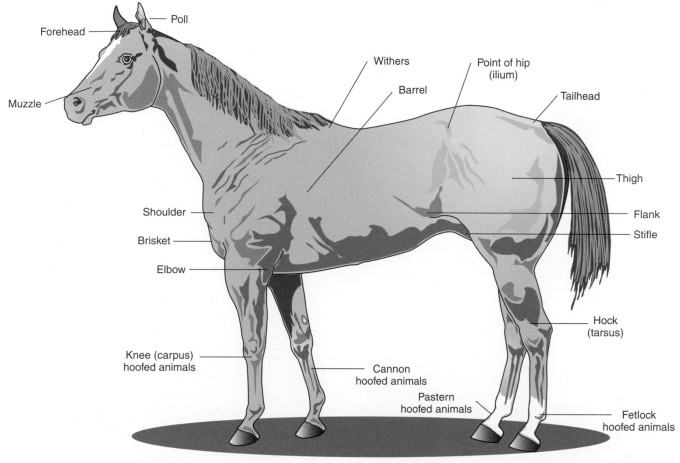

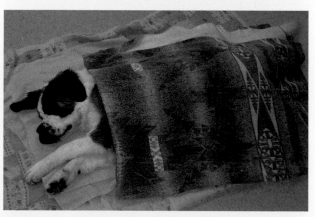

• **Fig. 1.7** Sternal recumbency.

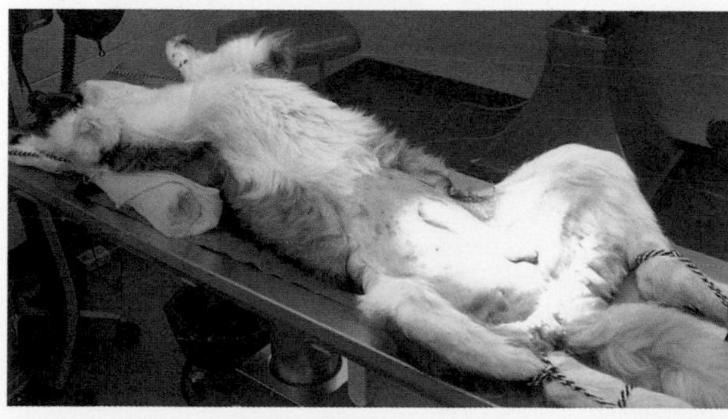

• **Fig. 1.6** Dorsal recumbency.

• **Fig. 1.8** Right lateral recumbency.

• BOX 1.5 Dental Terms

Mandible The lower jaw
Maxilla The upper jaw
Dental arch The complete arched arrangement of the maxilla and the mandible; also known as the dental arcade
Quadrant The left or right half of each dental arch
Incisor teeth The most rostral group of teeth
Canine teeth The teeth located just lateral to the incisor teeth
Premolar teeth The rostral cheek teeth
Molar teeth The caudal cheek teeth
Crown The exposed part of a tooth above the gum line
Root The hidden part of a tooth below the gum line
Coronal Toward the crown of a tooth
Apical Toward the tip of the root of a tooth
Gingival Toward the gingiva (gum)
Furcation The base of the root trunk on a tooth where two or more roots meet (bifurcation or trifurcation)
Periodontal fibers Connective tissue attached to the root of a tooth and the lining of the tooth socket
Mesial For canine, premolar, and molar teeth, the surface or edge facing toward the rostral end of the mouth; for the incisor teeth, the surface or edge facing toward the center (midline)
Distal For canine, premolar, and molar teeth, the surface or edge facing toward the caudal end of the mouth; for the incisor teeth, the surface or edge farthest from the center (midline)
Buccal Surface of a tooth facing the cheeks
Palatal Surface of an upper tooth facing the hard palate
Labial Surface of a tooth facing the lips
Lingual Surface of a lower tooth facing the tongue
Incisal edge The cutting edge of a sharp tooth's crown
Occlusal surface The flat grinding surface of molar teeth
Interproximal space Space between adjacent teeth
Interproximal surface Surface of a tooth that faces an adjacent tooth

Dental Arch, Dental Arcade, Quadrant

The **dental arch,** or dental arcade, is the U-shaped arrangement of all the teeth in the maxilla (upper jaw) or mandible (lower jaw). The left or right half of each dental arch is called the **quadrant**. Therefore, each animal has two dental arches (upper and lower) and four quadrants (upper left, upper right, lower left, and lower right).

Incisor, Canine, Premolar, and Molar Teeth

The teeth in each dental arch are divided into four general types of teeth (Fig. 1.9). **The incisor teeth** are the most rostral teeth in the arch. Ruminant animals do not have upper incisor teeth. They have a dental pad in their place. The **canine teeth,** if present, are located just lateral to the incisor teeth. Not all animals have canine teeth. (Note: vampires supposedly have very long canine teeth!) **Premolar teeth** are just caudal to the canine teeth if present. They are referred to as the "rostral cheek teeth" because they are on the sides of the jaw inside the rostral cheek area. The **molar teeth,** located just caudal to the premolars, are the "caudal cheek teeth."

Crown and Root

The terms crown and root refer to the two main parts of an individual tooth. The **crown** of a tooth is normally exposed above the gum line. It is the part of the tooth that does the actual grasping, tearing, or grinding. The **root** of the tooth is normally hidden beneath the gum line. It is anchored in the bone of the jaw by connective tissue called periodontal fibers. The size of the tooth root gives us an in-

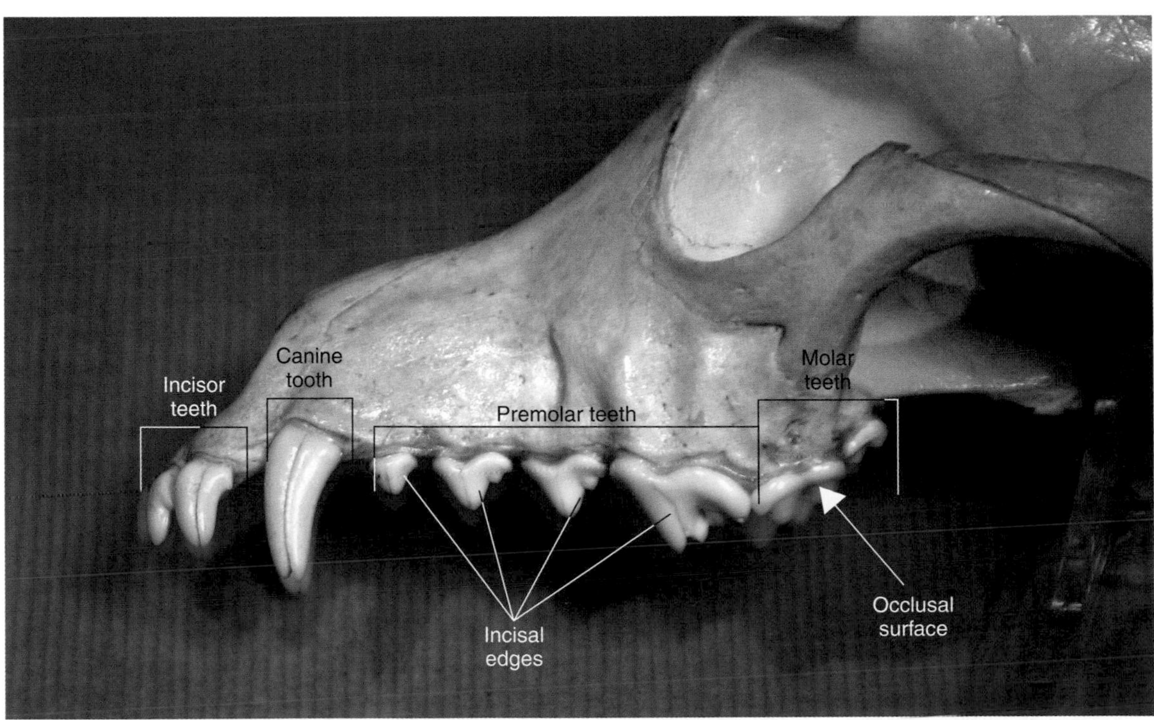

• Fig. 1.9 Canine upper teeth, left side.

dication of the amount of force applied by the tooth. Teeth with large roots generally withstand greater force than teeth with smaller roots.

Mesial and Distal

These terms indicate directions or surfaces in each quadrant of the dental arch (Figs. 1.10 and 1.11). It is easiest to grasp their meanings if you imagine the teeth of a dental arch all in a straight line instead of in the U shape of the actual jaw. In our straight line of teeth, the incisors (I) are in the center, the canines (C) are on both sides of them, then the premolars (P) and molars (M). This would be the straight-line arrangement of upper teeth for a dog:

M M P P P P C I I I | I I I C P P P M M

The vertical line between the center incisors denotes the center of the arch and divides it into left and right quadrants. **Mesial** means the direction, or tooth surface, that is toward that center line. **Distal** means the direction, or tooth surface, that is away from that center line. An example looks like this:

← Distal Distal →
Mesial → ← Mesial

M M P P P P C I I I | I I I C P P P M M

If we imagine the teeth arranged back in their normal arched shape, mesial and distal still refer to that center line between the two center incisors. For canine, premolar, and molar teeth, the mesial surface faces the rostral end of the mouth.

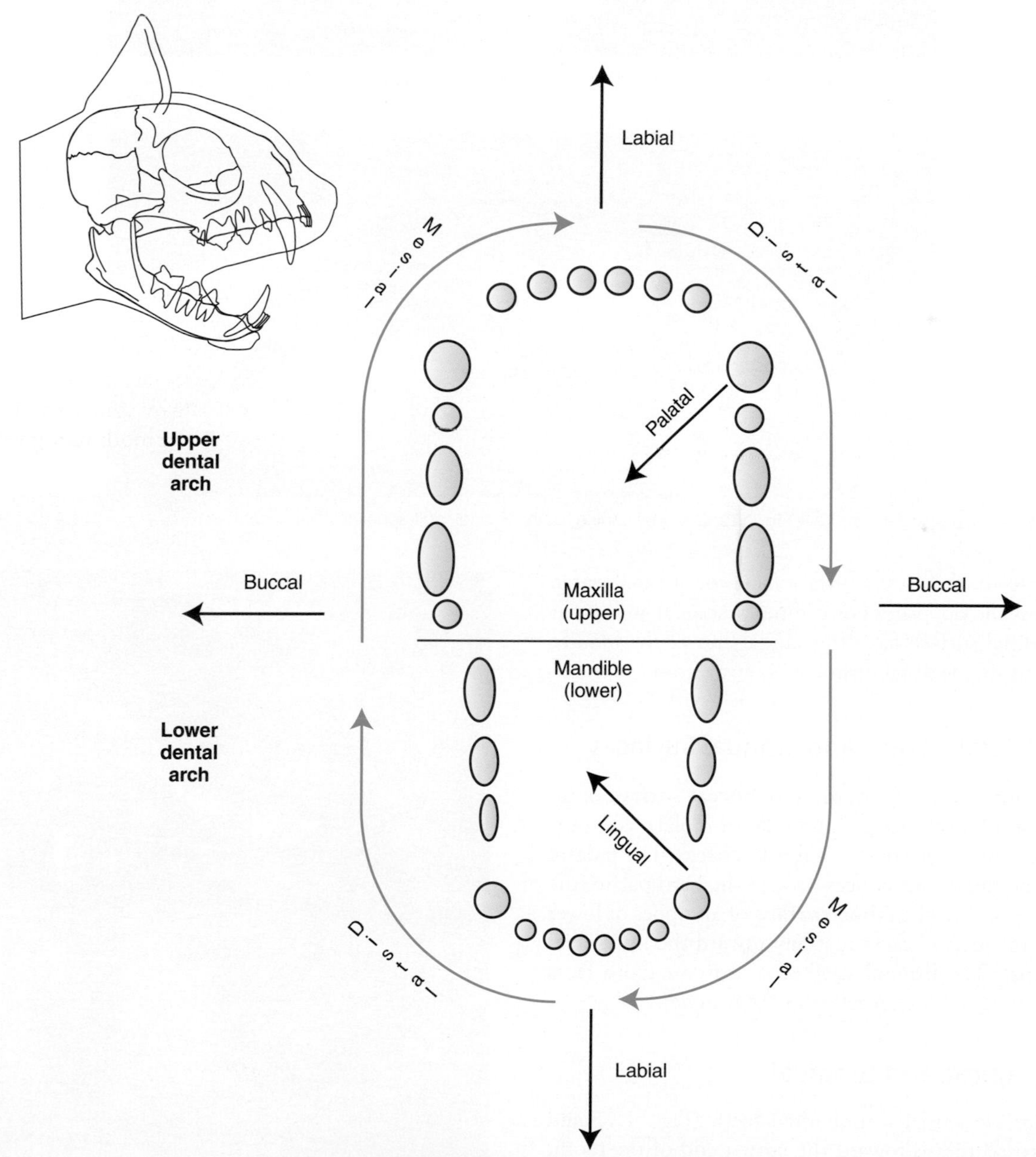

• **Fig. 1.10** Positional terminology: the oral road map.

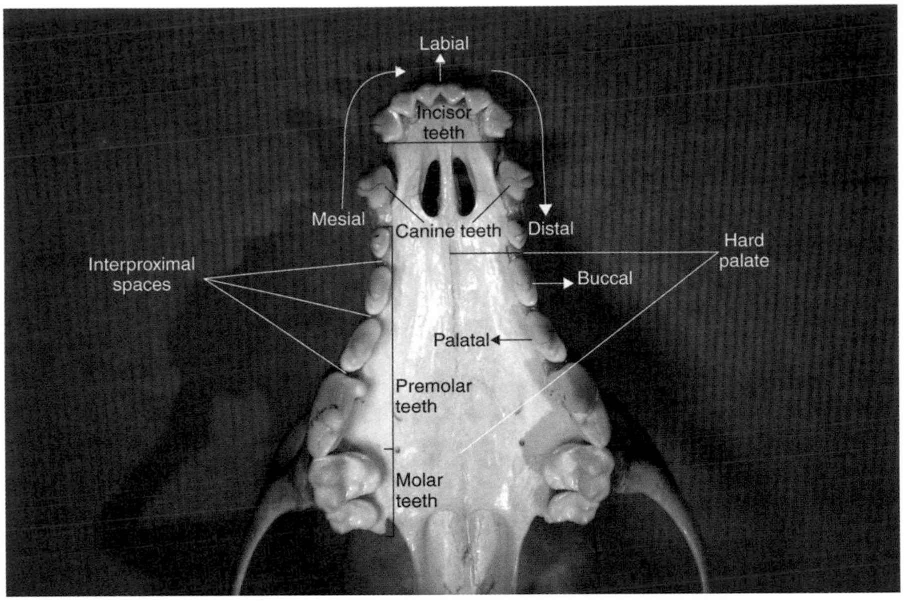

• **Fig. 1.11** Upper dental arch of the canine skull. Compared to the upper half of Fig. 1.10.

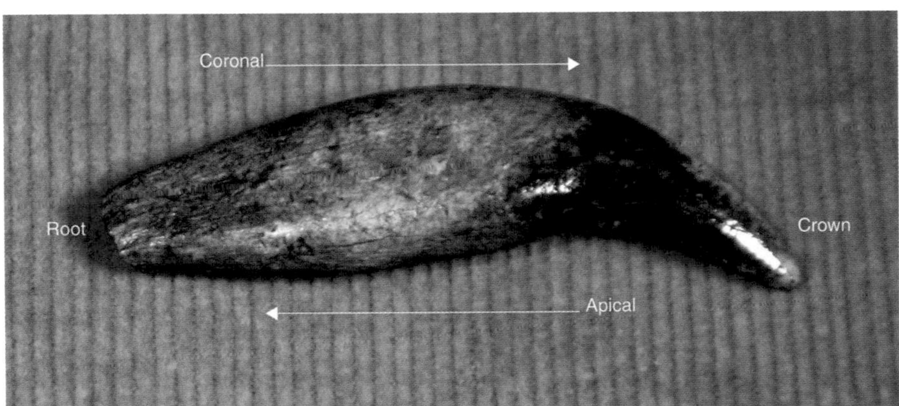

• **Fig. 1.12** Dire wolf canine tooth. (Extinct wolf species *Canis dirus*.)

For incisor teeth, the mesial surface faces toward the center. Distal means the opposite. For canine, premolar, and molar teeth, the distal surface faces the caudal end of the mouth. For incisor teeth, the distal surface faces away from the center.

Buccal, Palatal, Labial, and Lingual Surfaces

These are quite straightforward. The **buccal surface** of an upper or lower "cheek" tooth (premolar or molar) faces outward toward the cheek (buccal refers to cheek). The **palatal surface** of an upper tooth faces toward the hard palate (the roof of the mouth). The **labial surface** of an upper or lower "front" tooth (incisor) faces rostrally toward the lips (labial refers to lips). The **lingual surface** of a lower tooth faces toward the tongue (lingual refers to the tongue).

Coronal, Apical, and Gingival

These terms are used for individual teeth (Figs. 1.12 and 1.13). **Coronal** means toward the crown end of the tooth, and **apical** means toward the root end of the tooth. **Gingival** means toward the gingiva (gum).

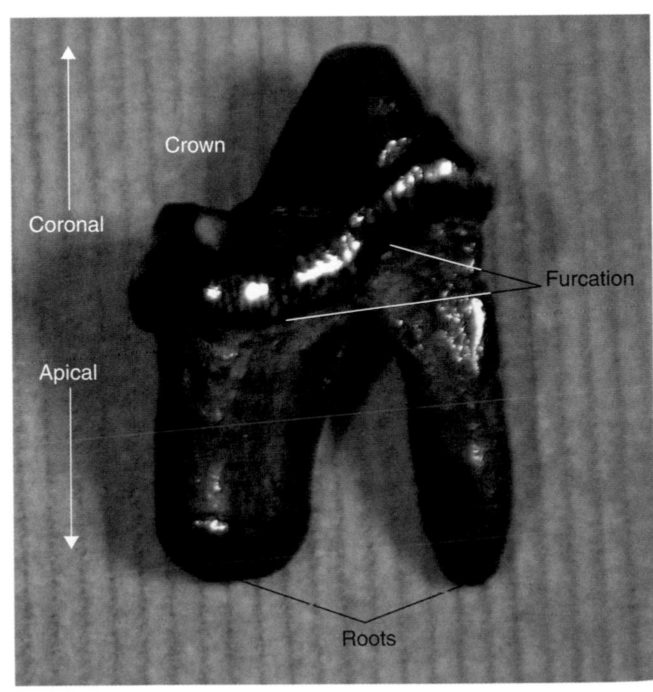

• **Fig. 1.13** Dire wolf molar tooth. (Extinct wolf species *Canis dirus*.)

Incisal Edge and Occlusal Surface

These describe the "business end" of a tooth, where the actual cutting and grinding of food take place. An **incisal edge** is the cutting edge of a sharp tooth, such as a canine or premolar tooth. An **occlusal surface** is the flat, grinding surface of a molar tooth (Fig. 1.14).

Interproximal Spaces and Surfaces

The word interproximal refers to the area between adjacent teeth. The **interproximal space** is between two adjacent teeth. The **interproximal surfaces** of a tooth are the surfaces that face toward adjacent teeth.

Furcation

Furcation is the area of a multirooted tooth (such as a molar) where the root trunk divides. Bifurcation refers to a tooth with two roots, and trifurcation refers to a tooth with three roots.

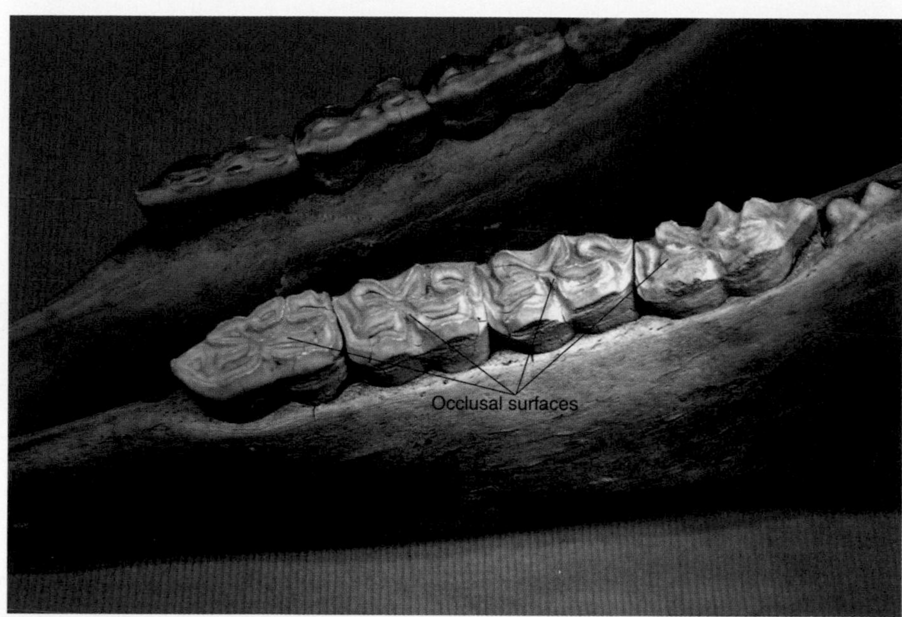

• **Fig. 1.14** Equine mandible.

EXERCISES

Anatomic, Common, and Position Terms

Exercise 1

Write the Right Word

Our first patient was a cat that got a chunk taken out of the tip of his nose by a feisty parrot. That wound was on the most (1) ____________ part of the cat's head. He was not happy when I inserted the rectal thermometer in his (2) ____________ end. I'm glad my assistant had a good hold of a scruff of skin over his shoulder blades in his (3) ____________ area.

A good way to avoid forgetting to clip the dewclaws when doing a nail trim is to always start with the dewclaw. It is located on the inside or (4) ____________ side of the paw. Then work out to the outermost nail on the (5) ____________ side of the paw.

I saw a cat give a cow a backrub today. The cow was lying on its ventral surface in (6) ____________ recumbency. The cat was on the cow's back, or (7) ________________ surface. Periodically the cat would slowly walk toward the cow's head in a (8) ____________ direction, stopping occasionally to knead the cow's back. When the cat reached the cow's neck, it would turn around and do the same thing toward the cow's tail, or (9) ____________ end. The cow seemed happy.

In the United States, dog and cat spay incisions are usually made on the midline of the belly. This is called a (10) ____________ midline incision and the animal must be positioned in (11) ____________ recumbency. In the United Kingdom, cat spay incisions are often made on the side of the abdomen. This is called a (12) ______________ incision, and the animal must be positioned in (13) ____________ recumbency.

Continued

Exercise 1—cont'd

Write the Right Word

When radiographing limb bones, we should include the joints above, or (14) ___________, and below, or (15) ___________, to the target bone to be sure we get the whole bone on the film. For a radiograph of the tibia (shinbone) and its trusty sidekick the fibula, we would have to include the (16) ________ joint (17) ___________ to the tibia and fibula, and the (18) ___________ joint (19) ___________ to the bones.

When an animal stands squarely on all four feet, the surfaces of its front feet that are on the ground are the (20) _______________ surfaces. The surfaces of its hind feet that are on the ground are the (21) ___________ surfaces. The top/front surfaces of all four feet are the (22) ___________ surfaces.

To position a cat for a ventral midline surgical incision into the abdomen, the animal's ventral surface must face upward. It must be in (23) ___________ recumbency. For a dorsal midline spinal surgery incision in a dog, the animal's dorsal surface must face upward. It must be in (24) ___________ recumbency. For surgical repair of a superficial laceration on the left side of a ferret's chest, the animal must be positioned on its right side with its left side facing upward. It is in (25) ___________ recumbency.

A ventral midline surgical incision is made along part of the (26) ___________ plane of the animal's body. A surgical incision made 2 inches to the left of the ventral midline would be along part of a (27) ___________ plane.

If a horse waded into a pond until the water was about midchest high, the surface of the water would represent a (28) ___________ plane through the animal's body. After cooling off in the pond, if the horse stood in the doorway of the barn so its front, or (29) ___________, end was inside the barn and its back, or (30) ___________, end was outside, the doorway would represent a (31) ___________ plane through the animal's body.

Exercise 2

Definitions

1. ____________________ Toward the median plane.
2. ____________________ Common term for tarsus.
3. ____________________ Toward the center of the body or body part.
4. ____________________ Side of abdomen between last rib and hind leg.
5. ____________________ Toward the belly.
6. ____________________ Toward the body (referring to an appendage).
7. ____________________ Equivalent to human knee.
8. ____________________ Toward the head.
9. ____________________ Away from the median plane.
10. ____________________ Proximal phalanx area of a horse.
11. ____________________ Top of the head between the ears.
12. ____________________ Toward the backbone.
13. ____________________ Dorsal part of the base of the tail.
14. ____________________ Plane that divides the body into equal left and right halves.
15. ____________________ Away from the body (referring to an appendage).
16. ____________________ Toward the tail.
17. ____________________ Toward the side of the body, away from the median plane.
18. ____________________ Plane parallel to the cranial-caudal midline, but not on the midline.
19. ____________________ Area over the cranial end of the sternum.
20. ____________________ Toward the tip of the nose.
21. ____________________ Toward the outer surface of the body or body part.
22. ____________________ Ground or rear surface of hindlimb distal to tarsus.
23. ____________________ Plane that divides the body into cranial and caudal portions.

Exercise 2—cont'd

Definitions

24. ______________________ Main trunk of the body.
25. ______________________ Rostral part of the face formed by the nose and upper jaw.
26. ______________________ Area dorsal to shoulder blades.
27. ______________________ Plane that divides the body into dorsal and ventral portions.
28. ______________________ Ground or rear surface of front limb distal to carpus.
29. ______________________ Joint between cannon bone and proximal phalanx of a horse.
30. ______________________ Carpus of a horse.

Exercise 3

Identification

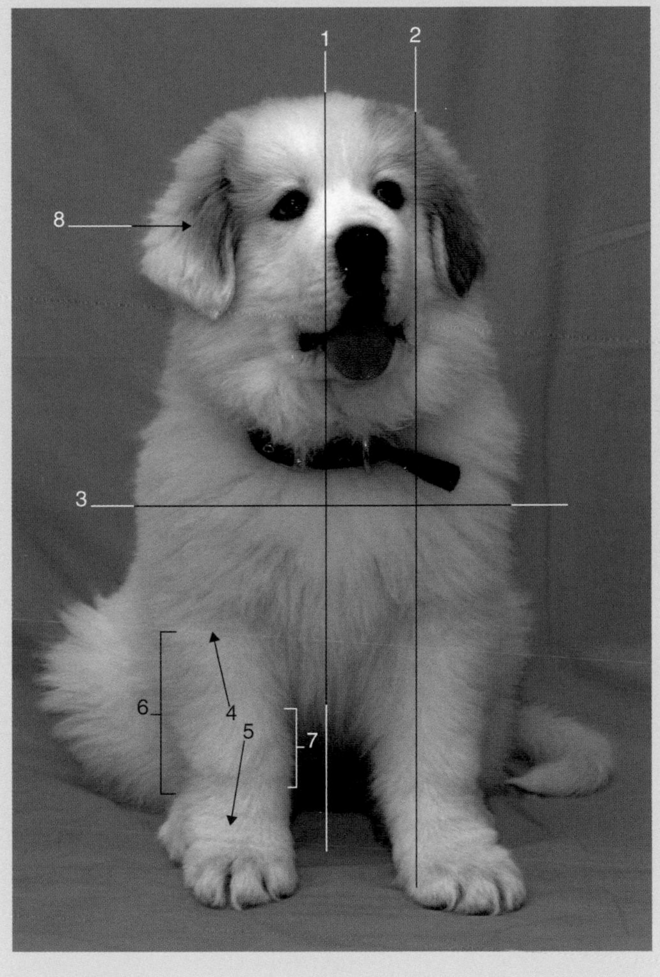

1. ______________________(Anatomic plane)
2. ______________________(Anatomic plane)
3. ______________________(Anatomic plane)
4. ______________________(Direction)
5. ______________________(Direction)
6. ______________________(Surface of leg)
7. ______________________(Surface of leg)
8. ______________________(Which ear is this?)

Continued

Exercise 3—cont'd

Identification

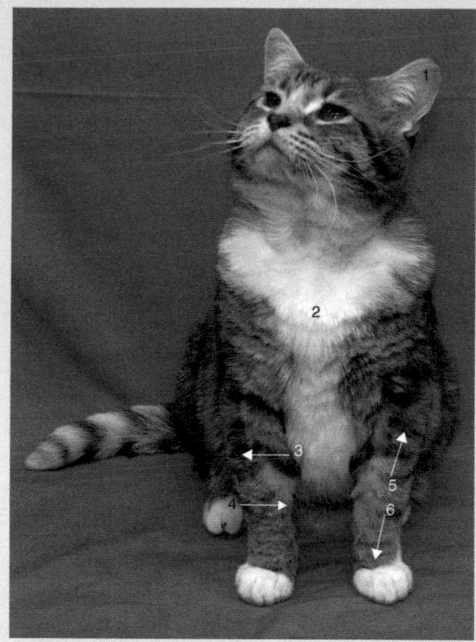

1. ______________________ (Which ear is this?)
2. ______________________ (Region)
3. ______________________ (Direction)
4. ______________________ (Direction)
5. ______________________ (Direction)
6. ______________________ (Direction)

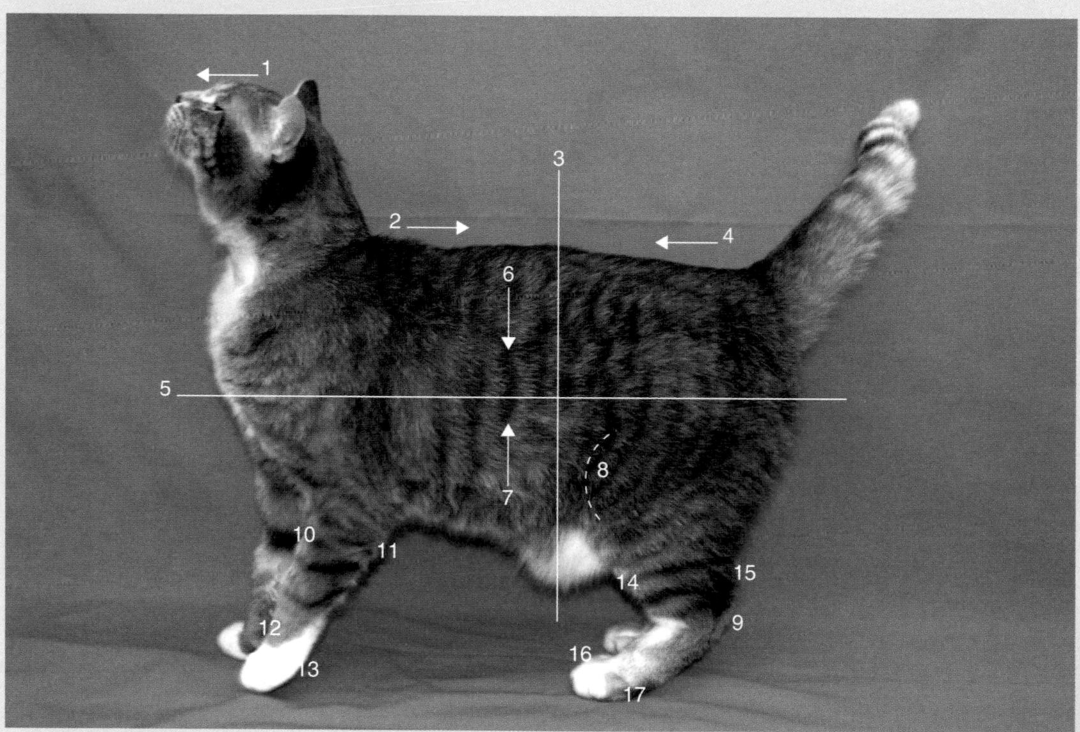

1. ______________________ (Direction)
2. ______________________ (Direction)
3. ______________________ (Anatomic plane)
4. ______________________ (Direction)
5. ______________________ (Anatomic plane)
6. ______________________ (Direction)
7. ______________________ (Direction)
8. ______________________ (Joint)
9. ______________________ (Joint)
10. ______________________ (Surface of leg)
11. ______________________ (Surface of leg)
12. ______________________ (Surface of leg)
13. ______________________ (Surface of leg)
14. ______________________ (Surface of leg)
15. ______________________ (Surface of leg)
16. ______________________ (Surface of leg)
17. ______________________ (Surface of leg)

Exercise 3—cont'd

Identification

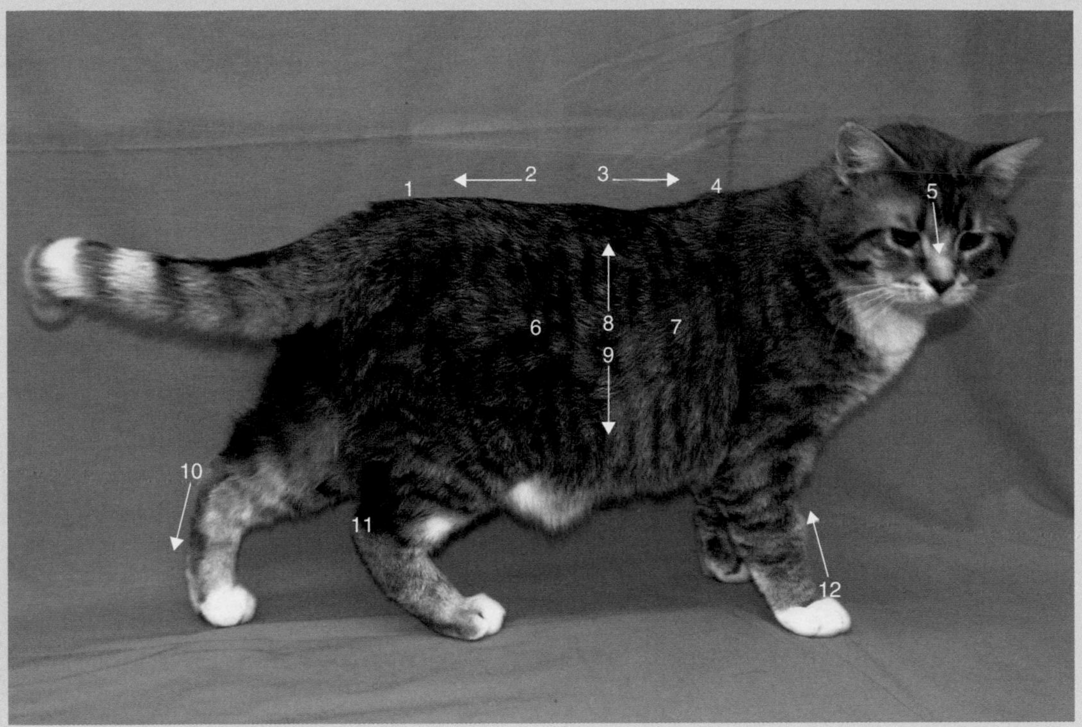

1. ______________________ (Region)
2. ______________________ (Direction)
3. ______________________ (Direction)
4. ______________________ (Region)
5. ______________________ (Direction)
6. ______________________ (Region)
7. ______________________ (Region)
8. ______________________ (Direction)
9. ______________________ (Direction)
10. ______________________ (Direction)
11. ______________________ (Joint)
12. ______________________ (Direction)

Continued

Exercise 3—cont'd

Identification

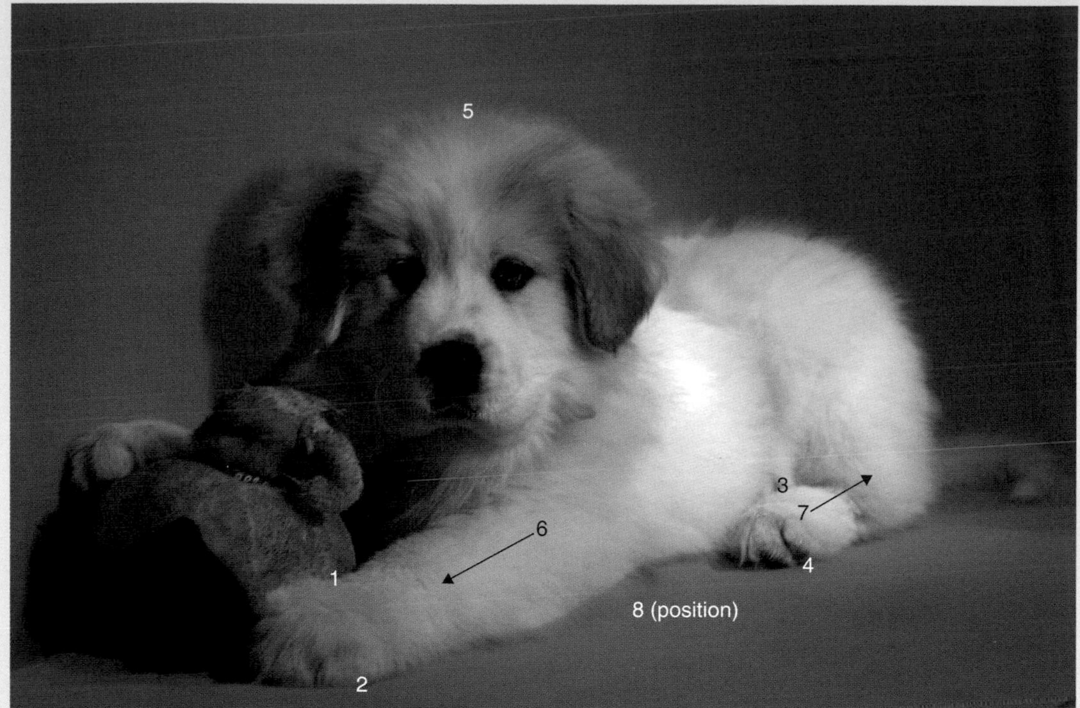

1. ______________ (Surface of paw)
2. ______________ (Surface of paw)
3. ______________ (Surface of paw)
4. ______________ (Surface of paw)
5. ______________ (Region)
6. ______________ (Direction on leg)
7. ______________ (Direction on leg)
8. ______________ (Position of dog)

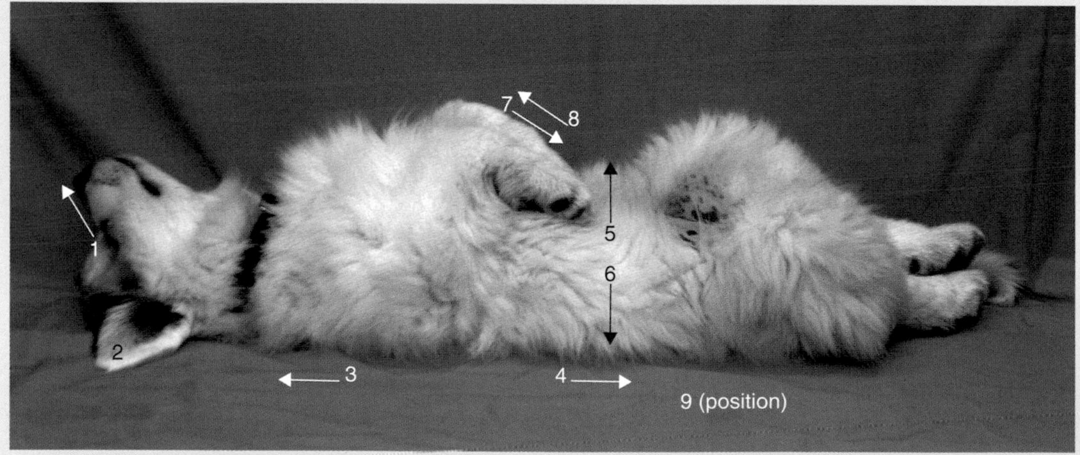

1. ______________ (Direction)
2. ______________ (Which ear is this?)
3. ______________ (Direction)
4. ______________ (Direction)
5. ______________ (Direction)
6. ______________ (Direction)
7. ______________ (Direction on leg)
8. ______________ (Direction on leg)
9. ______________ (Position of dog)

Exercise 3—cont'd

Identification

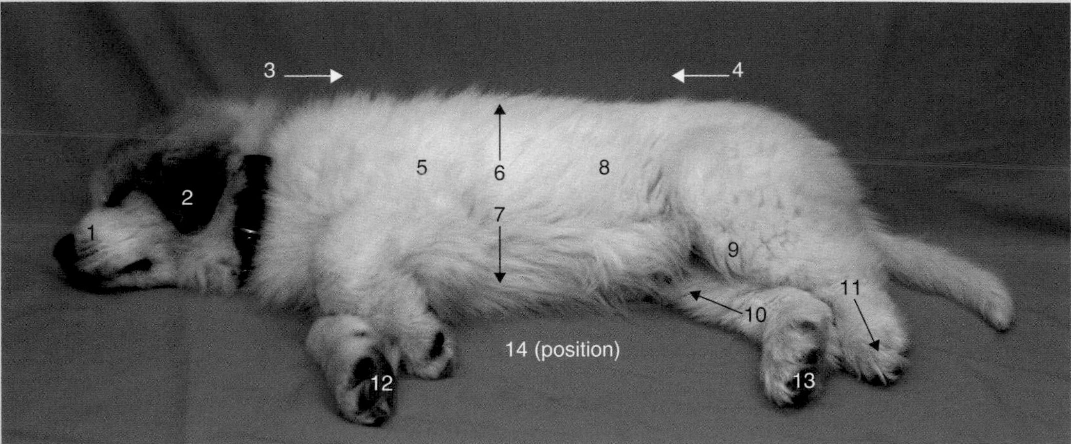

1. ______________________ (Region)
2. ______________________ (Which ear is this?)
3. ______________________ (Direction)
4. ______________________ (Direction)
5. ______________________ (Region)
6. ______________________ (Direction)
7. ______________________ (Direction)
8. ______________________ (Region)
9. ______________________ (Joint)
10. ______________________ (Direction on leg)
11. ______________________ (Direction on leg)
12. ______________________ (Surface of paw)
13. ______________________ (Surface of paw)
14. ______________________ (Position of dog)

Exercise 4

Suggested In-Class Activities

Plane and Simple

The instructor places rubber bands on stuffed animals to represent different anatomic planes. Students identify the planes.

Location Designation

Students work in groups with live animals. One student places a sticker on an animal. The other students in the group write a description of the location or direction indicated by the sticker using only anatomic terms.

X-Ray-Ted

The instructor describes common radiographic positions (e.g., ventrodorsal, left lateral, dorsopalmar). Students simulate an x-ray table with a light source simulating the x-ray beam and a piece of cardboard simulating the cassette. Write common radiographic positions on slips of paper and place them in a hat. Two students at a time draw slips of paper from the hat and position an animal appropriately on the cardboard "cassette."

Dental Terms

Exercise 5

Write the Right Word—Definitions

1. ______________________ Caudal cheek teeth.
2. ______________________ All of the upper or lower teeth.
3. ______________________ Surface of an incisor tooth facing toward the midline.
4. ______________________ Facing the tongue.

Continued

Exercise 5—cont'd

Write the Right Word—Definitions

5. ____________________ Toward the tip of a tooth's root.
6. ____________________ "Fangs" of a dog.
7. ____________________ Left or right half of the upper or lower teeth.
8. ____________________ Tooth surface facing an adjacent tooth.
9. ____________________ The part of a tooth an animal bites with.
10. ____________________ Facing the hard palate.
11. ____________________ Cutting edge of a sharp tooth.
12. ____________________ The part of a tooth that anchors it in the jaw.
13. ____________________ Surface of a premolar tooth facing toward the caudal end of the mouth.
14. ____________________ Facing the cheeks.
15. ____________________ Toward a tooth's crown.
16. ____________________ Flat surface of a grinding tooth.
17. ____________________ Rostral cheek teeth.
18. ____________________ Space between teeth.
19. ____________________ Surface of an incisor tooth facing away from the midline.
20. ____________________ Where the root trunk of a tooth divides into tooth roots.
21. ____________________ Facing the lips.
22. ____________________ Most rostral teeth.
23. ____________________ Surface of a molar tooth facing the rostral end of the mouth.

Exercise 6

Identification

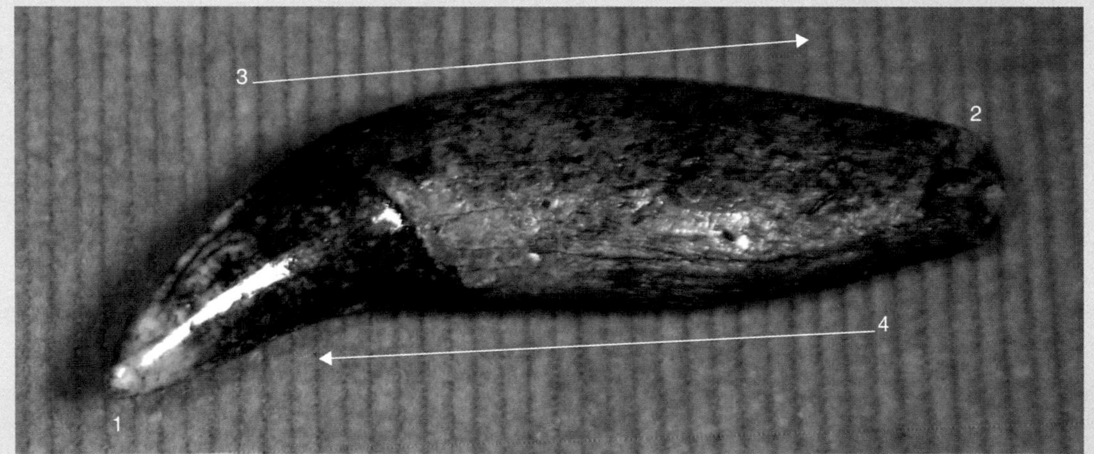

Canine tooth. Dire wolf.

1. ____________________ (Area of tooth)
2. ____________________ (Area of tooth)
3. ____________________ (Direction)
4. ____________________ (Direction)

Exercise 6—cont'd

Identification

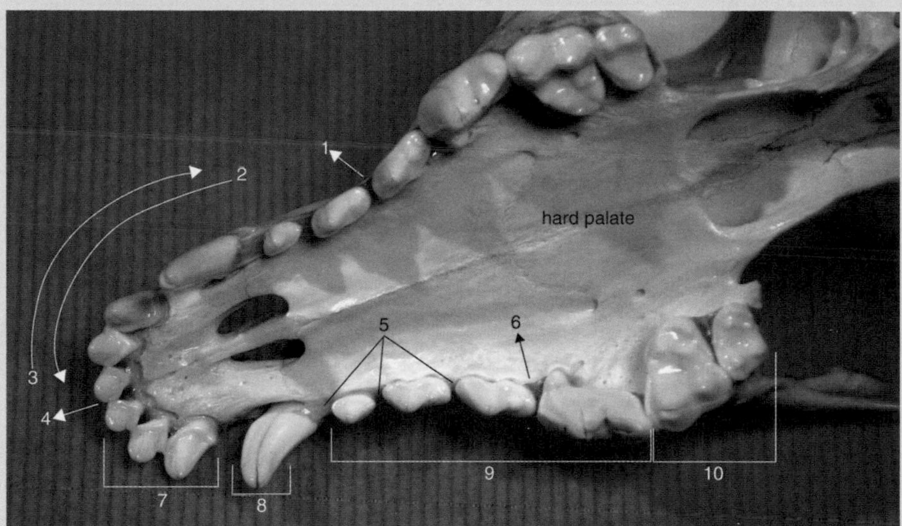

Upper dental arch of the canine skull.

1. ______________________ (Direction)
2. ______________________ (Direction)
3. ______________________ (Direction)
4. ______________________ (Direction)
5. ______________________ (Spaces)
6. ______________________ (Direction)
7. ______________________ (Group of teeth)
8. ______________________ (Tooth)
9. ______________________ (Group of teeth)
10. ______________________ (Group of teeth)

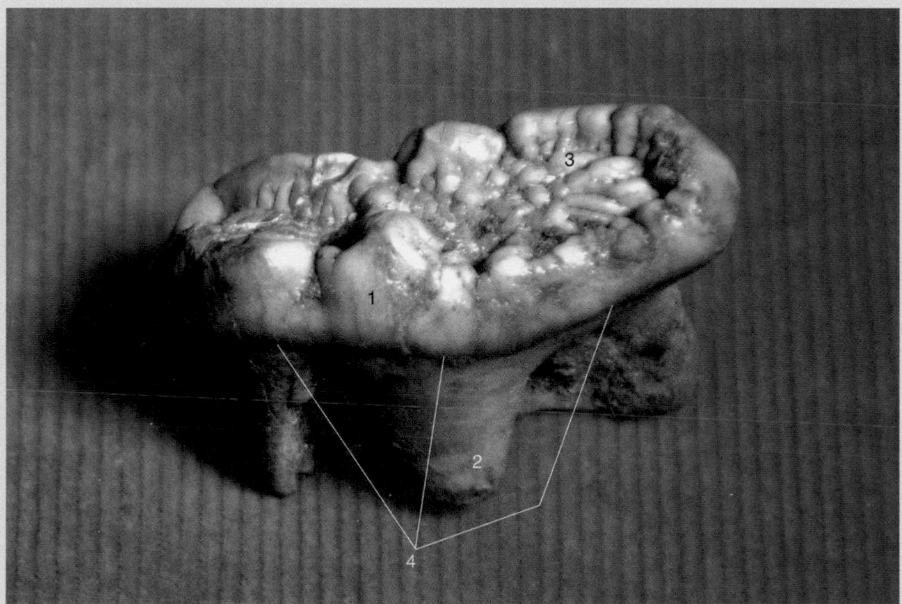

Molar tooth. Cave bear. (Extinct bear species *Ursus uralensis*.)

1. ______________________ (Area of tooth)
2. ______________________ (Area of tooth)
3. ______________________ (Surface of tooth)
4. ______________________ (Area of tooth)

Critical and Clinical Thinking

Exercise 7

Clinical Thinking Challenge

Support each of the following correct statements with appropriate rationale, stating why or in what way each statement is correct.

1. Anatomy and physiology describe two complementary but different ways to look at the animal body.

____

____

2. Terms such as *up, down, above, below,* and *beside* are not very useful in describing anatomic locations.

____

____

3. A radiograph of a horse's front fetlock joint is called a *dorsopalmar (DP) view.*

____

____

4. There are a few differences between human directional terms and those of nonhuman animals.

____

____

5. When performing surgery on the digestive tract, we must take care to suture it securely closed.

____

____

6. Oblique positions are sometimes used in radiography.

____

____

Exercise 8

Lab Partner Experience

A. With a lab partner, point to various body parts on Diagram 1. The partner is to describe the body part using directional terms. Switch roles. Using Diagram 2, follow the same exercise.

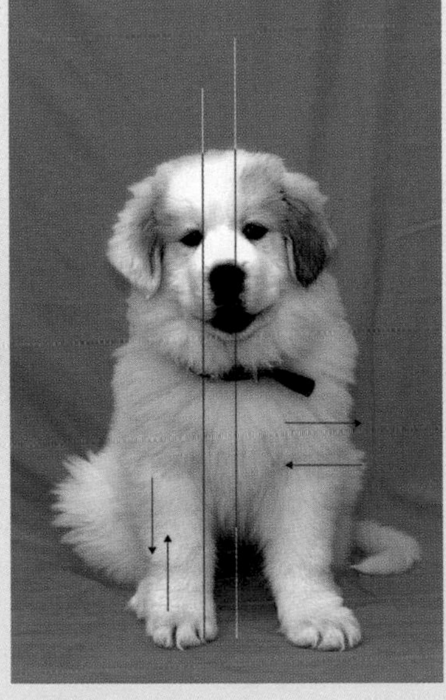

Exercise 8—cont'd

Lab Partner Experience

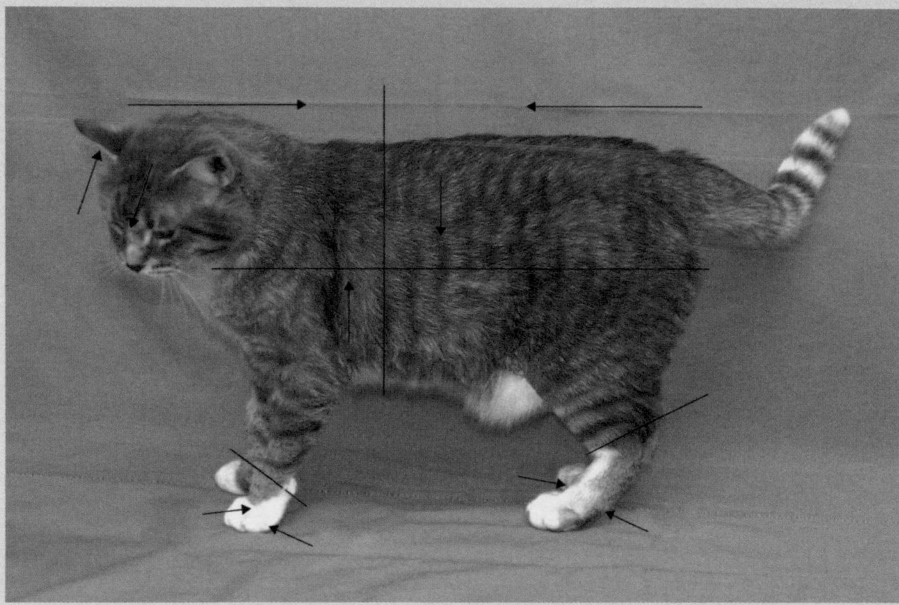

B. Lab Partner 1: Identify the contents of the dorsal and ventral body cavities.

C. Lab Partner 2: Compare and contrast the thorax and caudal abdominal cavities.

2 Microscopy[a]

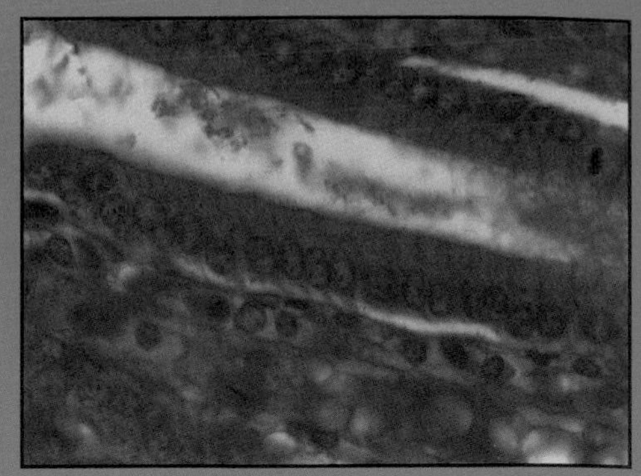

OVERVIEW AT A GLANCE

Identification of Parts of the Microscope 21

Care of the Microscope 25

Exercises 26–32

Parts of the Microscope 26–27

1. Label the Parts of the Microscope 26

2. Match the Parts of the Microscope With the Corresponding Definition 27

Use of the Compound Microscope 27–30

3. Procedure: Measure and Calculate Magnification 27

4. Procedure: Calculate Field Size 29

5. Procedure: Estimate Size of Objects 30

Critical and Clinical Thinking 32

6. Clinical Thinking Challenge 32

LEARNING OBJECTIVES

In this laboratory, students will learn:

- The location, name, and function of each part of the compound microscope, and how to use, adjust, and maintain these parts.
- To use the microscope to view the letter "e".
- To calculate the field size of the various magnifications.
- To estimate the sizes of objects viewed using a stained blood film.

CLINICAL SIGNIFICANCE OF LIGHT MICROSCOPY

Light microscopy is best suited to viewing very thin, stained specimens, such as sections of tissue, blood smears, and droplets of liquid containing bacteria. It is also useful for the examination of living, unstained specimens, such as mites, parasitic eggs from fecal flotations, and cellular and noncellular components of urine sediments. The following is a list of specimens that might be observed in practice using light microscopy.

- Stained bacteria from culture (1000×) (Fig. 2.1)
- Stained tissue sections (100×, 400×), thin sections with condensed chromosomes, or specially stained organelles (1000×)
- Stained blood smears—numbers and morphology of blood cells, presence of blood parasites (400×, 1000×)
- Wet mounts of feces (flotation or direct smear)—large protists—(100×), protozoan oocysts (100×, 400× occasionally), nematode eggs (100×)
- Wet mounts of ear debris or skin scrapings—mites and yeast (100×) (Fig. 2.2)
- Stained smears from wounds and infections—fungal elements and bacteria (400×, 1000×)
- Urine sediment, stained or unstained—presence of crystals, blood cells, casts, or bacteria (100×, 400×)
- Stained vaginal smear—stage of estrus is determined by the maturation of epithelial cells (100×, 400×) (Fig. 2.3)

INTRODUCTION

In veterinary practices and laboratories, the compound light microscope is used by veterinarians and veterinary technicians daily in the course of diagnosing and treating animal diseases. A series of lenses is used to form an image from light passing through the specimen. In this way, the image can be magnified as much as 1000 times. In veterinary practices, compound light microscopes are used for a wide variety of reasons, including:

- To examine the morphology and numbers of blood cells (Fig. 2.4)
- To check for the presence of intestinal parasites in feces
- To examine the contents of urine sediment
- To examine an ear swab for the presence of infectious agents such as bacteria, mites, and fungi

[a]The authors and publisher wish to acknowledge Mary Ann Seagren for previous contributions to this chapter.

The ability to use a microscope properly is essential to ensure the accuracy of these important laboratory tests.

In a standard compound light microscope, light from an incandescent source is aimed towards a lens, called the condenser, which is located beneath the stage (Fig. 2.5). The condenser concentrates the light before it passes through a hole in the stage where it then penetrates the specimen. From here the light passes through an objective lens, before being magnified a second time by the ocular, or eyepiece. Finally, the light reaches the eye so that what was too small to be seen is now made clearly visible. Some microscopes have a built-in illuminator as shown in Fig. 2.5A, whereas others use a mirror to reflect light from an external source (see Fig. 2.5B).

MATERIALS NEEDED

- Compound light microscope
- Prepared microscope slide of newsprint letter "e"
- Prepared microscope slide of a stained blood film
- Prepared slide of a grid, ruled in millimeters (grid slide)
- Immersion oil
- Millimeter ruler
- Lens paper
- Lens cleaner

TERMS TO BE IDENTIFIED

- Eyepiece or ocular (each 10× or 5×)
- Arm
- Stage
- Opening of the stage
- Fine adjustment knob
- Coarse adjustment knob
- Base
- Illuminator or light source
  - Light on or off switch
  - Rheostat for light source
- Iris diaphragm
  - Iris diaphragm lever
- Condenser
  - Condenser knob
- Stage clips
  - Control knob of mechanical stage clips
- Objective lenses
  - Scanning objective (3.2×, 3.5×, or 4×)
  - Low-power objective (10×)
  - High-power or high dry objective (40×, 43×, or 45×)
  - Oil immersion (97× or 100×)
- Nosepiece
- Body tube

Identification of Parts of the Microscope

A labeled photograph of a compound microscope is shown in Fig. 2.6. Observe the labeled parts as you read the description and function of each part.

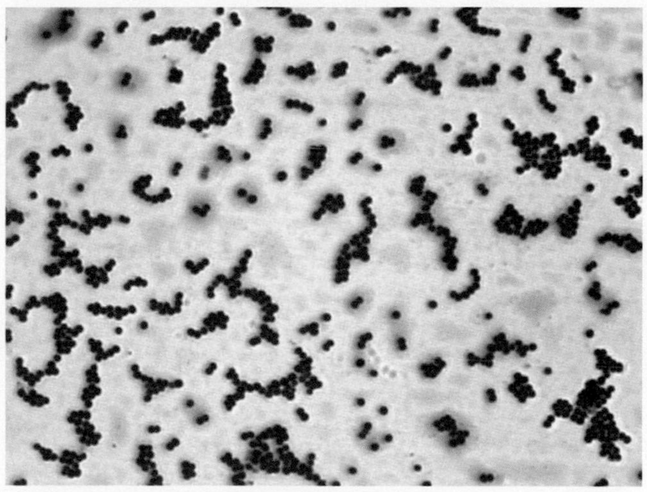

• Fig. 2.1 Stained bacteria. This photomicrograph is of a smear of *Staphylococcus aureus* bacteria stained with Gram stain. Bacteria that absorb the purple Gram stain are called "gram positive." Staphylococci are common infectious agents in mastitis and skin infections of all species.

Oculars (Eyepieces)

A compound light microscope can either be binocular (containing two eyepieces) or monocular (containing one eyepiece). The usual magnification of the eyepiece is 10×. It is important periodically to remove the eyepieces and clean them with lens cleaner and lens paper.

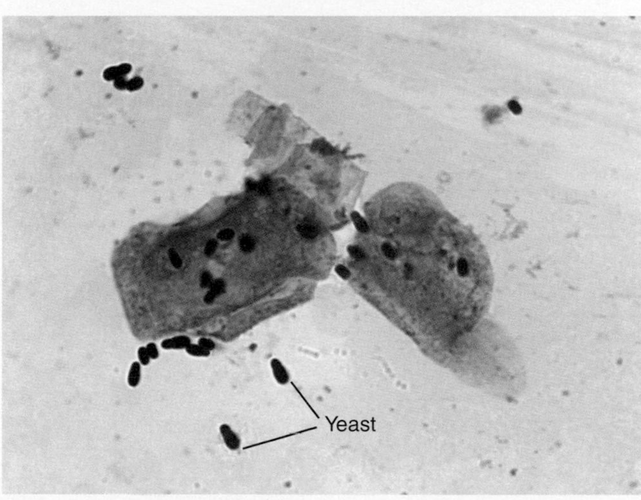

• Fig. 2.2 Yeast. This photomicrograph shows yeast cells (oval and peanut-shaped) along with squamous epithelium from the ear canal. This is a common finding in a smear from a dog with a yeast ear infection.

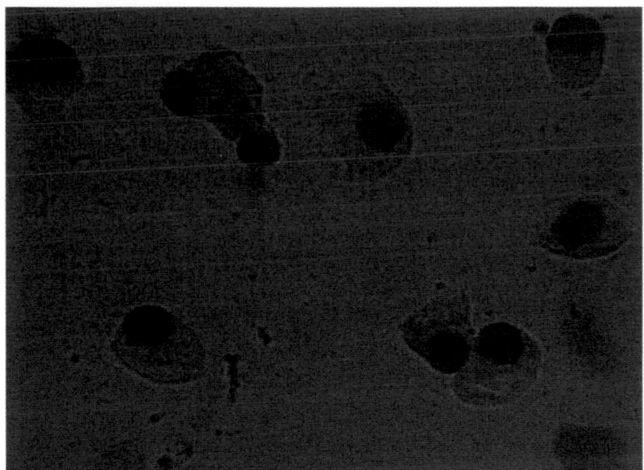

• Fig. 2.3 Vaginal smear. This photomicrograph shows epithelial cells that have sloughed from the lining of the vagina. The appearance of the cells is used to gauge the stage of the dog's heat cycle. (From Bassert J: Images for veterinary technician educators, Summer 2001.)

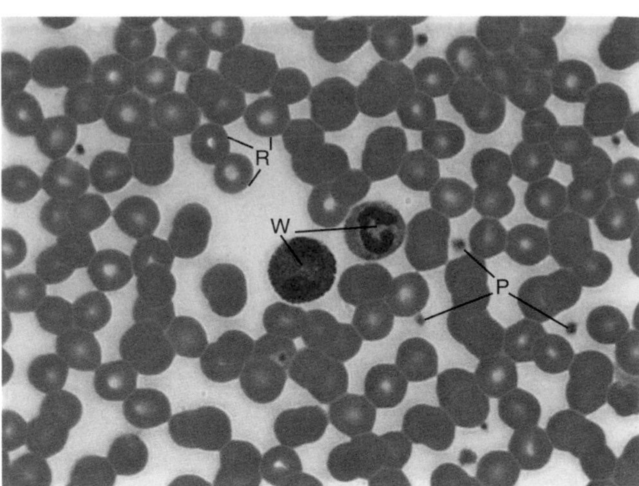

• Fig. 2.4 Blood smear. This is a photomicrograph (a photograph of a microscopic field) of a smear of stained canine blood. Note the presence of two white blood cells. Each has a purple multilobed nucleus. They are surrounded by doughnut-like red blood cells, which have no nuclei. Platelets are seen interspersed among the red blood cells and they appear as pale cell fragments or small dots. *P,* platelets; *R,* red blood cells; *W,* White blood cells. (Photo courtesy Manor College.)

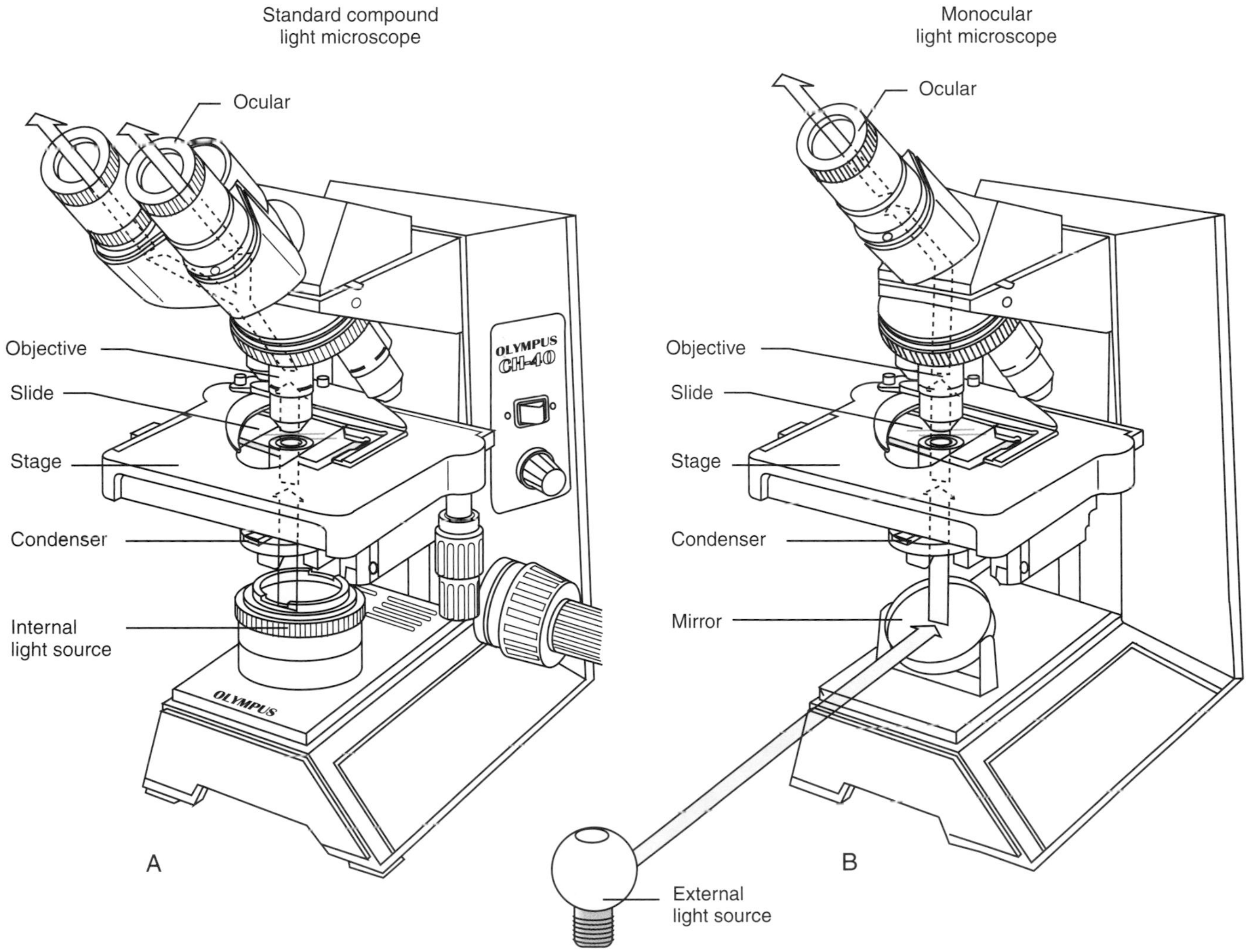

• Fig. 2.5 (A) Standard compound light microscope. Some microscopes have a built in illuminator. (B) Monocular light microscope. Others use a mirror to reflect light from an external source.

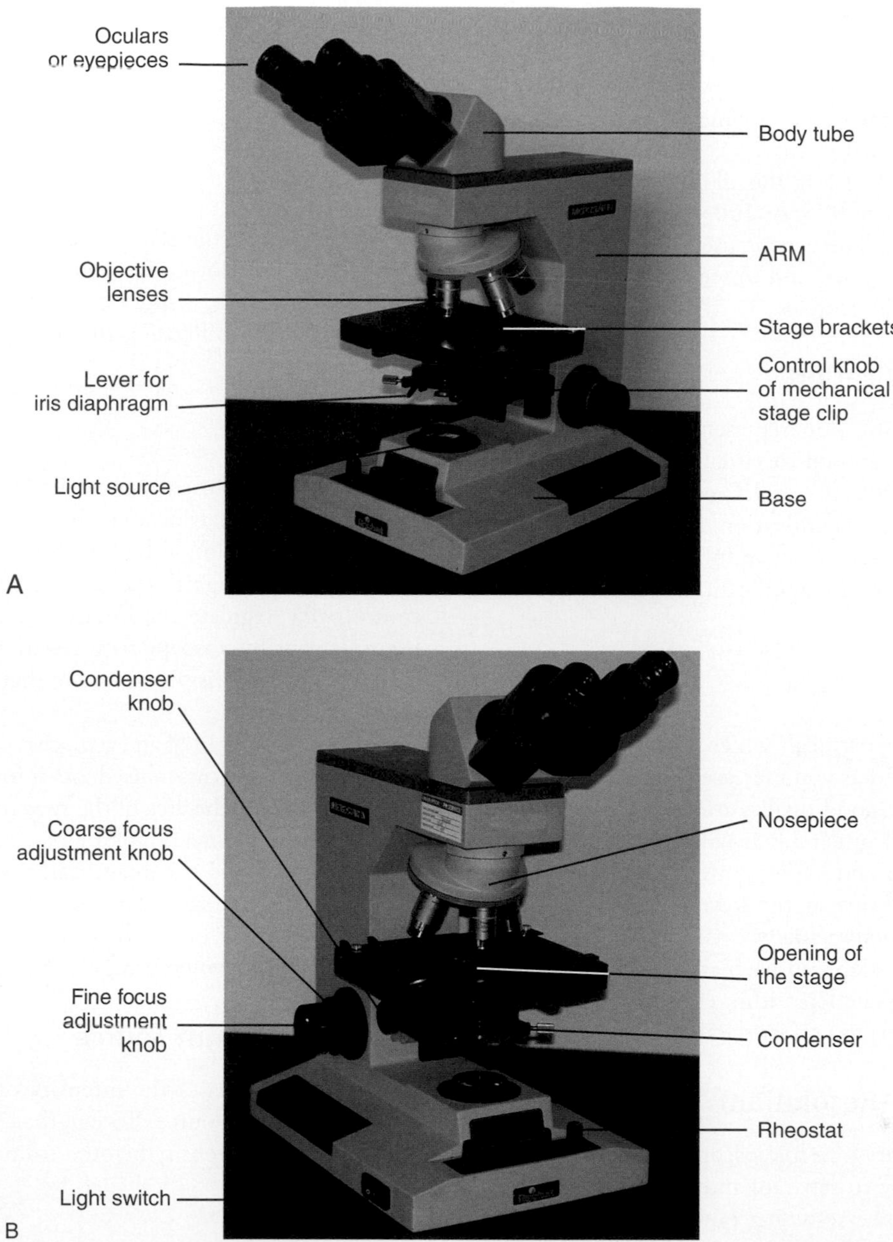

• **Fig. 2.6** (A and B) The most common microscope used in light microscopy is the compound light microscope. The compound light microscope has at least two magnifying lenses. One is in the eyepiece (ocular), and one is in the objective.

Binocular vision offers greater clarity, detail, and a wider field of view than monocular vision, but some adjustments to the microscope will need to be made to reap the benefits of binocular vision. First, the distance between pupils (in the eye) varies from person to person, so the distance between the oculars will need to be adjusted to match your interpupillary distance. Second, one or both of the eyepieces may be "a telescoping ocular," which allows it to be focused. Most people see better using one eye than the other. So, the focusing of one or both eyepieces allows the visual acuity in both eyes to be matched. Because our visual acuity is measured in units called diopters, this focusing process is called the diopter adjustment.

Objective Lenses

The objective lenses are attached to a revolving nosepiece. The power of each lens is engraved on the side of the objective. The smallest power lens may be 3.2×, 3.5×, or 4×, and is used when first locating and viewing a specimen. Because some specimens can be quite tiny and difficult to find on a comparatively large glass slide, this objective is sometimes called the "scanning lens."

The next lens is called the low power (LP) objective and is at 10× magnification. It is used for initial, coarse focusing and for the examination of large specimens such as nematode eggs.

The high power (HP) objective, or the high dry lens, offers high magnification without the use of oil. HP lenses may magnify 40, 43, or 45 times, depending upon the objective, and are used for small specimens, such as protists, large yeasts, and urine sediments.

The highest power lens is in the oil immersion objective. It has a magnification of 97× or 100×. It is used with oil to improve resolution. This lens is used for viewing blood smears and bacterial smears, and to see details (such as cell organelles) in histologic samples.

Degree of Magnification

The degree of magnification represents the *total amount* of magnification that is used to visualize a specimen. It is calculated by multiplying the ocular magnification (usually 10×) by the objective magnification. For example, if you are using the high-power objective (40×) to view a group of cells, the total degree of magnification would be equal to 10× × 40× or 400×.

Parfocal

Most microscopes are parfocal, which means that the image will remain focused as you increase magnification. This is a characteristic of a good quality microscope. When the microscope is focused under LP, it will remain in focus as you switch to a higher and higher power. It is good practice to begin light microscopy at the lowest power and move up in magnification incrementally, even if the microscope is parfocal. This step-by-step approach allows you the opportunity to center the specimen within each new field and to use the fine adjustment to perfect the image.

Resolving Power (Resolution)

Resolution is the ability of a microscope to produce a clear image. It is the ability to separate and distinguish fine details of a specimen. The resolving power is the minimum distance by which two points must be separated and still be perceived as two distinct points. Better microscopes have higher resolution, that is, objects in the specimen can be closer together and still be seen as distinct from one another.

Working Distance

When a specimen is in sharp focus, the working distance is the distance between the objective lens that is in use and the specimen. As stronger lenses are used, the working distance decreases. The specimen and the glass slide on which it rests become closer and closer to the objective as you move from scanning to LP to HP. Caution should be taken when using high dry and oil immersion objectives in particular because there is a risk of lowering these objectives too far when focusing and jamming the objectives into the glass slide. Carefully prepared slides may be broken in this way, not to mention the potential for damaging the lens in the objective. Therefore, be very cautious when focusing with high-powered objectives. Observe the working distance when using LP, HP, and oil immersion. The distance should approximate 16, 4, and 1.8 mm, respectively.

Arm and Base

The arm connects the base, stage, and body tube. The base is the bottom platform of the microscope, which holds the illuminator. Always be sure to carry a microscope by its arm with one hand, while using the other hand to support the base.

Light Source

The light source is usually built into the base. A good light source will have a wide dynamic range to provide high-intensity illumination at high magnifications and lower intensities at low magnifications. The best microscopes have controls that regulate the intensity and shape of the light beam. If your microscope requires an external light source, make sure the light is positioned so that it strikes the middle of the condenser.

The apparent field of an eyepiece is constant regardless of the level of magnification used. So, it follows that, as magnification increases, the area of the specimen that is visible decreases. Because you are looking at a smaller area, less light reaches the eye, and the image darkens. With an LP objective, you may have to cut down on illumination intensity. When using an HP objective, you will need all the light you can get, especially when using a less expensive microscope.

Rheostat for Light Source

The rheostat regulates the intensity of light coming from the lamp or light source. To lengthen the life of the bulb, reduce the light intensity before turning off the light.

Condenser

The condenser is located directly above the light source. It focuses the incoming light into a narrow beam that passes through the specimen and then enters the objective. Although some condensers are fixed in position and cannot be adjusted, adjustable ones can be moved up and down to improve the resolution and contrast of the image. Lowering the condenser away from the stage increases contrast, which is helpful when viewing unstained specimens such as urine sediments (Fig. 2.7). Raising the condenser, on the other hand, decreases contrast and is helpful when viewing thin stained specimens.

Iris (Aperture) Diaphragm

Most condensers contain an iris (aperture) diaphragm, a device that controls the diameter of the light beam coming up through the condenser. When the diaphragm is stopped

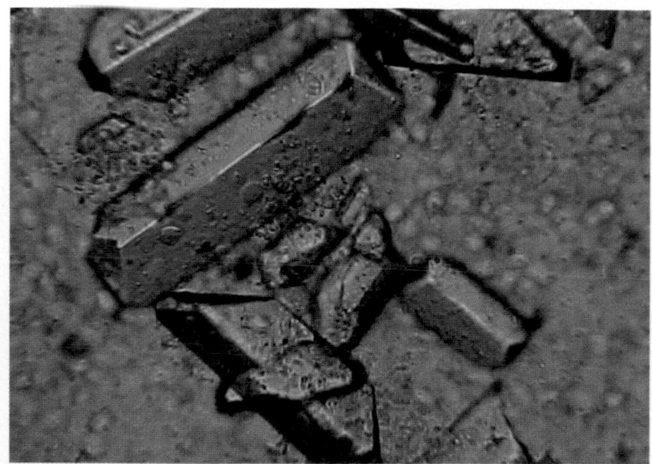

• **Fig. 2.7** Urine sediment. This photomicrograph of dog urine shows crystals that are typically present when the dog has a bacterial infection of the urinary bladder. An unstained specimen such as this is most easily viewed using high contrast (low condenser position). The illumination may need to be increased when the condenser is lowered. (From Bassert J: Images for veterinary technician educators, Summer 2001.)

down (nearly closed), the light comes straight up through the center of the condenser lens and contrast on the specimen is high, but you lose resolution. When the diaphragm is wide open, resolution improves, but the light may glare, and contrast is decreased. The optimum position of the iris diaphragm is an intermediate position.

Coarse and Fine Adjustment

The adjustment knobs located on the arm of the microscope change the distance between the stage and the objectives. The coarse adjustment knob is used during LP work and moves the stage quickly up or down to bring the specimen into view. To fine-tune this image and to focus specimens under HP and oil immersion objectives, the fine adjustment knob is used carefully to move the stage minute distances. *Never* use the coarse adjustment knob when working under high magnification because there is a risk of breaking the slide and scratching the objective.

Stage and Stage Brackets or Clips

The stage is the platform below the objectives upon which a glass or plastic specimen slide is placed. There is a hole in the stage through which the light from the condenser passes. A bracket holds a slide in place on a mechanical stage. Knobs, located below and to the right side of the stage, direct the brackets to move the slide to the right and left, and forward and backward. If a mechanical bracket is not present, stationary stage clips are used and the slide must be moved manually. Stage clips are found on older microscopes without mechanical stages. They are flexible pieces of metal that rest on the slide. Slides must be moved manually to change fields.

Care of the Microscope

Every part of a good-quality microscope is expensive, so be careful when moving, handling, and using one. Adhering to the following recommendations will help ensure the health of your microscope:

1. Always carry the microscope in an upright position with two hands: one under the base and the other on the arm. Never grab a microscope by any part other than the arm!
2. When placing the microscope on a tabletop, be sure that the entire base is in contact with the counter surface. The edge of the base should be no less than 10 cm from the edge of the table.
3. Make sure the stage and objectives are as far apart as possible and that the lowest power objective is in position.
4. Unwind the lamp cord carefully, avoiding damage to any parts of the microscope. Hold the plug, not the cable, when plugging in and unplugging the illuminator.
5. When using the focus adjustment knobs, focus carefully. Don't speed through the focusing process, particularly when using the coarse focus adjustment.
6. Apply immersion oil *only* to the oil immersion objective. Never apply oil to the high dry or any other objective. The oil immersion lens has a protective seal that prevents oil from leaking into the objective; the other objectives lack this protective seal.
7. Remove immersion oil immediately after use. Don't let it dry on the lens. The oil can degrade the glue that holds the lens in place.
8. *Always* use good-quality lens paper on all optical surfaces. Never use paper towels or other tissue paper products to clean the lenses. Only use appropriate lens cleaner or distilled water to clean the lenses. Organic solvents may separate or damage the lens elements or coatings.
9. Because bulbs are expensive, and have a limited life, turn the illuminator off when you are not using the microscope.

Putting the Microscope Away

1. Move the scanning objective into position and lower the stage as far as possible.
2. Always make sure the stage and all of the objectives are *thoroughly* cleaned before putting away the microscope. Remember that oil can damage the lenses.
3. Unplug the illuminator cord and wrap it *carefully* around the base of the microscope, being cautious with the illuminator.
4. Cover the instrument with a dust jacket when not in use.

EXERCISES

Parts of the Microscope

Exercise 1

Label the Parts of the Microscope

Below is an illustration of a compound microscope (Fig. 2.8). Match the terms with the corresponding parts on the drawing.

Oculars
Nosepiece
Objective lenses
Base
Arm
Light source
Condenser
Iris diaphragm
Light switch
Rheostat
Coarse adjustment knob
Fine adjustment knob
Stage
Stage adjustment knobs

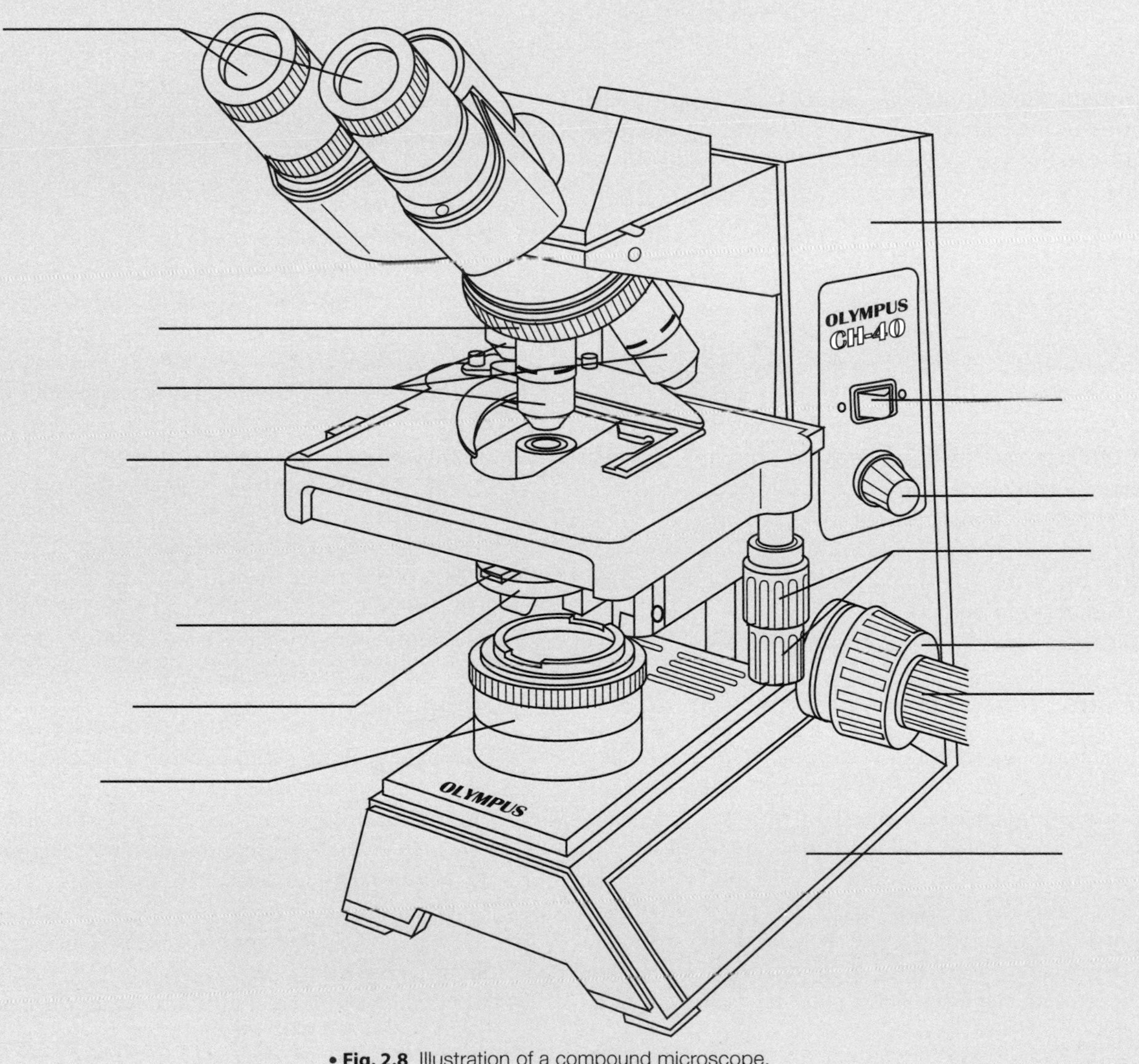

• **Fig. 2.8** Illustration of a compound microscope.

Exercise 2

Match the Parts of the Microscope With the Corresponding Definition

_____ Oculars
_____ Objective lenses
_____ Arm
_____ Condenser
_____ Iris diaphragm
_____ Rheostat
_____ Coarse adjustment knob
_____ Fine adjustment knob
_____ Stage

a. Focuses the image. Can move the stage quickly a large distance.
b. Focuses the light into the objectives. Adjustment can change contrast.
c. Controls the intensity of the illumination.
d. Magnifying lenses that are closest to the specimen. Can be changed to increase magnification.
e. Platform for holding the slide.
f. You carry the microscope by this part.
g. Focuses the image. Moves the stage in very small increments.
h. Controls the diameter of the light beam.
i. Magnifying lenses that are closest to your eye. Usual magnification is 10×.

Use of the Compound Microscope

Exercise 3

Procedure: Measure and Calculate Magnification

1. Carefully unwind the cord from around the base, making sure not to damage any parts of the microscope. Plug in the cord.
2. Make sure the stage and objectives are as far apart as possible and that the lowest power objective (scanning objective) is in position.
3. Clean the oculars and objective with lens paper, if needed.
4. Turn on the light source by pushing the light switch to the "on" position.
5. Adjust the oculars to match your interpupillary distance (distance between your eyes).
6. Carefully place the prepared slide of the newsprint letter "e" on the stage and secure it in place with stage clips or mechanical brackets, if present.
7. Move the slide so that the letter "e" is centered over the stage's hole.
8. While looking from the side, use the coarse adjustment knob to lower the lowest powered objective carefully as close to the slide as possible. Do not allow the objective lens to touch the slide.
9. Look through the oculars and use the coarse focus knob to raise the objective slowly away from the slide. When the image becomes clear, switch to the fine adjustment knob to perfect the image.
10. Using the condenser knob, raise the condenser so that it is almost touching the bottom of the microscope slide. If the condenser has selectable options, set it to "bright field." Start with the iris (aperture) diaphragm in a closed position. Slowly move the diaphragm lever so that the aperture gradually opens. You will see increasing amounts of light coming through the specimen as you move the aperture diaphragm lever to a more open position.
11. Take a moment to adjust the oculars. Make a diopter adjustment by adjusting the movable eyepiece(s) so that both of your eyes see through the oculars equally well. Look at the image with each eye individually and then together to confirm balanced vision.
12. Calculate the degree of magnification by multiplying the magnification of the ocular by the magnification of the objective. Enter this Fig. into the table on next page. Use the millimeter ruler to measure the working distance from the top of the slide to the bottom of the objective and enter this measurement in millimeters (mm) in Table 2.1.
13. Turn the 10× objective until it is over the microscope slide. Turn the fine adjustment knob to sharpen the image. Sketch the image you see in the circle provided.

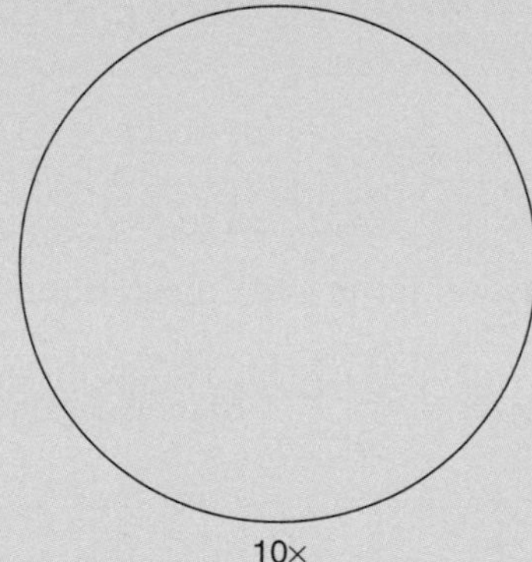
10×

1. Calculate the degree of magnification and enter the figure in Table 2.1. Using the millimeter ruler, measure the working distance from the top of the slide to the bottom of the objective and enter this number in millimeters (mm) in the chart (see Table 2.1).
2. Next, move the 40× objective into position. Turn the fine adjustment knob to sharpen the image. Remember never to use the coarse adjustment to focus when using high magnification. Scan the slide by using the mechanical

Continued

Exercise 3—cont'd

Procedure: Measure and Calculate Magnification

stage knobs to move the slide left and right and backward and forward while looking through the oculars. If you do not have a mechanical stage, you will need to move the slide on the stage by hand. Sketch the image in the corresponding circle below. You may need to adjust the lighting and contrast to generate the best possible image.

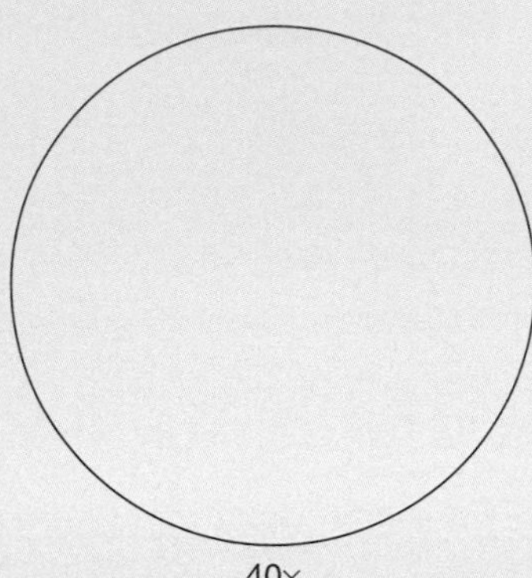

40×

1. While using the 40× objective, calculate the degree of magnification and enter it in Table 2.1. Using the millimeter ruler, measure the working distance from the top of the slide to the bottom of the objective in millimeters and enter the figure in Table 2.1.
2. Rotate the 100× objective (oil immersion lens) slightly, but do not click it into position. At this point, no objective should be in position. Carefully place one drop of immersion oil on the portion of the slide that is directly over the condenser and stage hole. Do not get oil on your hands or on any part of the microscope. Rotate the 100× objective into position, being careful not to rotate any other lens into the oil. While looking into the oculars, use only the fine adjustment to focus the 100× (oil immersion) objective. Using the coarse adjustment could break the slide and damage the lens. Adjust illumination and contrast as needed. Sketch the image that you see in the corresponding circle below.

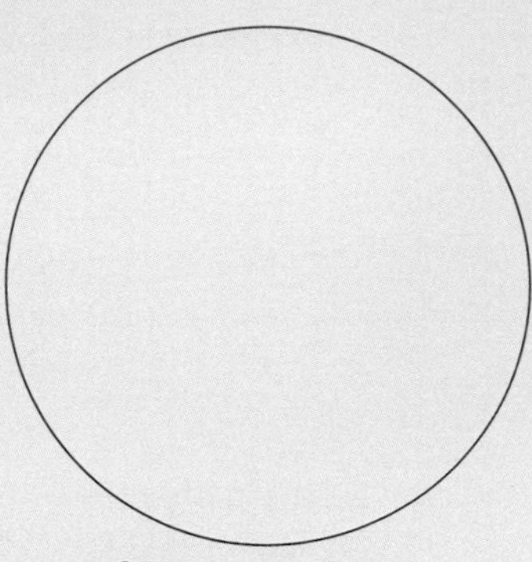

Oil immersion (100×)

1. Calculate the degree of magnification and enter it into Table 2.1. Using the millimeter ruler, measure the working distance from the top of the slide to the bottom of the objective and enter this figure into the table as well.
2. Rotate the 100× objective to the side and rotate the 4× objective into place (not the 40× objective because it would touch the oil). Carefully remove the slide without getting oil on your fingers or on any part of the microscope. Clean the slide with lens paper. Discard the oily paper right away. If you have oil on your fingers, you will need to wash your hands. Next, clean the 100× objective with fresh lens paper and lens cleaner to remove all traces of oil.
3. Move the lowest power objective into position. Separate the objectives from the stage so that they are as far apart from one another as possible
4. Re-examine the stage and lenses to ensure that they are thoroughly cleaned.
5. Turn off the microscope light and unplug the illuminator cord. Wrap it carefully around the base of the microscope.
6. Cover the microscope with a dust cover.

TABLE 2.1 Measurements and Calculations for Each Magnification

Objective Power	Magnification	Working Distance	Field Diameter
4×	________	________	________
10×	________	________	________
40×	________	________	________
100× (oil)	________	________	________

Exercise 4

Procedure: Calculate Field Size

It is useful to be able to estimate the size of objects viewed under the microscope. For instance, the oocyst of *Isospora canis* looks similar to the nematode egg *Toxascaris leonina.* The major difference between the two is that *I. canis* is half the size of *T. leonina.* Being able to estimate the size of both *I. canis* and *T. leonina*, therefore, is important in making a correct identification. But how is the size of a specimen calculated? The answer is that it is not calculated directly, but indirectly, by first calculating the field size. Field size refers to the amount of a specimen that is visible through the microscope. As the magnification of a specimen *increases,* the field size *decreases.* By knowing the total field size, you can estimate the size of the specimen inside the field.

Here Is How It is Done. . .

The diameter of the microscope field and the objects in it are measured in millimeters (abbreviation: mm, 1/1000th of a m) and micrometers (abbreviation: μm, 1/1,000,000th of a meter). More importantly (and more relevant to microscopy), a micrometer (μm) is 1/1000th of a millimeter (mm) or 0.001 mm. To measure the diameter of a microscopic field, you will need a grid slide. A grid slide is a special microscope slide that contains ruled millimeter squares. Each square is 1 mm by 1 mm. Once a grid slide is acquired, complete the following steps:

1. Center the grid slide on the stage of the microscope. Using the 4× objective, adjust focus, brightness, and contrast until the image is clear and sharp.
2. Move the grid slide until one line of the grid is lined up along the left-hand side of the field. Count the number of squares that extend across the diameter of the microscopic field. If the last square is only partially in the field, estimate the fraction of the square that is visible. For example, in Fig. 2.9 there are three squares in the diameter of the field and approximately half of the fourth square is showing. So, the length of the diameter of the field is 3.5 mm. Calculate the length of the diameter of *your* field using the 4× objective and enter your result into Table 2.1.

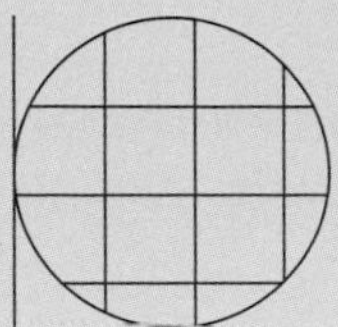

• **Fig. 2.9** A 3.5-mm microscope field.

3. Move the 10× objective into position and again calculate the length of the diameter of the field in millimeters. Enter your result in Table 2.1.
4. We could keep going and directly measure the length of the high-power field (HPF, 40× objective) and oil immersion field (100× objective) as you have been doing. But you can also calculate these fields by using the measurements you already have of the low power field (LPF, 10× objective). Calculating these fields is easier and faster than measuring them directly. Use the following formula to calculate the diameter of the fields seen under 40× and 100× objectives. Enter your results in Table 2.1.

$$\text{Diameter of HPF} = \frac{\text{Diameter of LPF}' \text{ degree of magnification of the LP objective}}{\text{Degree of magnification of the HP objective}}$$

Example:
What would be the diameter of the HPF if the diameter of the LPF is equal to 2 mm? The degree of magnification of the low-power objective is 100 (10× objective × 10× ocular) and the degree of magnification of the high-power objective is 400 (40× objective × 10× ocular). Therefore:

$$\text{Diameter of HPF} = \frac{2\text{ mm} \times 100}{400} = 0.5\text{ mm} = 500\ \mu\text{m}$$

Exercise 5

Procedure: Estimate Size of Objects (using a prepared blood film)

To estimate the size of objects in the field, simply estimate the percentage of the diameter of the field that is occupied by the object. For example, if a field is 1 mm in diameter and an oocyst takes up half of the field size, then the object is approximately 0.5 mm in diameter. Refer to Fig. 2.10 for another example.

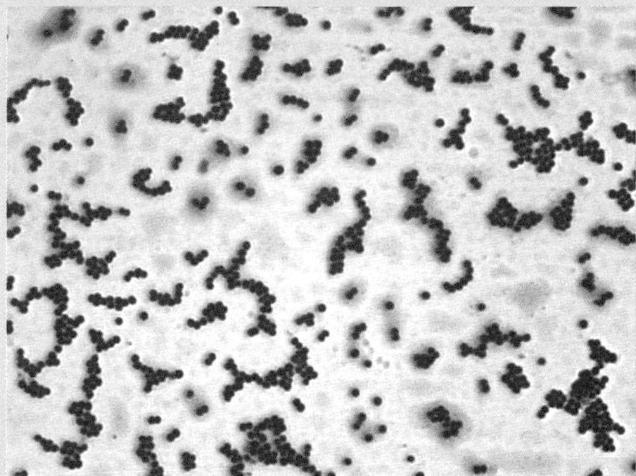

Set Up for Viewing

Clean the oculars and objective with lens paper as needed. Move the 4× objective into position. Adjust the oculars to your interpupillary distance (distance between your eyes).

Carefully place a slide of a blood smear on the stage. If there is no coverslip, be sure that the blood film is facing upward.

Optimize the Lighting

Turn on the illuminator and adjust it so that the field is bright without hurting your eyes. The higher the magnification, the more light you will need.

Adjust the Condenser

Adjust the condenser using the condenser knob so that the condenser is almost touching the bottom of the microscope slide. This is the ideal setting for viewing stained smears. Start with the iris (aperture) diaphragm stopped down (high contrast). You should see the light that comes up through the specimen increase in brightness as you move the aperture diaphragm lever to a more open position. Adjust the aperture diaphragm to optimize viewing.

Focus, Locate, and Center the Specimen

Start with the lowest magnification objective lens (4×), to find the specimen and/or the part of the specimen you wish to examine. Start with the specimen out of focus so that the stage and objective must be brought closer together. Use the coarse focus knob to bring the stage and objective closer together. Once you have found the specimen, adjust the contrast and intensity of illumination, and move the slide around on the stage until you have a good area for viewing. Find an area where the cells are close together but not touching. Use the fine focus knob to sharpen the image.

Adjust Eyepiece Focus

Look with the appropriate eye into the fixed eyepiece and focus with the microscope focus knob. Next, look into the adjustable eyepiece (with the other eye of course), and adjust the eyepiece, not the microscope focus knob.

Move the 10× objective into position over the microscope slide. Turn the fine adjustment to sharpen the image.

Locate a specific red blood cell in the field. Referring to Table 2.1, find the field size for the 10× objective that you calculated earlier. Using this number, estimate the diameter of the red blood cell. Draw the cell and write the diameter in the space provided below.

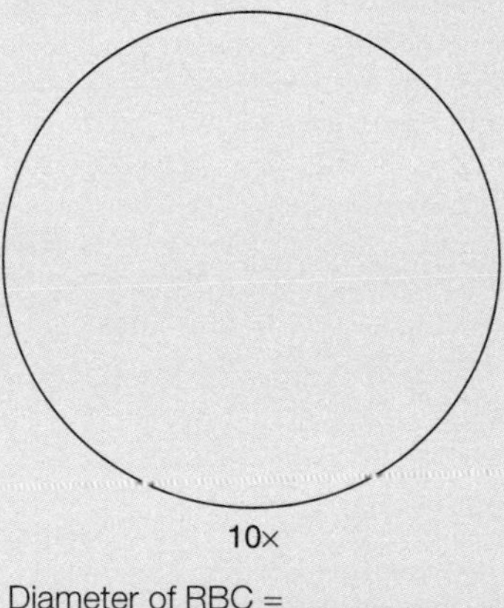

10×

Diameter of RBC = ___________

Locate a specific white blood cell in the smear and estimate its diameter. Draw the cell and write the diameter in the space provided below.

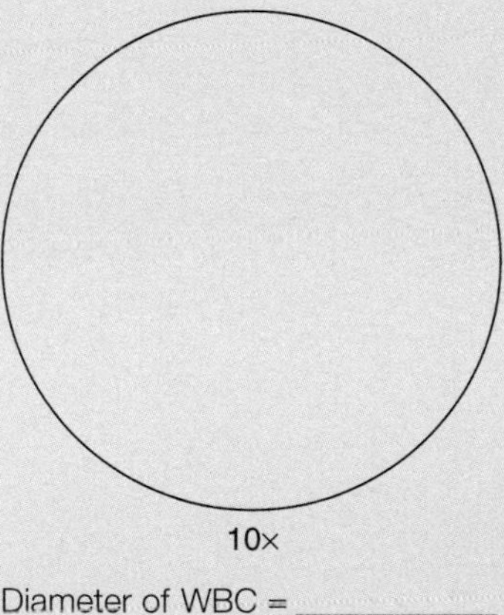

10×

Diameter of WBC = ___________

Turn the 40× objective into position above the microscope slide. Use the fine adjustment to sharpen the image. Scan the slide using the mechanical stage knobs to move the slide on the stage, while looking through the oculars. Adjust illumination if necessary.

Exercise 5—cont'd

Procedure: Estimate Size of Objects (using a prepared blood film)

Locate a red blood cell in the smear and estimate its diameter using the field size for the 40× objective that you previously calculated. Draw the cell and record its diameter in the space provided below.

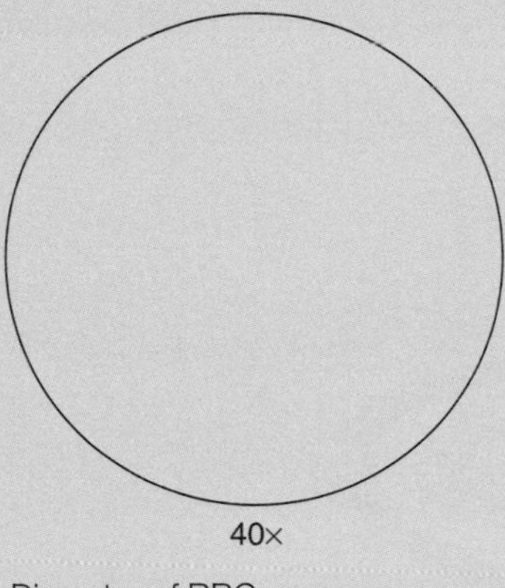

40×

Diameter of RBC = ___________

Locate a white blood cell in the smear and estimate its diameter. Draw the cell and write its diameter in the space provided below.

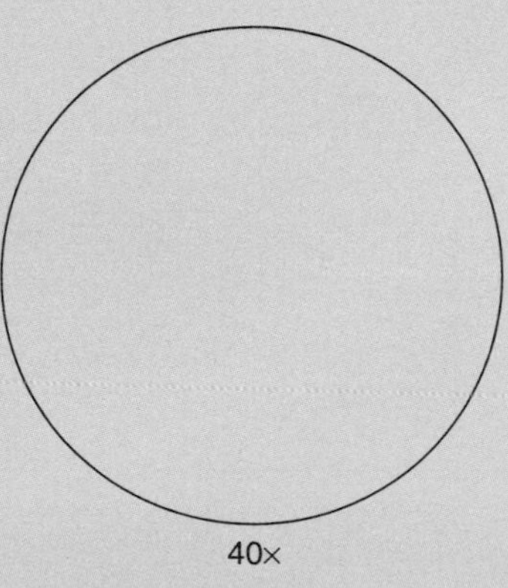

40×

Diameter of WBC = ___________

Rotate the 100× objective (oil immersion lens) to the side slightly (so that no objective is in position). Place one drop of immersion oil on the portion of the slide that is directly over the condenser. Rotate the 100× objective into position, being careful *not* to rotate any other lens into the oil. While looking into the oculars, use only the fine adjustment to focus the 100× (oil immersion) objective. Using the coarse adjustment could break the slide or damage the lens. Adjust illumination if necessary.

Locate a specific red blood cell in the smear and, referring to the field size for the 100× objective that you previously calculated, estimate the diameter of the red blood cell. Draw the cell and write its diameter in the space provided below.

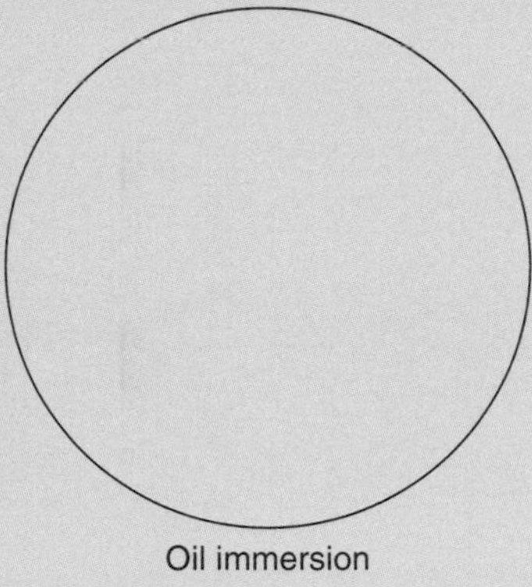

Oil immersion

Diameter of RBC = ___________

Locate a specific white blood cell in the smear and estimate its diameter. Draw the cell and write its diameter in the space provided below.

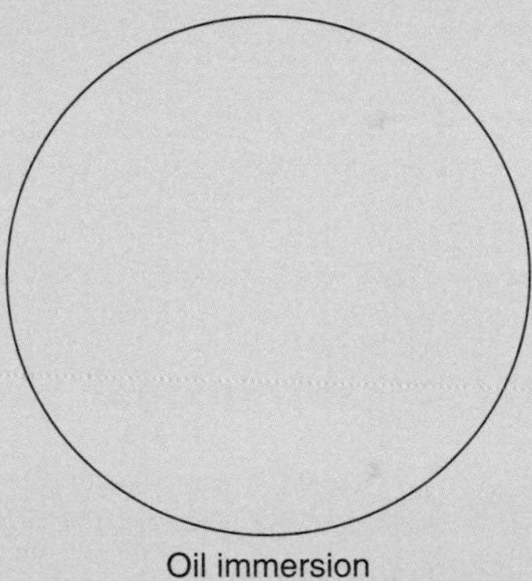

Oil immersion

Diameter of WBC = ___________

Move the 4× objective into position (*not* the 40× objective because it would touch the oil). Carefully remove the slide, without getting oil on your fingers or on any part of the microscope. Clean the slide with lens paper. Discard the oily paper right away. If you have oil on your fingers, you will need to wash your hands. Next, clean the 100× objective with fresh lens paper and lens cleaner to remove all traces of oil.

Continued

Exercise 5—cont'd

Procedure: Estimate Size of Objects (using a prepared blood film)

Separate the objectives from the stage so that they are as far apart from one another as possible.

Re-examine the stage and lenses to ensure that they are *thoroughly* cleaned.

Turn off the microscope light and unplug the illuminator cord. Wrap it *carefully* around the base of the microscope.

Cover the microscope with a dust cover.

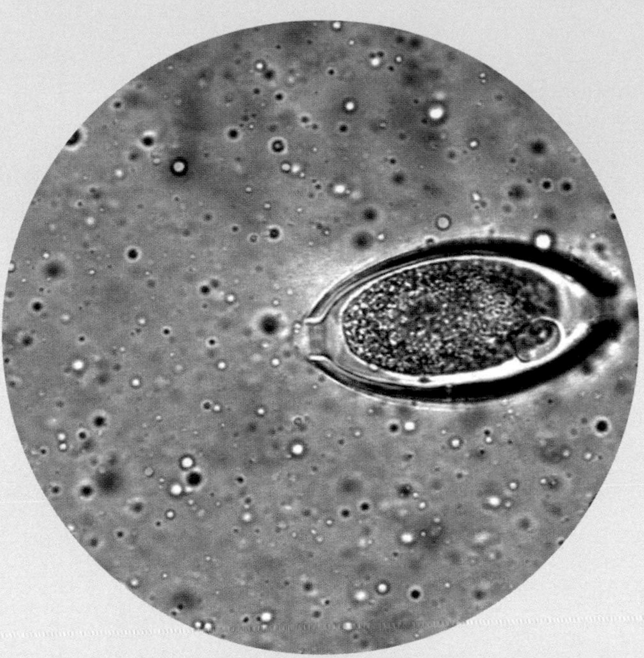

• **Fig. 2.10** Fecal flotation. This photomicrograph of a fecal flotation specimen shows an egg from the nematode *Trichuris*. The field size is 140 μm, and the egg takes up half of the field diameter. So, we estimate the egg length to be 70 μm.(From Bassert J: Images for veterinary technician educators, Summer 2001.)

Critical and Clinical Thinking

Exercise 6

Clinical Thinking Challenge

Support each of the following correct statements with appropriate rationale, stating why or in what way each statement is correct.

1. Oil should be cleaned off the oil immersion lens before it dries.

____

____

2. Oil cannot be used with any objective other than the oil immersion objective.

____

____

3. As you change to a higher degree of magnification, you have to increase the illumination.

____

____

4. The distance between the oculars on a microscope needs to be adjusted for each user.

____

____

5. Adjustments need to be made to both oculars.

____

____

Exercise 6—cont'd

Clinical Thinking Challenge

6. The highest power lens is used with oil.

7. The objective lens is sometimes referred to as the scanning lens.

8. Caution should be observed when using the high dry and oil immersion objective lenses.

9. One should never use the coarse adjustment knob when working under high magnification.

10. One should turn off the illuminator when the microscope is not in use.

11. It is useful to be able to estimate the size of objects viewed under the microscope.

12. The elements nitrogen, oxygen, hydrogen, and carbon are essential to life.

13. Ongoing blood loss results in iron deficiency anemia.

14. Colloids appear translucent or milky.

15. More chemicals can be dissolved in water than any other known solvent.

16. Water is an ideal transport medium.

17. Acids and bases are called electrolytes.

18. A pH of 7 is considered neutral.

19. Proteins can be considered the worker molecules of the body.

20. Hyperthermia can result in death.

3
Cell Anatomy

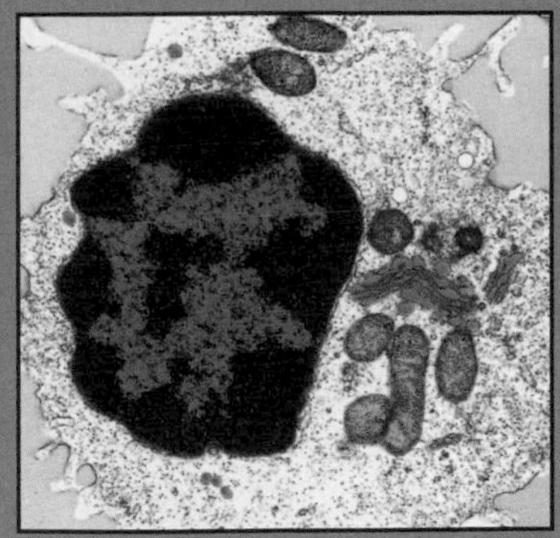

OVERVIEW AT A GLANCE

The Anatomy of the Cell 35

Stages of Cell Division 42

Exercises 44–53

Cell Anatomy 44–45
- *1. Color and Label Plasma Membrane 44*
- *2. Match Definitions and Terms 45*

Cellular Microscopy 46–49
- *3. Cell Diagram and Observations 46*
- *4. Color and Label Cellular Components 48*
- *5. Prepare and Examine a Wet Mount Slide 49*

Cell Division 49–51
- *6. Diagram of Stages of Mitosis 49*
- *7. Identify Stages of Mitosis 50*
- *8. Diagram of Stages of Meiosis 51*

Fluid Therapy 52
- *9. Determining Type of Fluid Administration 52*
- *10. Estimate the Percent of Dehydration in Dogs 52*

Critical and Clinical Thinking 53
- *11. Clinical Thinking Challenge 53*

LEARNING OBJECTIVES

Upon completion of this lab you will be able to:

1. Identify the various organelles of the cell.
2. Understand the function of each organelle.
3. Discuss the anatomic relationships between the various parts of the cell.
4. Compare the shape of a cell with its function.
5. List in order the stages of mitosis and describe what occurs during each stage.
6. Recognize the stages of mitosis in cells from a white fish blastula.
7. Understand the differences that occur in the division of sex cells (meiosis) versus somatic cells (mitosis).

CLINICAL SIGNIFICANCE

To understand the cell as the basic structural, functional, and biologic unit of all living organisms is to understand the basis of life. Veterinary medicine depends on knowledge of anatomy and physiology; foundational to that base of knowledge is the study of the cell.

INTRODUCTION

The cell is the structural and functional unit of all living organisms. As you can imagine, the cell is very complex. Differences in the sizes, shapes, and internal compositions of cells reflect their diverse functions within the animal. Even though cells may have distinctive anatomic characteristics and specialized functions, there are generalizations that can be made about cells as a whole. For example, most of the cells in an animal maintain their boundaries, absorb and digest nutrients, dispose of waste, grow in size, reproduce, and respond to various stimuli. This chapter focuses on the structural components of the *typical* cell and examines the miracle of cell division.

MATERIALS NEEDED

To complete this laboratory, you will need the following:

- Model of an animal cell or a laboratory chart of cell anatomy
- Compound microscope
- Prepared slides of the following:
  - Skeletal muscle
  - Adipose tissue
  - Tracheal mucosa (ciliated columnar)
  - Lung alveoli (simple squamous)
  - Blood smear
  - Whitefish blastula
- Models or drawings of cell division
- Microscope slides and cover slips
- New methylene blue stain
- Cotton-tipped applicator sticks
- Colored pencils

TERMS TO BE IDENTIFIED

Plasma membrane
- Internal membrane surface
- External membrane surface
- Phospholipid
  - Polar head (hydrophilic)
  - Nonpolar tails (hydrophobic)
- Glycolipid
  - Carbohydrate portion
  - Phospholipid portion
- Integral proteins: globular proteins
  - Channel proteins
  - Carrier proteins
- Receptor proteins: glycoprotein
  - Carbohydrate portion
  - Protein portion
- Peripheral proteins
- Cholesterol

Nucleus
- Nuclear pores
- Nucleoli
- Chromatin
  - Chromosomes
  - Chromatids
  - Centromere

Cytoplasm and its organelles
- Centriole
- Golgi apparatus
- Endoplasmic reticulum (smooth and rough)
- Lysosome
- Peroxisome
- Mitochondria
- Cytoskeletal elements
  - Microtubules
  - Intermediate filaments
  - Microfilaments
- Ribosomes
- Inclusion bodies

The Anatomy of the Cell

A cell is composed of three primary parts, two of which can be easily identified with the compound microscope (Fig. 3.1):

- The plasma membrane (not visible with a light microscope)
- The nucleus
- The cytoplasm (which contains the organelles)

The plasma membrane surrounds the internal structures of the cell, forming a flexible barrier between the intracellular and extracellular environments. At the heart of the cell is the large darkly staining nucleus.

Within the cytoplasm are numerous components called **organelles** (little organs). These organelles are highly organized and metabolically active structures that have their own characteristic shape and function. It has only been since the advent of the electron microscope that the structures of the plasma membrane and the organelles have been identified and studied.

Plasma Membrane

The **plasma membrane** separates the cell contents from the surrounding environment (Fig. 3.2). It is composed of **phospholipids** and various globular and structural proteins, which are arranged into a bilayer (two layers) called the *fluid mosaic*. The phospholipids have phosphate heads, which are polar and **hydrophilic** (water-loving), and two fatty acid tails, which are nonpolar and **hydrophobic** (water-fearing). The **nonpolar tails** of each layer face each other and form the inner world of the plasma membrane. The **polar heads** face away from one another, forming a single row of phosphate heads on the outside of the cell and another similar row on the inside of the cell. Embedded within the phospholipid bilayer are globular proteins called **integral proteins,** which span the entire width of the membrane and serve many functions. **Channel proteins**, for example, allow certain substances to pass through pores within them and in this way connect the inside and the outside of the cell. Small molecules such as water can pass through the pores easily, whereas large molecules cannot. **Carrier proteins** use active transport to move substances from one side of the plasma membrane to the other. **Receptor proteins** contain specific receptor sites that bond only to specific molecules such as hormones. In addition, the plasma membrane is composed of **cholesterol** molecules that wedge themselves between phospholipids to assist in the stabilization of the cell membrane. Refer to Chapter 3 of the textbook for more details about the plasma membrane.

Besides providing a protective barrier for the cell, the plasma membrane acts as a gatekeeper for the cell, determining what can and what cannot enter or leave. It has been

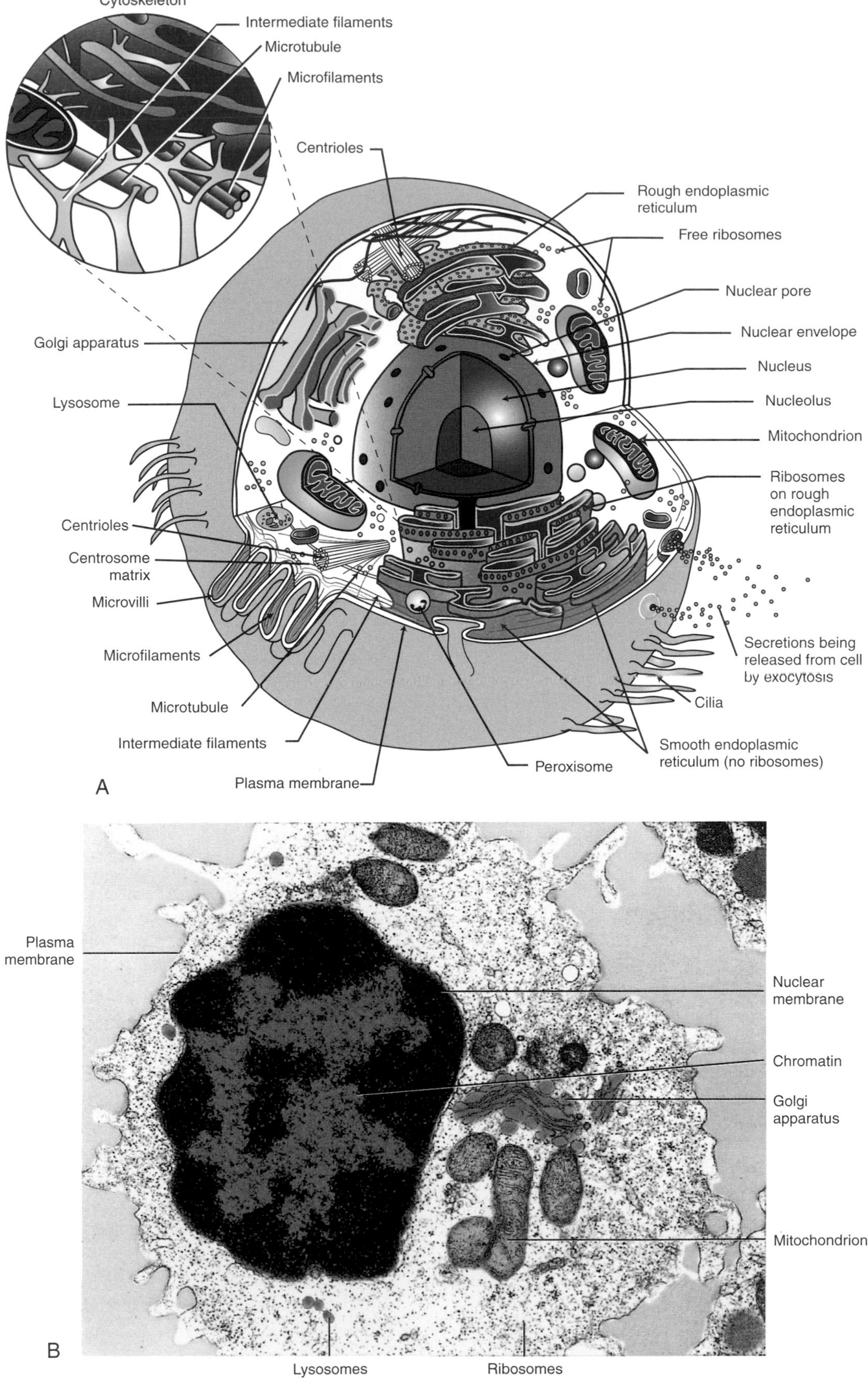

• Fig. 3.1 (A) The generalized cell and cellular components. (B) Electron micrograph of a cell that has been color enhanced to distinguish cellular components. (B, Courtesy A. Arlen Hinchee.)

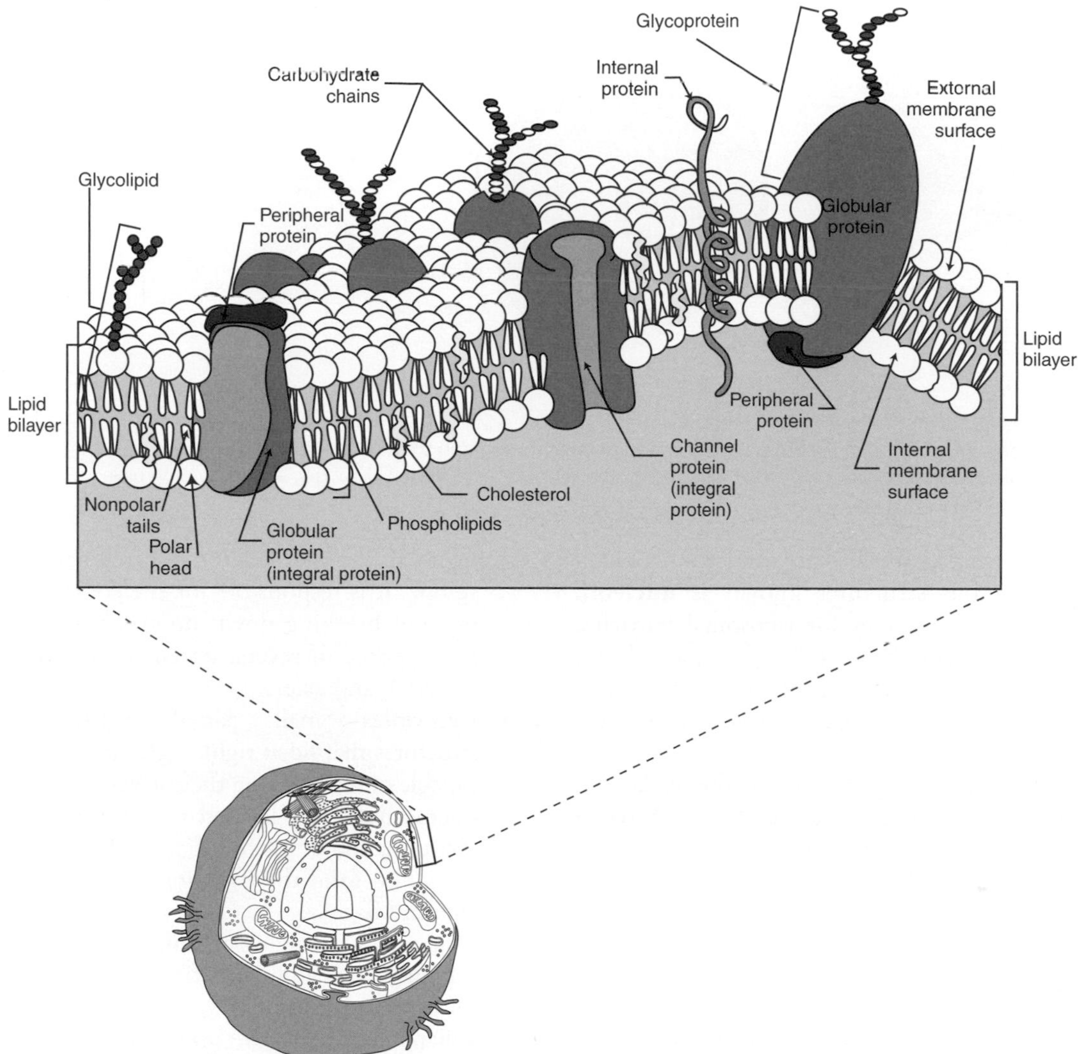

• **Fig. 3.2** Plasma membrane. Section of cellular membrane showing the phospholipid bilayer and various transmembrane channels that allow substances to pass in and out of the cell.

compared with a "picket fence," allowing certain things into the cell while keeping others out. For example, it allows many lipid-soluble molecules and very tiny molecules, such as gases, to pass through the cell membrane easily, just like air moving through the pickets of a fence. The hydrophobic tails of the phospholipids and the cholesterol molecules, however, prohibit water-soluble molecules from moving passively into or out of the cell.

In some cells, the plasma membrane is thrown into fingerlike folds called **microvilli,** which act to increase the surface area of the cell for absorption or secretion. Cilia and flagella are also extensions of the cell membrane, whose movements require a great deal of energy.

Nucleus

The **nucleus** is one of the largest structures in the cell (Fig. 3.3). It can be found in a wide variety of places in the cell depending on the cell's shape and function. Some cells, such as skeletal muscle cells, have multiple nuclei. The nucleus is often described as the control center of the cell and is necessary for protein synthesis and reproduction because it contains the vital genetic instruction, DNA. A mature red blood cell, for example, lacks a nucleus and therefore cannot survive for long without the ability or instructions needed to make protein. If a cell cannot make the protein needed to repair and maintain itself, it will inevitably die. When viewed under the compound microscope, the nucleus is a spherical or oval structure and usually is the most prominent intracellular structure due to its dark appearance. The nucleus normally stains dark purple or blue.

When the cell is not dividing, the genetic material in the nucleus is dispersed throughout the nucleus as small threadlike or granular forms called **chromatin.** As the cell prepares to divide, the chromatin condenses to form coiled rodlike bodies called **chromosomes.**

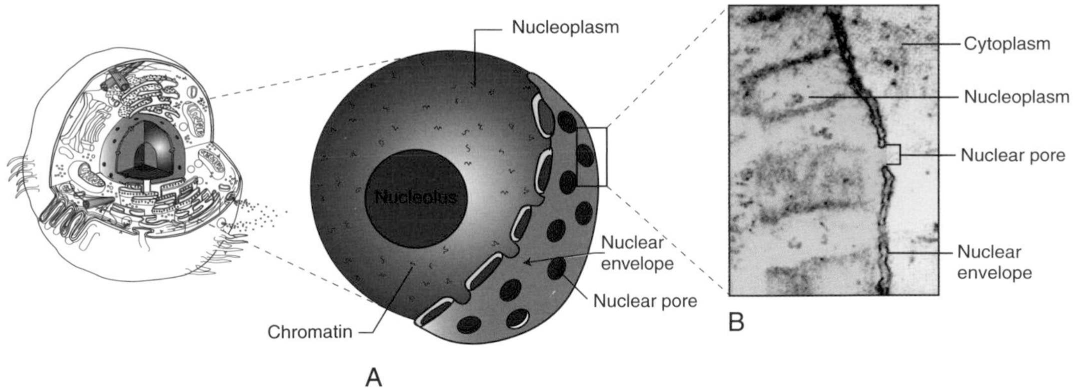

• **Fig. 3.3** (A) Cell nucleus. A double membrane nuclear envelope surrounds the internal nucleolus, nucleoplasm, and chromatin. (B) Color-enhanced electron micrograph showing the double membrane structure of the nuclear envelope. Note the nuclear pores. (B, Courtesy Charles Flickinger, University of Virginia.)

Also located within the nucleus are one or more small round nonmembranous structures known as **nucleoli.** The nucleoli are assembly sites for ribosomal particles. The nucleoli will therefore be much larger in a cell that manufactures larger quantities of proteins, such as muscle and liver cells, than in cells that are less metabolically active.

The nucleus is surrounded by a porous double-layered membrane, much like the plasma membrane. **Nuclear pores** allow the export of large nucleic acid molecules such as messenger RNA (mRNA).

Cytoplasm: Cytosol, Cytoskeleton, and Organelles

The cytoplasm consists of the cell contents other than the nucleus and therefore is the site of most metabolic activities. The cytoplasm is made up of a gelatinous fluid called **cytosol,** cytoskeletal elements, and many small structures termed **organelles**.

- **Cytoskeletal elements**—Internal scaffolding located within the cell that acts to support and move substances through the cell. These small elements or fibers consist of **microtubules, intermediate filaments,** and **microfilaments** and make up the three-dimensional framework within the cell. **Microtubules** are hollow tubules made up of protein. They direct the forming of the mitotic spindle during cell division and act to move other organelles and substances throughout the cell. **Intermediate filaments** are twisted protein strands that act as internal guy wires to resist pulling forces that may act on the cell. **Microfilaments** are thin strands of twisted contractile proteins that have the ability to shorten and then relax to assume a more elongated form. They are termed the "cellular muscle" of the cell because as they contract they can cause shortening of the cell. Microfilaments are very important in muscle cells. The **centrosome** is an important region of the cytoskeleton, located near the nuclear envelope. It is responsible for the coordination of building and breaking down microtubules in the cell and is composed of several parts: centrioles, pericentriolar material, and asters.
- **Centrioles**—Small, paired, rod-shaped, cylindrical structures that lie at right angles to one another and are capable of reproducing themselves. They are made up of microtubules, are located near the nucleus, and direct the formation of the mitotic spindle during cell division. They also form the basis for cell projections called the cilia and flagella.
- **Organelles** are highly organized structures that perform the major metabolic functions of the cell. They include mitochondria, ribosomes, endoplasmic reticulum, Golgi apparatus, lysosomes, proteasomes, peroxisomes, and vaults.
- **Mitochondria**—Small rod-shaped bodies located in the cytosol of the cell (Fig. 3.4). The inner wall of this double-walled organelle has folds, or cristae, that extend into its interior. The cristae increase surface area and contain enzymes that are used to make energy for the cell. Energy is stored in the phosphate bonds of adenosine triphosphate (ATP). The mitochondria are considered to be the powerhouses of the cell. Cells can have as few as 100 mitochondria or as many as several thousand. The mitochondria can self-replicate when increased energy demands are placed on the cell.
- **Ribosomes**—Densely staining small spherical bodies that are composed of ribosomal RNA and protein and serve as the site for protein synthesis. Refer to Chapter 3 in the textbook for a review of protein synthesis. Ribosomes may be free floating in the cytosol or attached to the outside of the endoplasmic reticulum or the nucleus. Membrane-bound ribosomes such as these make protein for use in the cell membrane or for export to other cells. Free-floating ribosomes make protein to be used within the cell.

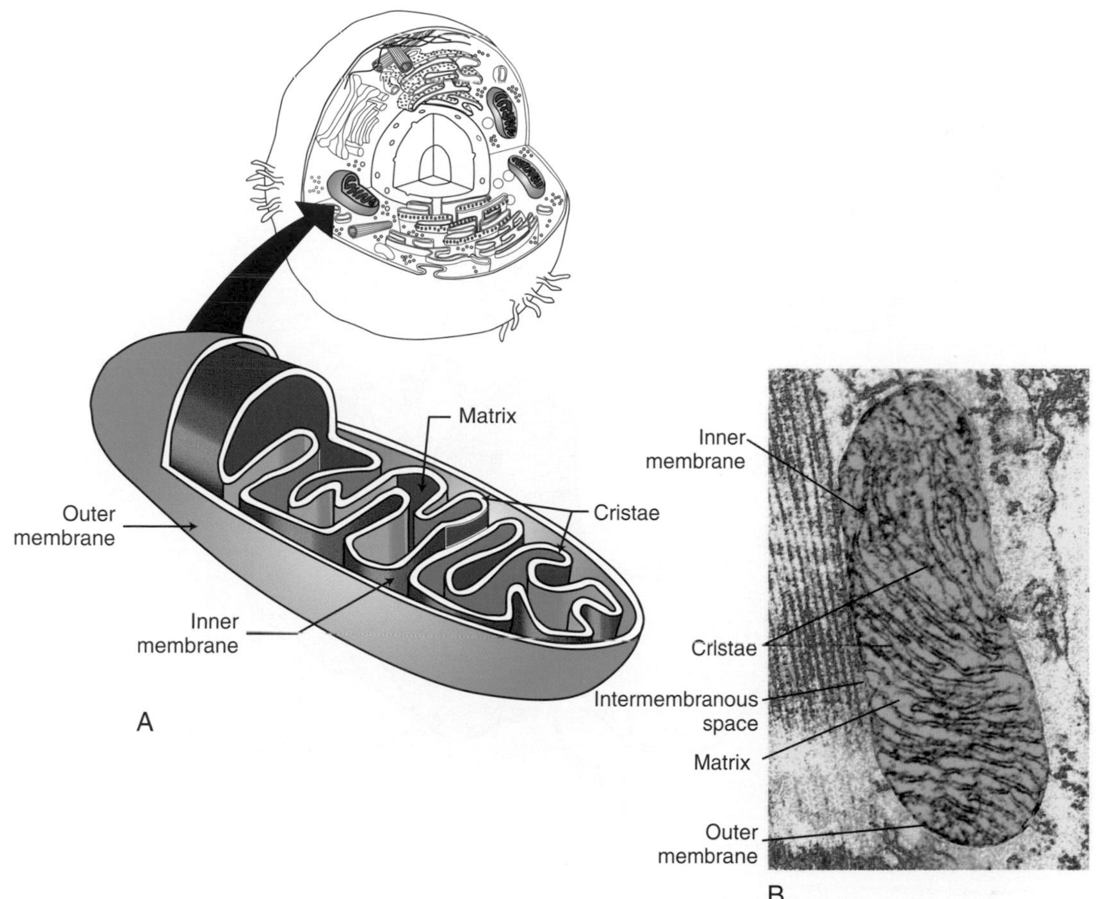

• **Fig. 3.4** (A) Mitochondrion. The inner and outer mitochondrial membranes are evident. The inner membrane forms numerous folds called cristae that contain enzymes used for energy production. (B) Transmission electron micrograph of a mitochondrion. (B, Courtesy Brenda Russell.)

- **Endoplasmic reticulum (ER)**—A membranous network of tubules and flattened sacs that are in contact with the nuclear envelope and are continuous with the Golgi apparatus and the plasma membrane (Fig. 3.5). It is thought that the ER functions as a miniature circulatory system because proteins and other substances can move through its inner canals. The ER exists in two forms within the cell. It may have ribosomes attached to it and is termed **rough ER**, or it may have no ribosomes attached to it and is called **smooth ER**. The rough ER is thought to manufacture, store, and transport proteins to be used outside the cell, whereas the smooth ER is highly active in lipid metabolism and drug detoxification activities.
- **Golgi apparatus**—A membranous organelle consisting of tiny, flattened sacs stacked on top of each other (Fig. 3.6). It is generally found close to the nucleus. The Golgi apparatus processes and packages protein molecules for export from the cell. Proteins from the rough ER are presented to the Golgi apparatus where they may be modified by the attachment of sugar groups and then placed in vesicles that travel to the cell periphery and attach to the plasma membrane for release.
- **Lysosome**—An organelle that has membranous walls like the ER and Golgi apparatus (Fig. 3.7). Lysosomes are vesicles that have pinched off from the Golgi apparatus, carrying potent digestive enzymes. The enzyme hydrolase, for example, which is found in most lysosomes, digests worn-out cell structures and foreign bodies that enter the cell through phagocytosis. The lysosomes are often called "suicide sacs" because of their potential ability to digest and therefore destroy the entire cell.
- **Proteasomes**—Small cylindrical structures composed of protein subunits that digest and break down old proteins one at a time, unlike lysosomes which can digest large amounts of cellular debris. Linear ubiquitin protein attaches to old protein and pulls it into the proteasome where the old protein is broken down into short chain amino acids. These are expelled from the distal cap into the cytosol, where they are further broken down and recycled into new proteins. When the proteasome system is

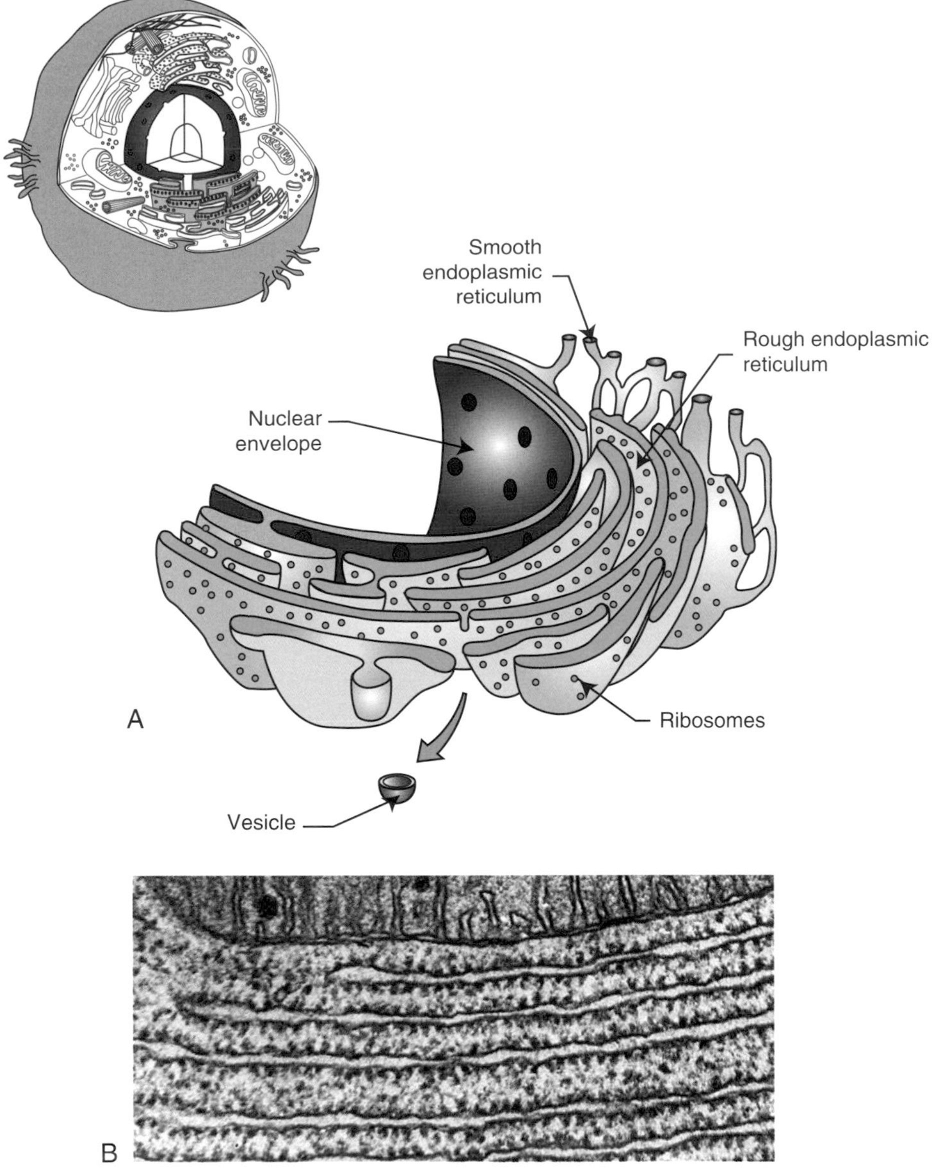

• **Fig. 3.5** (A) Rough endoplasmic reticulum with countless ribosomes attached to its surface. (B) Electron micrograph of rough endoplasmic reticulum showing numerous pinpoint ribosomes located on the surface of the folded ER membrane.(B, From Thibodeau GA, Patton KT: Anatomy and physiology, ed. 8, St Louis, 2013, Mosby.)

not functioning properly, an accumulation of misfolded proteins can kill cells, for example, those in the brain that regulate muscle function (e.g., Parkinson's disease in humans).

- **Peroxisomes**—Enzyme-containing membranous sacs similar to lysosomes; however, peroxisomes contain oxidase enzymes, which use oxygen to detoxify a number of harmful substances such as free radicals. They also contain catalase enzymes that are important in breaking down hydrogen peroxide, which is a by-product of cell metabolism. They are often seen in great numbers in kidney and liver cells.
- **Vaults**—Recently discovered, this tiny organelle is thought to play a role in transporting molecules to and from the cell nucleus, sliding rapidly from one end of the cell to another. Their small size enables them to dock in nuclear pore complexes where they can open up into a rosette shape that echoes the nuclear pore complex. They are numerous, tiny, and made of protein and a small amount of RNA (vRNA or vtRNA).
- **Inclusion bodies**—The cell cytoplasm also contains storage granules that may contain glycogen, water, pigments such as melanin, and ingested foreign material. These substances are termed inclusion bodies.

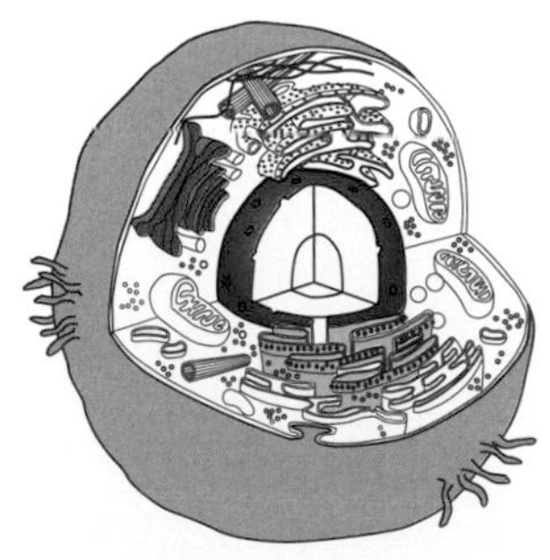

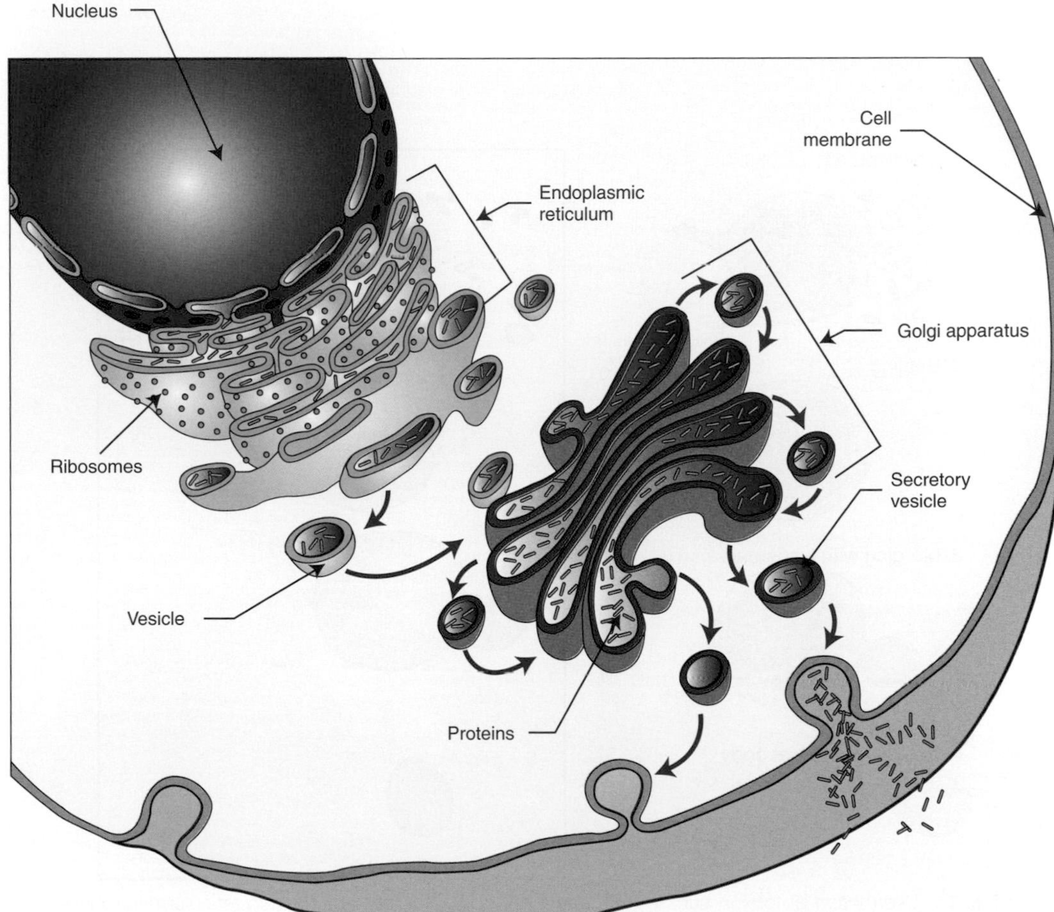

• **Fig. 3.6** Golgi apparatus. Substances are transported out of the cell for use in other parts of the body.

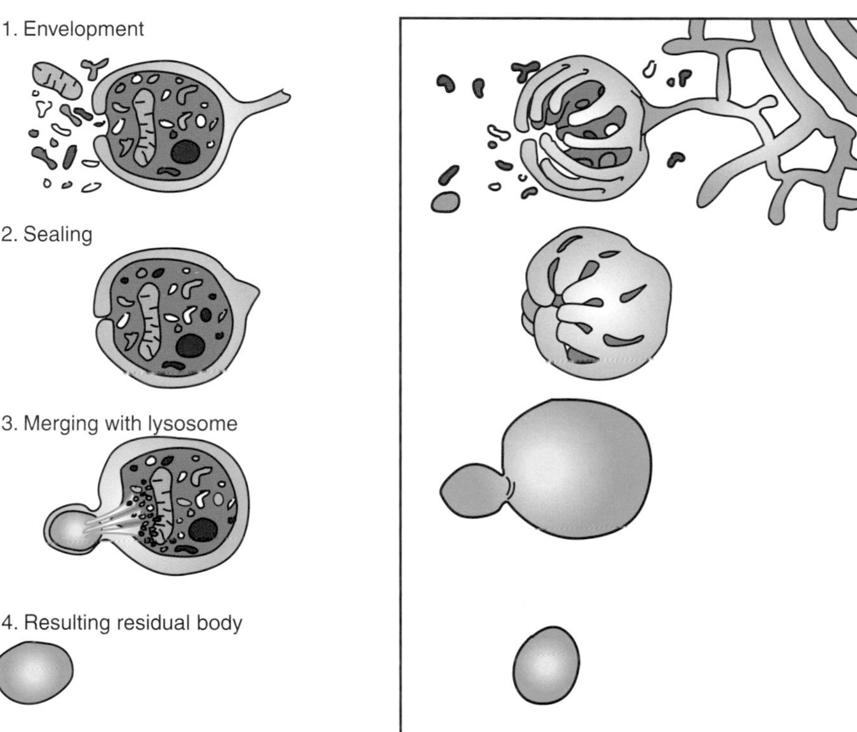

• Fig. 3.7 Destruction of foreign substances. The Golgi apparatus or endoplasmic reticulum surrounds foreign debris, trapping it. A lysosome containing digestive enzymes merges with the vesicle to cause a chemical breakdown of the foreign debris. A residual body is all that remains.

Stages of Cell Division

Cells in animals and humans divide to produce more cells of the same type (Fig. 3.8). A cell's life cycle is the series of changes it goes through from the time it is formed until the time it reproduces. In multicellular animals, cells are divided into two broad categories based on the way in which they divide. Reproductive cells (found in ovaries and testicles) divide by **meiosis**. Somatic cells (all the rest of the cells in the body except reproductive cells) divide by **mitosis**.

The lifecycle of a cell is divided into two major periods: **interphase**, when the cell is growing, maturing, and differentiating, and the **mitotic phase**, when the cell is actively dividing.

Interphase

Interphase is the period between cell divisions, and for the vast majority of cells, it is the stage in which the cell spends the greatest portion of its life and might more accurately be called the metabolic phase. The interphase is divided into three subphases: growth one (G1), synthesis (S), and growth two (G2). Although interphase is divided into distinct stages, the events contained within them flow from one to another as a smooth and continuous process.

During the G1 phase:

- intensive metabolic activity and cellular expansion contribute to the cell doubling in size,
- the number of organelles doubles,

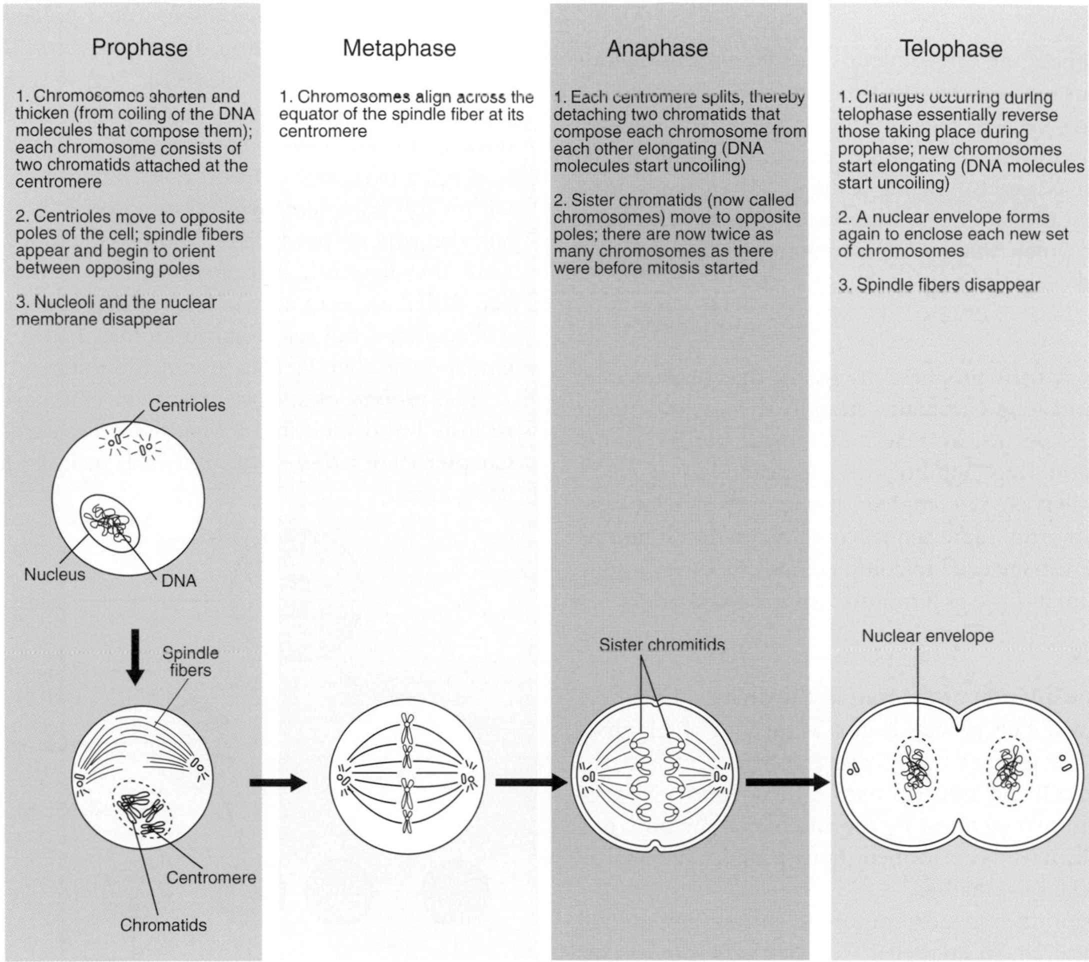

Prophase
1. Chromosomes shorten and thicken (from coiling of the DNA molecules that compose them); each chromosome consists of two chromatids attached at the centromere
2. Centrioles move to opposite poles of the cell; spindle fibers appear and begin to orient between opposing poles
3. Nucleoli and the nuclear membrane disappear
Centrioles
Nucleus
DNA
Spindle fibers
Centromere
Chromatids
Metaphase
1. Chromosomes align across the equator of the spindle fiber at its centromere
Anaphase
1. Each centromere splits, thereby detaching two chromatids that compose each chromosome from each other elongating (DNA molecules start uncoiling)
2. Sister chromatids (now called chromosomes) move to opposite poles; there are now twice as many chromosomes as there were before mitosis started
Sister chromitids
Telophase
1. Changes occurring during telophase essentially reverse those taking place during prophase; new chromosomes start elongating (DNA molecules start uncoiling)
2. A nuclear envelope forms again to enclose each new set of chromosomes
3. Spindle fibers disappear
Nuclear envelope

• **Fig. 3.8** Identification of each stage of mitosis showing the reproduction and division of chromosomes that result in each daughter cell being genetically identical to the original cell.

- cytoplasm expands,
- and centrioles begin to replicate in preparation for cell division.

The synthetic phase is marked by:

- DNA replication.

The final phase, growth phase 2 (G2) includes:

- The synthesis of enzymes and proteins necessary for cell division on future cell growth.

Towards the end of interphase, before the cell begins the division phase, the DNA material in the nucleus is duplicated so that it can be evenly distributed between the two "daughter" cells. Once replication of the DNA has occurred, cell division can proceed to produce two identical daughter cells.

The Stages of Mitosis

Cell division consists of a series of events that occur in a specific order. **Mitosis** or nuclear division occurs first and this happens in four distinct stages: prophase, metaphase, anaphase, and telophase. Towards the end of mitosis, the cytoplasm will divide in a process called **cytokinesis.**

Prophase

The nuclear membrane and the nucleolus break down and disappear during prophase. The **chromatin** threads that were found in the nucleus coil and shorten to form densely staining, tiny, rodlike bodies called **chromosomes.** By the time the cell is halfway through prophase, the chromosomes have taken on an X shape. The X is composed of two **chromatids** held together at their midpoint by a small structure known as a **centromere.** Centrioles, which are found in the cytoplasm, move toward one another and pair up. The two pairs move apart from one another, generating spindle fibers as they go. In this way, the mitotic spindle needed in cell division is rapidly constructed. The spindle fibers act as scaffolding to which the chromosomes are attached. Movement of the spindle fibers will cause the separation of the chromatids from one another to form two new chromosomes.

Metaphase

This brief stage is characterized by the alignment of the chromosomes along the midline (or metaphase plate) of the spindle. Each centromere is attached to a single spindle fiber. When properly assembled with correctly aligned spindles occurs, the cell can move forward into anaphase.

Anaphase

During anaphase the centromeres split and the chromatids separate from one another. In this way, two chromosomes are born from one. The new chromosomes are pulled by the spindle fibers toward the opposite poles of the cell. At the end of anaphase, each pole has a full set of chromosomes. The chromosomes at one pole are exactly the same as those at the other pole. Anaphase is complete when the movement toward the poles ceases.

Telophase

This stage is actually prophase in reverse; the chromosomes uncoil to form long chromatin strands, the spindle breaks down and disappears, a nuclear membrane forms around each chromatin mass, and nucleoli reappear.

Nuclear division is complete at the end of telophase. Mitosis follows the same sequence of events in all animal cells, but the time needed to complete mitosis varies among cell types from as little as 5 minutes up to several hours.

Cytokinesis

Following the division of the nuclei, the division of the cytoplasm occurs. This process begins at the end of telophase and is called cytokinesis. A *cleavage furrow* begins at the center of the cell and eventually splits the original cytoplasmic mass into two sections. By the end of cell division, two daughter cells have been formed, both genetically equal to the mother cell but smaller.

Cell division is extremely important during growth and periods of healing. In epithelial tissue, cell division occurs relatively rapidly. Skeletal muscle, cardiac muscle, and nervous tissue lose much of their ability to divide after puberty and if injured in adults may not be repaired well.

Cell Division in Sex Cells (Meiosis)

Mitosis occurs in the cells of the body known as somatic cells. However, the cells found in the testes and ovaries, which generate sperm and eggs, respectively, are not somatic cells. They are called sex cells and their process of dividing is very different from mitosis. When sex cells divide, the result is the formation of sperm and eggs that contain half as many chromosomes as the somatic cells (Fig. 3.9). To produce sperm and eggs (known as gametes), the parent cells undergo a two-stage division called **meiosis.** A somatic cell with a full complement of chromosomes is called diploid and the gametes produced by meiosis are called haploid because they have one-half of the somatic chromosome number. When a sperm and an egg join together, the offspring will acquire a full set of chromosomes, half from each parent, and will then be able to undergo mitosis.

The process of meiosis occurs in two stages known as meiosis I and meiosis II. Meiosis is discussed in detail in Chapter 19 of *Clinical Anatomy and Physiology for Veterinary Technicians*.

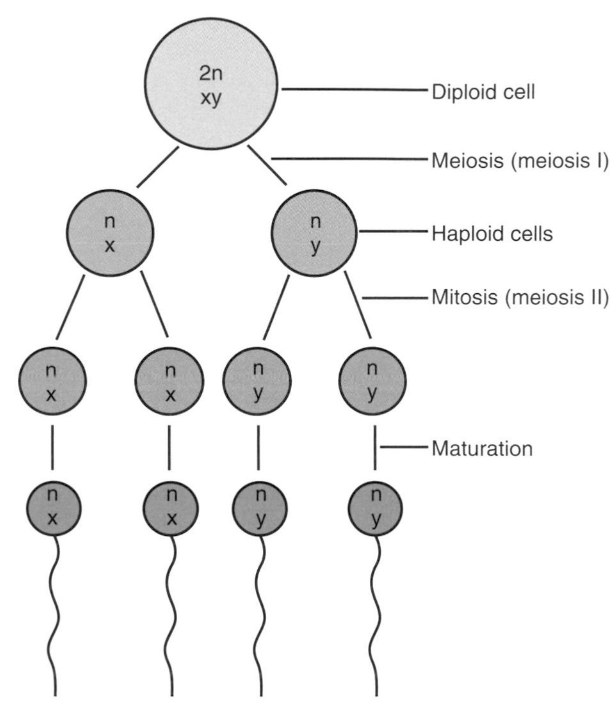

• Fig. 3.9 Meiosis and mitosis.

EXERCISES

Cell Anatomy

Exercise 1

Color and Label Plasma Membrane

Use colored pencils to color in the various components of the plasma membrane in Fig. 3.10. Match the term with the corresponding cell structure by placing the number of the term in the corresponding blank, coloring the structure, and underlining the term with the same color. Use a different color for each structure.

_____ Carbohydrate chains

_____ Channel protein

_____ Cholesterol

_____ Integral protein

_____ Peripheral protein

_____ Phospholipid, nonpolar tail

_____ Phospholipid, polar head

Exercise 1—cont'd

Color and Label Plasma Membrane

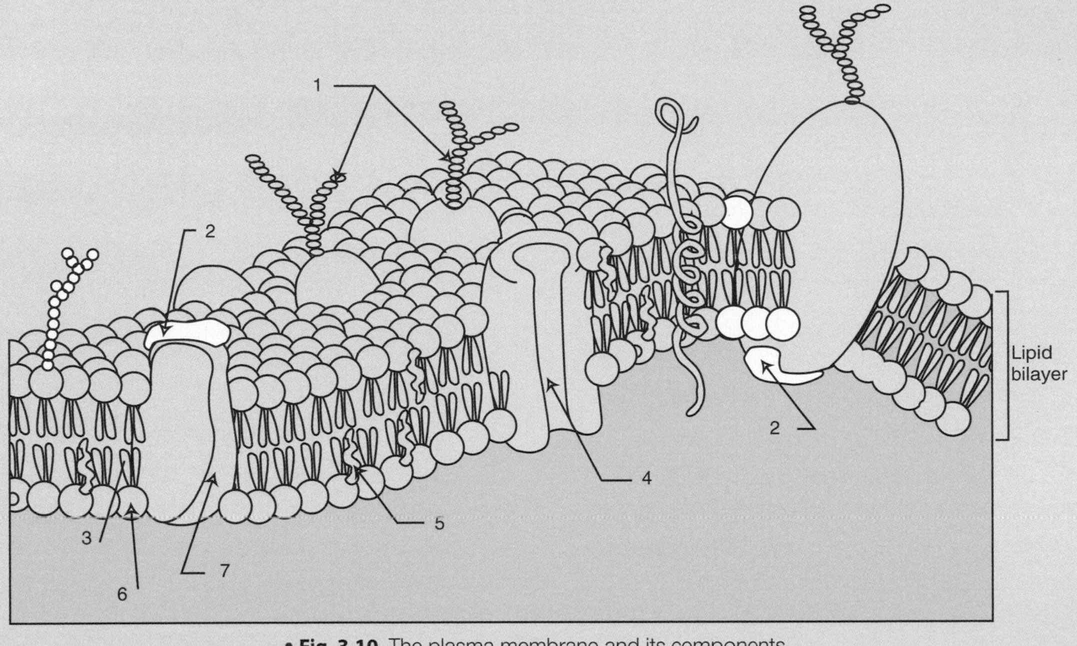

• **Fig. 3.10** The plasma membrane and its components.

Exercise 2

Match Definitions and Terms

Using the word bank below, match the correct cellular term with its corresponding function.

_____	Chromatin	a.	Highly organized subcellular living system
_____	Cytosol	b.	Nonliving structures within the cytoplasm
_____	Endoplasmic reticulum	c.	Threadlike granules dispersed throughout the nucleus
_____	Golgi apparatus	d.	Fingerlike folds in the plasma membrane that act to increase the surface area for absorption
_____	Haploid	e.	Control center for cell, chromosomes are found within this structure
_____	Inclusions	f.	Protein channels within the plasma membrane that allow certain substances to enter the cell
_____	Integral proteins	g.	Arranged in two layers in the plasma membrane
_____	Lysosomes	h.	Assembly sites for ribosomal particles—found within the nucleus
_____	Meiosis	i.	Gelatinous fluid that contains organelles
_____	Microfilaments	j.	Site of protein synthesis
_____	Microvilli	k.	Found in the cytoplasm and is a transport system within the cell—can be smooth or rough
_____	Mitochondria	l.	Contractile protein with the ability to shorten; found within cytosol
_____	Mitosis	m.	Membranous sacs found within the cytoplasm containing oxidase enzymes
_____	Nucleoli	n.	Manufactures energy for cellular use
_____	Nucleus	o.	Processes and packages protein molecules for export
_____	Organelles	p.	Membranous structure that contains potent digestive enzymes
_____	Peroxisomes	q.	Cellular reproductive process that results in offspring with half as many chromosomes as the cell they originated from
_____	Phospholipids	r.	Cellular reproductive process that results in two "daughter" cells that are exactly like the cell they originated from
_____	Ribosomes	s.	One-half the chromosome number

Cellular Microscopy

Exercise 3

Cell Diagram and Observations

1. Obtain the following prepared slides:
   - Skeletal muscle (skeletal myocytes or muscle cells)
   - Adipose tissue (adipocytes or fat cells)
   - Tracheal mucosa (ciliated columnar epithelium)
   - Lung alveoli (simple squamous epithelium)
   - Blood smear (red and white blood cells)
   - White fish blastula
2. Carefully set up your compound microscope using the instructions from the previous chapter. Use the high dry or oil immersion objective.
3. Starting with the blood smear, carefully examine the cells on the feather edge (the thinnest part on the slide). Examine the red, doughnut-shaped red blood cells. Notice that the centers of the cells are lighter in color than the perimeters.
4. Using the colored pencils, make a careful drawing of what you actually see in the corresponding circle on p. 47. Be sure to look carefully and draw exactly what you see. Do not draw what you think you should be seeing. As you make your observations, consider the following:
   - Cell shape and size
   - The relative position of the cells to one another
   - The presence or absence of nuclei
   - If nuclei are present, think about these questions:
     - Are nucleoli visible within the nuclei?
     - What are the number and position of the nuclei in each cell?
     - Why does a cell have more than one nucleus?
     - Why might a cell have no nucleus?
5. Examine each of the other prepared slides and make drawings of the cells found there. Make your drawing in the corresponding circle on p. 47 and consider the questions above as you work.
6. Answer the following questions:

Questions

Describe the unique features of the cell types listed below (e.g., shape, size).

1. Red blood cell, or erythrocyte

   ____

2. Fat cell, or adipocyte (adipose tissue)

   ____

3. Ciliated columnar epithelial cell (in tracheal mucosa)

   ____

4. Skeletal muscle cell, or myocyte

   ____

5. Simple squamous epithelial cell (lung alveoli)

   ____

For each cell type below, describe the relationship between its shape and its function.

1. Red blood cell, or erythrocyte

   ____

2. Fat cell, or adipocyte (adipose tissue)

   ____

3. Ciliated columnar epithelial cell (in tracheal mucosa)

   ____

4. Skeletal muscle cell, or myocyte

   ____

5. Simple squamous epithelial cell (lung alveoli)

   ____

Which of the five cells have cell membrane projections?

____

How do the projections affect the function of the cell?

____

Exercise 3—cont'd

Cell Diagram and Observations

Do any of these cells lack a cell membrane? Why or why not? Given that you cannot actually see the cell membrane with a compound microscope, your answer must be based on logic. ____________________

____

Do all of these cells have nuclei?

____

Which cells are not nucleated?

____

Why do you think these cells gave up their nuclei and all of their organelles, too, for that matter?

____

Can you see the nucleoli in the nuclei of the cells?

____

Can you see the organelles within the cytosol of the cells?

____

Why or why not?

____

____

____

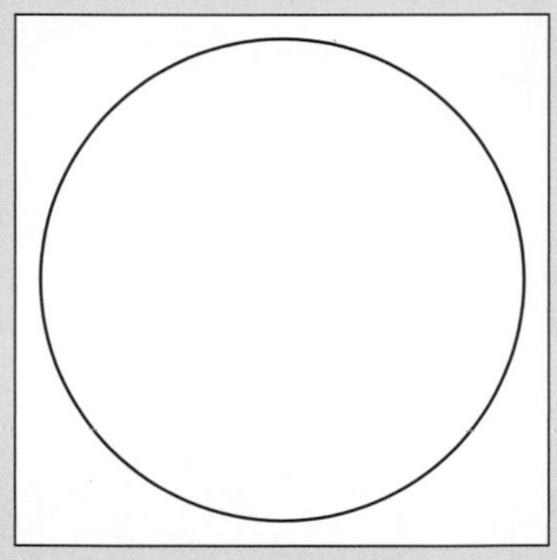

Skeletal muscle cells

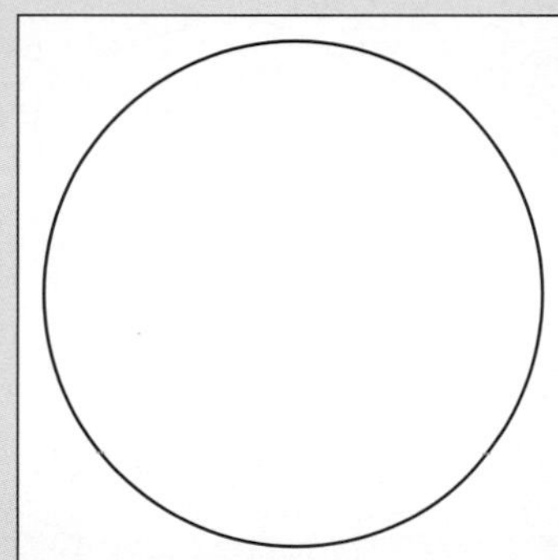

Adipose tissue

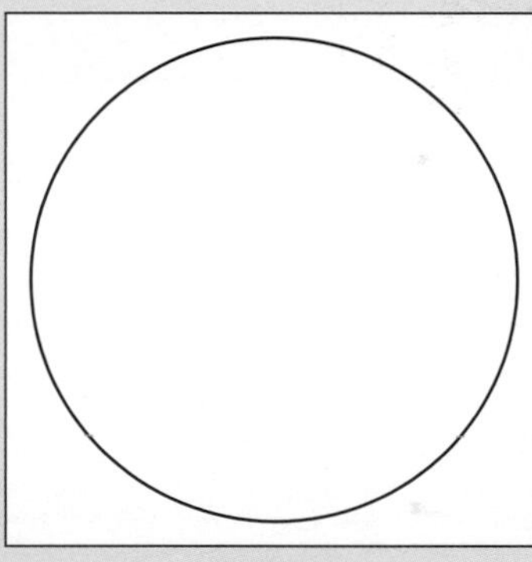

Trachea

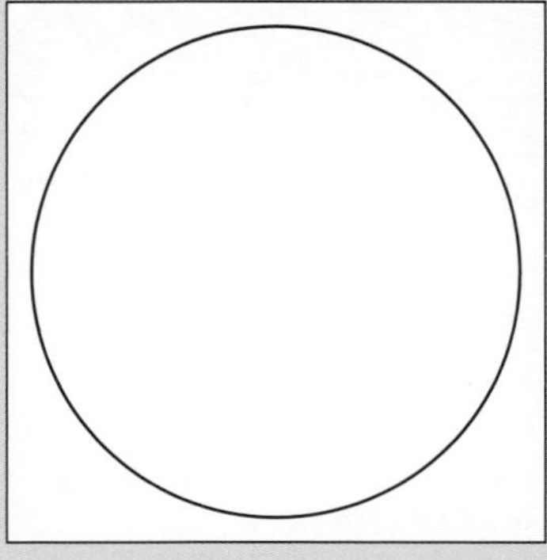

Lung alveoli

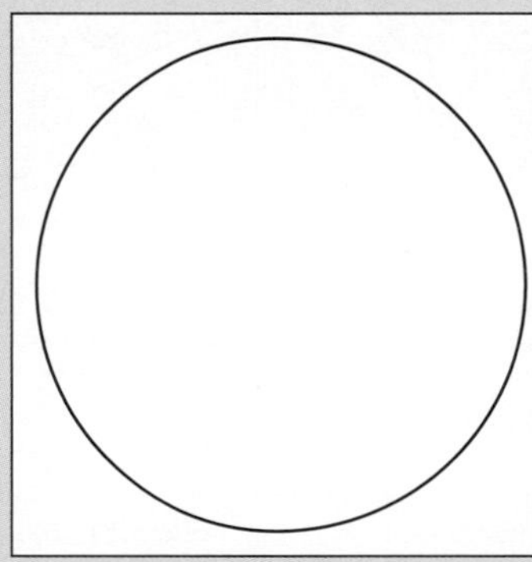

Blood cells

Exercise 4

Color and Label Cellular Components

Using colored pencils, color in the various organelles and other cellular components that are visible in the diagram of the cell (Fig. 3.11). Underline each term with the same color as the corresponding structure. Use a different color for each structure. Then match the number in the drawing below with the corresponding term.

_____ Centrioles
_____ Centrosome
_____ Golgi apparatus
_____ Lysosome
_____ Microvilli
_____ Mitochondrion
_____ Nuclear envelope
_____ Nucleolus
_____ Nuclear pore
_____ Plasma membrane
_____ Ribosomes
_____ Rough endoplasmic reticulum
_____ Smooth endoplasmic reticulum

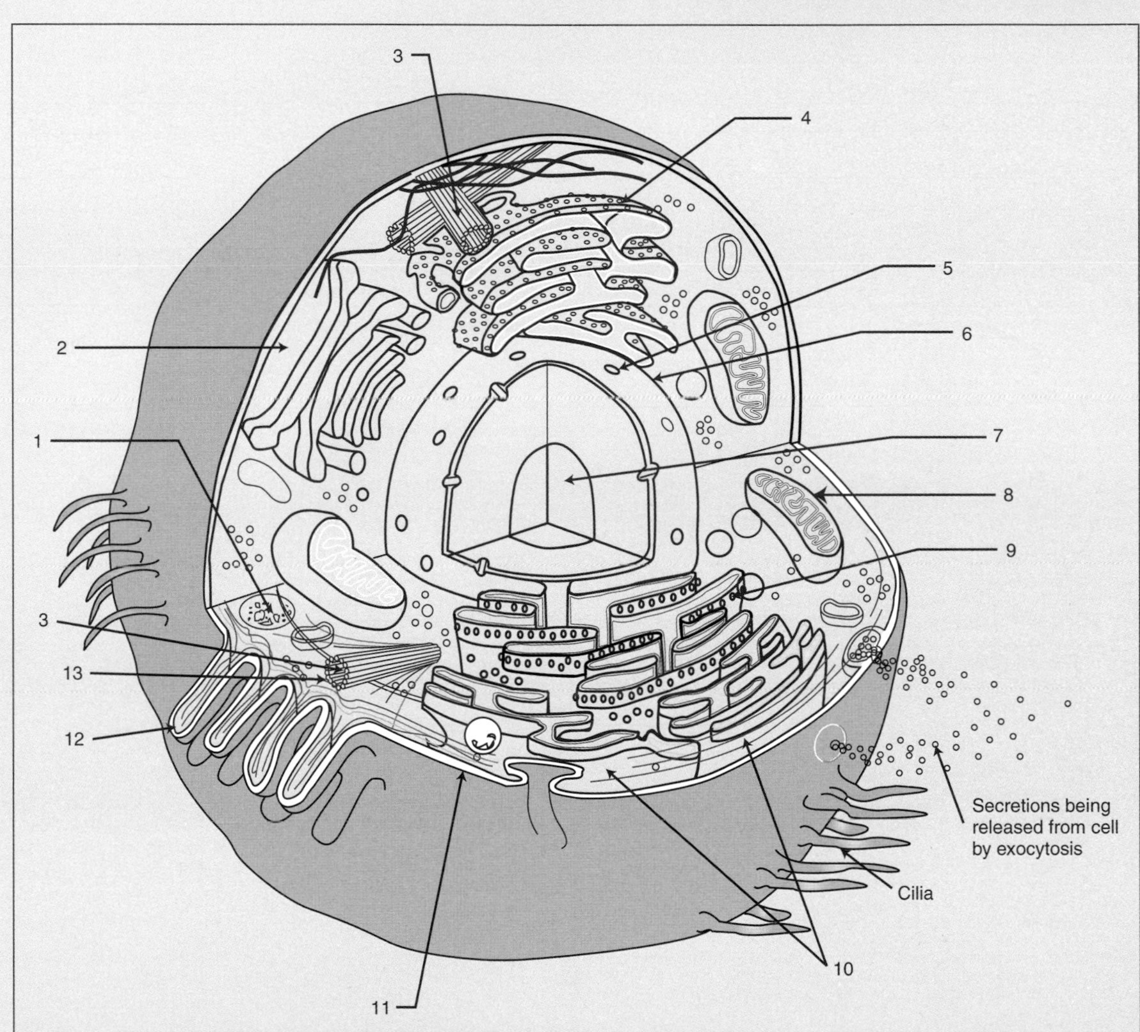

• **Fig. 3.11** The cell and its organelles.

Exercise 5

Prepare and Examine a Wet Mount Slide

Prepare a wet mount slide using cells from your own mouth. A wet mount slide is one on which a wet specimen is placed and examined under the microscope.

Steps

1. Using a cotton-tipped applicator, scrape the inside of your cheek and roll the cotton swab across the slide several times to form several rows. This will leave a thin layer of cells from the scraping on the slide.
2. Apply one drop of methylene blue stain to the scrapings on the slide.
3. Next, apply a coverslip to the slide by placing one edge of the coverslip next to the specimen and allowing it to drop slowly over the drop of stain.
4. Examine the cells under the microscope and draw what you observe in the circle below. Again, be sure to draw exactly what you see, not what you think you should be seeing.

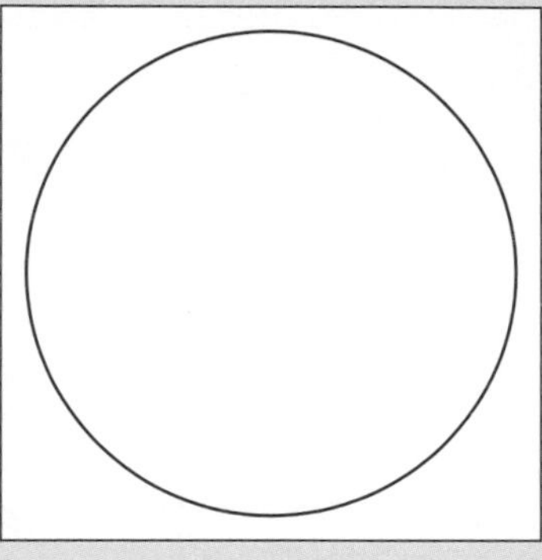

Cheek cells

Do these cells differ from the prepared slides you looked at previously?

____

What differences do you see?

____

Cell Division

Exercise 6

Diagram of Stages of Mitosis

Use your colored pencils to color in the brackets and intracellular structures in Fig. 3.12. Use the same color to underline the corresponding term. Use a different color for each term. Then match the number from the figure to the correct term below.

_____ Anaphase
_____ Cell membrane
_____ Centrioles
_____ Centromere
_____ Chromatin/chromosome
_____ Cytokinesis
_____ Interphase
_____ Metaphase
_____ Mitosis
_____ Nuclear membrane
_____ Nucleolus
_____ Prophase
_____ Telophase

Continued

Exercise 6—cont'd

Diagram of Stages of Mitosis

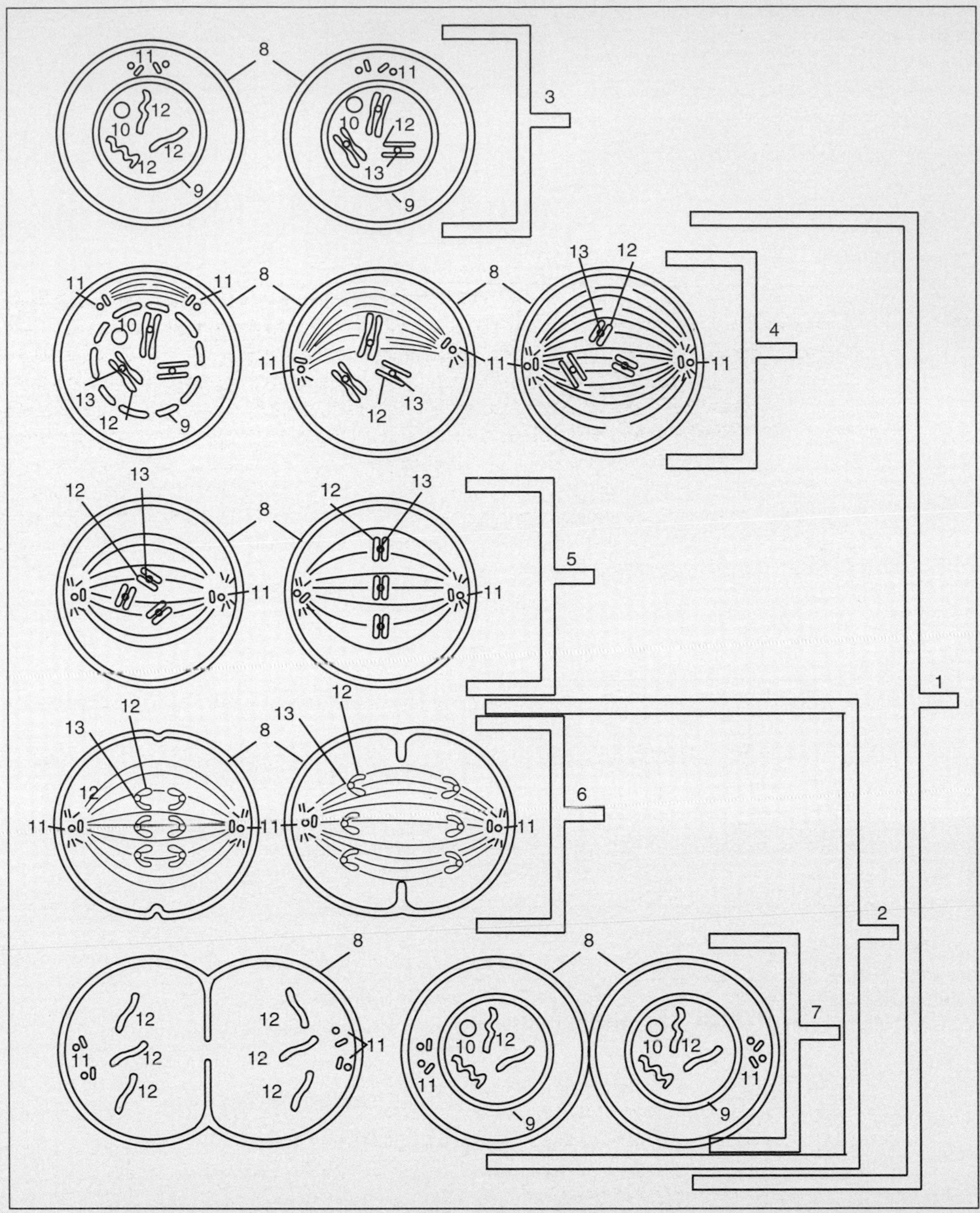

• **Fig. 3.12** Mitosis. Stages of cell division, which result in an identical copy of the mother cell.

Exercise 7

Identify Stages of Mitosis

Using the prepared white fish blastula slide, find the various stages of mitosis. Use the low power objective to find the groups of cells that have been placed on the slide. After you have located the cells, move to the high power objective and identify the various stages of cell division we have discussed. Because the cells are at approximately the same embryonic stage it may be necessary to look at more than one blastula.

What is a blastula? A blastula is an early stage of embryonic development where the cells undergoing change form a hollow sphere of these cells.

Exercise 8

Diagram of Stages of Meiosis

Use your colored pencils to color in the brackets and intracellular structures listed in Fig. 3.13. Use the same color to underline the corresponding term. Use a different color for each term. Then match the number in Fig. 3.13 with the correct term below.

_____ Anaphase 1
_____ Anaphase 2
_____ Centrioles
_____ Centromere
_____ Chromatids
_____ Chromosome
_____ Cleavage site
_____ Two diploid cells
_____ Four haploid cells
_____ Meiosis I (first division)
_____ Meiosis II (second division)
_____ Metaphase 1
_____ Metaphase 2
_____ Nucleus
_____ Prophase 1
_____ Prophase 2
_____ Spindle fibers
_____ Telophase 1
_____ Telophase 2

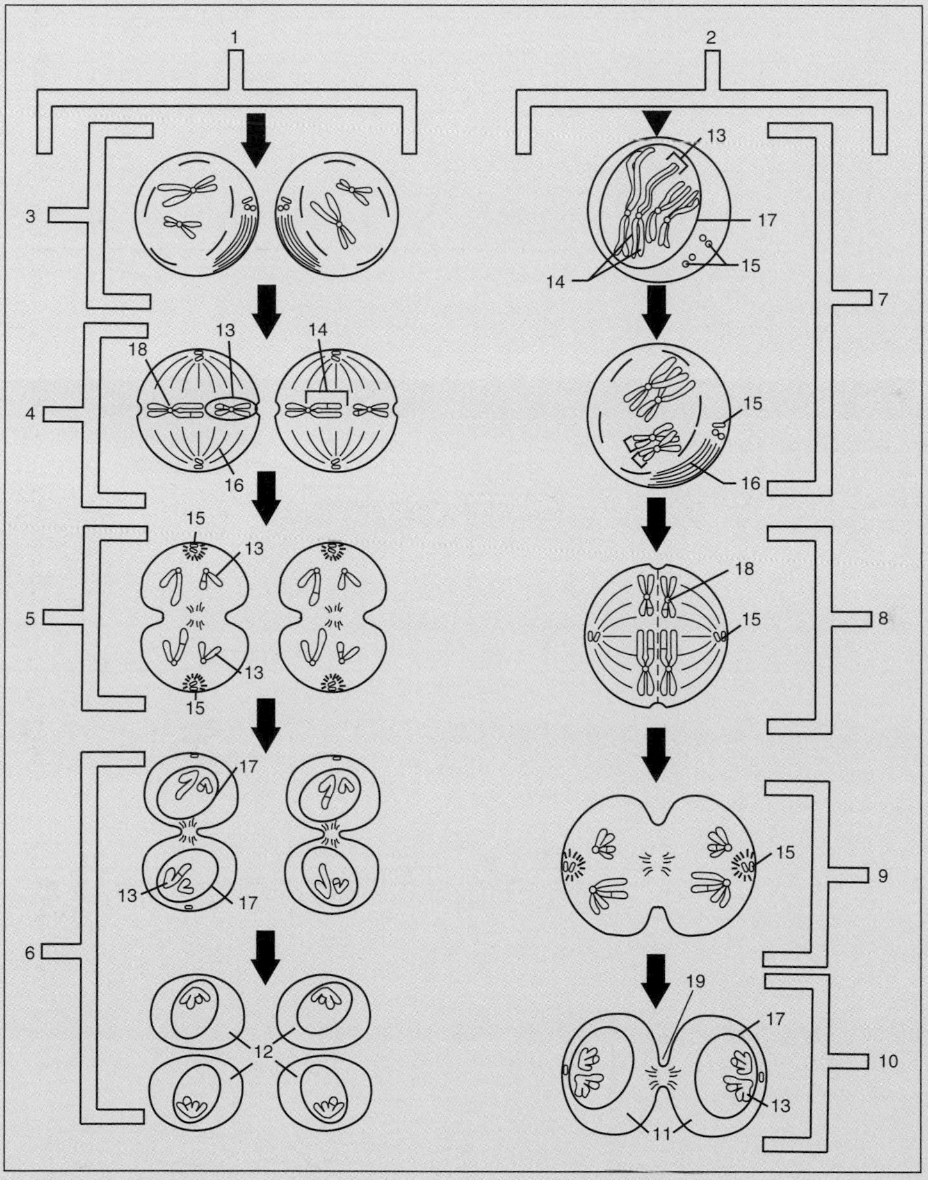

• **Fig. 3.13** Meiosis. Division of sex cells occurs in two distinct phases called meiosis I and meiosis II. Four daughter cells are produced from meiosis I, with each one having one-half the chromosome number of the mother cell. Each of the four daughter cells produces two identical cells from meiosis II (mitosis), with each one having the same chromosome number (one-half the mother cell's chromosome number).

Fluid Therapy

Exercise 9

Determining Type of Fluid Administration

For each of the conditions listed, indicate the phase of fluid administration and the appropriate type of fluid.

	FLUID ADMINISTRATION				
Condition	**Resuscitation**	**Replacement**	**Maintenance**	**Colloid**	**Crystalloid**
Quickly raise the blood pressure					
Increase fluid from loss					
Shock					
Correct dehydration					
Ongoing fluid loss from vomiting, urination, diarrhea					
No drinking but no signs of dehydration					

Exercise 10

Estimate the Percent of Dehydration in Dogs

For each of the physical conditions listed, indicate the percent of dehydration.

Condition	**Percentage Dehydration**
Animal is recumbent and unconscious, in cardiovascular shock. Pulse is very rapid and thready. Eyes are severely sunken and recessed in the orbits. MM very dry and contracted, tongue is dry and contracted, CRT ∇ 5–8 s. Skin remains tented with no skin turgor.	________
Patient is quiet. MM tacky, CRT = 2.5 s. Skin turgor is slightly delayed.	________
No clinical signs of dehydration are evident. Mentation is normal. MM wet or moist, CRT <2 s. Skin turgor: strong snap, ≤1 s return.	________
Patient is depressed and recumbent but conscious. Pulse is rapid and weak. Eyes are slightly sunken and recessed into the orbits. MM dry, dry tongue, CRT 4–5 s. Skin turgor severely delayed: 5–8 s.	________

MM, Mucous membranes; r.u. CRT

CRT, Capillary refill time.

Critical and Clinical Thinking

Exercise 11

Clinical Thinking Challenge

Support each of the following correct statements with appropriate rationale, stating why or in what way the statement is correct.

1. The plasma membrane acts as a protective barrier for the cell.
2. The lysosomes are often called "suicide sacs."
3. The first, primitive, cells are called prokaryotes.
4. The size of most animal cells is restricted to a range of 10–30 μm in diameter.
5. Cardiac and skeletal muscle tissues have two or more nuclei.
6. The AFM (atomic force microscope) has led to a greater understanding of the causes of some diseases that have devastated both humans and animals.
7. Prions can generate grossly visible holes in brain tissue.
8. The cell membrane is not visible using light microscopy.
9. Insulin stimulates glucose uptake.
10. Flagella and cilia, extensions of the plasma membrane, are structurally identical but function differently.
11. The fluid of the cell is called cytosol and has a thick jelly-like consistency.
12. Mitochondria are known as the powerhouses of the cell.
13. Animals, even inactive ones, must consume water or they will die in a relatively short time.
14. Crystalloids are good for rehydrating extravascular spaces.
15. Colloids are good for raising blood pressure.
16. The cell membrane is considered to be selectively permeable.

4

Exploring Tissues

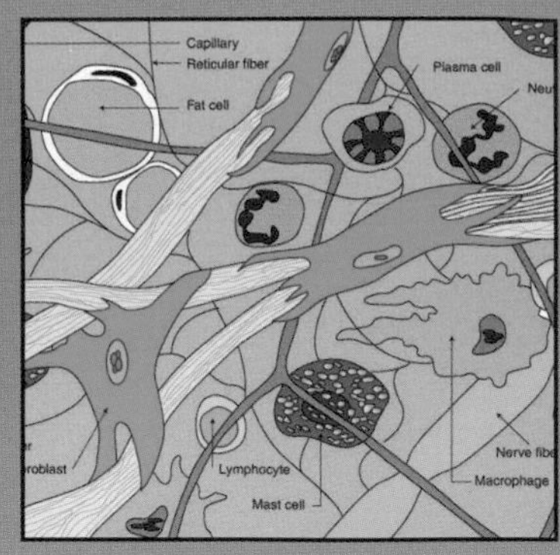

OVERVIEW AT A GLANCE

Identification of Tissues 55

Exercises 55–69

Epithelial Tissue 55–57

1. Label, Identify, and Classify Epithelial Tissue 55

2. Match Figures to Type of Epithelial Tissue 57

3. Exocrine Gland Classification 57

Connective Tissue 58

4. Classify, Identify, and Locate Connective Tissue 58

Muscle Tissue 59–60

5. Identify, Locate, and Classify Muscle Tissue 59

Nervous Tissue 60

6. Label and Describe Nervous Tissue 60

Critical and Clinical Thinking 60–69

7. Clinical Application—Histopathology 61

8. Histologic Preparation of Tissues 62

9. Microscope Exercise 63

10. Clinical Thinking Challenge 66

11. Case Application—The Healing Process 67

12. Mucous Membranes and Clues in Diagnoses 69

13. Capillary Refill Time 69

14. Case Application—Arrhythmogenic Right Ventricular Cardiomyopathy 69

LEARNING OBJECTIVES

1. To review and understand the process of preparing tissues for histologic examination.
2. To become familiar with the microscopic appearance of the four primary tissue types and their subcategories.
3. To be able to classify the tissues by name.
4. To understand the function of each tissue type.
5. To become familiar with the process of preserving and preparing tissues for microscopic examination.
6. To identify specified cellular layers and microscopic structures within each tissue specimen.
7. To apply histology to a clinical scenario.
8. To demonstrate an understanding of tissue structure and function through both written and illustrated examples.
9. To visualize the histologic structure of various tissues using a compound microscope.

CLINICAL SIGNIFICANCE

The importance of microanatomy or histology in the field of veterinary medicine is demonstrated every time a tissue **biopsy** is obtained from a patient. Histologic examination of a tissue biopsy can aid in the identification of disease processes such as inflammation, infection, and neoplasia.

INTRODUCTION

To understand how an animal's body functions (and how our own human body functions, for that matter), we must examine all of the tissues that compose it, both at the macroscopic and the microscopic level. Macroscopic anatomy is also known as gross anatomy and refers to the study of tissues, organs, and structures that can be seen with the unaided eye. During the dissection of animals, students are exposed to the macroscopic organization of body cavities and organs, such as the heart, lungs, and liver. On the other hand, microscopic anatomy, or histology, is the study of structures too small to be seen without magnification. The careful preparation and staining of tissues and the cells that compose them, as well as the use of a good microscope, are essential to see minute anatomic structures adequately.

This chapter will give you a better visual understanding of tissues at the microscopic level. It will allow you to apply the knowledge you acquire to understanding the function of each tissue type. Here are some key points about tissues:

- A tissue is composed of cells that are similar in shape and function.
- There are four primary tissue types:

Epithelial	Muscle
Connective	Nervous

INTRODUCTION—cont'd

- Each tissue type has a primary function:
  Epithelial tissue is responsible for *covering* or *lining* other tissues and organs.
  Connective tissue is responsible for *supporting* and *connecting* other tissues.
  Muscle tissue is responsible for *movement* and *contraction.*
  Nervous tissue is responsible for *controlling work* through electrical and chemical signals.

READING ASSIGNMENT

This laboratory chapter corresponds to Chapter 5 in *Clinical Anatomy and Physiology for Veterinary Technicians*. Be sure to read this chapter before beginning this lab.

MATERIALS NEEDED

Pencil or pen
Colored pencils
Compound light microscope
Lens paper
Lens cleaner
Microscopic slides of the following tissues:
- Elastic cartilage
- Intestinal mucosa
- Skeletal muscle
- Adipose tissue
- Compact bone
- Cardiac muscle

TERMS TO BE IDENTIFIED

Epithelium
- Squamous, cuboidal, and columnar
- Simple, stratified, pseudostratified, and transitional
- Basal lamina

Connective tissue
- Dense regular or irregular
- Compact bone
- Adipose tissue
- Cartilage: hyaline, elastic, and fibrocartilage
- Loose (areolar) connective tissue
- Blood

Muscle tissue
- Skeletal
- Smooth
- Cardiac

Nervous tissue
- Parts of the neuron
- Cell body
- Axon
- Dendrites

IDENTIFICATION OF TISSUES

Using the information from Chapter 5 in *Clinical Anatomy and Physiology for Veterinary Technicians*, complete the following exercises. Examine each figure carefully and familiarize yourself with the structure and function of each tissue type.

EXERCISES

Epithelial Tissue

Exercise 1

Label, Identify, and Classify Epithelial Tissue

A.

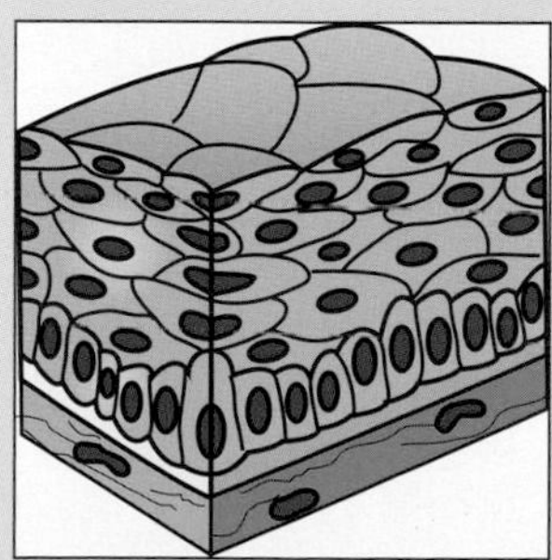

1. On the drawing, label the basement membrane *(basal lamina)*.
2. In the blank, write the name of the cell type on the luminal surface. ______________________
3. Classify the tissue as *simple* or *stratified*. ______________________
4. Based on your responses to 2 and 3, classify the epithelium. ______________________

Continued

Exercise 1—cont'd

Label, Identify, and Classify Epithelial Tissue

B.

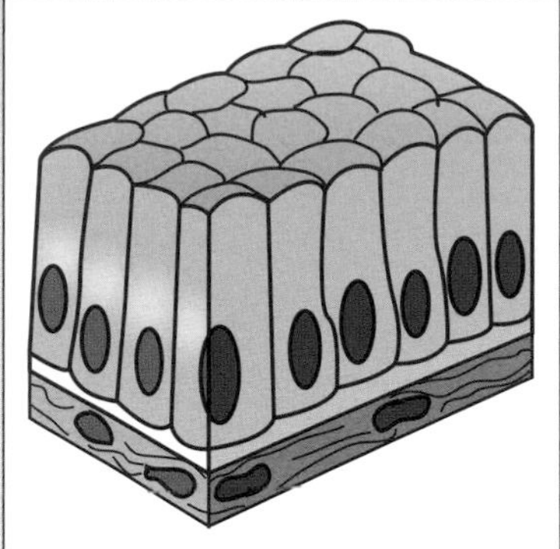

1. On the drawing, label the basement membrane *(basal lamina)*.
2. Identify the cell type on the luminal surface. ______________________
3. Classify the tissue as *simple* or *stratified*.______________________
4. Based on your response to 2 and 3, classify the epithelium. ______________________
5. Give an example of where this type of epithelium is found. ______________________

C.

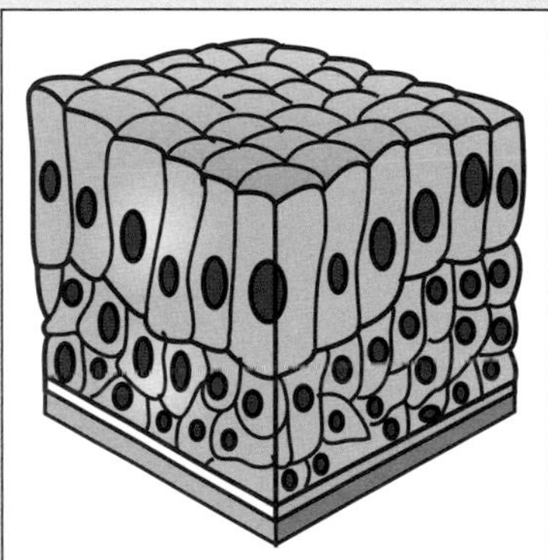

1. On the drawing, label the basement membrane *(basal lamina)*.
2. Identify the cell type on the luminal surface. ______________________
3. Classify the tissue as *simple* or *stratified*. ______________________
4. Based on your response to 2 and 3, classify the epithelium. ______________________
5. Give an example of where this type of epithelium is found. ______________________

D.

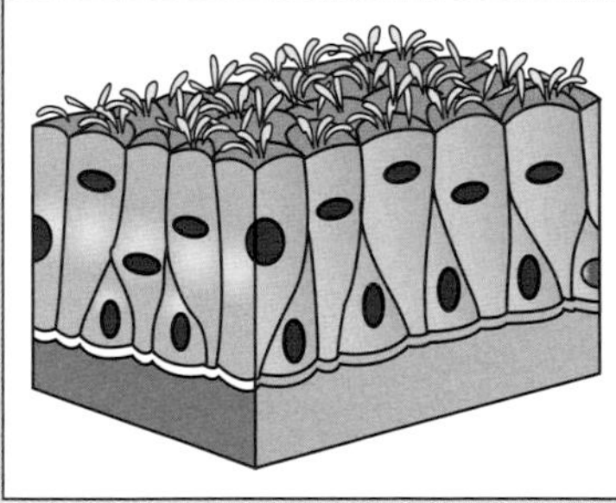

1. On the drawing, label the basement membrane *(basal lamina)*.
2. Identify the cell type on the luminal surface. ______________________
3. Classify the tissue as *simple* or *stratified*. ______________________
4. Based on your response to 2 and 3, classify the epithelium. ______________________
5. Give an example of where this type of epithelium is found.______________________

Exercise 2

Match Figures to Type of Epithelial Tissue

Identify the type of epithelial tissue by matching the figure to the type's description.

A. Simple squamous
B. Stratified squamous
C. Simple cuboidal
D. Pseudostratified
E. Simple columnar

1. ______________________

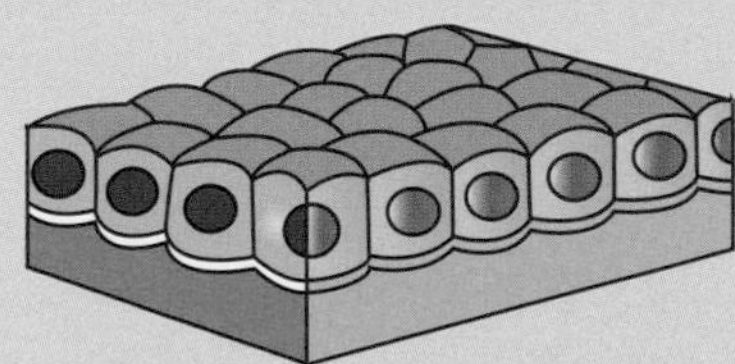

2. ______________________

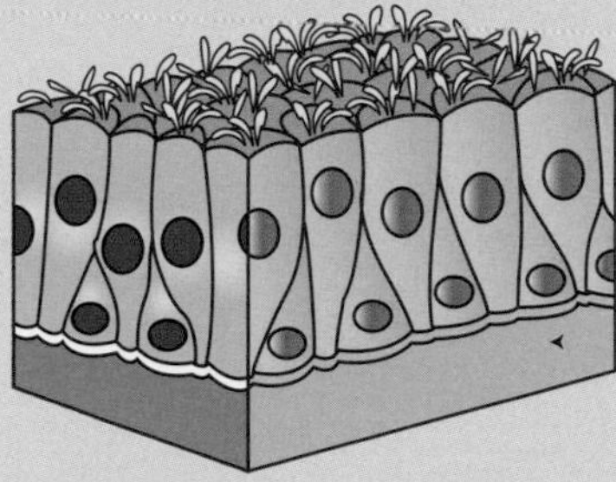

3. ______________________

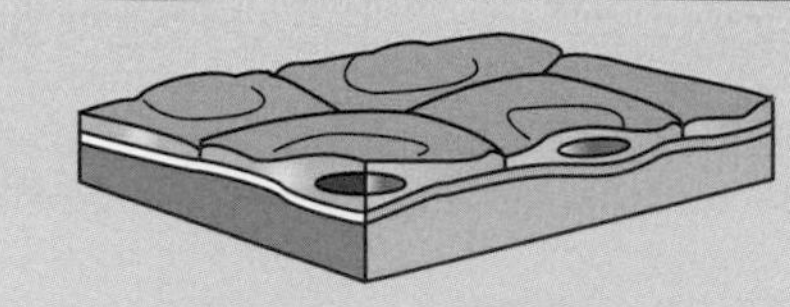

4. ______________________

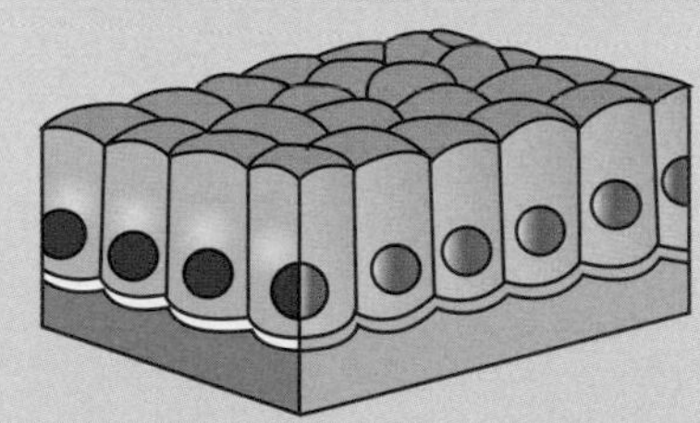

5. ______________________

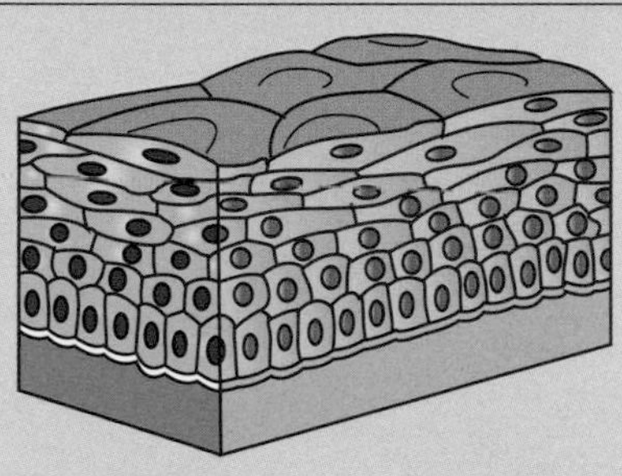

Exercise 3

Exocrine Gland Classification

Classify the type of exocrine gland by matching the figure to the description.

A. Simple tubular
B. Simple coiled tubular
C. Simple branched tubular
D. Simple alveolar
E. Branched alveolar (acinar)
F. Compound tubular
G. Compound alveolar (acinar)
H. Compound tubuloalveolar

1. ______________

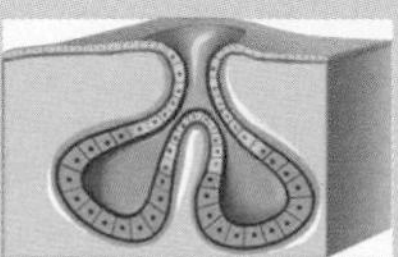

2. ______________

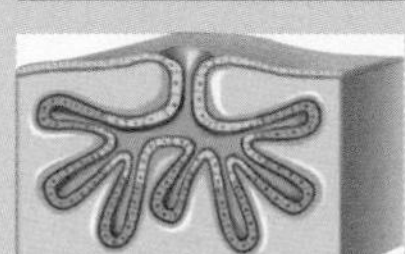

3. ______________

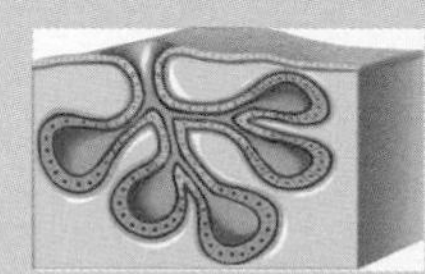

4. ______________

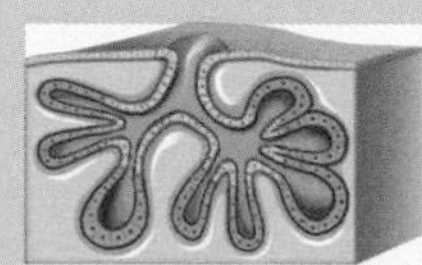

5. ______________

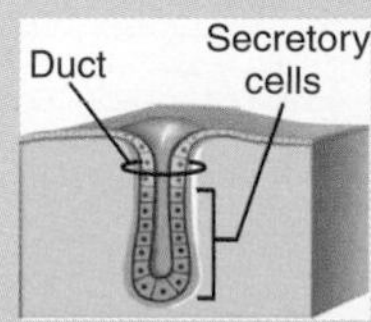

6. ______________

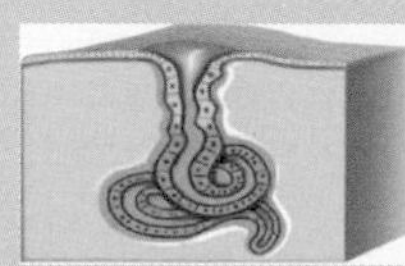

7. ______________

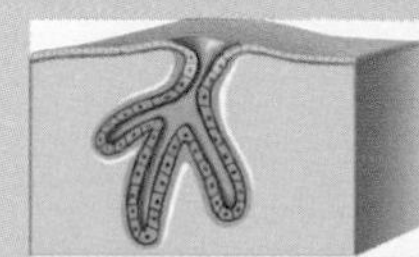

8. ______________

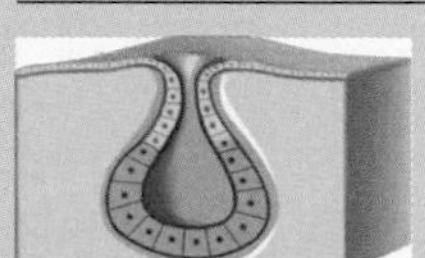

Connective Tissue

Exercise 4

Classify, Identify, and Locate Connective Tissue

A.

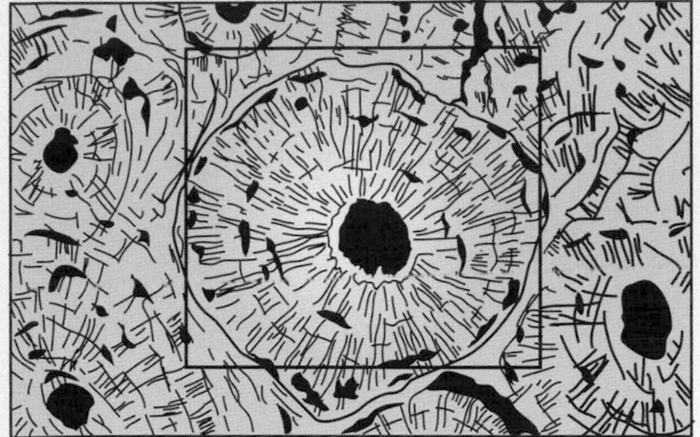

1. Classify the tissue as *connective tissue proper or specialized connective tissue.* ___________
2. Identify the type of connective tissue shown (be as specific as possible). ___________
3. Where in the body is this connective tissue found? ___________

B.

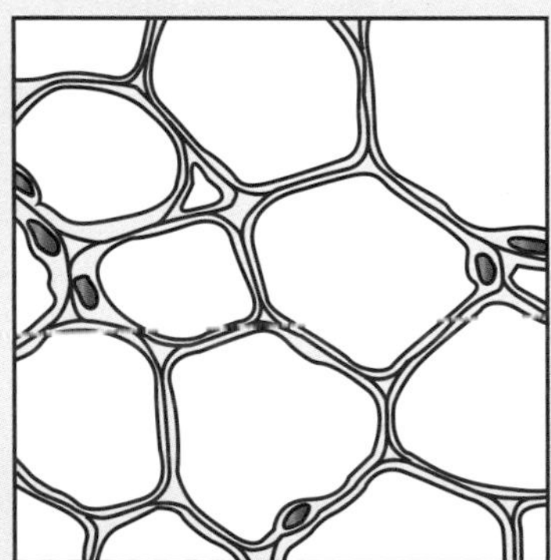

1. Classify the tissue as *connective tissue proper or specialized connective tissue.* ___________
2. Identify the type of connective tissue shown (be as specific as possible). ___________
3. Where in the body is this connective tissue found? ___________

C.

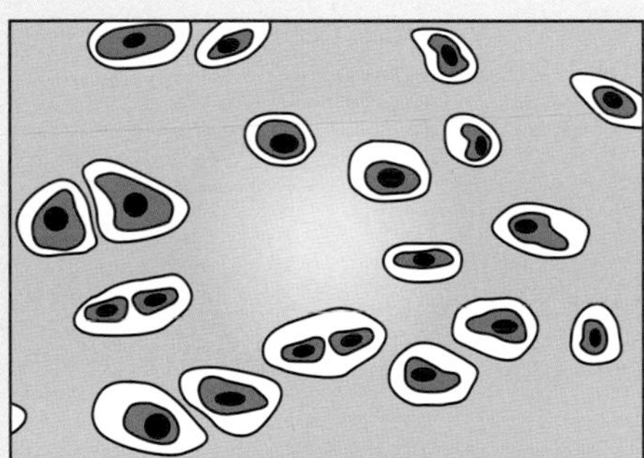

1. Classify the tissue as *connective tissue proper or specialized connective tissue.* ___________
2. Identify the type of connective tissue shown (be as specific as possible). ___________
3. Where in the body is this connective tissue found? ___________

D.

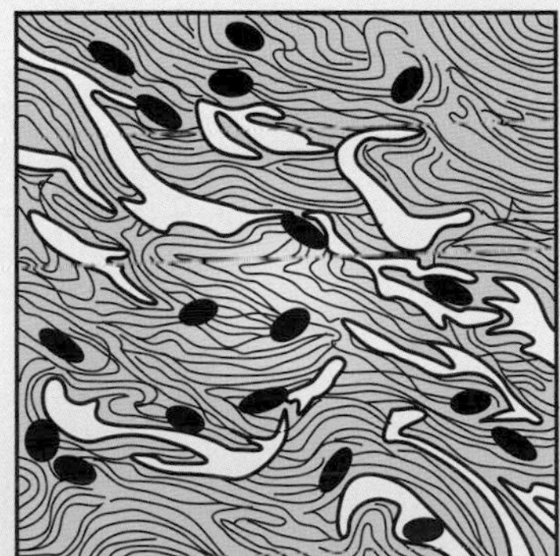

1. Classify the tissue as *connective tissue proper or specialized connective tissue.* ___________
2. Identify the type of connective tissue shown (be as specific as possible). ___________
3. Where in the body is this connective tissue found? ___________

Muscle Tissue

Exercise 5

Identify, Locate, and Classify Muscle Tissue

A.

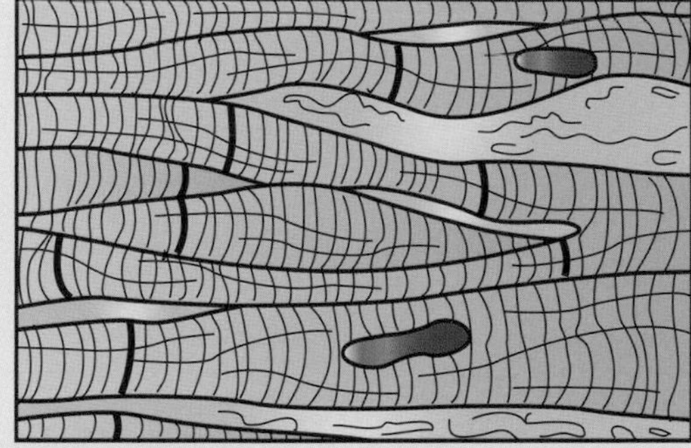

1. Identify the type of muscle tissue. ______________________
2. Where in the body is this muscle tissue found? ______________________
3. Indicate whether this type of muscle is under voluntary or involuntary control. ______________________

B.

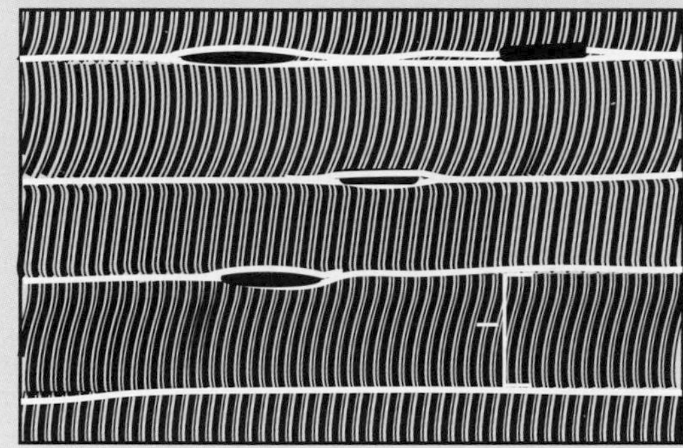

1. Identify the type of muscle tissue. ______________________
2. Where in the body is this muscle tissue found? ______________________
3. Indicate whether this type of muscle is under voluntary or involuntary control. ______________________

C.

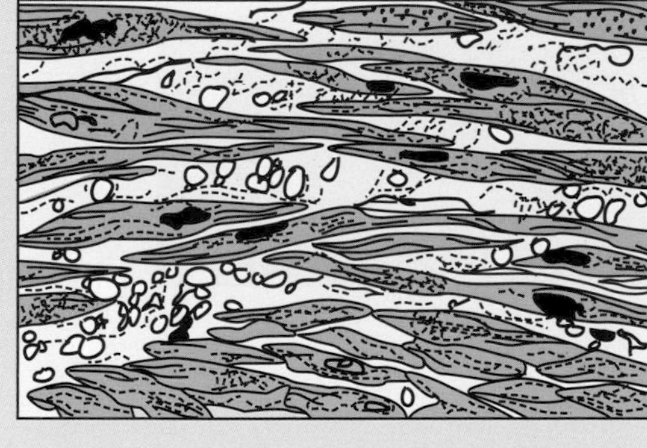

1. Identify the type of muscle tissue. ______________________
2. Where in the body is this muscle tissue found? ______________________
3. Indicate whether this type of muscle is under voluntary or involuntary control. ______________________

Nervous Tissue

Exercise 6

Label and Describe Nervous Tissue

A.

Use the labeled figures as a guide to label the histologic image of a neuron from a pig (below left) and the immunocytochemistry image of a neuron from a rat (below right). Label the following structures: **cell body, axon,** and **dendrites**.

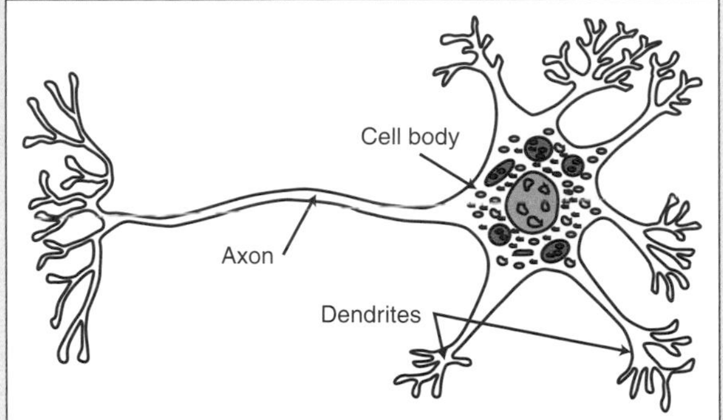

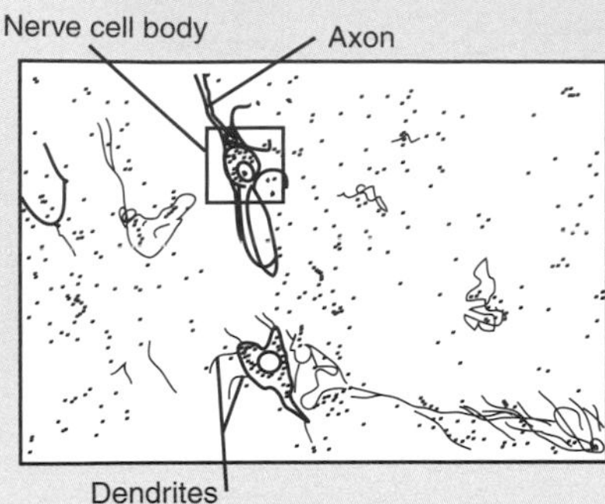

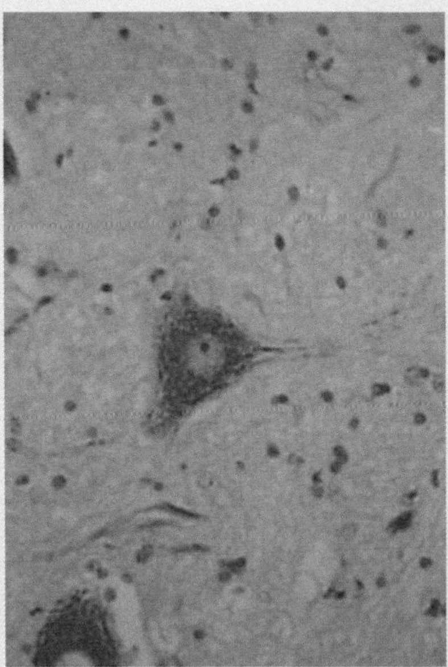

(From Banks WJ: Applied veterinary histology, ed. 3, St Louis, 1993, Mosby.)

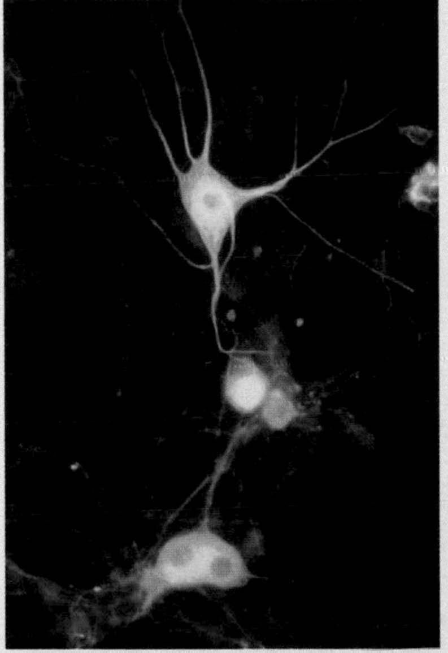

(From Gartner LP, Hyatt JL: Color textbook of histology, ed. 3, Philadelphia, 2006, Saunders.)

B.

Describe the function of each of the neuronal structures.

Cell body: ______________________________

____

Axon: ______________________________

____

Dendrites: ______________________________

____

Critical and Clinical Thinking

Each of the following questions focuses on a clinical scenario and an associated disease process. The questions will direct you to complete the exercise using illustrations and written explanations of the histologic changes to the tissue. As a veterinary technician, it is important to understand the microscopic alterations that occur in diseased tissue. This will give you more appreciation for the **pathogenesis** of the disease and the prognosis and treatment of the affected patient.

Exercise 7

Clinical Application—Histopathology

The mixed animal practice for which you work receives a phone call from a local swine operation. The owner tells you that his 4-week-old piglets are depressed, **anorectic,** and have developed diarrhea characterized by a yellow color. Dr. Davis, the head veterinarian at the clinic, asks you to come to the swine farm with her to evaluate the piglets. She tells you that this swine operation has had an outbreak of rotavirus infection in the past, and she suspects the piglets are afflicted with the disease. You ask Dr. Davis what rotavirus is and how it causes diarrhea. She explains that rotavirus infection is ubiquitous (i.e., widespread) in the environment. When piglets are exposed, the virus replicates in their small intestines. The small intestines contain fingerlike projections called villi, which help in absorption of nutrients. The villi have even smaller projections on their **brush border** called **microvilli.** Digestion and absorption are facilitated by these structures. Rotavirus infects the epithelial cells of the villi, causing destruction of these cells and the brush border. The result is villous **atrophy,** a blunting and deterioration of the villi. The atrophy leads to an inability of the small intestines to absorb and digest nutrients, causing malabsorption and diarrhea.

Following is a drawing of a healthy intestinal villus (singular of villi), and two photomicrographs of small intestinal villi infected with rotavirus also appear. Using your understanding of tissue structure and the apparent effects of rotavirus (based on the photomicrographs of the infected villi and the description above), please draw a rotavirus-infected villus in the corresponding box. Label the villus/villi, microvilli, and epithelial cells.

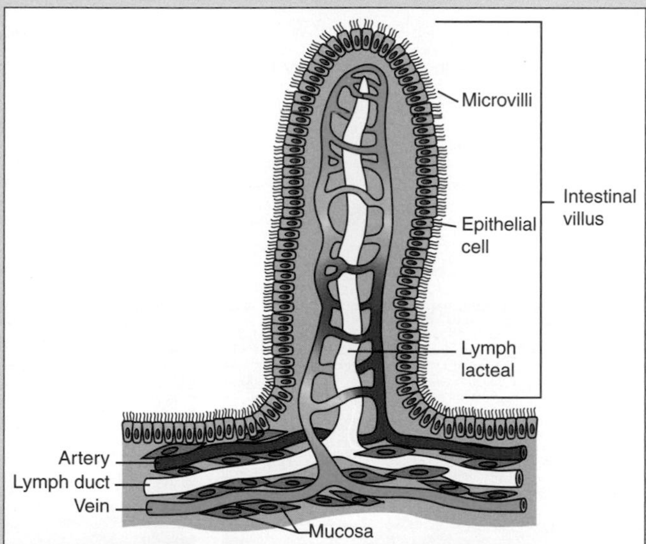

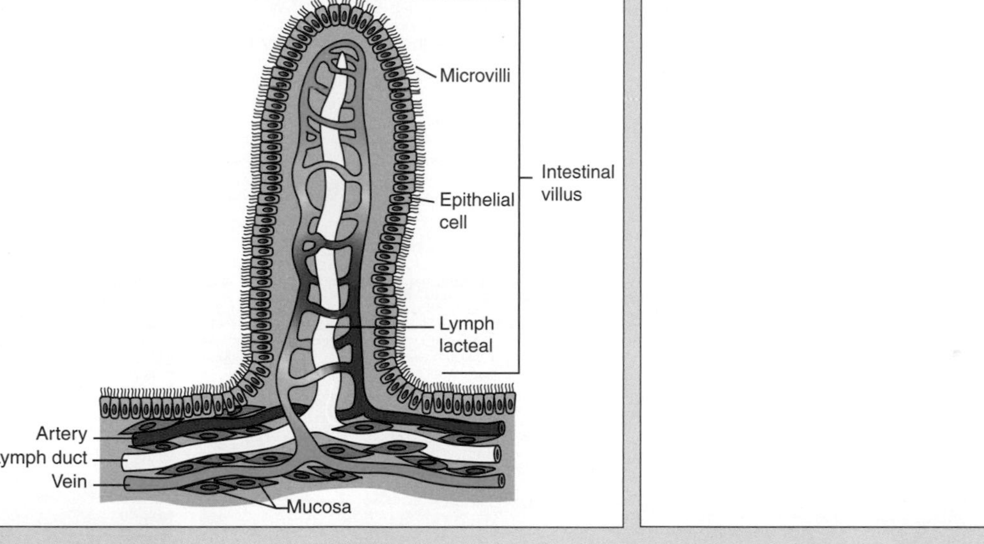

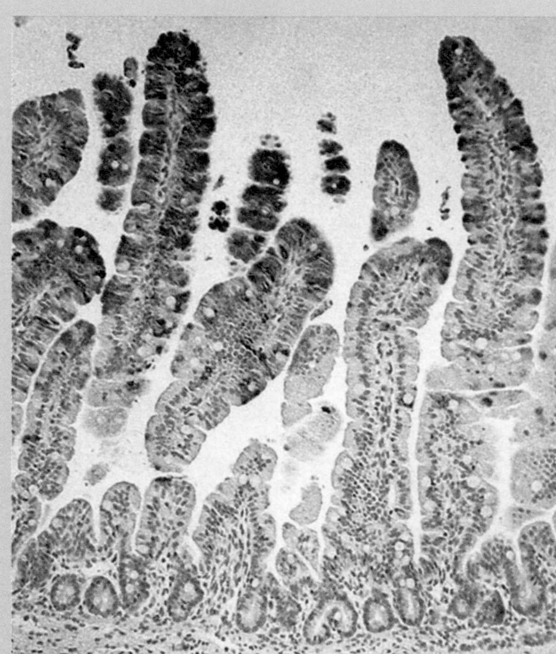

(Courtesy Dr. H. Gelberg, College of Veterinary Medicine, Oregon State University.)

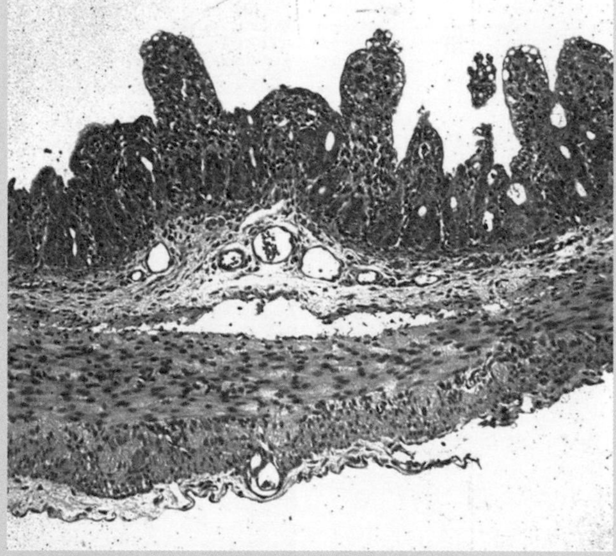

(Courtesy Dr. H. Gelberg, College of Veterinary Medicine, Oregon State University.)

Exercise 8

Histologic Preparation of Tissues

Read the steps for the histologic preparation of tissues in Chapter 5 of the textbook. Match the following steps to the corresponding photograph. There are fewer photos than there are steps, so not all of the steps will have matches.

Step 1: Tissue is placed in a fixative solution, such as formalin. The ratio of the volume of formalin to the volume of tissue is 10:1. This step is called **fixation.**

Step 2: Tissues are examined, sectioned, and placed in cassettes, which are numbered for identification. They are then placed in an automatic tissue processor to be treated overnight. Under a vacuum system, the tissues are dehydrated and infiltrated with paraffin.

Step 3: The tissue cassettes are removed from the processor, and the contents transferred to rectangular metal molds, which are filled with liquid paraffin. The paraffin hardens into a soft white wax.

Step 4: Just before being sliced, the block of paraffin is chilled with ice to facilitate slicing.

Step 5: Using a special cutting device called a microtome, extraordinarily thin slices (4–8 μm) are made of the tissue.

Step 6: Several slices are completed serially, forming a paper-thin strip, which is carefully placed on the surface of a water bath.

Step 7: Carefully, the thin sections are collected onto labeled glass microscope slides.

Step 8: The slides are transferred to a warm incubator, which speeds the drying process and helps the paraffin-infused tissue to adhere to the glass slide.

Step 9: The tissues are transferred to a machine that deparaffinizes and rehydrates them so that aqueous stains can react with them. They are then stained and subsequently dehydrated again.

Step 10: A small amount of Permount and a protective cover slip are applied to each slide.

Step 11: Finished slides are logged in a journal before being examined microscopically by a veterinary pathologist.

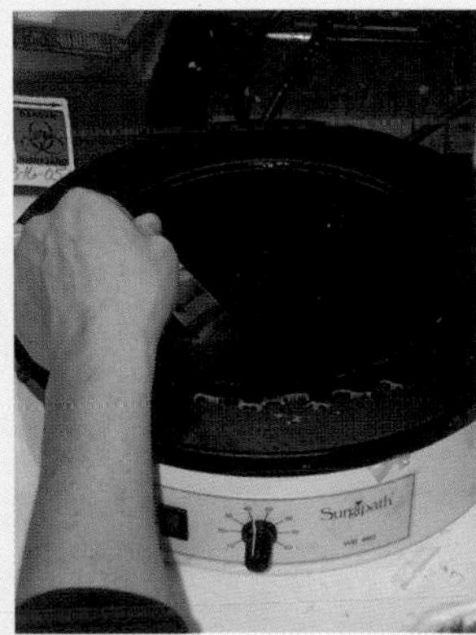

Step ____________

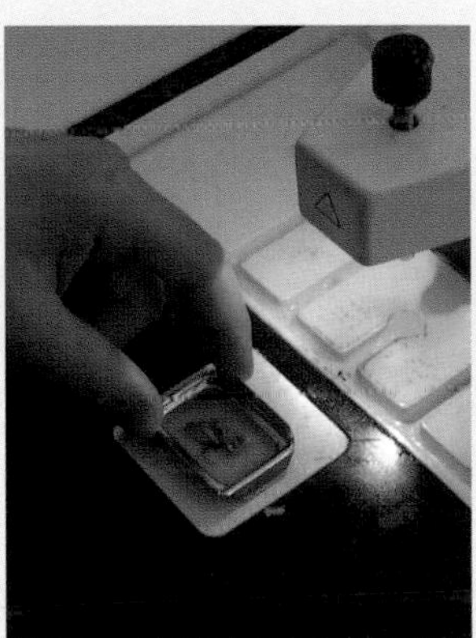

Step ____________

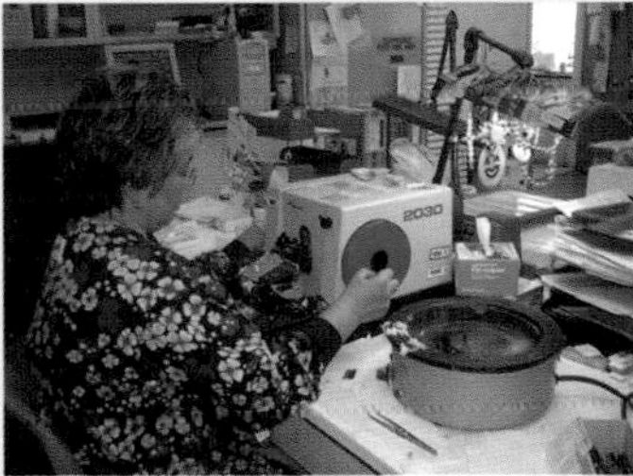

Step ____________

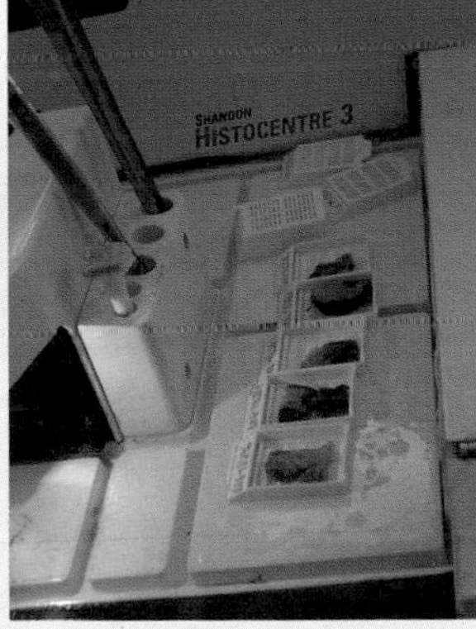

Step ____________

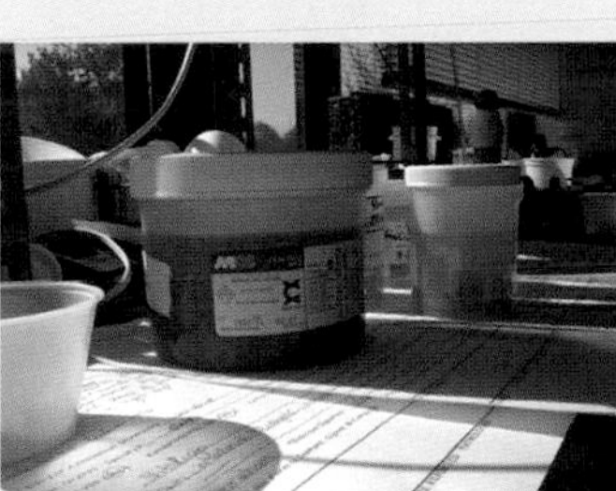

Step ____________

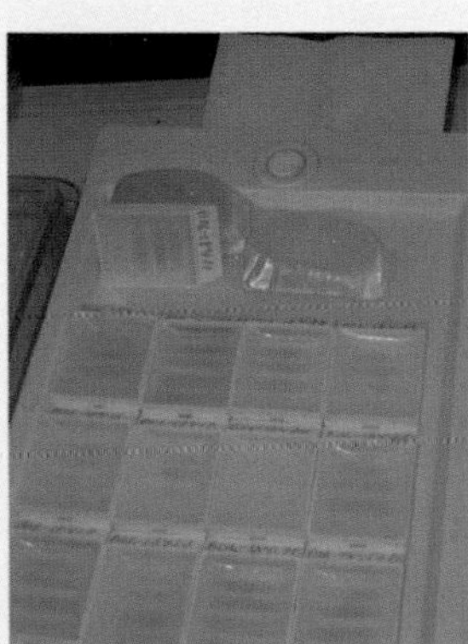

Step ____________

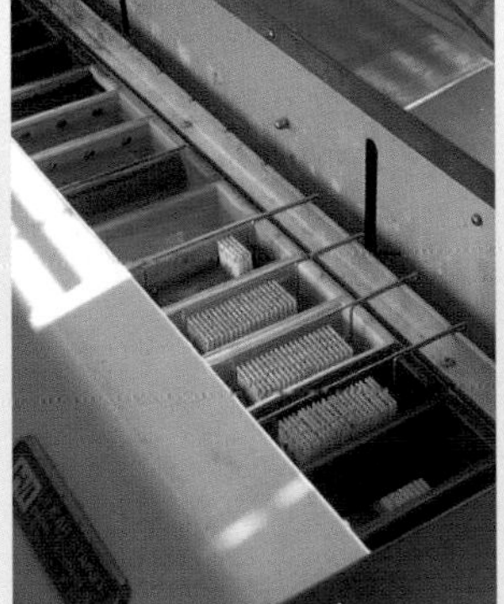

Step ____________

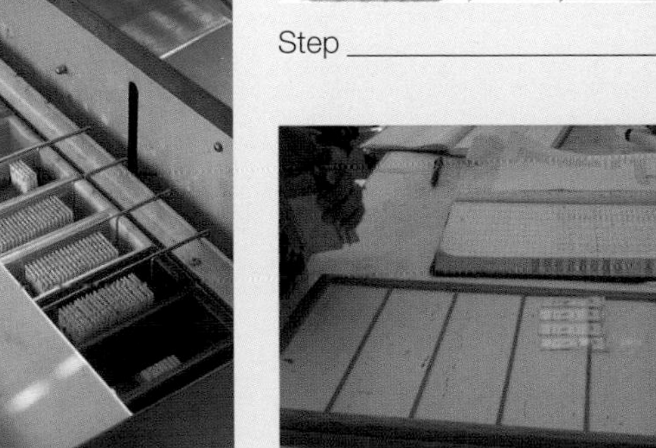

Step ____________

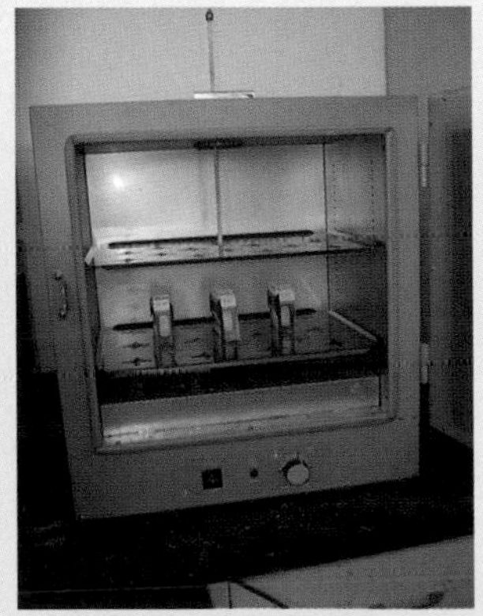

Step ____________

Exercise 9

Microscope Exercise

Description of Exercise

Photomicrographs of various tissues are featured in each question. A corresponding histology slide should be viewed as a supplement to each image. Examine the histology slides under the microscope. Use the corresponding box for each question to draw a portion of the image you observe upon microscopic examination. Make sure to note the magnification of the microscope's objective lens (10×, 40×, and so on) that you used as a basis for your illustration. Label any histologic structures that you are able to identify (e.g., basal lamina, cells, cellular structures). If you do not have access to the corresponding histology slides, use the photomicrograph provided to draw the tissue sample and label any identifiable histologic structures.

A.

Elastic cartilage

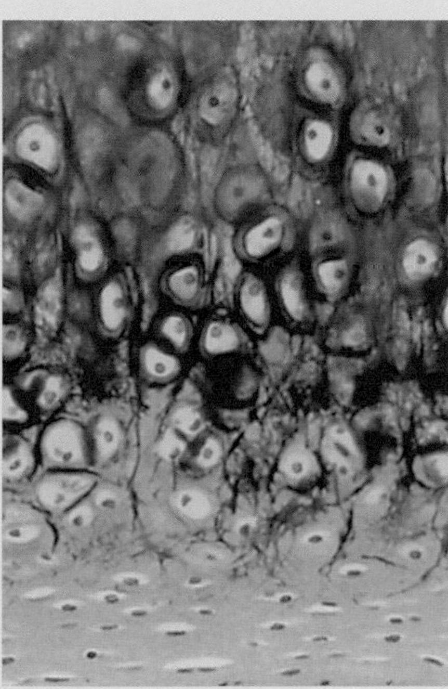

Section of elastic cartilage. (From Banks WJ: Applied veterinary histology, ed. 3, St Louis, 1993, Mosby.)

B.

Intestinal mucosa

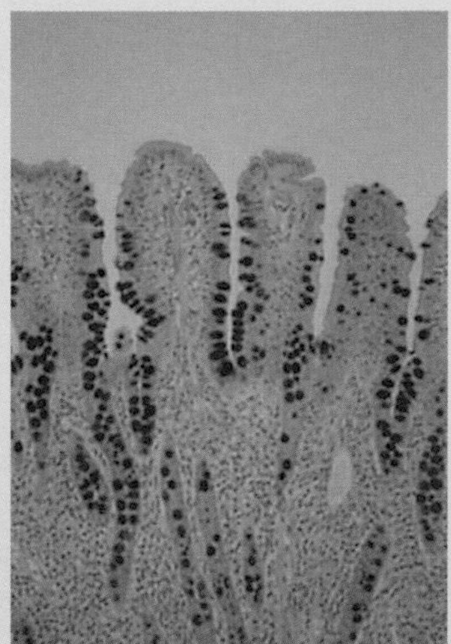

Equine intestinal mucosa. (From Banks WJ: Applied veterinary histology, ed. 3, St Louis, 1993, Mosby.)

Continued

Exercise 9—cont'd

Microscope Exercise

C.

Skeletal muscle

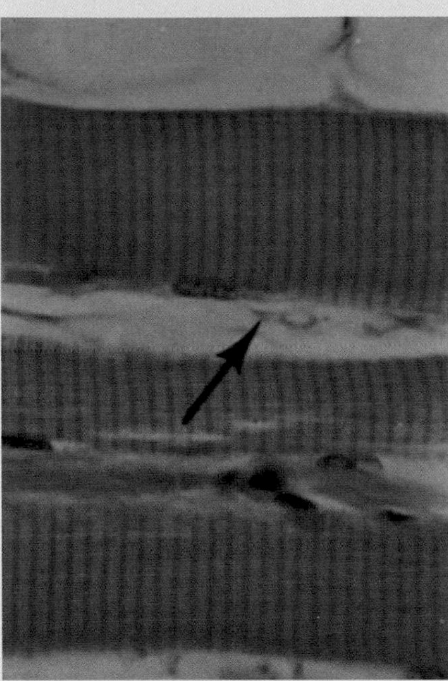

Longitudinal section of skeletal muscle. (From Banks WJ: Applied veterinary histology, ed. 3, St Louis, 1993, Mosby.)

D.

Adipose tissue

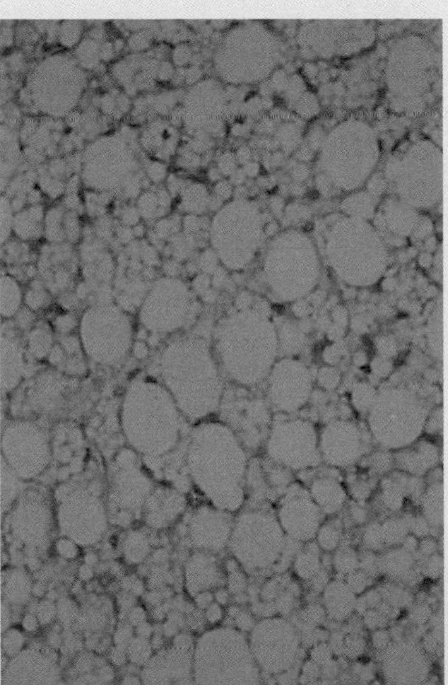

Adipose tissue. (From Banks WJ: Applied veterinary histology, ed. 3, St Louis, 1993, Mosby.)

Exercise 9—cont'd

Microscope Exercise

E.

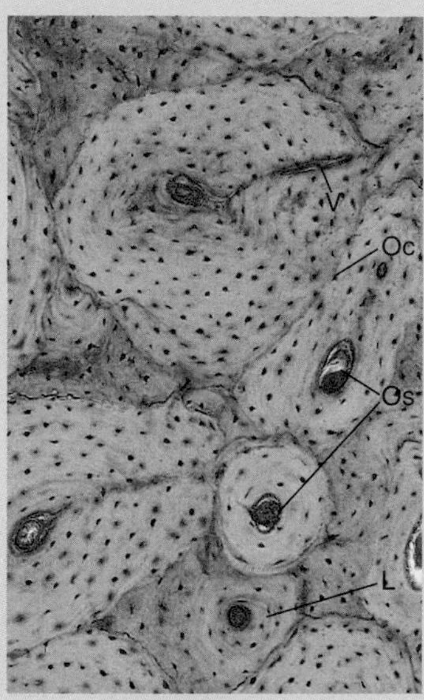

Decalcified compact bone. (From Gartner LP, Hyatt JL: Color textbook of histology, ed. 3, Philadelphia, 2006, Saunders.)

Compact bone

F.

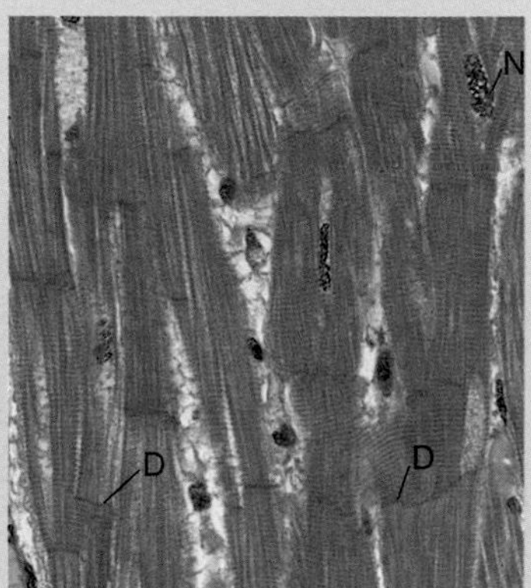

Cardiac muscle. (From Gartner LP, Hyatt JL: Color textbook of histology, ed. 3, Philadelphia, 2006, Saunders.)

Cardiac muscle

Exercise 10

Clinical Thinking Challenge

Support each of the following correct statements with appropriate rationale, stating why or in what way each statement is correct.

1. A unicellular organism, such as a paramecium, can live as an individual. However, the cells that compose multicellular organisms cannot survive independently of communities.
2. The body substances, excretions, and secretions differ.
3. Although the size and shape of the cells vary, epithelia share certain common characteristics.
4. A brush border is found on epithelia in the intestinal and urinary tracts.
5. In animals that contract parvovirus, mortality is high when the disease is untreated, particularly in young animals.
6. Two types of cells make up the gut lining.
7. Transitional epithelium is found in portions of the urinary tract.
8. Mucus functions in two ways.
9. Exocrine glands can be classified in four distinct ways.
10. Connective tissue is composed of three distinct components.
11. Connective tissue is composed of three distinct fibers.
12. The good news is that some white blood cells have the ability to produce hyaluronidase.
13. Cartilage can withstand a great deal of compression without causing pain to the animal.
14. Cartilage is slow to heal.

Exercise 10—cont'd

Clinical Thinking Challenge

15. Elective surgery is avoided in unhealthy animals.

16. There are four stages of healing and repair.

17. Both gross anatomy and microanatomy are important in animal care.

18. There are four primary tissue types.

19. There are three types of muscle tissue.

20. Neurons are the longest cells in the body and may reach up to a meter in length. They are composed of three primary parts.

Exercise 11

Case Application—The Healing Process

"Cupcake" Johnson, a 5-year-old spayed female Toy Poodle, presents to Four Paws Small Animal Clinic unable to bear weight on her right forelimb. You assist the veterinarian with Cupcake's examination, which reveals a shard of glass protruding from the skin on the right forelimb. The veterinarian removes the glass shard and asks you to take Cupcake into the treatment area so you can clean and bandage the wound.

After you are finished, you bring Cupcake to the reception area where the Johnsons are waiting for her. You ask them if they have any questions. The Johnson's 13-year-old daughter asks you what happens during the healing process. Understanding how important client education is, you sit down with the Johnsons and reach for a pad of paper to give them a visual explanation of Cupcake's healing process.

Following are the four stages of tissue healing and repair. For each stage, please draw an image of the physiologic process and write a corresponding description. The image for Stage 1: Injury is already provided as an example.

Stage 1

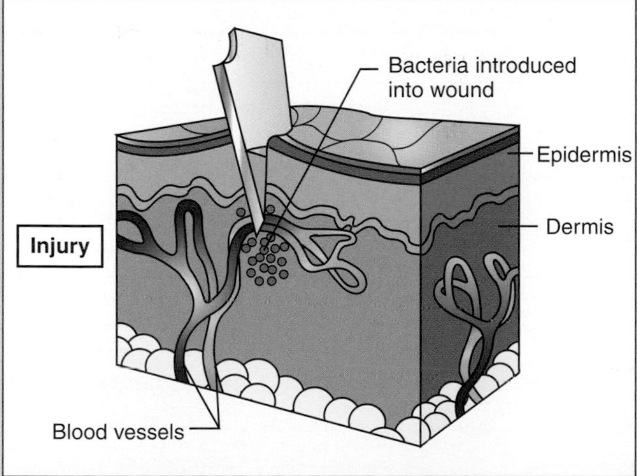

Description: INJURY

Continued

Exercise 11—cont'd

Case Application—The Healing Process

Stage 2

Drawing: INFLAMMATION	Description: INFLAMMATION

Stage 3

Drawing: ORGANIZATION	Description: ORGANIZATION

Stage 4

Drawing: REGENERATION	Description: REGENERATION

Exercise 12

Mucous Membranes and Clues in Diagnoses

When animals are sick, they show signs of illness in many ways, one of which is a change in the appearance of their mucous membranes.

A veterinarian or veterinary technician can gain clues about the general state of the animal through an examination and observation of the oral mucous membranes, including the gingiva (gum tissue). Fill in the chart below with the missing information.

Physical Condition	Result	Observation of Mucous Membranes	Terminology
Vomiting, diarrhea, no intake of solids or fluids	Depression and lethargy	________	________
Liver failure, hemolytic anemia	________	________	Icterus
________	Inadequate oxygenation of tissues	Blue mucous membranes	________
Febrile, hypertensive, or allergic reaction	________	________	Hyperemia
Anemia, shock, hypothermia	Decreased blood flow to peripheral tissues	Pale or white mucous membranes	N/A

Exercise 13

Capillary Refill Time

A clinician may gain additional clues about the state of the circulatory system by examining the gingival tissues (gums). If pressed firmly, the pink region of an animal's gingiva blanches white. When released, the gingiva changes from white back to pink relatively quickly. The time it takes for blood to return to the capillaries and turn the gum pink again is called the capillary refill time (CRT). **For each of the conditions described below, indicate whether the CRT is normal (N), delayed (D), or shortened (S), and the possible underlying cause(s).**

Observation of Gingival Coloration	CRT	Possible Cause(s)
>2 s delay in gingiva returning to normal coloration	____	________
1–2 s delay in gingiva returning to normal coloration	____	________
<1 s delay in gingiva returning to normal coloration	____	________

Exercise 14

Case Application—Arrhythmogenic Right Ventricular Cardiomyopathy

Brownie, a 6-year-old male Boxer, has been brought to the Companion Care Veterinary Center by the Truitt family. They are very concerned because Brownie doesn't seem to be as active as he usually is, and he seems to pant quite a bit with any exercise. Dr. Pritchett tells you he wants to rule out ARCV. List the tests that will be necessary, including the physical examination.

1. ________
2. ________
3. ________
4. ________

The Truitts are concerned and ask that you explain what ARCV is and how it affects their Brownie. Give them an overview of cardiomyopathy and why ACRV is suspected in Brownie's case.

____

____

____

5 The Integumentary System[a]

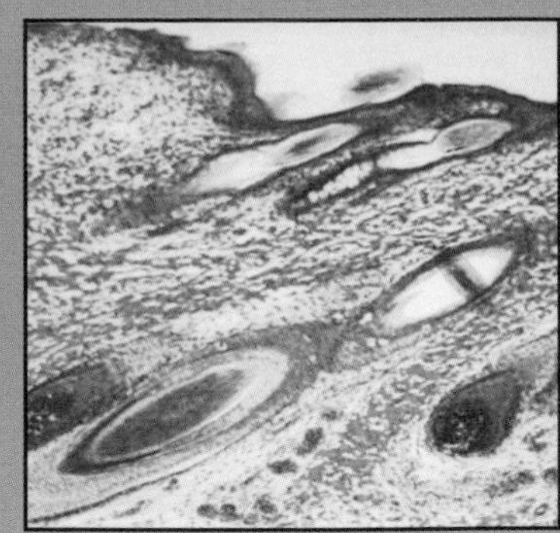

OVERVIEW AT A GLANCE

The Layers of the Integument 71

Special Features of the Integument 76

Associated Structures 80

Exercises 84–96

Layers of the Integument 84–86

1. *Describe Tissue Differences 84*
2. *Compare and Contrast Thick and Thin Skin 84*
3. *Microscopic Exam of Thick and Thin Skin 84*
4. *Histologic Description of the Epidermis 85*
5. *Observation of Feline Skin 86*

Special Features of the Integument 86–87

6. *Draw Nose and Paw Pads of Dog 86*
7. *Identify Location of Chestnuts and Ergots 87*

Hair 88–90

8. *Label and Color Pig Skin 88*
9. *Describe Types of Hair 88*
10. *Color Structures of a Hair Follicle 89*
11. *Microscopic Exam of Hair Follicles 90*

Assorted Structures 90–93

12. *Function and Location of Corium Layers in the Equine Foot 90*
13. *Color Structures in a Feline Claw 91*
14. *Label an Equine Foot 91*
15. *Color Structures in the Ruminant Horn 93*

Critical and Clinical Thinking 93–96

16. *Appearance of Cancer of the Skin 93*
17. *Exploring Allergy and Mange 94*
18. *Matching Terms and Definitions 95*
19. *Clinical Thinking Challenge 96*

LEARNING OBJECTIVES

The student will learn to identify the histologic layers of thick and thin skin, and the components of associated structures of the skin, including hair, glands, nails, hooves, and horns.

CLINICAL SIGNIFICANCE

Knowledge of the anatomy of the **integumentary system** is important for the veterinary technician because skin-related problems are common among animals. The skin is the largest organ of the body, and plays the vital role of protecting the body from desiccation and infection. It provides sensations relating to the surrounding environment through touch and is one of the few organs that we can directly visualize. In veterinary practice, a great deal of time is spent treating infectious diseases of the skin and glands. Injuries to the hooves of horses and cows are common and can be life-threatening if the animal cannot support its weight in a standing position. Knowledge of the anatomy of the skin is essential to understanding dermatologic disorders and the process of wound healing. In addition, problems with the growth of hair can signal an internal metabolic disease. Knowledge of anatomy is helpful when assisting with dehorning and declawing procedures and with closure of incision sites and wounds. Thus a thorough knowledge of the anatomy of the skin and associated structures can lead to the successful treatment of many serious animal illnesses.

INTRODUCTION

The integument, covering and protecting the underlying structures, forms a critical barrier between the internal structures or systems and the environment. The integumentary system, one of the largest and most extensive organ systems, covers every millimeter of an animal's external surface, and includes the hooves, hair, horns, claws, skin, and related glands. Of all organ systems, the integument has a vigorous ability to regenerate and heal.

[a]The authors and publisher wish to acknowledge Mary Ann Seagren for previous contributions to this chapter.

READING ASSIGNMENT

This laboratory chapter corresponds to Chapter 6 in *Clinical Anatomy and Physiology for Veterinary Technicians.* Be sure to read that chapter before beginning this lab.

MATERIALS NEEDED

- Compound light microscope
- Prepared slide: epidermis of thick skin (example: paw pads)
- Prepared slide: epidermis of thin skin, including hair follicles and associated structures
- Preserved cat for dissection
- Live dog
- Model of equine foot if available
- Colored pencils

TERMS TO BE IDENTIFIED

- Layers of the skin
  - Epidermis
  - Dermis
  - Hypodermis or subcutaneous layers of skin
- Layers of the epidermis (in thick skin)
  - Stratum basale or stratum germinativum
  - Stratum spinosum
  - Stratum granulosum
  - Stratum lucidum
  - Stratum corneum
- Layers of the epidermis (in thin skin)
  - Stratum basale
  - Stratum spinosum
  - Stratum corneum
- Layers of the dermis
  - Papillary layer
  - Reticular layer
- Structures associated with the skin
  - Dermal papilla
  - Hair follicle
- Hair shaft
  - Medulla
  - Cortex
  - Cuticle
- Hair bulb
- Meissner's corpuscle
- Arrector pili muscle
- Tactile elevation
- Glands
  - Sebaceous glands
  - Eccrine sweat glands
- Structures associated with the nose and paw
  - Planum nasale
  - Planum nasolabiale
  - Polygonal plates in the canine planum nasale
  - Conical papillae of canine paw pads
- Equine structures
  - Ergots
  - Chestnuts
- Equine hoof
  - Toe
  - Wall
  - White line
  - Sole
    - Angle of the sole
  - Quarters
  - Heel
    - Bulbs of the heel
- Frog (and underlying digital cushion)
  - Apex of the frog
  - Central sulcus or commissure
  - Collateral sulcus or commissure
- Bars
- Periople
- Coronary band (coronet)
- Corium (sensitive and insensitive)
  - Laminar corium
  - Coronary corium
  - Sole corium
  - Frog corium
- Bones of the hoof and lower leg
  - Equine species walk on digit 3; ruminants walk on digits 3 and 4
  - Equine: metacarpal/tarsal 3 or cannon bone
  - Ruminants: fused metacarpal/tarsal 3 and 4
  - Proximal phalanx (P1)
  - Middle phalanx (P2)
  - Distal phalanx (P3) or coffin bone (equine term)
  - Distal sesamoid or navicular bone (equine term)
- Structures in the bovine horn
  - Cornual process (horn process)
  - Cornual sinus

The Layers of the Integument

The integument is made up of three layers: the epidermis, the dermis, and the hypodermis or subcutis. The **epidermis** is the outermost layer and is composed of stratified squamous epithelium. It is waterproof and provides external protection to the body. Under the epidermis is the **dermis,** a tough layer of fibroelastic connective tissue. Fibroblasts are the main cell type present in the dermis and they are surrounded by the collagen and elastin fibers, which they produce. The dermis contains many blood vessels, hair follicles, and glands. The **hypodermis, or subcutaneous layer,** lies below the dermis. It is composed primarily of adipose tissue and helps regulate the animal's body temperature, acts as a shock absorber, and allows the skin to move freely over the underlying muscle and bones. Fig. 5.1 is a photomicrograph of pig skin showing all three layers.

Layers of the Epidermis

The outermost layer of the skin, the **epidermis,** is composed of three to five layers of stratified squamous epithelial cells

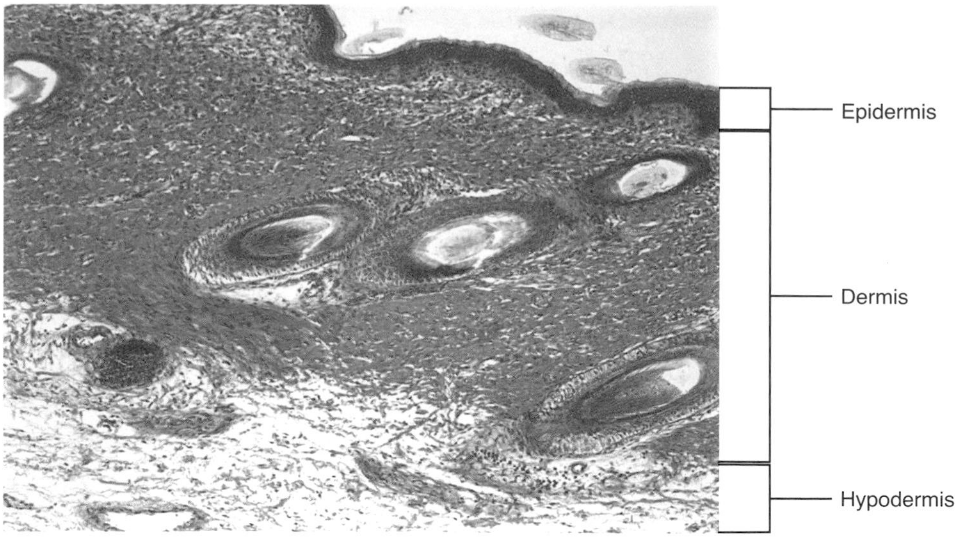

Epidermis
Dermis
Hypodermis

• **Fig. 5.1** Pig skin. The three main components of the integument are shown. The epidermis is the thin, darker staining band in the top right of the photo. The dermis is the layer under the epidermis. It contains transverse sections of hair follicles. The hypodermis or subcutaneous layer is the pale staining area in the bottom left of the photo.

called **keratinocytes.** Other cells present in the epidermis include **melanocytes,** which produce pigment called **melanin; Langerhans cells,** which are macrophages specific to the epidermis; and **Merkel cells,** which are associated with sensory nerve endings. **Thick skin** contains five layers and is usually present on areas of the body that receive a lot of wear and tear, such as the palms and paw pads. Fig. 5.2 contains photomicrographs and a diagram of thick skin in which the five standard layers are identified. Study the photos while reading about each layer.

The lowest layer of keratinocytes is called the **stratum germinativum or stratum basale** (basal layer) and consists of a single layer of cells along the basement membrane of the epidermis. These cells are actively dividing and are the parent cells of all the other cells in the epidermis. The melanocytes and the Merkel cells are also in this layer. The next layer is the **stratum spinosum** (spiny layer). This consists of about three layers of squamous epithelial cells. There is some evidence of cell division in this layer and the cells still contain their nuclei. The next layer is the **stratum granulosum** (granular layer). The cells in this layer begin to become diamond shaped or elongated. The nuclei and cellular organelles in these cells are starting to degenerate. Keratin is being created and is starting to fill the cytoplasm of the cells. The **stratum lucidum** (clear layer) is next and is composed of elongated dead cells, which are mostly filled with keratin and have lost their nuclei. The cells appear to be clear when they are stained. The topmost layer is the **stratum corneum** (horny layer). This is a layer of dead remnants of squamous epithelial cells. The material remaining forms very flat layers of keratin. In thick skin this layer is quite large and protects the underlying tissues from abrasion.

The skin is thinner in some areas of the body than in others. For example, the back of the neck and between the shoulder blades has thicker skin than the eyelids, groin, and axilla, where the skin is quite thin. **Thin skin** is composed of only three layers: the **stratum basale**, **stratum spinosum**, and **stratum corneum**. Fig. 5.3 contains photomicrographs of the epithelium of thin skin showing the layers that compose it.

Epidermis of the Nose and Paw Pads

The epidermis of the nose and paw pads has a specialized morphology. The nose of the dog, cat, sheep, and pig is called the **planum nasale**. The nose of the horse and cow, commonly called the muzzle, is technically known as the **planum nasolabiale**. If you look closely at the skin of the nose of the dog as shown in Fig. 5.4, you will see **polygonal plates** or plaques packed together. This pattern is caused by the presence of deep grooves in the epidermis. Note the epidermal grooves in the diagram of the planum nasale in Fig. 5.5.

The paw pads of the dog are the weight-bearing surface of the foot, and therefore have many special features. Fig. 5.6 shows a photo of the palmar surface of a dog's foot. The pads closest to the nails are called the digital pads and support the weight placed on the phalanges. The large central pad is called the metacarpal (forelimb) or metatarsal (hindlimb) pad and supports the body's weight as it comes down through the metacarpal and metatarsal bones. The small pad proximal to these is called the carpal (forelimb) or tarsal (hindlimb) pad and is not used for weight bearing, but is a vestigial pad.

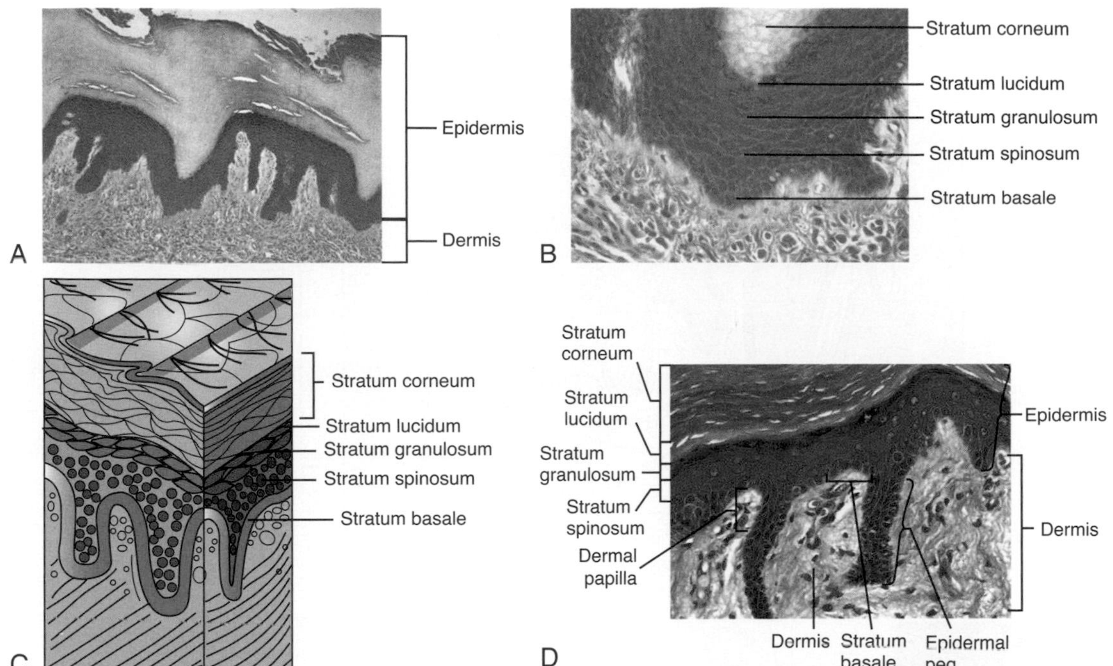

• **Fig. 5.2** Thick skin—monkey's palm. (A) This is a photomicrograph of the skin of a monkey's palm. Note the very thick stratum corneum. Also note the deep interdigitations of the epidermis with the dermal papilla. These extensions of the dermis provide a strong connection between the epidermis and dermis in areas that receive a lot of friction and stress, such as the palm or the plantar surface of the foot. (B) This higher power photomicrograph shows all five layers of epidermis. Note the difference in the morphology of the cells in each layer. (C) A diagram of the skin layers. (D) Light micrograph of integument.

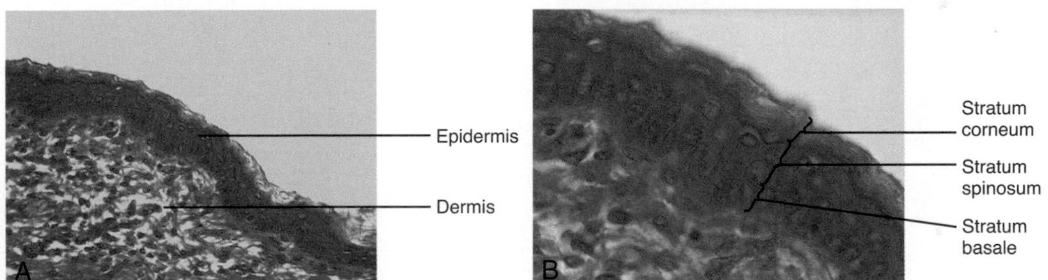

• **Fig. 5.3** Thin skin—pig. (A) This photomicrograph shows the epidermis and underlying dermis of the thin skin of a pig. (B) This higher magnification shows the three layers of squamous cells that are usually present in thin skin. (Photos courtesy Manor College.)

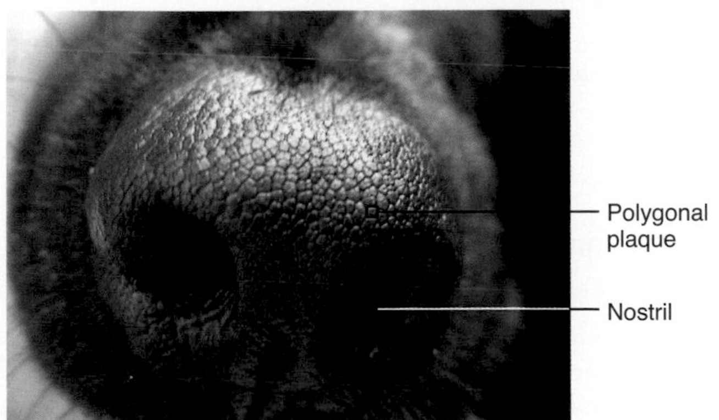

• **Fig. 5.4** Polygonal plates—dog nose. This photo shows the surface of the skin of a dog's nose. Note the grooves in the epidermis that make the surface appear like plates or plaques. It is actually a continuous layer of epidermis.

The integument of the paw pad is quite specialized. Fig. 5.7 is a photo of the surface of a dog's pad. The surface is composed of **conical papillae**. These add extra protection to the pad and can become fairly abraded without causing the foot any harm. Occasionally, if a dog spends too much time walking on rough surfaces, the conical papillae will become worn down and the dog will experience pain. I have seen a group of dogs that became very excited while their owners were swimming in the backyard pool. The dogs ran around and around the pool for hours and the paws became abraded. In addition to the specialized conical papillae of the epithelium, paw pads also have a thick layer of subcutaneous adipose tissue to provide insulation and cushioning (Fig. 5.8).

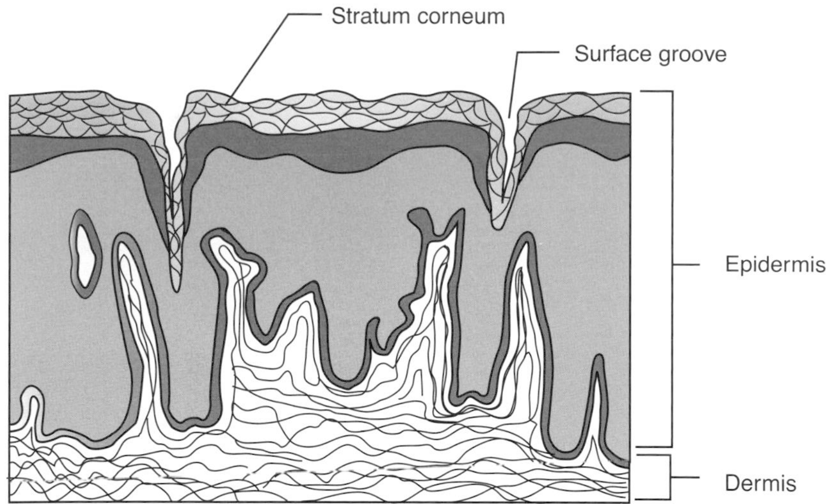

• **Fig. 5.5** Epidermis—dog nose. This diagram of the epidermis of a dog's nose shows the grooves in the epidermis that create the look of polygonal plates.

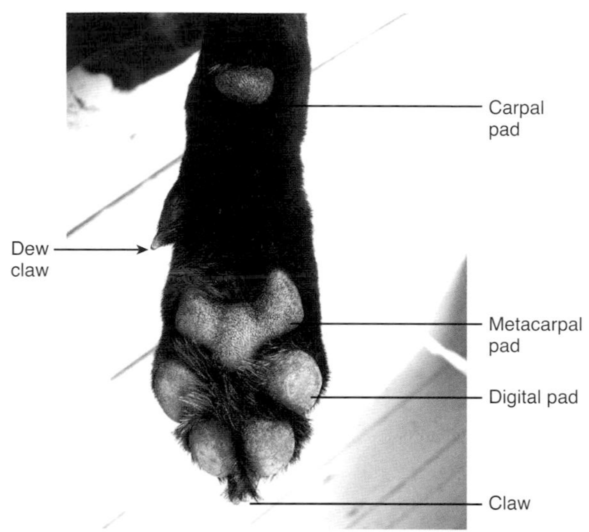

• **Fig. 5.6** Foot pads—dog. The palmar surface of this dog's foot has four digital pads, a metacarpal pad, and a carpal pad.

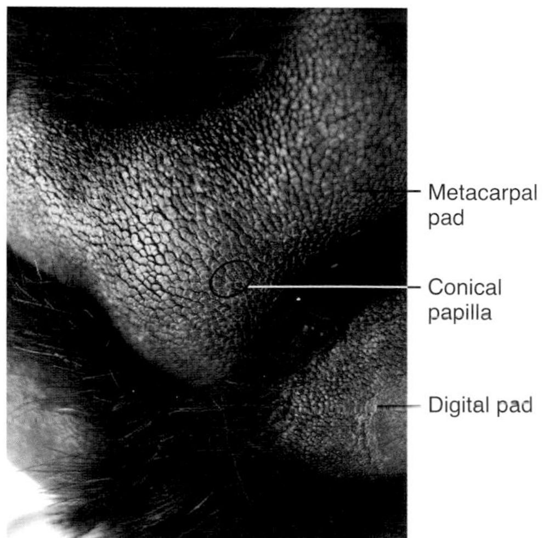

• **Fig. 5.7** Conical papillae—dog pad. This close-up of a dog's pad shows the conical papillae that make up the surface of the pad. These papillae can be worn down (circle) if the dog is walked on hard surfaces such as concrete.

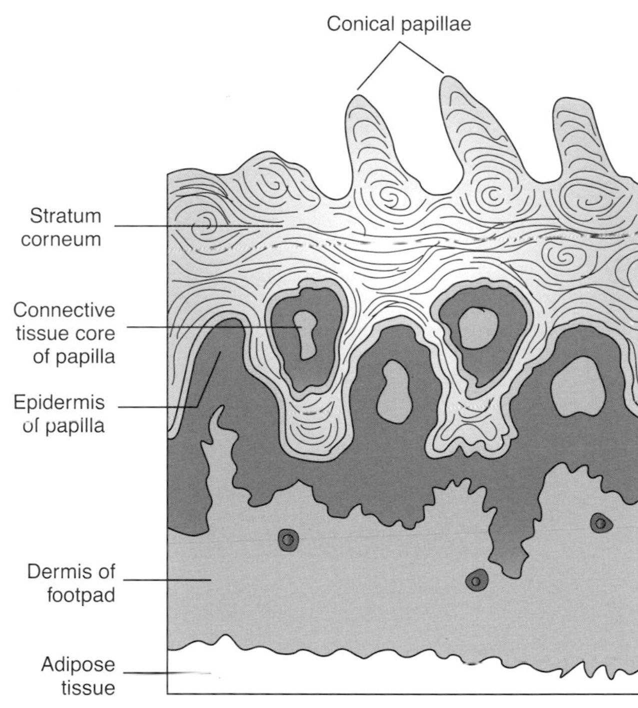

• **Fig. 5.8** Epidermis—paw pad. In this diagram, note that the conical papillae are extensions of the stratum corneum of the epidermis.

Ergots and Chestnuts

Chestnuts and ergots are dark horny layers of epidermis that are present on the legs of members of the equine family. They are thought to be remnants of foot pads. Fig. 5.9 shows photographs of chestnuts and ergots on a horse. **Chestnuts** are brown, tan, or gray (depending on the pigmentation of the horse) structures on the medial side of the knee (carpus) and hock (tarsus). They are vestiges of carpal and tarsal pads. **Ergots** are horny tissue found in the long hairs below the fetlock joint. They are thought to be vestiges of pads of the second and fourth digits.

CLINICAL APPLICATION

Proud Flesh

When skin is injured, cells migrate from the stratum basale over the surface of the open wound. When a layer of these germinal, basal cells lies over the wound, this tissue is called **granulation tissue.** In most cases the granulation tissue will proceed to grow new layers of epithelium, leading eventually to the development of all the strata of skin, including the stratum corneum (the keratinized layer). In horses, especially with wounds over joints that receive a lot of physical motion, sometimes the granulation tissue is broken down repeatedly and has to regrow. This phase of regrowth can get out of control and the granulation tissue can multiply and thicken without producing more mature skin layers. This granulation tissue can become quite large. It is referred to as exuberant granulation tissue or **proud flesh.** It can become so large that it inhibits wound healing and must be removed surgically or cauterized for the wound to heal. The accompanying figure shows an example of proud flesh in a horse.

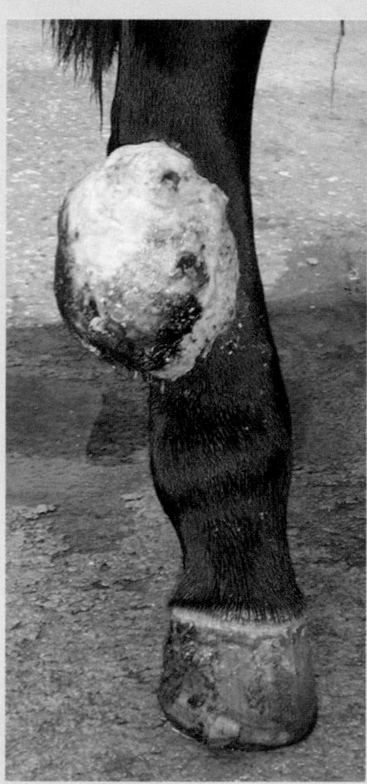

Proud flesh. In this photo, note the exuberant granulation tissue (proud flesh) on the metatarsus of a horse. (From McCurnin DM, Bassert JM: Clinical textbook for veterinary technicians, ed. 6, St Louis, 2006, Saunders.)

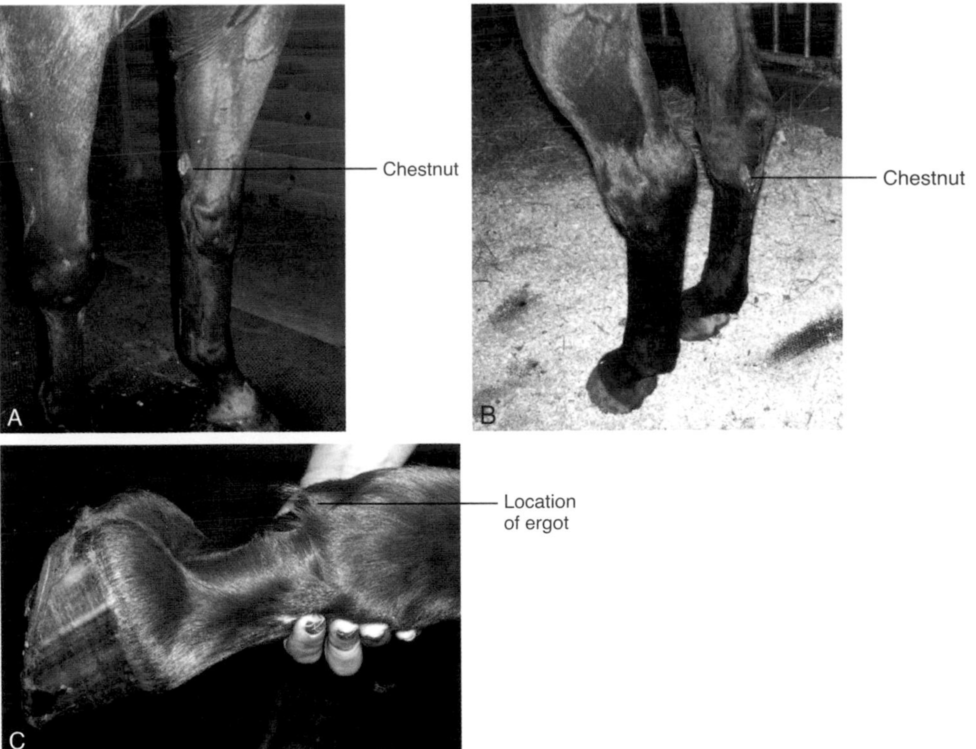

• **Fig. 5.9** Chestnuts and ergots. (A) In the forelimb the chestnut is located on the medial side of the limb and just above (proximal to) the knee (carpus). (B) In the hindlimb, the chestnut is also on the medial side of the limb, just below (distal to) the hock (tarsus). The ergots are located behind (caudal to) the fetlock joints. (C) In this photo, the ergot is covered by a spike of hair.

Special Features of the Integument

Identify the Structures Associated with the Dermis

Using the light microscope, examine the prepared slides of skin. Begin with low power examination of thin skin. Notice the three major layers of the skin:

1. Epidermis
2. Dermis
3. Hypodermis (or subcutis)

Beneath the epidermis is the layer of the integument called the dermis. The dermis is divided into two layers. The uppermost layer is called the **papillary layer** and is composed of loose irregular connective tissue. It is called the papillary layer because there are various **dermal papillae** that project into the epidermis. You may need to use higher magnification to visualize the details of the papillary layer. Notice that the wavelike dermal papillae help connect the epidermis to the dermis and prevent it from tearing off when under stress, particularly the stress of a shearing force. Skin that is subjected to a lot of stress has numerous dermal papillae, which extend deeper into the dermal layer than those found in skin that is stressed less frequently.

The lower layer of the dermis is called the **reticular** layer and is composed of dense irregular connective tissue. There are many collagen and elastin fibers in both layers. In the reticular layer, the fibers line up parallel to one another. In addition, they are oriented in the same direction as the forces (stresses) that routinely act upon that particular region of skin. The collagen and elastin fibers and their directionality give skin its strength and elasticity.

Other structures found in the three major layers of skin may be evident in the model exhibited in Fig. 5.10 and in your prepared slides. Compare the model of the integument in Fig. 5.10 with Fig. 5.11. One of the most prominent structures found in the dermis is a **hair follicle.** Look for a longitudinal cross section of the hair shaft and the root in the hair follicle. The root is the portion of the hair that is within the skin. The **hair bulb** is the expansion of the hair follicle at the base of the root. Connected to the hair follicle is a small band of muscle called the **arrector pili muscle.** When this muscle contracts, it raises the hair to a vertical position, fluffing out the hair coat either for warmth or to make the animal appear larger and fiercer.

Sebaceous glands are also associated with hair follicles. Cells within the glands rupture and release the white, oily **sebum** that they contain. Sebum is important in lubricating the hair shaft. **Eccrine sweat glands** can also be seen in the model. They consist of a curled tube in the dermis that connects to the surface of the epidermis. In the dermal papilla are nerve endings called **Meissner's corpuscles**, which are receptors for touch. Blood vessels are in the dermis, and loops of these vessels protrude into the dermal papillae to provide nourishment for the epidermis. **Pacinian corpuscles** are touch receptors found in the hypodermis. They are sensitive to deep touch, whereas the Meissner's corpuscles are sensitive to light touch.

CLINICAL APPLICATION

Skin Infection: Crusts, Pustules, and Papules

Dermatologic cases make up a large part of small animal practice. A very common diagnosis is bacterial skin infection in the dog. Some practitioners estimate that 95% of the canine infectious skin disease presented is bacterial infection due to *Staphylococcus* bacteria. The other 5% of infections include other bacterial skin infections, fungal infections, such as ringworm or yeast, and parasitic infestations, such as demodectic or sarcoptic mange. Bacterial infection has a very classic look. The skin of the dog shows the presence of papules, pustules, or crusts. The accompanying photo shows an example of these lesions. Papules are raised reddened areas; pustules are raised lesions with pus showing through the overlying epidermis; crusts occur after the pustules rupture and serum, pus, and sebum collect on the skin surface. These lesions are all a result of bacterial infection of the hair follicle (bacterial folliculitis). Bacteria that normally inhabit the skin (commensal organisms) overgrow in response to some underlying irritation of the skin—often allergic disease. The hair of the dog sometimes falls out in a circular pattern as the infection spreads, leading to lesions called "cookie cutter lesions" because it looks as though someone stamped out the hair with a round cookie cutter. Usually a short course of an appropriate antibiotic and treating the underlying irritation clears up this condition.

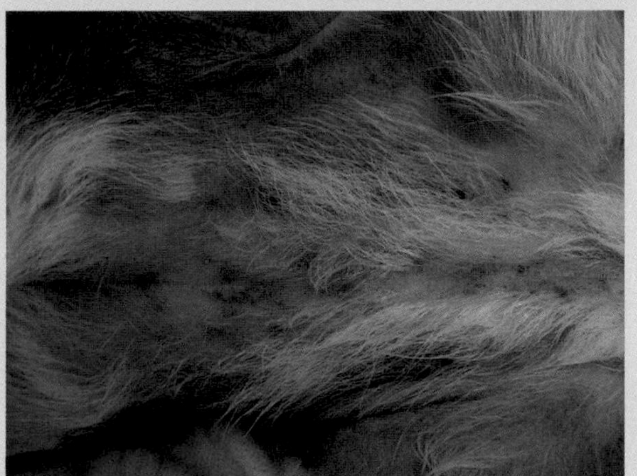

Bacterial skin infection. This photo shows the abdomen of a Beagle with multiple crusts, papules, and pustules of the skin around the midline. If you look carefully, you can see some crusts and papules in the skin of the inner thigh also.

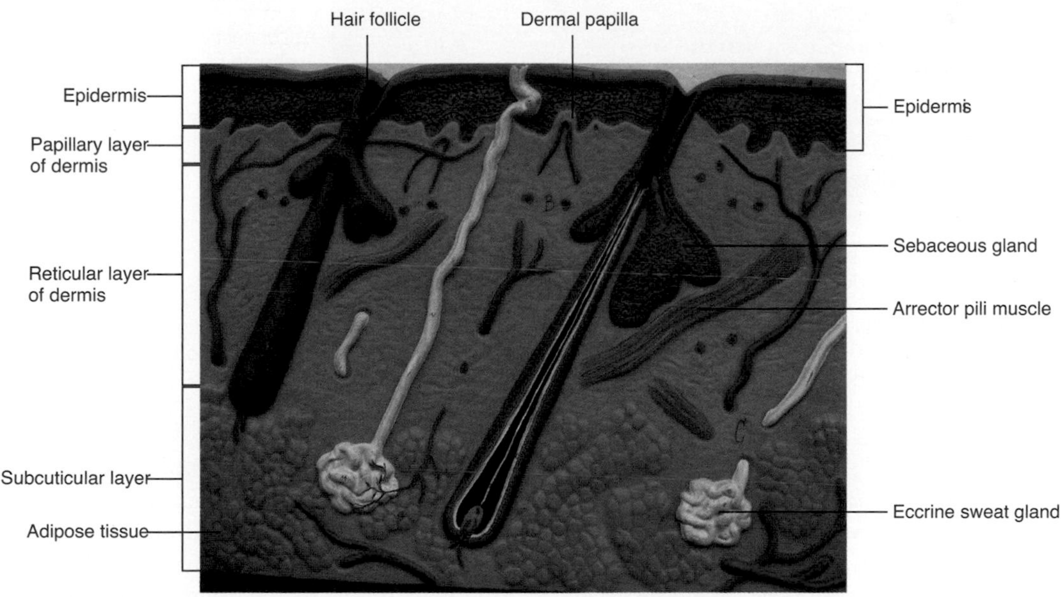

• **Fig. 5.10** Model of the integument. This photo shows a plastic model of the integument with the associated structures labeled.

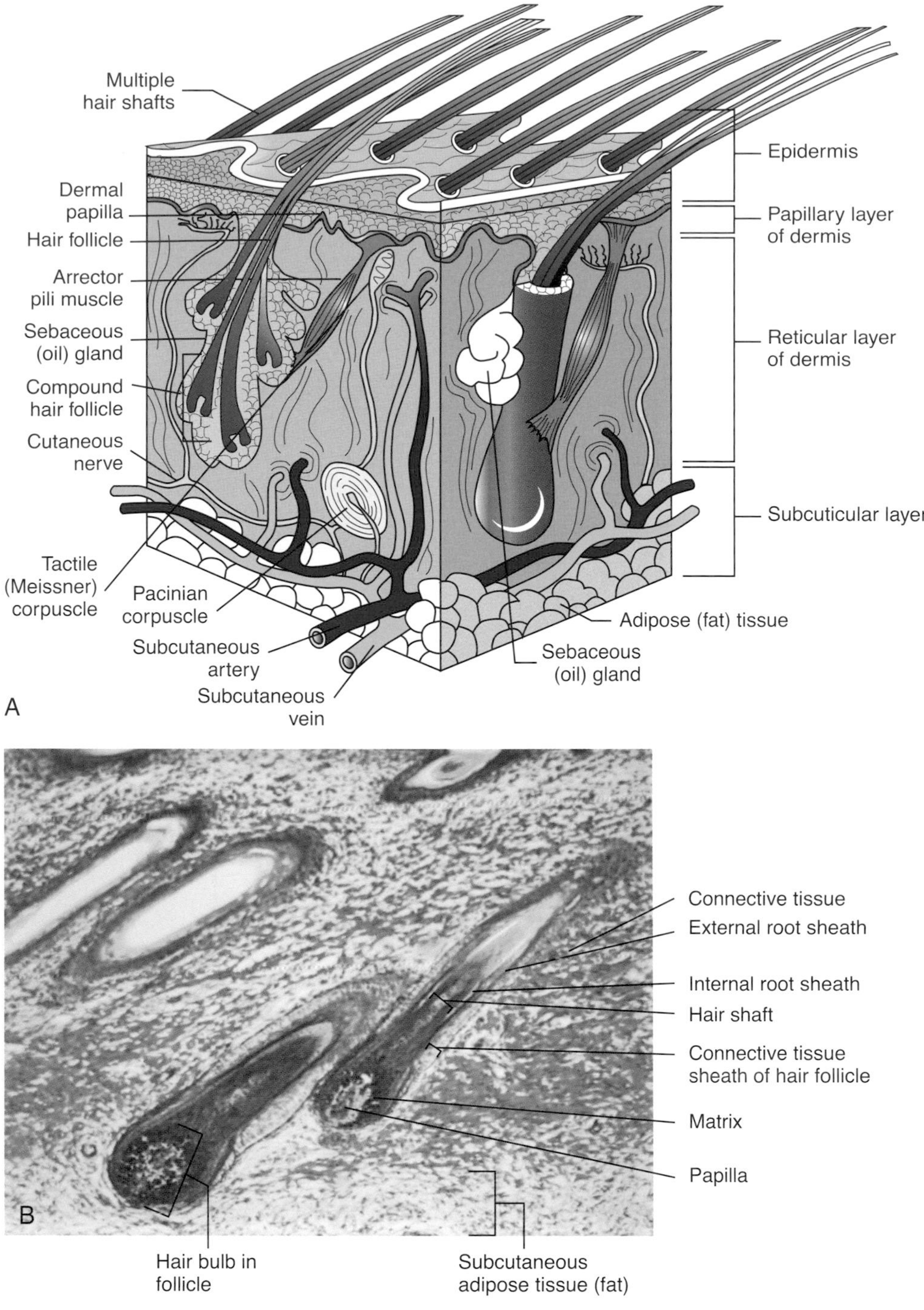

• **Fig. 5.11** Canine skin. (A) Cubed section of canine skin, underlying subcutaneous tissue, and structural details discussed in this chapter. Notice that epidermis of canine skin includes folds from which compound hairs arise. (B) Light photomicrograph of two hair follicles in the dermis of hairy skin.(Photo courtesy J.M. Bassert.)

Structure of Hair

The hairy skin of animals has scalelike folds that cover the surface of the epidermis. **Hair shafts** emerge from under the scales in the same direction that the scales are layered. Dogs have a cluster of three hair shafts per scale. There are generally two types of hair on animals: the undercoat, which consists of softer, finer hairs; and the topcoat, which consists of thick, longer hairs. These latter hairs are often called guard hairs. The topcoat grows when the animal reaches maturity.

Another type of hair that you may see in animals is a **tactile** hair. It is a special hair that emerges from an elevation in the skin called a **tactile elevation**. These hairs are connected to specialized nerves and allow the animal to "touch" objects in its environment. You can see these hairs especially around the muzzle or on the face of animals where they are referred to as **whiskers.**

The hair shaft is made of three layers of dead keratinized cells: the medulla, the cortex, and the cuticle. The **medulla** is in the middle of the hair shaft. The **cortex** is the next layer and contains various amounts of melanin, which determines the color of the hair. The **cuticle** is the outermost layer, composed of cells that lie, like the scales of a fish, in a longitudinal direction over the cortex.

The **hair root** is the part of the hair that is secured within the skin (Fig. 5.12). The region of epidermis that has invaginated to accommodate the formation of a hair shaft is called the hair follicle. The hair bulb is the expansion of the hair follicle at the base of the root. The **matrix** is the layer of live germinal epithelial cells analogous to the basal layer of the epithelium. These cells are actively dividing and as they move away from the hair bulb they fill with keratin and die to form the layers of the hair shaft. Along the inside of the hair follicle are layers of epithelial cells called the **internal root sheath** and **external root sheath.** These are part of the root of the hair, but do not become part of the hair shaft as it grows out of the follicle. The **connective tissue root sheath** is a continuation of the dermis, which helps anchor the hair root. Within the hair bulb is a section of the papillary layer of the dermis called the **connective tissue papilla.**

CLINICAL APPLICATION

Skin: A Signal of Internal Disease

Sometimes changes in the skin or hair coat can be an important clue that the animal has an internal disease. For example, many endocrine diseases cause a bilaterally symmetric alopecia—a symmetric loss of hair on both sides of the trunk. In hypothyroidism, the decreased level of thyroid hormone in the dog signals the hair follicles to stay in the telogen phase (resting stage) for a longer period of time. It can also cause the hair follicles to atrophy. Cushing disease in the horse causes the hair coat to become long and shaggy. Cushing disease in the dog can cause calcification of the hair follicles, a condition called calcinosis cutis. Many nutritional and metabolic diseases can cause the hair to become dry and brittle and the skin dry and scaly. Any abnormality in the hair or skin should be explored with a thorough physical examination and screening blood work. When the hair follicles are injured, the cells that produce pigment may be damaged. The hair can grow back with no pigment (see accompanying figure).

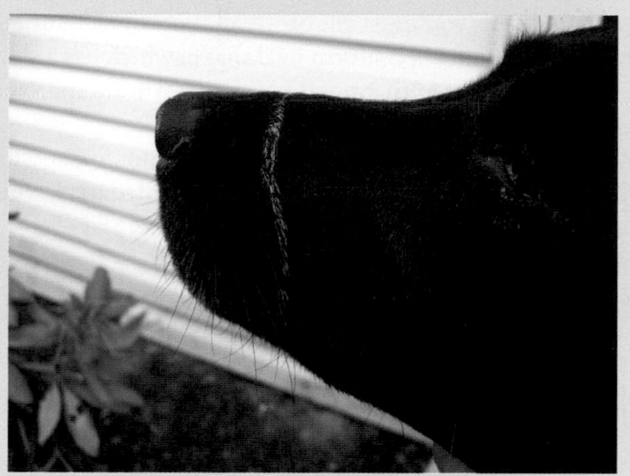

Hair pigment changes. When this Labrador Retriever was a puppy, he caught his muzzle in the bars of his crate and received a circumferential injury to the skin around his muzzle. The hair continues to grow without pigment 6 years later.

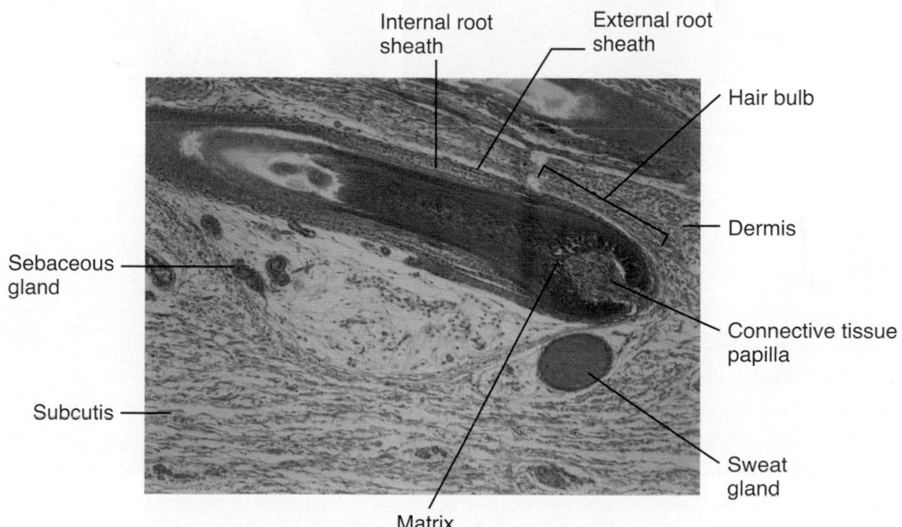

• **Fig. 5.12** Hair follicle. This photomicrograph of pig skin shows a longitudinal section of a hair shaft and its root.

Associated Structures

Structure of Canine and Feline Claws

The **claw** or **nail** of the dog and cat is composed of specialized keratinized epithelium. The germinal cells that create the keratinized cells are contained in a thin layer of modified dermis called the **corium.** The corium is similar to other dermal tissue in that it is vascular and has nerves and is sensitive to pain. It provides the nutrients to the germinal cells. The corium is commonly known as the "quick." If you cut the horny part of the nail, the animal will not feel pain, but if you trim too far proximally and cut the quick, the vessels will bleed, and the animal will feel pain. The corium is tightly adherent to a bony projection of the **distal phalanx** called the **ungual process.** Note in Fig. 5.13 that some claws or nails are pigmented, and some are not. In unpigmented nails you are able to visualize the quick and avoid cutting it. In pigmented nails you must cut off small slices of nail until the cut surface becomes a uniform oval shape, which has a shiny, fleshy appearance. At that point you know you are approaching the quick and the nail is fully trimmed.

Most dogs and cats have five toes on the front feet and four on the rear feet, but some dogs and cats are **polydactyl,** which means they have extra toes on one or more feet (Fig. 5.14).

Inspect the Retractable Nails of the Cadaver

Press on the second phalanx of the cat cadaver. This should extrude the retractable claw of the compressed digit. Find an unpigmented claw. Note the area of claw that contains the quick. Also note the area of the claw that is free of quick and safe to trim without causing bleeding or pain to the animal.

The Equine Foot

The equine foot can be divided into three structures: the hoof, the corium, and the bones of the foot. Fig. 5.15 shows a diagram of the equine foot and hoof. Use the diagrams and the equine foot model to identify the structures as they are described.

Like the claw of the dog and cat, the outer hoof wall of all ungulates (hoofed animals) is an insensitive, dead, keratinized structure. As in the claw, the germinal cells that create the keratin structure (the hoof wall) are contained in a thin layer of modified dermis called the corium. The corium (like other dermal tissues) is vascular, has nerves, is sensitive to pain, and contains the germinal cells that create the outer hoof wall. The corium attaches strongly to the

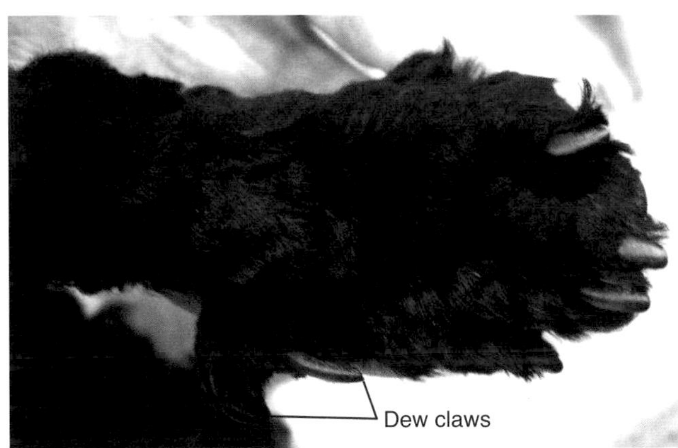

• **Fig. 5.14** Polydactyl dog. Note that this dog has two dew claws, for a total of six digits on its rear foot.

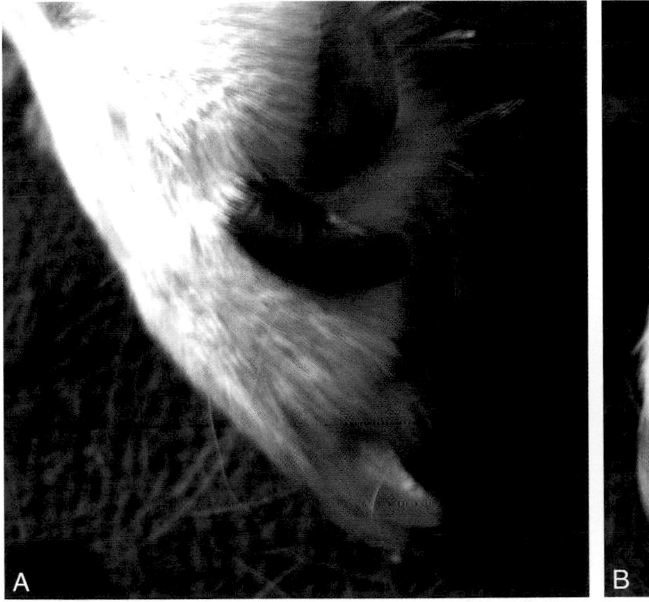

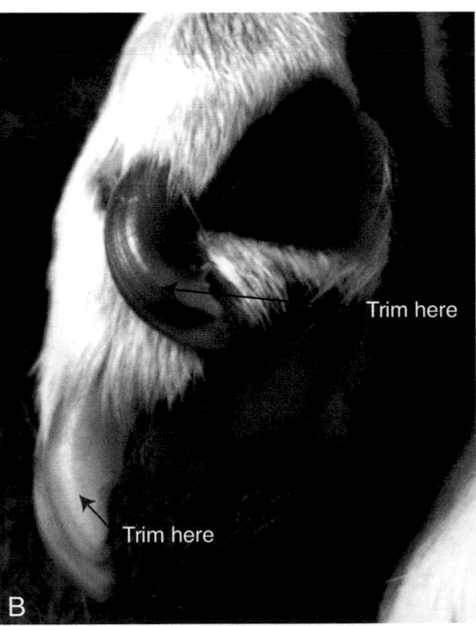

• **Fig. 5.13** Dog nails. (A) The uppermost nail is pigmented and it is impossible to visualize the quick. The lower nail is unpigmented. (B) The quick can be seen in both the upper nail, which is partially pigmented, and the lower nail, which is unpigmented. There is an arrow at the spot where the nail can be safely trimmed.

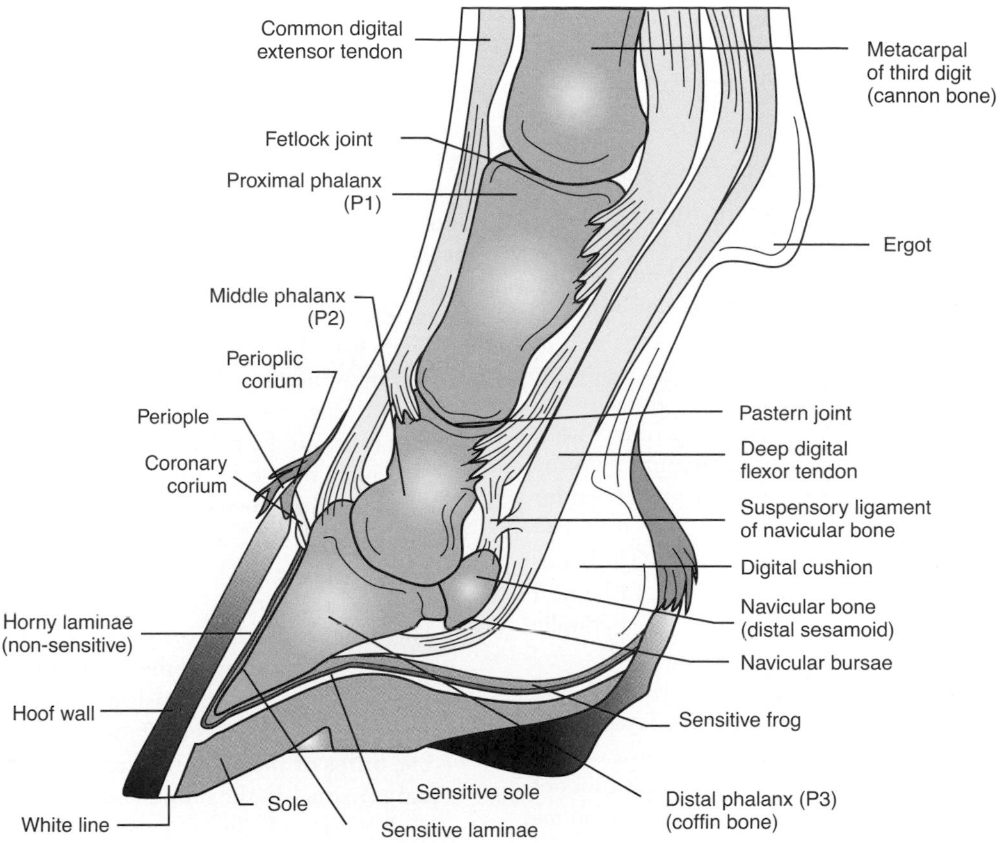

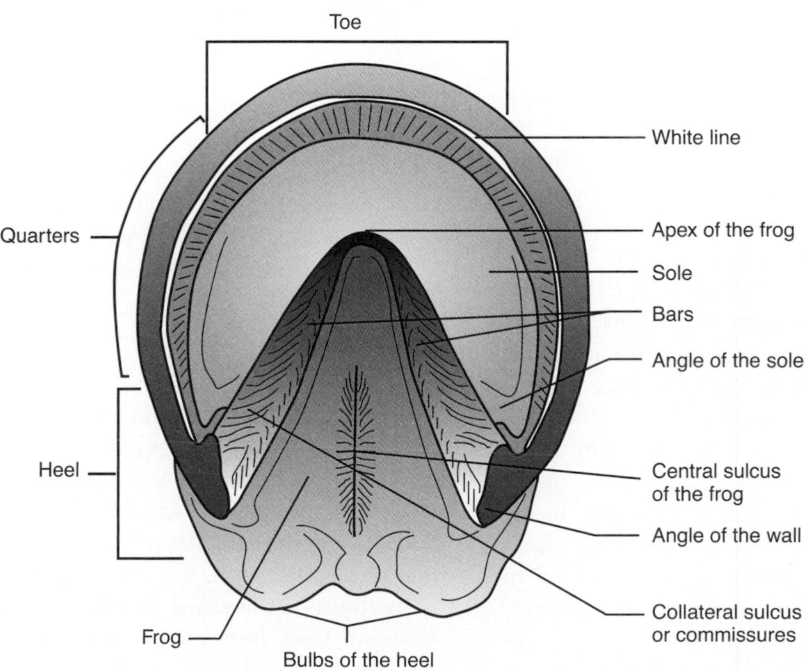

• **Fig. 5.15** The equine foot.

inner surface of the hoof and also attaches strongly to the periosteum of the underlying coffin bone. Therefore, it is the essential "glue" that holds the hoof onto the foot.

The Skeleton

Horses walk on their **third digit,** which is analogous to our middle finger. The bones that make up the equine foot are:

1. The distal end of the second phalanx (P2).
2. The entire third phalanx, called the **coffin bone or P3.**
3. The distal sesamoid bone, called the **navicular bone.**

The Corium

As previously stated, the corium is innervated and contains blood vessels. The corium also contains the germinal cells, which produce the keratinized structures that make up the hoof. There are five types of coria, and they are named for the area of the hoof they create.

The **perioplic corium** lies under the periople. The periople is the most proximal area of the hoof that can be seen and is a thin band of soft, light-colored horn. The perioplic corium generates the periople.

The **coronary corium** lies deep to the periople and perioplic corium. The coronary corium is the layer of corium that produces the **hoof wall** (the hard convex outer portion) of the hoof. These germinal cells produce tubes of keratin, which grow downward from the coronary band toward the ground. This is analogous to a human fingernail, which grows outward from a band of germinal tissue under the cuticle.

The **laminar corium** covers the periosteum of the coffin bone and is also called the **sensitive lamina** because it is rich with nerve endings and blood vessels. The hoof lamina lies underneath the hoof wall and is called the **insensitive lamina** because it lacks innervation. Both the sensitive and insensitive laminae are composed of tight vertical waves (laminae) that interdigitate with one another. In this way, the interdigitations of the laminae hold the hoof wall onto the foot. During laminitis, a serious disease in horses, the interdigitating sensitive laminae become inflamed and swollen. Pressure rises within the inflexible hoof, which decreases blood flow to the foot. This, in turn, can cause tissue death (necrosis) because of the loss of oxygen provided to the tissues (ischemia). Severe laminitis can cause breakdown of the interdigitations, resulting in the separation of the hoof wall from the coffin bone. In the most severe cases of laminitis, all four hooves slough from the coffin bones. Horses are usually spared this level of suffering through euthanasia, but extraordinarily valuable horses have survived with intensive nursing care at specialized equine hospitals, such as the New Bolton Center at the University of Pennsylvania.

The **sole corium** lies beneath the sole of the hoof and the **frog corium** lies beneath the **frog**. These layers attach the overlying keratinized structures to the foot.

The Hoof

The hoof wall is the portion of the hoof visible while the horse is standing. The most proximal edge of the hoof is called the **coronary band** or the **coronet.** It is seen as a swelling under the distal edge of the haired skin. The hoof is divided roughly into the **toe** or cranial portion, the medial and lateral **quarters** on the sides, and the medial and lateral **heels** or rear portion of the hoof.

On the bottom of the foot (the palmar and plantar surfaces), the following structures can be observed.

- The **white line** is just inside the edge of the horny hoof. It is the innermost layer of the hoof wall and central to it are deeper sensitive tissues. When shoeing the horse, nails must not be placed central to this white line.
- The angle of the wall is where the wall turns in at the heels, forming the **bars,** which are extensions of the wall leading toward the **apex of the frog**.
- The **sole** is the thick, horny tissue between the wall, the frog, and the bars.
- The **frog** is thick, horny, triangle-shaped tissue that comes to a point toward the cranial direction of the hoof. There is a thick **digital cushion** under the frog that aids in shock absorption as the foot hits the ground.
- The **bulbs of the heel** are softer structures that lie caudal and proximal to the horny hoof wall on each side of the hoof, both medially and laterally. They contain a continuation of the digital cushion.
- **Collateral cartilages** lie lateral to the bulbs and are attached to the caudodorsal aspect of the coffin bone. As the horse places weight on the foot, the frog and digital cushion become compressed. This pressure is also absorbed by outward movement of the bars and the collateral cartilages. Like a pump, the compression of the softer structures of the foot against the rigid hoof wall and sole forces blood out of the vascularized soft tissue and up into the veins in the horse's legs. Blood flows freely back into the foot when the weight and pressure are removed.

The Bovine Horn

The horns of domestic ruminants (cows, sheep, goats) are composed of layers of highly keratinized specialized epidermis over a bony projection. Fig. 5.16 shows a cow skull and a close-up of the junction between the frontal bone and the horn bone. Under the keratinized horn is a thin layer of epithelium that produces keratin. Under the epithelium, there is a layer of modified dermis called the corium. Like the corium of the claw and hoof, horn corium is a vascular, innervated tissue that supplies blood and nutrients to the germinal cells that create the keratinized stratum corneum of the horn. The corium covers an outgrowth of the frontal bone of the skull called the **cornual process** or horn process. Within the cornual process is a **sinus** that communicates with the frontal sinus.

CLINICAL APPLICATION

Dehorning

As you have learned, in the adult ruminant there is a sinus in the cornual process that is continuous with the frontal sinus. For this reason, it is better to dehorn ruminants when they are young—either before the sinus develops or, better yet, before the horn develops. Dehorning before the horn develops (in animals less than 1 month old) is achieved by destroying the germinal layers of cells by burning the epidermis and dermis around the horn bud (see accompanying figure). In somewhat older calves and kids, the small yet growing horn must be cut off, ensuring that the surrounding skin and corium are removed (see accompanying figure). This may be more painful owing to the necessity of cutting through bone as well as soft tissue. In any case, when the dehorning is complete, local anesthetic should be administered. The corneal nerve is blocked with an injection of local anesthetic midway between the horn base and the lateral canthus of the eye. In older calves and goats, a ring block around the base of the horn should also be given to prevent discomfort during the procedure.

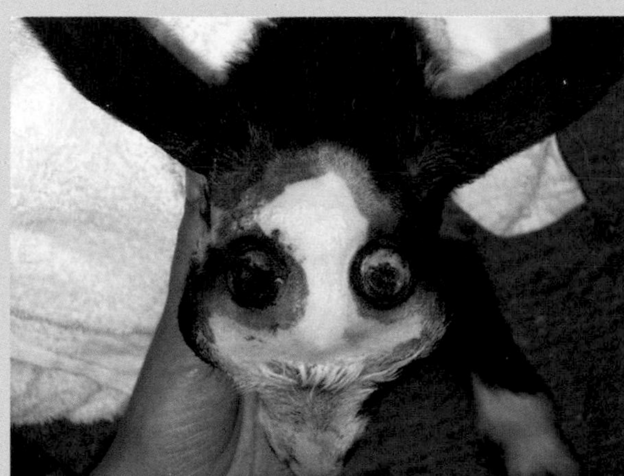

To debud a kid, the disbudding iron is placed over the horn bud. The heat from the iron will burn the epidermis and dermis (corium) around the bud, killing the germinal cells. This tissue will slough off after a few days. (From McCurnin DM, Bassert JM: Clinical textbook for veterinary technicians, ed 6, St Louis, 2006, Saunders.)

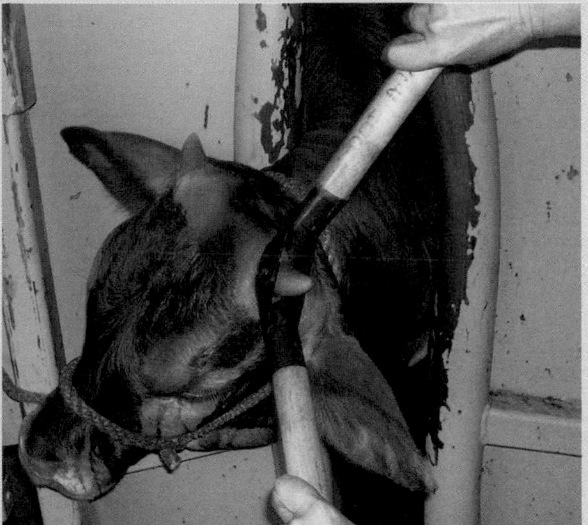

To dehorn a calf, a nerve block is administered and a Barnes scoop dehorner is used to clip off the small horn of an older calf. Care should be taken to ensure the surrounding epidermis and corium are removed as well. (From McCurnin DM, Bassert JM: Clinical textbook for veterinary technicians, ed 6, St Louis, 2006, Saunders.)

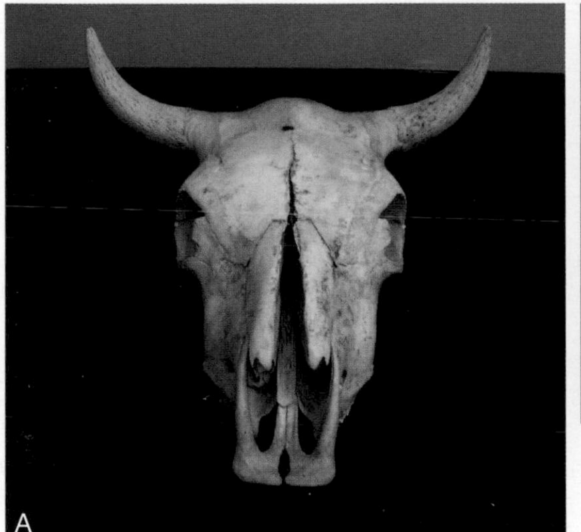

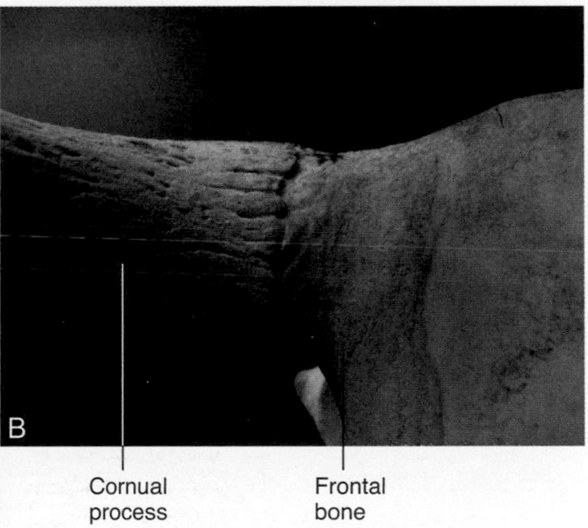

• **Fig. 5.16** Cow skull and horn. (A) The skull of a cow with attached horn bones (cornual processes). Horns are found on male and female cattle, sheep, and goats, and are made of highly keratinized stratum corneum of the epidermis. The medullary cavity of the horn is continuous with the frontal sinus in the skull. Variations in nutrition affect the rate at which horns grow. (B) Close-up of the junction between the frontal bone and the cornual process. Horns form from the os cornua, or horny process, which is an outgrowth of the frontal bone. The horny process is covered with a thick layer of modified dermis called corium, which gives rise to the epidermal cells that make up the horn.

EXERCISES

Layers of the Integument

Exercise 1

Describe Tissue Differences

Refer to Fig. 5.1. Observe the differences in the tissue of the three layers and describe what you see in each layer. Take particular note of the types of cells present in each layer, of noncellular elements, and of differences in staining.

Epidermis: ______________________________

____

____

Dermis: ______________________________

____

Hypodermis: ______________________________

____

Exercise 2

Compare and Contrast Thick and Thin Skin

Color the layers of thick and thin skin in the diagram in Fig. 5.17. Label the layers of the epidermis in each view and color the layers, following the key:

Stratum basale: green

Stratum spinosum: blue

Stratum granulosum: orange

Stratum lucidum: red

Stratum corneum: yellow

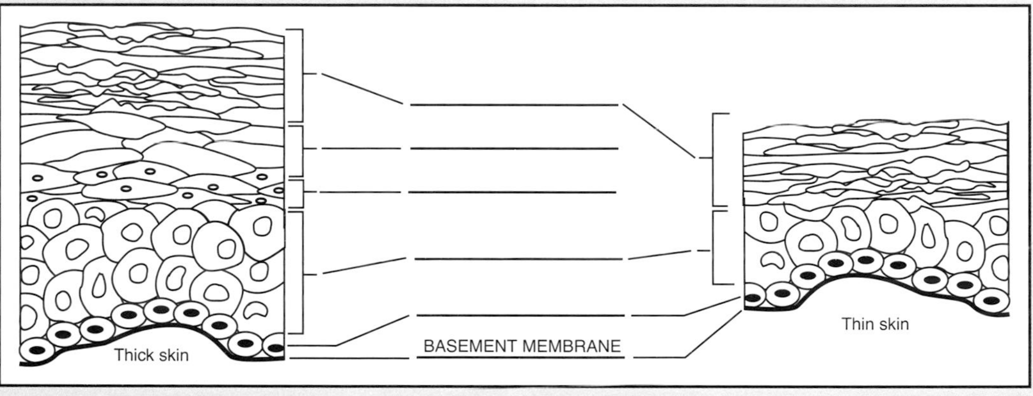

• **Fig. 5.17** In this diagram, the epidermal layers of thick and thin skin are shown side by side.

Exercise 3

Microscopic Exam of Thick and Thin Skin

Using the microscope, view the prepared slides of thick and thin skin with the high-power objective. Draw what you see and label the layers of the epidermis in each drawing.

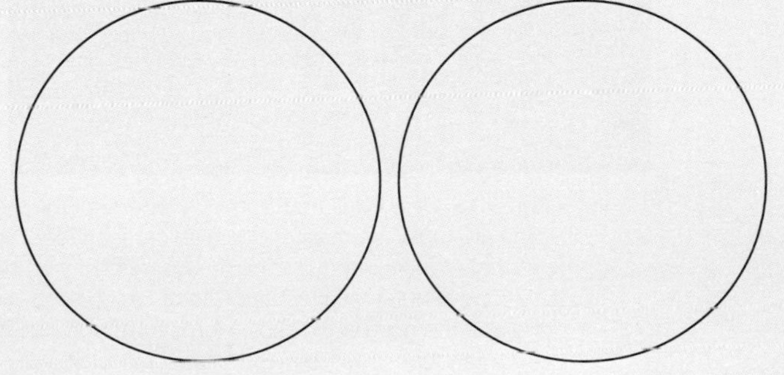

Exercise 4

Histologic Description of the Epidermis

List the distinct epidermal layers found in humans and animals, from deepest to outermost layer. Indicate the Latin name, the common name, the histologic presentation, the cells common to each layer, and whether the layer is present in animals.

Layer Latin Name	Common Name	Histologic Presentation	Cells Common to the Layer	Present in Animals (A Always) (B Rarely)
Stratum germinativum or Stratum basale	______	• ______ ______ ______ ______ • ______ ______ ______ ______	______ ______ ______ ______ ______	______
Stratum spinosum	______	• ______ ______ ______ ______ • ______ ______ ______ ______	______ ______ ______ ______ ______	______
Stratum granulosum	______	• ______ ______ ______ ______ • ______ ______ ______ ______	______ ______ ______ ______ ______	______
Stratum lucidum	______	• ______ ______ ______ ______ • ______ ______ ______ ______	______ ______ ______ ______ ______	______
Stratum corneum	______	• ______ ______ ______ ______ • ______ ______ ______ ______	______ ______ ______ ______ ______	______

Exercise 5

Observation of Feline Skin

Reflect the skin covering most of the preserved cat. You do not need to skin the tail or paws. Notice that the skin on the back of the neck and covering the jowls is much thicker than the skin covering the abdominal muscles. Inspect the cadaver for other areas of thick and thin skin. How thin or thick are the following areas of skin?

Paw pads: ______________________________

Eyelids: ______________________________

Chest: ______________________________

As you separate the skin from the underlying tissue, look for a very thin muscle that typically stays attached to the underside of the dermis. This is the **cutaneous trunci** muscle most easily found on the back, sides, and flanks of the cat. Notice that the cutaneous trunci consists of thin strands of muscle fibers that run in a longitudinal direction. It is attached to the dermis above the shoulder blades and continues along the entire length of the trunk of the animal. The cutaneous trunci plays an important role in the lives of animals that cannot slap at a fly or scratch in an unreachable place. It is the muscle responsible for twitching the skin when insects such as fleas or flies bite the skin or tickle the hairs. Clinically, it is a valuable tool for assessing the extent of paresis in patients with spinal cord injury. To do so, the skin is pinched progressively along the trunk in a caudal direction. If at any point the cutaneous trunci does not contract or twitch, spinal cord damage can be suspected.

Special Features of the Integument

Exercise 6

Draw Nose and Paw Pads of Dog

Inspect the nose and paw pads of a live dog. Draw the planum nasale and paw pads in the two boxes.

Planum nasale.

Paw pads.

Exercise 7

Identify Location of Chestnuts and Ergots

Identify the location of the chestnuts and ergots on the horse in Fig. 5.18 by drawing and labelling.

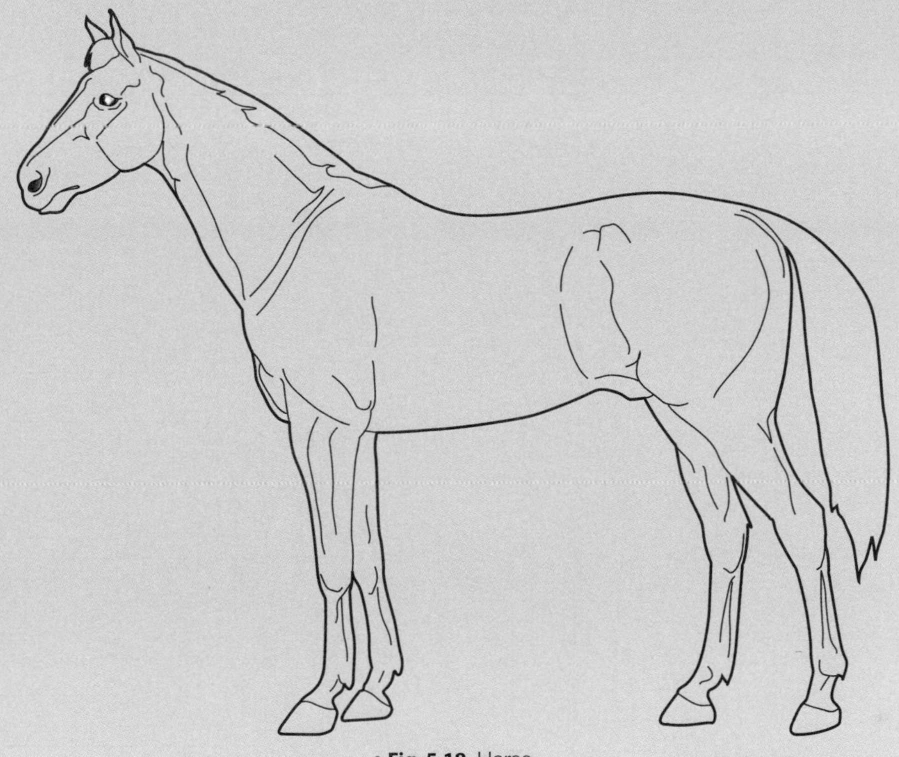

• **Fig. 5.18** Horse.

Hair

Exercise 8

Label and Color Pig Skin

Color in this drawing of pig skin (Fig. 5.19), then label the structures indicated.

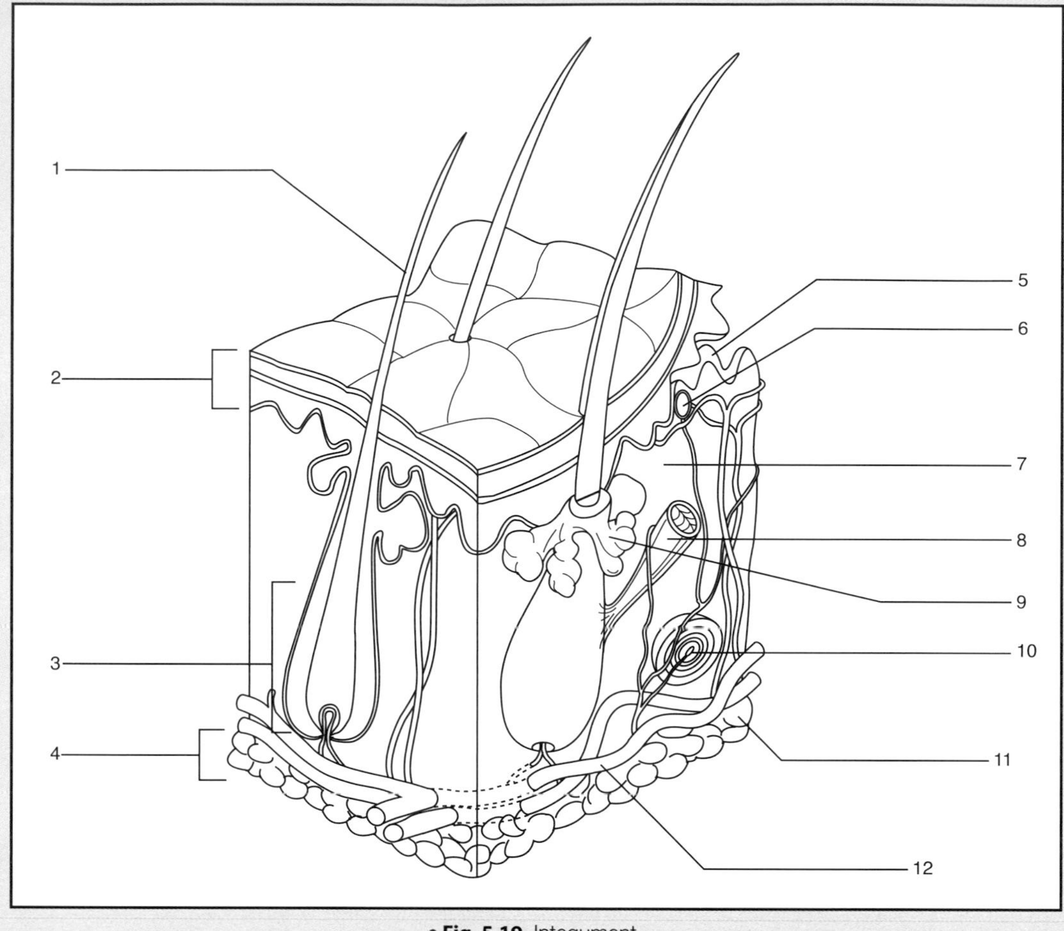

• **Fig. 5.19** Integument.

Exercise 9

Describe Types of Hair

Animal hair has been classified into three broad groups or categories. Identify each, their characteristic or quality, and their quantity.

Name	Quality	Quantity

Exercise 10

Color Structures of a Hair Follicle

In the diagram in Fig. 5.20, color the identified structures as indicated by the key:

Internal root sheath (green)

External root sheath (red)

Connective tissue root sheath (yellow)

Matrix (dark blue)

Connective tissue papilla (purple)

Sebaceous gland (pink)

Arrector pili muscle (brown)

Hair shaft

- Medulla (light blue)
- Cortex (gray)
- Cuticle (orange)

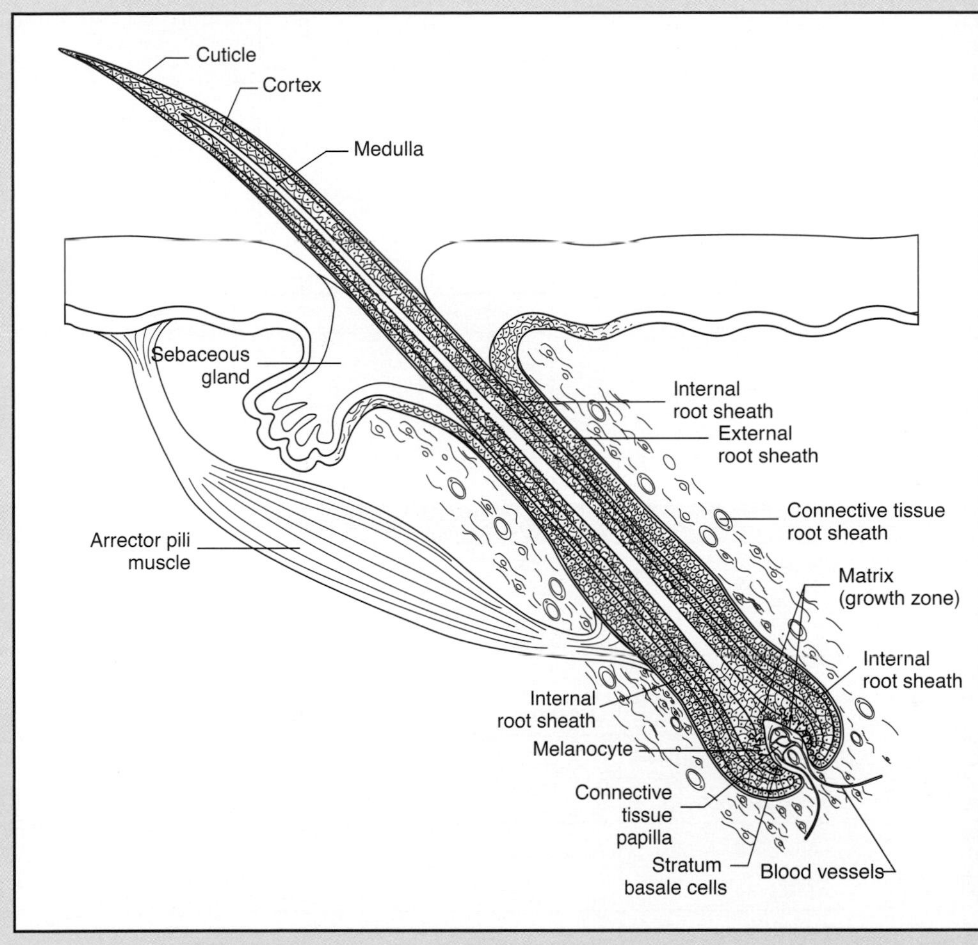

• **Fig. 5.20** This drawing shows the structure of hair and hair follicles in pig skin.

Exercise 11

Microscopic Exam of Hair Follicles

Using the microscope, view the prepared slide of thin skin that contains hair follicles in the dermis. Find a representative longitudinal section of a hair follicle and draw what you can see, labeling as many layers of cells and structures as possible.

Assorted Structures

Exercise 12

Function and Location of Corium Layers in the Equine Foot

Claws and hooves rest on underlying sensitive tissue called the corium. For each of the five types of corium in the equine foot, identify the location and function.

Layer	Location	Function
Laminar corium	______________	______________
Perioplic corium	______________	______________
Coronary corium	______________	______________
Sole corium	______________	______________
Frog corium	______________	______________

Exercise 13

Color Structures in a Feline Claw

Color the structures of a cat claw in Fig. 5.21 according to the key provided.

Bones (gray)

Corium (pink)

Claw (yellow)

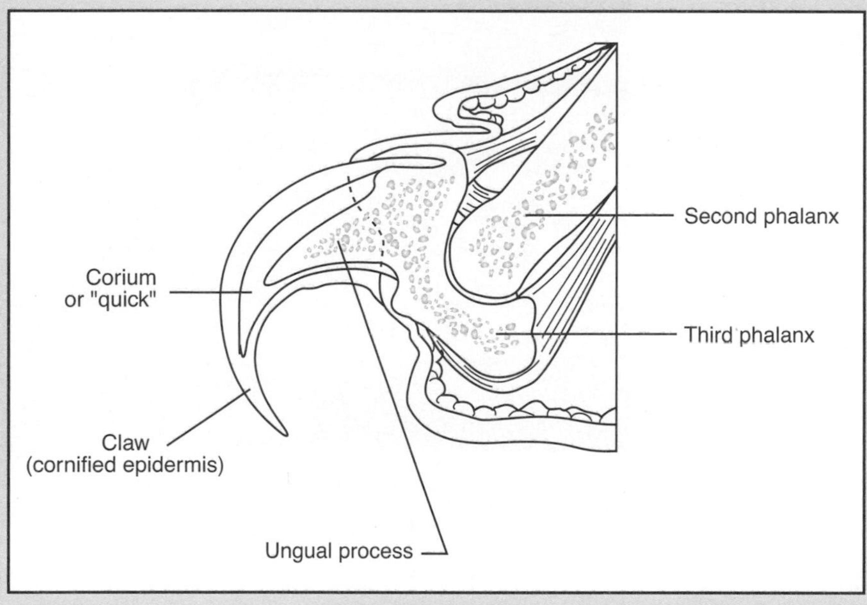

• **Fig. 5.21** Cat claw.

Exercise 14

Label an Equine Foot

A. Match the number on the figure with one of the following labels:

_____ Heel

_____ Quarters

_____ Toe

_____ Periople

_____ Coronet (coronary band)

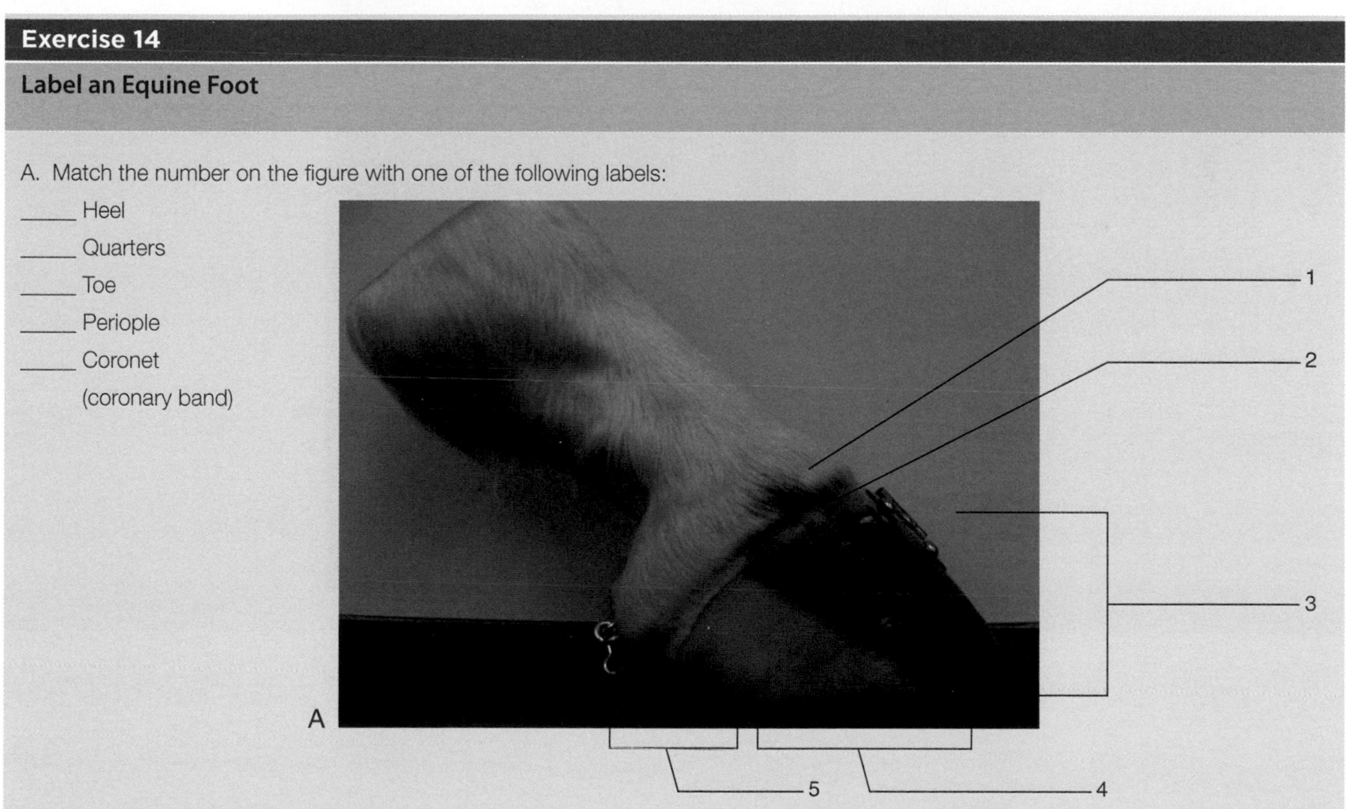

Continued

Exercise 14—cont'd

Label an Equine Foot

B. Match the number on the figure with one of the following labels:

_____ Proximal phalanx
_____ Middle phalanx
_____ Distal phalanx—coffin bone
_____ Navicular bone
_____ Common digital extensor tendon
_____ Superficial flexor tendon
_____ Deep digital flexor tendon
_____ Hoof wall
_____ Area where the corium would be in a live specimen
_____ Digital cushion
_____ Frog

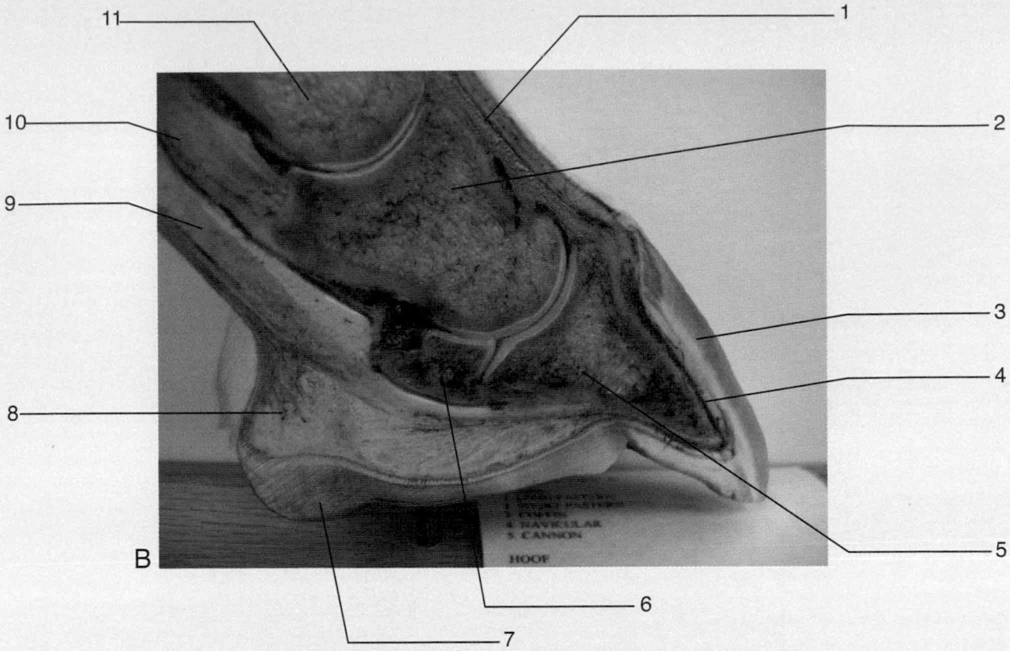

C. Match the number on the figure with one of the following labels:

_____ Sole
_____ Frog
_____ Bar
_____ White line
_____ Hoof wall

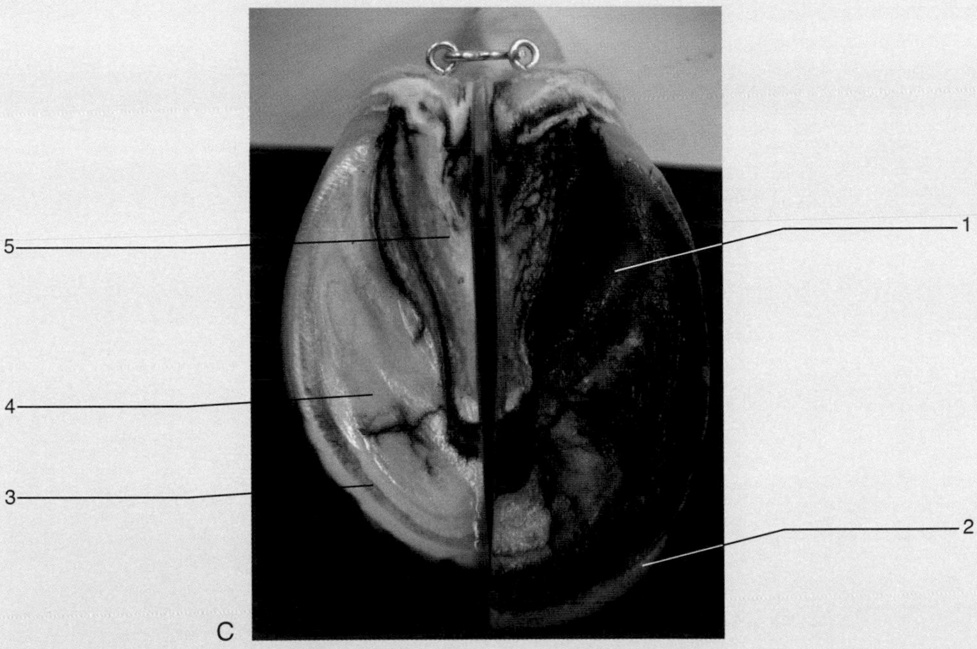

Exercise 15

Color Structures in the Ruminant Horn

Color the structures of the ruminant horn in Fig. 5.22 according to the following key:

Frontal sinus (yellow)
Cornual process (blue)
Corium (red)
Epidermis (green)
Keratinized horn (brown)

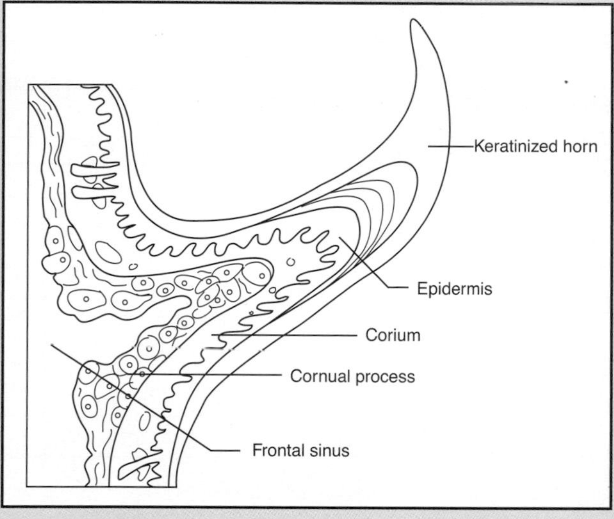

• **Fig. 5.22** Ruminant horn.

Critical and Clinical Thinking

Exercise 16

Appearance of Cancer of the Skin

For each of the clinical descriptions, indicate the *possible* type of neoplasm.

Clinical Presentation	Possible Neoplasm
A white cat presents with circular ulcerated lesions on its nose. Tissue has been eroded by the lesion.	________________
An aged grey horse presents with nodules under the tale base, the perianal area, and the scrotum. Nodules at first appeared small, then grew, ulcerated, and spread to internal organs.	________________
A dog presents with a tumor that can be palpated in its neck. The owner reports it has been present for some time without a change in size.	________________
A cow presents with a circular ulcerated lesion on its eye and surrounding eyelid.	________________
A Duroc-Jersey breed of pig presents with a tumor in the ocular orbit.	________________

Exercise 17

Exploring Allergy and Mange

For each of the clinical descriptions, an allergy or mange is suspected. Indicate the *possible* offending agent.

Clinical Presentation	Possible Condition
A dog presents with a black pigmented excoriated, hairless area on a front limb. The owner reports the dog has been constantly scratching the area for months.	______________
A rabbit presents with small hairless areas on its ears and small lesions beginning on its face.	______________
A Golden Retriever scoots its face along the carpet and repeatedly licks the tops of its paws.	______________
A cat presents with excessive licking, grooming, and face scratching with a hind leg.	______________
A Border Collie appears with red hairless patches on its eyebrow caps and the edges of its ears. The owner reports the dog cannot sleep and is constantly scratching and appears miserable.	______________
The medial sides of the hind legs of a Chow appear chewed in a corncob pattern.	______________
White fur on a cat appears yellow in discrete areas.	______________
An immunosuppressed dog presents with red, hairless patches. Microscopic examination reveals a long, thin organism living in the hair follicle.	______________

Exercise 18

Matching Terms and Definitions

Match the structure below with its description.

_____ Epidermis _____ Dermis _____ Subcutaneous layer (hypodermis) _____ Stratum basale _____ Stratum spinosum _____ Stratum granulosum _____ Stratum lucidum _____ Stratum corneum _____ Keratinocyte _____ Merkel cell _____ Melanocyte _____ Melanin _____ Langerhans cell _____ Papillary layer _____ Dermal papilla _____ Fibroblast _____ Meissner's corpuscle _____ Reticular layer _____ Hair follicle	a. Layer found only in thick skin consisting of a few rows of flattened dead cells. b. A dark pigment produced by melanocytes that protects the skin from ultraviolet radiation. c. Gland that secretes sweat directly onto the surface of the epidermis via a duct. d. Outermost layer of the epidermis. e. Uppermost, thin superficial layer of the dermis. f. Small muscle attached to each hair follicle. g. Makes up the greatest portion of the skin and is responsible for the structural strength of the skin. h. Touch receptor in the hypodermis that is sensitive to heavy pressure. i. Epidermal layer that still shows some cell division and contains a large number of Langerhans cells. j. Keratin-producing cell. k. Upward projections of the dermis that interdigitate with the epidermis to hold the layers together. l. A macrophage found in the epidermis. m. A layer made of a single row of actively dividing keratinocytes. n. Thick layer of the integument made of loose areolar connective tissue rich with adipose. o. Found in the basal layer of the epidermis and associated with sensory nerve endings. p. Invagination of the epidermis in which a hair is anchored. q. Main cell in the hypodermis and is filled with fat. r. The outermost layer of the skin.
_____ Sebaceous gland _____ Arrector pili muscle _____ Eccrine sweat gland _____ Adipocyte _____ Pacinian corpuscle	s. Epidermal layer that consists of multiple rows of keratinocytes that are beginning to fill with keratin and the nuclei are degenerating. t. Cell found in the epidermis that produces a dark pigment. u. Sebum-producing gland that secretes directly into the hair follicle. v. Cellular component of the dermis that manufactures fibers and ground substance. w. Deeper layer of the dermis that consists of dense, irregular connective tissue. x. Touch receptor in the hypodermis that is sensitive to light touch.

Exercise 19

Clinical Thinking Challenge

Support each of following correct statements with appropriate rationale, stating why or in what way each statement is correct.

1. The dermis is composed of two layers and differs from the epidermis.
2. Separations between the bundles in the reticular layer are called tension lines and are important to surgeons.
3. Most species have multiple foot pads.
4. Ergots are often overlooked.
5. There are three primary cutaneous pouch locations found in sheep.
6. In most animals, hair is essential for survival.
7. When an animal blows its coat, hair is lost to make room for new hair.
8. When frightened or cold, animals can make their hair stand up beyond the normal implantation angle.
9. Hair is kept soft, pliant, and semi-waterproof by the contraction of the arrector pili muscle.
10. Antlers grow and are shed annually.
11. Laminitis can be fatal.
12. There are five predisposing factors for laminitis.

6

The Skeletal System[a]

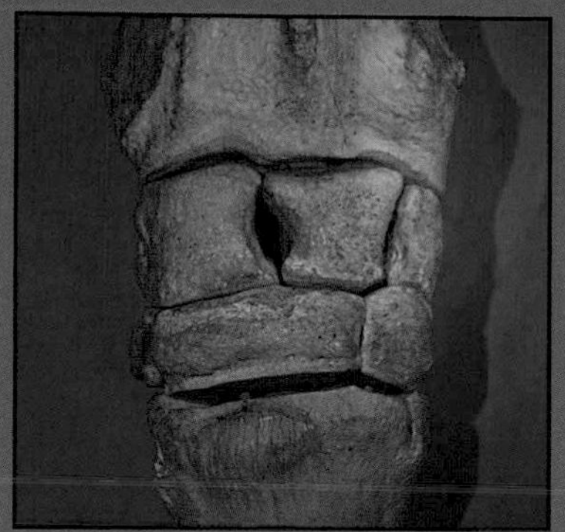

OVERVIEW AT A GLANCE

The Skeletal System 99

The Skeleton 112

Joints 130

Suggested In-Class Activities 132

Bone Shapes and Features 132

The Axial Skeleton 132

The Appendicular Skeleton 133

Exercises 134–146

The Skeletal System 134–136

1. *Identify Structures of Compact and Cancellous Bone 134*
2. *Identify Structures of Long Bone 135*
3. *Identify Bone Shape 136*

The Skeleton 137–142

4. *Identify Rabbit Skeletal Structures 137*
5. *Identify Rat Skeletal Structures 138*
6. *Identify Skeletal Features of the Cat Skull 139*
7. *Identify Bones and Processes of the Equine Thoracic Limb 140*
8. *Identify Bones, Joints, and Processes of the Equine Pelvic Limb 141*
9. *Label the Bones of the Horse Foot from Proximal to Distal 142*

Joints 143

10. *Identify Joint Type 143*

Critical and Clinical Thinking 144–146

11. *Defining Clinical Terms 144*
12. *Clinical Thinking Challenge 146*

LEARNING OBJECTIVES

When you finish this chapter, you will be familiar with bone shapes, common types of bones, bone features, and clinically significant bones. You will not be asked to learn all the bones in the body, but you will be able to name most of them. Luckily, the common domestic animal species generally have the same bones, so you'll have to learn them only once.

CLINICAL SIGNIFICANCE

Suppose you have been asked to take two radiographs of a patient's left femur—a lateral (side-to-side) view and a cranial-caudal view. To take the shots, you need to know a few things:

1. Which bone is the femur? (thigh bone)
2. What externally palpable (feelable) landmark can be used to identify the proximal end of the bone? (greater trochanter)
3. What externally palpable landmarks can be used to identify the distal end of the bone? (patella, medial and lateral condyles, and epicondyles)

Suppose you are doing a physical exam on a cat and as you palpate the hind legs, one leg seems to have a bump on a bone and the other leg doesn't have the same bump on the same bone. Is the bone supposed to have the bump or not? What do you write on the physical exam sheet?

When you listen to heart and lung sounds in animals, you place the stethoscope at various places on the animals' chests. Sometimes it's next to the costochondral junction and other times it's placed between the ribs more cranially or caudally. Specific sounds are heard at specific places. You will need to be able to locate these specific places by counting ribs and locating the area where the ribs attach to the cartilages that anchor them to the sternum.

Many other structures are named by which bones they are near. For example, the radial nerve is found by the radius bone in the front leg. The ulnar nerve is found by the ulna bone in the front leg. The femoral artery and vein run alongside the femur in the hind leg. If you know where the bone is located, you will have an easier time locating and identifying structures near it.

[a]The authors and publisher acknowledge Joann Colville and Amy Ellwein for previous contributions to this chapter.

Bones have many physical characteristics. You will need to know their normal anatomy before you can detect abnormalities.

As you study the bones, feel them on live animals. Figure out which parts can be palpated on the outside of various animals' bodies. Some things that are easily felt on a cat may be difficult or impossible to feel on a horse, and vice versa.

INTRODUCTION

The bones that make up an animal's skeleton (1) support and (2) protect the soft tissues of the body and (3) act as levers that the skeletal muscles use to move the body. They also (4) store minerals, particularly calcium.

- **Bones providing support.** The support function is often easy to visualize. The bones of the limbs support the rest of the body. Other bones perform their supporting roles more subtly. For example, the ribs help maintain the size and shape of the thoracic (chest) cavity. They help prevent the lateral walls of the thorax from collapsing in response to gravity. The lumbar (abdominal) vertebrae support the weight of the abdominal organs by serving as the attachment sites for the slinglike abdominal muscles.
- **Bones providing protection.** The best examples of bones playing protective roles are the bones of the cranium (the portion of the skull that surrounds the brain) and the vertebrae that make up the spinal column. The very important brain and spinal cord are soft and fragile. If you held an animal's brain in your hand, you could easily crush it between your fingers. The spinal cord has the same soft consistency. The bones of the cranium form a rigid case for the delicate brain. The arches of the vertebrae combine to form a bony canal (the spinal canal) that protects the fragile spinal cord. The individual joints between the vertebrae allow limited movement. These joints combine to allow the spine as a whole a considerable range of motion while still protecting the enclosed spinal column. Cats in particular give excellent demonstrations of spinal flexibility as they contort themselves.
- **Bones as levers.** The role of bones as levers is easy to visualize. The articular (joint) surfaces are the fulcrums for the levers, and the processes where the tendons attach muscles to bones are where the forces are applied. Note that the larger the process, generally the greater the force that can be applied there. Note also that, as a result of the body being sleek and compact, some bony levers have very poor mechanical advantage. This results in some muscles, such as the gluteals, having to be fairly large and powerful.
- **Bones as storage sites.** Bones act as reservoirs for important minerals, such as calcium. This storage capacity enables the body to deposit and withdraw vital minerals precisely as needed to maintain health.

As you examine skeletons and bones, try to imagine how the bones, joints, and muscles work together to make the body move. Look at the various bony processes, and try to infer what the muscles attached to them would do when they contracted. That's the kind of detective work paleontologists perform when they examine the fossilized bones of dinosaurs and other extinct beasts. They can make educated guesses about things such as muscle sizes, shapes, and strengths, body shapes, and even how the animal moved.

TERMS TO BE IDENTIFIED

- Bone shapes
  - Flat bones
  - Irregular bones
    - Sesamoid bones
    - Long bones
    - Short bones
- Types of bone
  - Cancellous bone
  - Compact bone
- General bone features
  - Articular surface
    - Condyle
    - Head
    - Facet
- Foramen
  - Nutrient foramen
- Fossa
- Processes
- Bones of the axial skeleton
  - Skull bones (external)
    - Frontal bones
      - Cornual process
    - Incisive bones
    - Interparietal bones
    - Lacrimal bones
    - Mandible
      - Ramus
      - Shaft
    - Maxillary bones
    - Nasal bones
    - Occipital bone
      - Foramen magnum
      - Occipital condyles
    - Parietal bones
    - Temporal bones
      - External acoustic meatus
      - Tympanic bullae
    - Zygomatic bones
  - Skull bones (internal)
    - Turbinates
  - Ribs
    - Costal cartilage
    - Costochondral junction
    - Head
  - Sternum
    - Manubrium (manubrium sterni)
    - Xiphoid (xiphoid process)
  - Vertebrae
    - Arch
    - Body
    - Processes
      - Articular processes
      - Spinous process
      - Transverse processes
    - Cervical vertebrae
      - Atlas
      - Axis
    - Thoracic vertebrae
    - Lumbar vertebrae
    - Sacral vertebrae (sacrum)
    - Coccygeal vertebrae
- Bones of the appendicular skeleton
  - Thoracic limb

- Scapula
  - Glenoid cavity
  - Neck
  - Spine
- Humerus
  - Condyle
  - Epicondyles
  - Greater tubercle
  - Head
  - Neck
  - Olecranon fossa
- Radius
  - Head
  - Neck
  - Styloid process
- Ulna
  - Anconeal process
  - Coronoid processes
  - Olecranon process
  - Radial notch
  - Styloid process
  - Trochlear notch
- Carpal bones (carpus)
  - Accessory carpal bone
- Metacarpal bones
  - Cannon bone (hoofed animals)
  - Splint bones (horse)
- Phalanges
  - Proximal sesamoid bones (hoofed animals)
  - Distal sesamoid bones (hoofed animals)

Pelvic limb
- Pelvis
  - Acetabulum
  - Ilium
  - Ischium
  - Obturator foramen
  - Pubis
- Femur
  - Condyles
  - Epicondyles
  - Greater trochanter
  - Head
  - Neck
  - Trochlea
  - Patella
  - Fabellae
- Tibia
  - Condyles
  - Tibial crest
  - Tibial tuberosity
  - Medial malleolus
- Fibula
  - Lateral malleolus
- Tarsal bones (tarsus, hock)
  - Calcaneus
- Metatarsal bones
  - Cannon bone (hoofed animals)
  - Splint bones (horse)
  - Phalanges
  - Proximal sesamoid bones (hoofed animals)
  - Distal sesamoid bones (hoofed animals)
- Joints
  - Cartilaginous
  - Fibrous
  - Synovial

MEDICAL WORD PARTS

Arthr/o = joint
Articular = joint
Chondr/o = cartilage
Cost/o = rib
Os = bone
Oste/o = bone

The Skeletal System

Types of Bone

Virtually all bones are made up of two types of bone: **cancellous bone**, which is light and spongy; and **compact bone**, which is heavy and dense (Figs. 6.1 and 6.2).

Bone Shapes

Long Bones

Long bones are so named because they are longer than they are wide (Fig. 6.3). Most of the bones of the limbs are long bones. The two bones in Fig. 6.3 are a feline femur *(A)* from the thigh area of the hind leg, and a canine humerus *(B)* from the upper front leg. The ends of long bones are called epiphyses. Each long bone has a proximal epiphysis and a distal epiphysis. The epiphyses are made of cancellous bone covered with a thin layer of compact bone. The long part of a long bone is the diaphysis. It is composed primarily of compact bone. Between the epiphyses and diaphysis, there are the areas where the bone grows longer in young animals. These growth plates are composed mainly of cartilage and are called the epiphyseal plates. The epiphyseal plates are the weakest part of the bone in young animals and are prone to fractures. Once an animal reaches its full size, the epiphyseal plates are replaced by solid bone through a process called ossification.

Short Bones

This equine carpus shows **short bones** that are shaped like cubes or marshmallows (Fig. 6.4). They are composed of an inner core of cancellous bone covered by a thin layer of compact bone. Carpal and tarsal bones are the most common short bones in the body (Fig. 6.5).

Flat Bones

Flat bones are mostly flat and thin (Fig. 6.6 and see Fig. 6.10). Their structure is like a "cancellous bone sandwich"—a central layer of cancellous bone covered on both sides by thin layers of compact bone. The pelvic bones and the scapula (shoulder blade) are prominent flat bones as are some of the skull bones (Fig. 6.7).

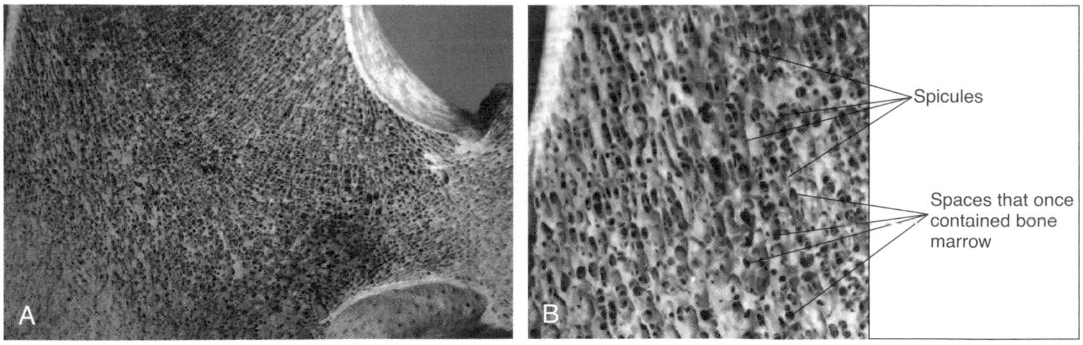

• **Fig. 6.1** Cancellous bone. (A) The gross spongy appearance of cancellous bone in the distal end of a horse femur. (B) A closer view that clearly shows the spicules of bone and the spaces between the spicules that once contained bone marrow.

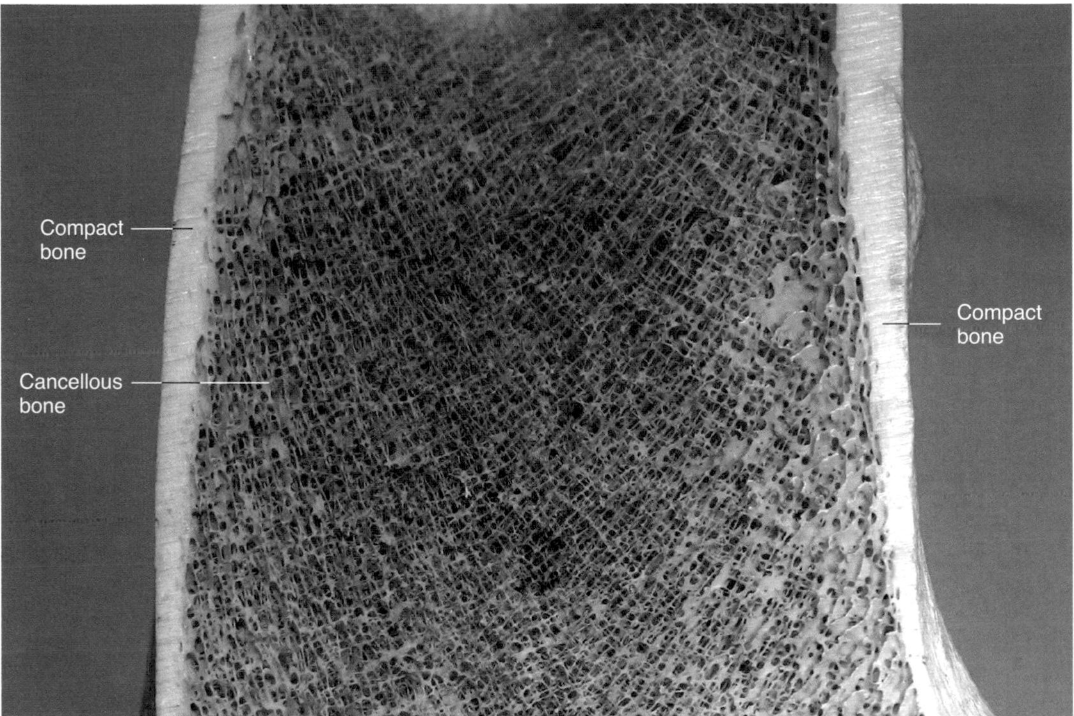

• **Fig. 6.2** Compact bone. Compact bone forms the outside layer of all bones and the shafts of long bones such as this horse femur.

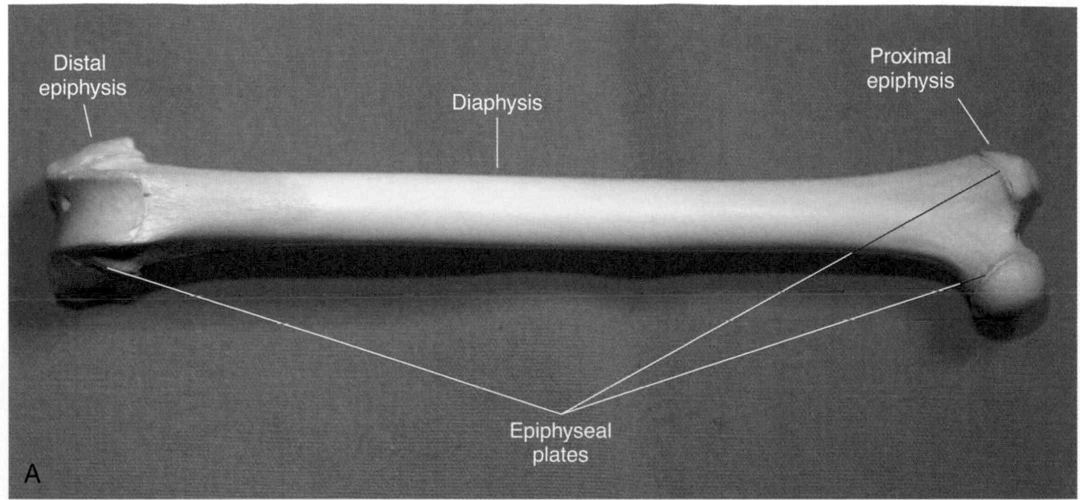

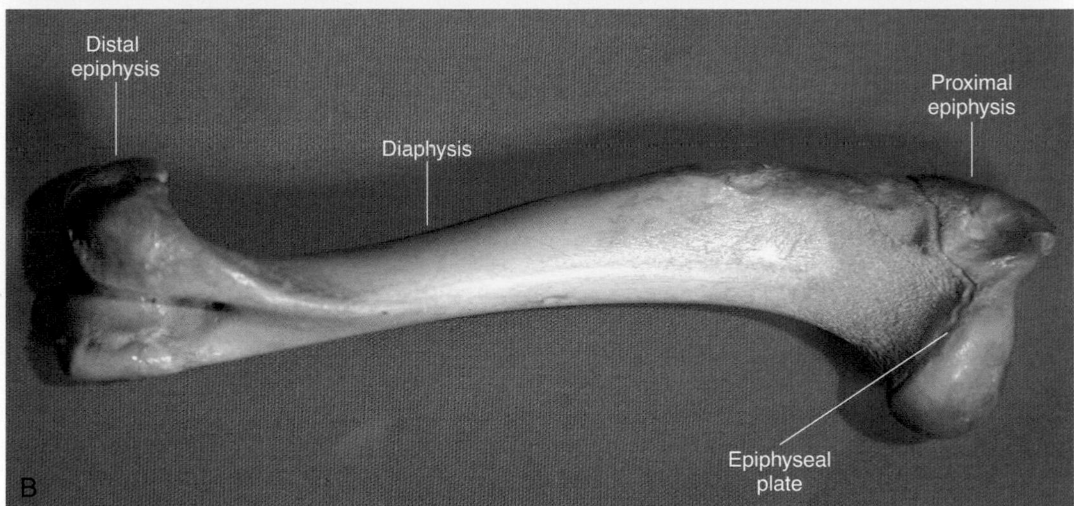

• **Fig. 6.3** (A and B), Long bones.

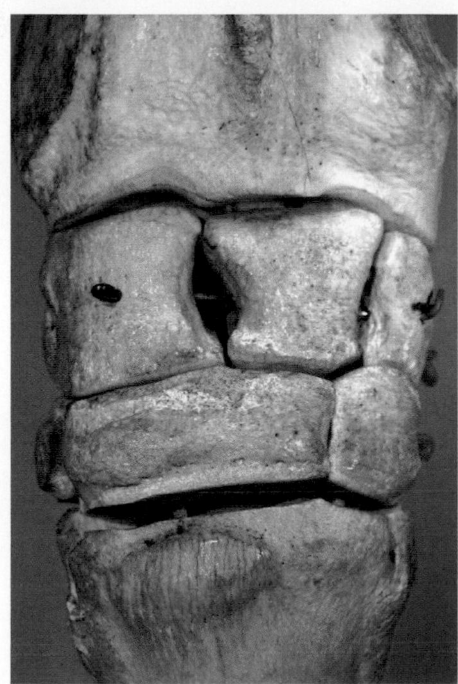

• **Fig. 6.4** Short bones in an equine skeleton.

Irregular Bones

Irregular bones are odd shaped and don't fit into any of the other three categories (Figs. 6.8–6.11).

Common Bone Features (Lumps, Bumps, Grooves, and Holes)

Articular Surfaces

Articular surfaces are smooth areas of compact bone that come in contact with smooth surfaces of another bone to form a joint. The articular surfaces are covered with hyaline cartilage (Fig. 6.12).

Condyles

A **condyle** is usually a large, round articular surface. The distal ends of the femur and humerus, and the occipital bone have the most prominent condyles (Figs. 6.13–6.15).

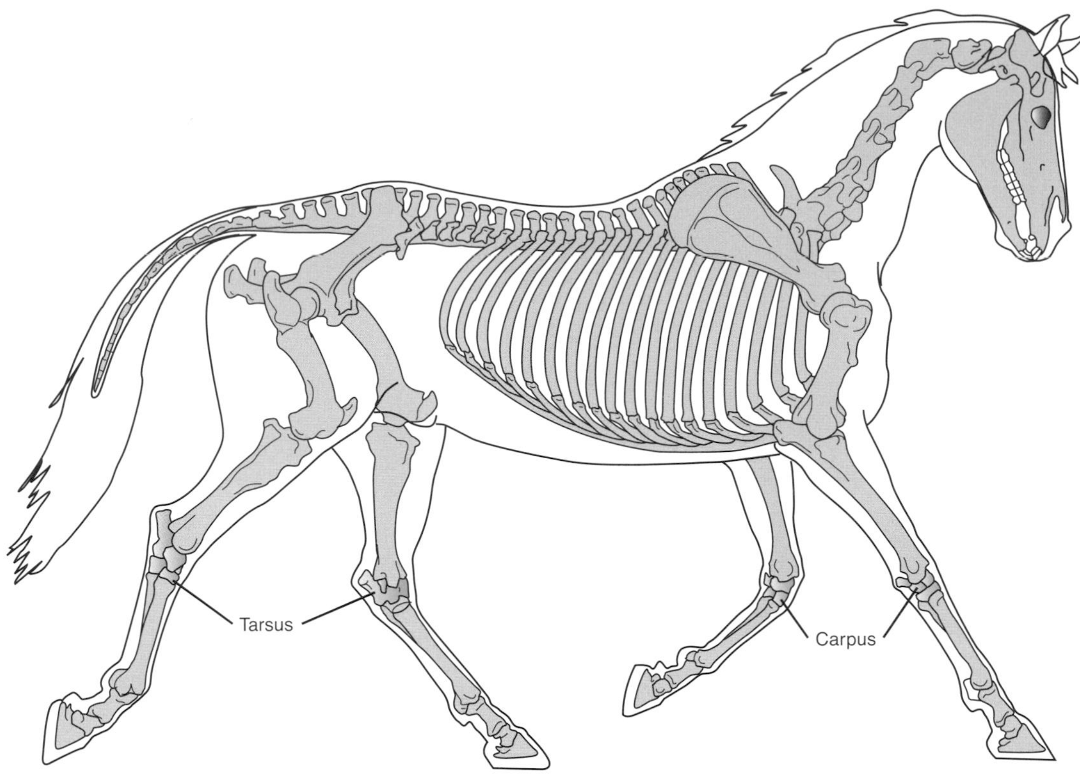

• **Fig. 6.5** Short bones. Equine carpal bones.

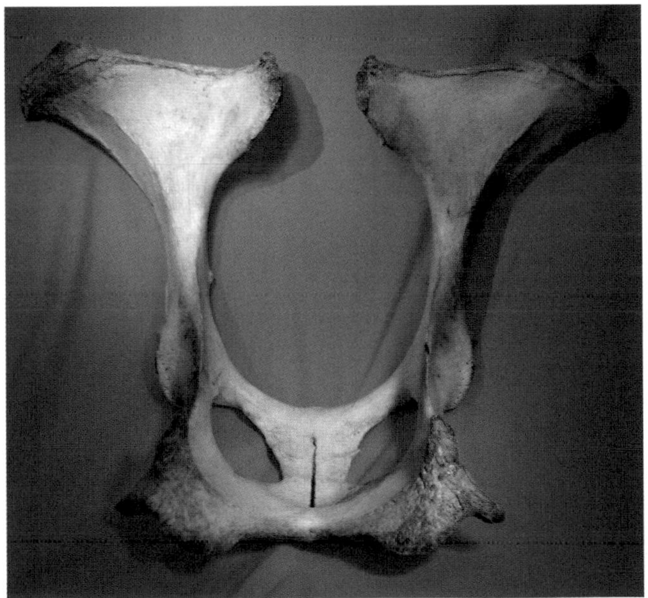

• **Fig. 6.6** Flat bones. Pelvis from a bovine skeleton (dorsal view).

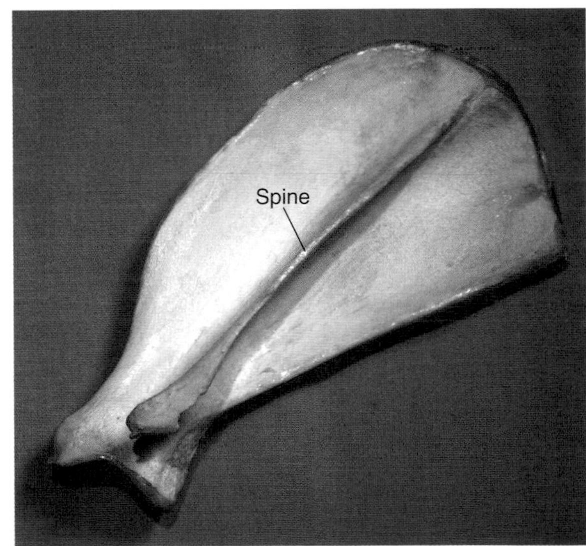

• **Fig. 6.7** Flat bone. Scapula from a canine skeleton (lateral view). Note the prominent spine facing toward us.

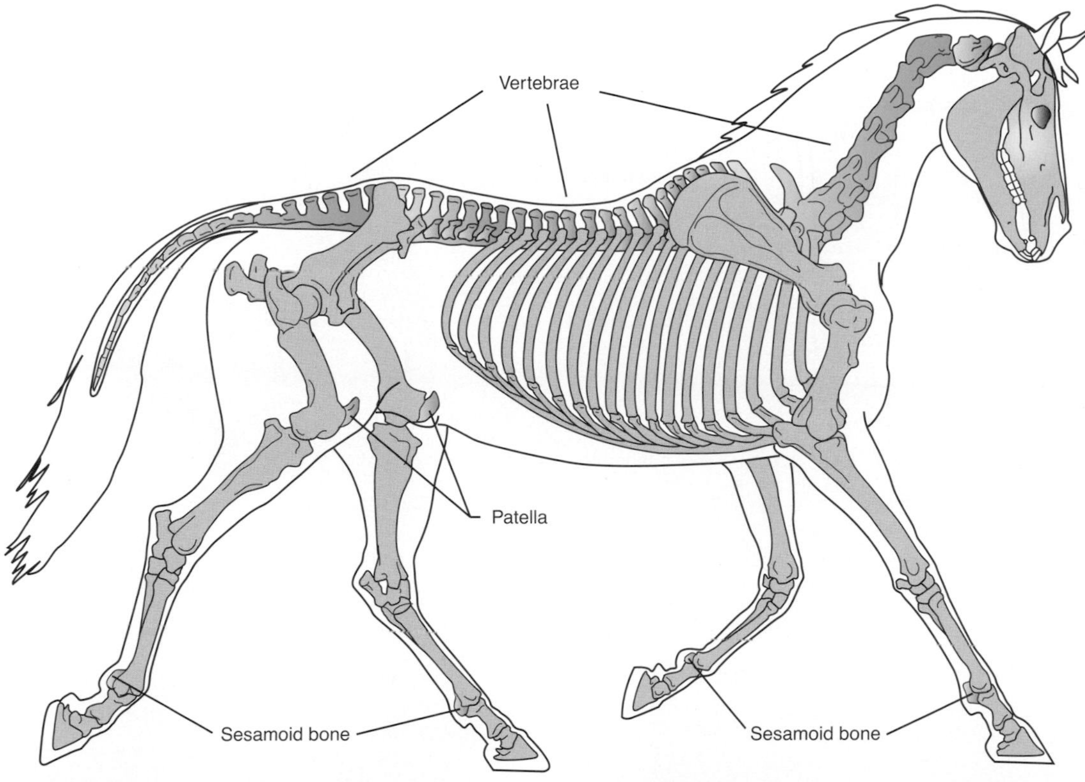

• **Fig. 6.8** Irregular bones in an equine skeleton.

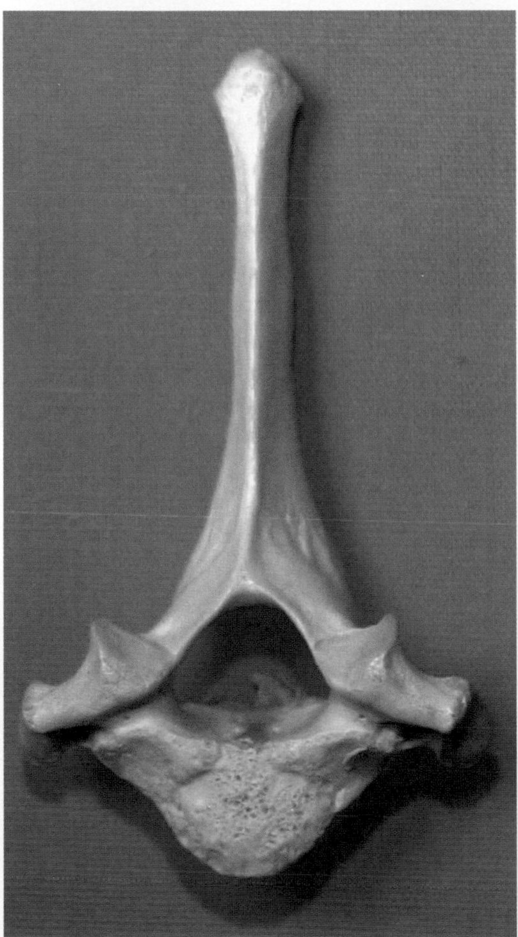

• **Fig. 6.9** Irregular bone. Canine vertebra. Vertebrae don't fit into the long bone, short bone, or flat bone categories.

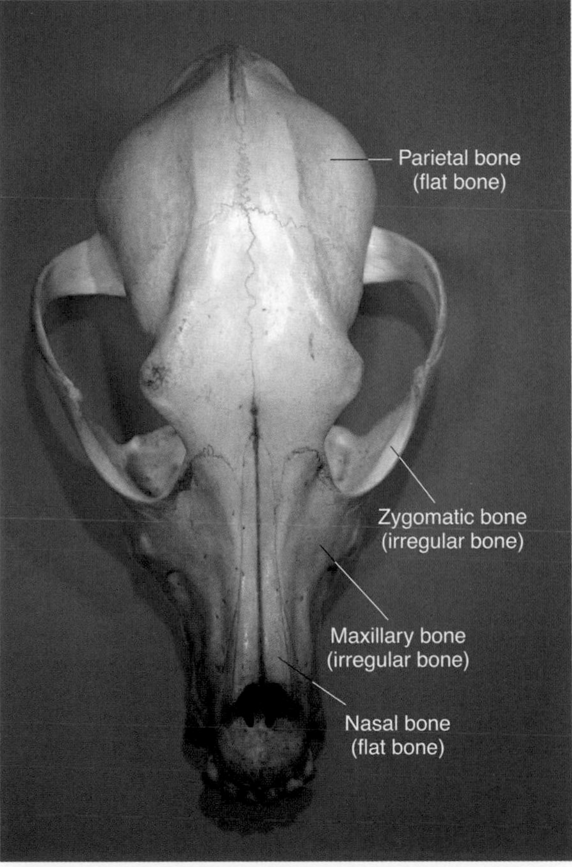

• **Fig. 6.10** Flat bones and irregular bones. Canine skull bones. Some skull bones are flat bones (e.g., parietal bones, nasal bones), whereas others have very irregular shapes (e.g., maxillary bones, zygomatic bones).

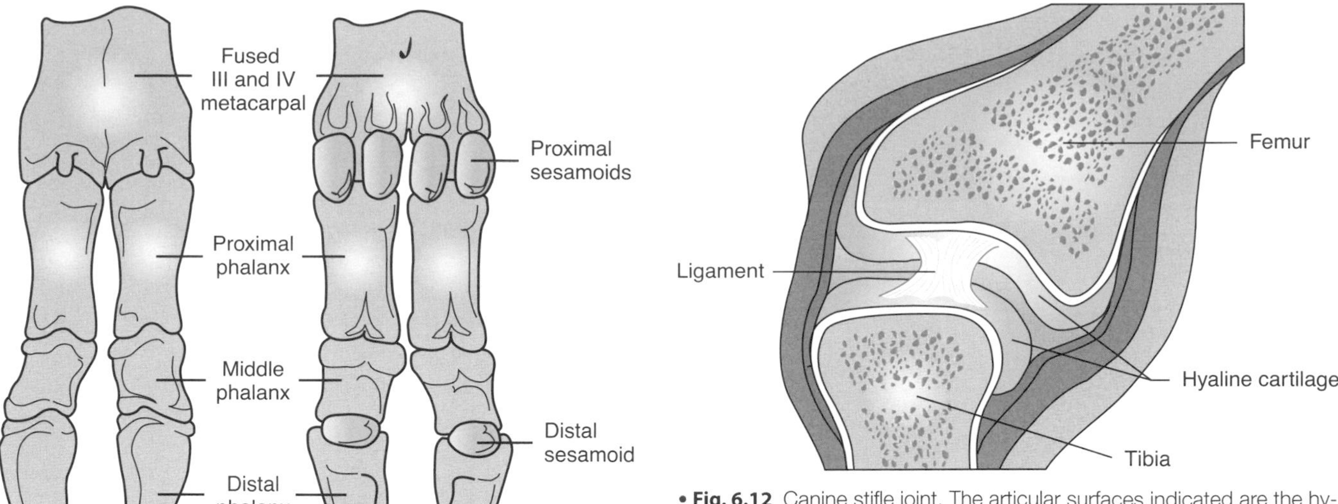

• **Fig. 6.12** Canine stifle joint. The articular surfaces indicated are the hyaline cartilage covering the distal articular surface of the femur and the proximal articular surface of the tibia.

Dorsal view Palmar/plantar view

• **Fig. 6.11** Irregular bones in a bovine skeleton. Sesamoid bones.

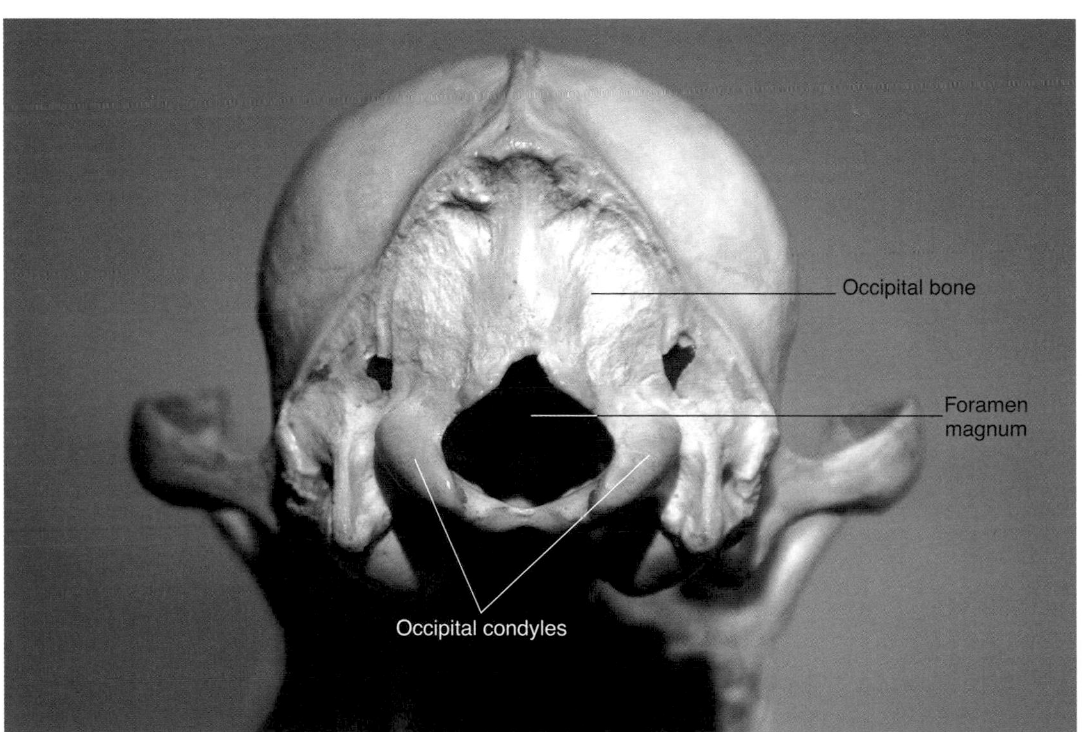

• **Fig. 6.13** The condyles of the occipital bone in the canine skull. These articular surfaces are where the skull joins the spinal column. It connects the head to the neck. (This joint is the one your mother meant when she said you would lose your head if it wasn't attached.)

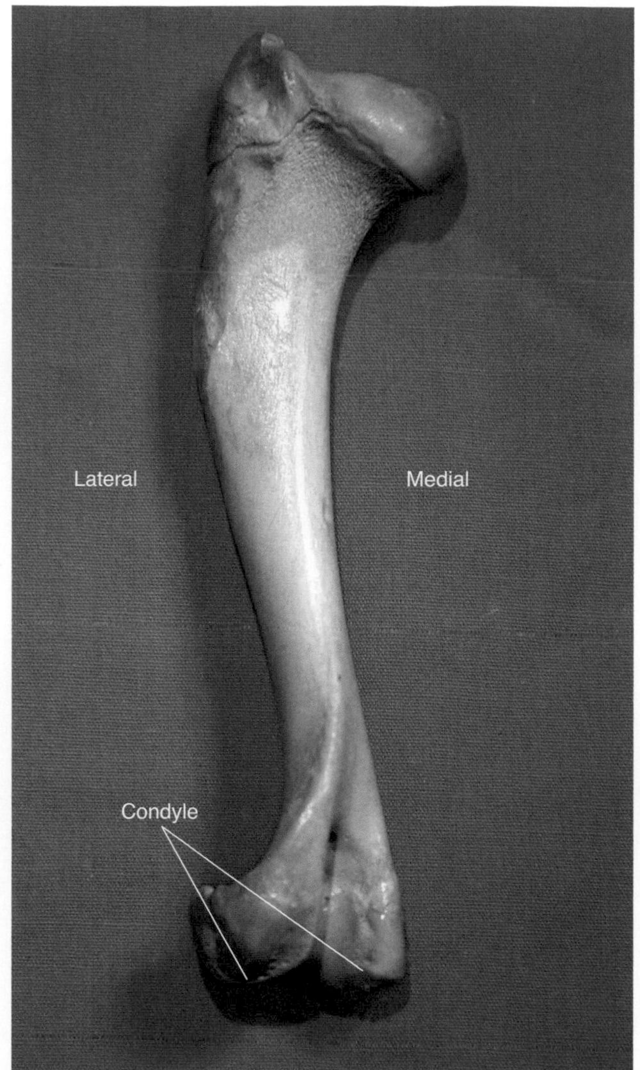

• **Fig. 6.14** The condyles of the canine humerus. These surfaces along with the proximal articular surfaces of the radius and ulna form the elbow joint (caudal view).

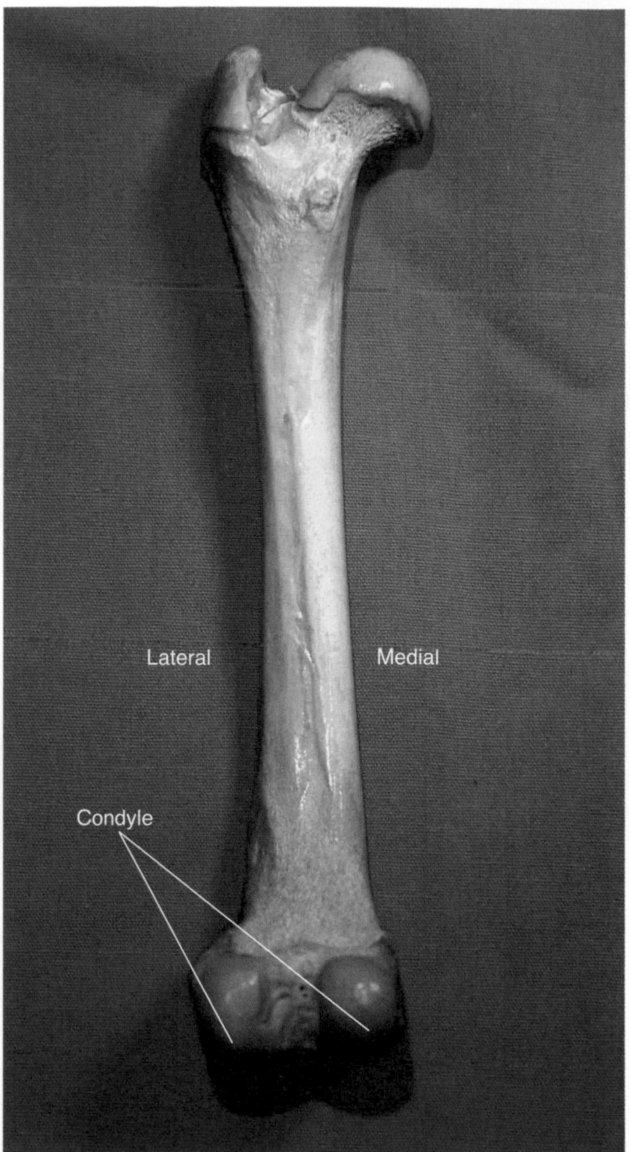

• **Fig. 6.15** Condyles of the canine femur. These condyles meet the proximal end of the tibia to form the stifle joint (caudal view).

Head

The **head** of a bone is found at the proximal end of a long bone. It is mostly spherical in shape. The proximal ends of the femur, humerus, and ribs have heads (Figs. 6.16–6.18). The head is usually joined to the rest of the bone by a narrowed region called the neck.

Facet

A **facet** is a flat articular surface. It is found on carpal bones, tarsal bones, vertebrae, and some long bones, such as the radius and ulna (Figs. 6.19 and 6.20).

Processes

Processes are the lumps and bumps on bones. Condyles and heads on long bones are considered processes, but they have a specific articular function, so they are classified as articular surfaces. Most of the other processes on bones are places where the tendons of muscles attach to the bone. Larger processes are where more powerful muscles attach. Processes are given different names on different bones. Some of the names used are trochanter (femur), tubercle (humerus), tuber (ischium), crest (tibia), olecranon (ulna), spine (scapula), and wing (atlas) (Figs. 6.21–6.27).

Holes and Depressed Areas

A hole in a bone is called a **foramen**. Usually, it is a passageway for blood vessels or nerves to enter and leave the bone (Figs. 6.28 and 6.29).

A **fossa** is a depressed, sunken area on the surface of a bone. Bone fossae are usually occupied by muscles or tendons (Figs. 6.30 and 6.31).

Text continued on page 112

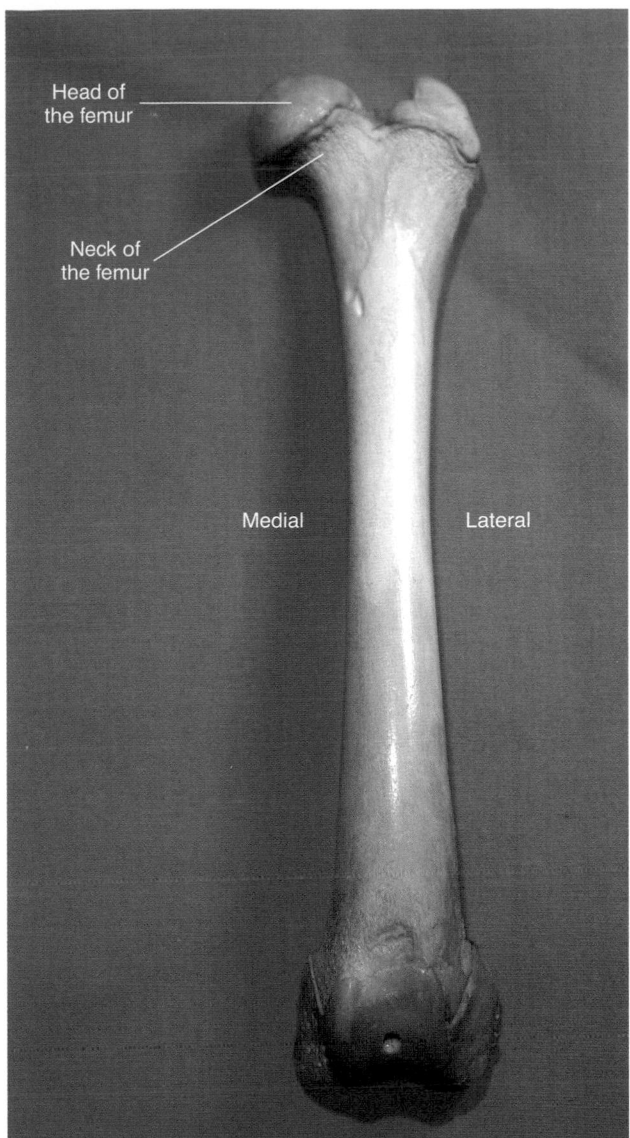

• **Fig. 6.16** Head of the canine femur. The head of the femur fits into a socket in the pelvis (the acetabulum) to form the hip joint. The neck is the narrow area between the head and the main part of the bone (cranial view).

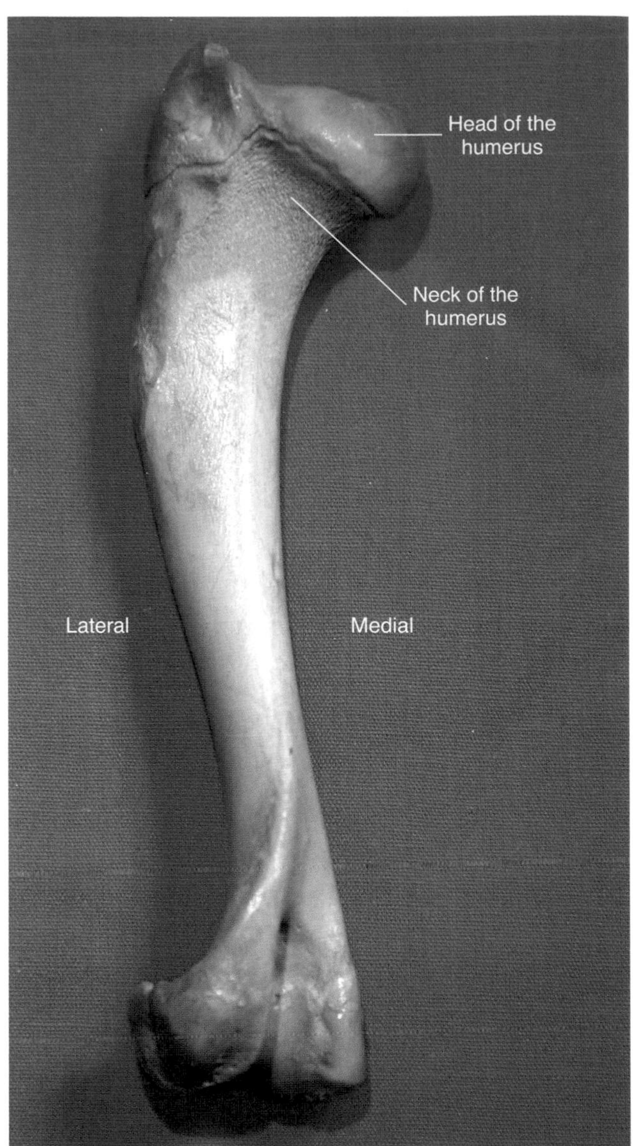

• **Fig. 6.17** Head of the canine humerus. The head of the humerus joins the glenoid cavity of the scapula to form the shoulder joint. The neck, which is just lateral to the head, is not as pronounced as in the femur (caudal view).

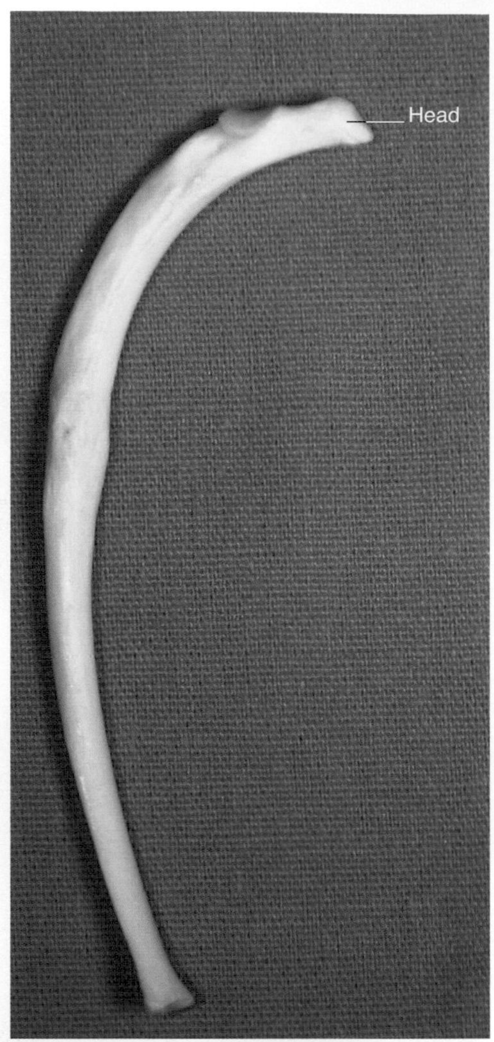

• **Fig. 6.18** Head of a rib. The heads of the ribs articulate with the thoracic vertebrae of the spinal column.

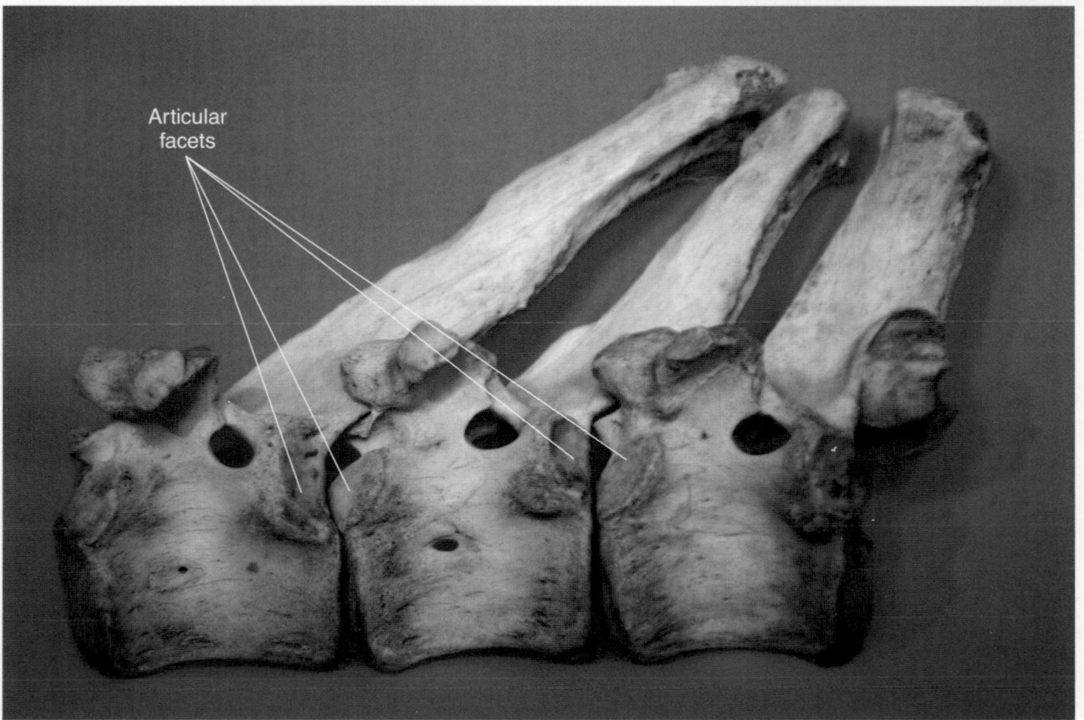

• **Fig. 6.19** Articular facets on bovine thoracic vertebrae. The heads of ribs articulate with these articular facets (lateral view).

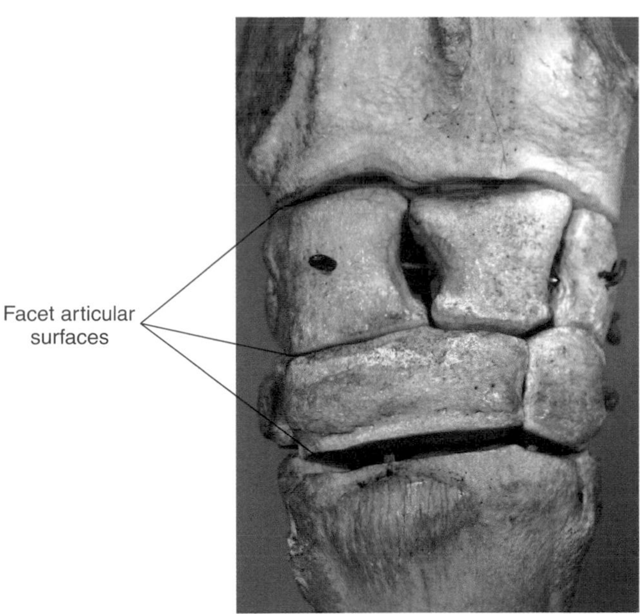

• **Fig. 6.20** Facet articular surfaces. Equine carpus. (Cranial view.)

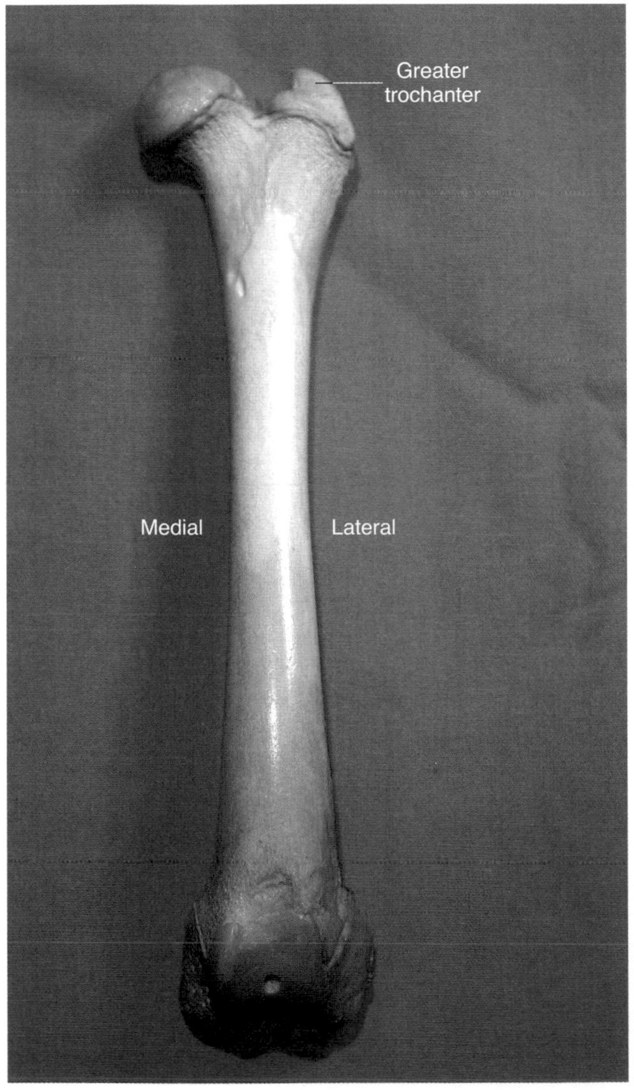

• **Fig. 6.21** Greater trochanter of the canine femur. (Cranial view.)

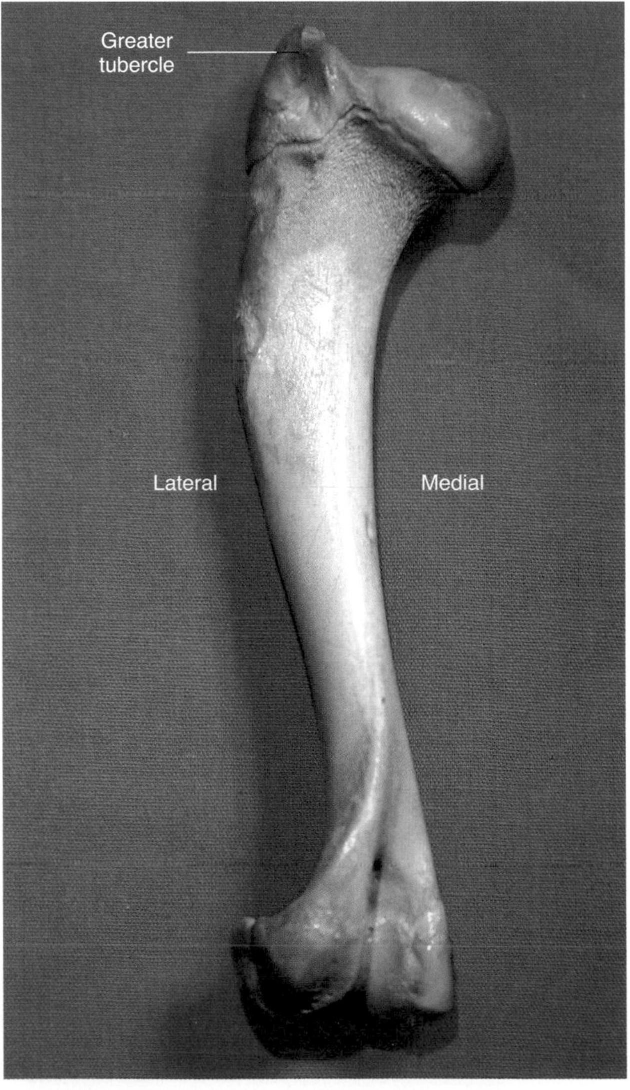

• **Fig. 6.22** Greater tubercle of the canine humerus. (Caudal view.)

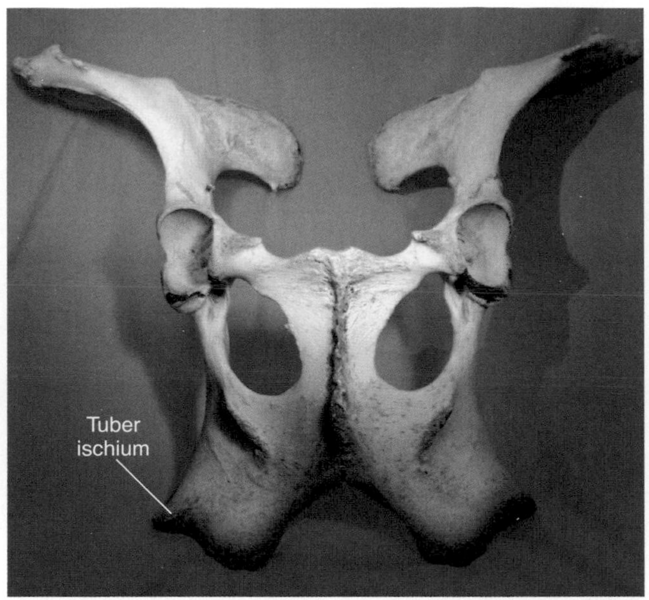

• **Fig. 6.23** Tuber ischium of the bovine pelvis. (Ventral view.)

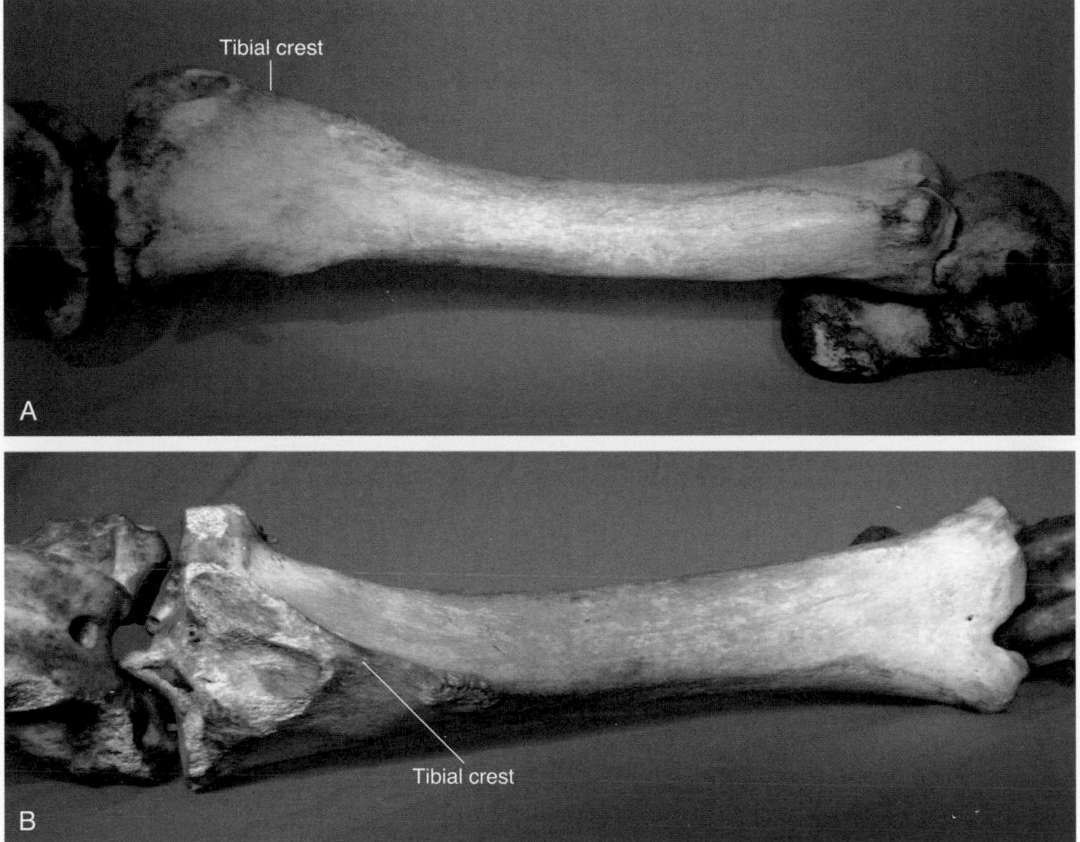

• **Fig. 6.24** Lateral (A) and cranial (B) views of the tibial crest of the equine tibia.

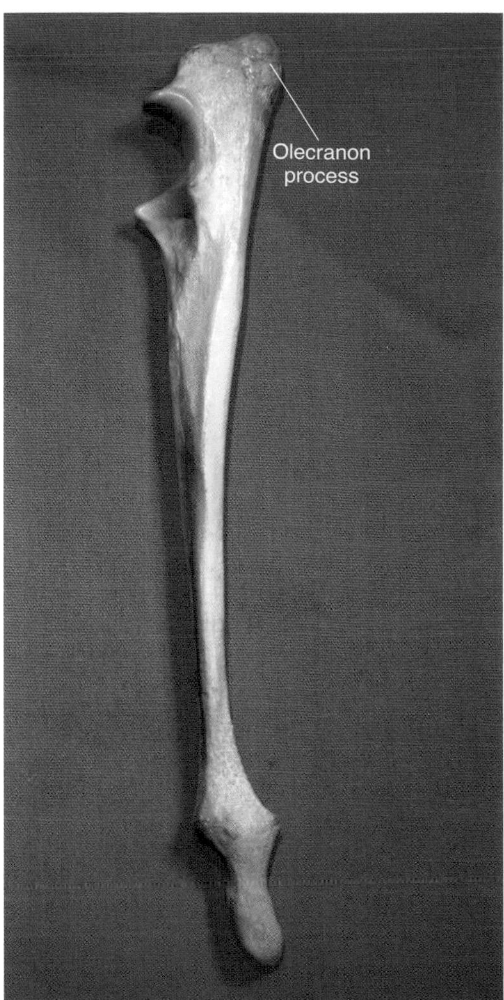

• **Fig. 6.25** Olecranon process of canine ulna. This is the "point" of the elbow where the powerful triceps brachii muscle attaches.

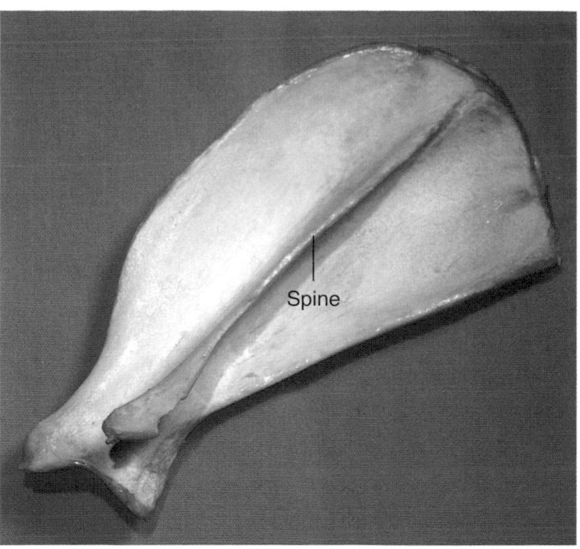

• **Fig. 6.26** Spine of the canine scapula. The spine runs along the lateral surface.

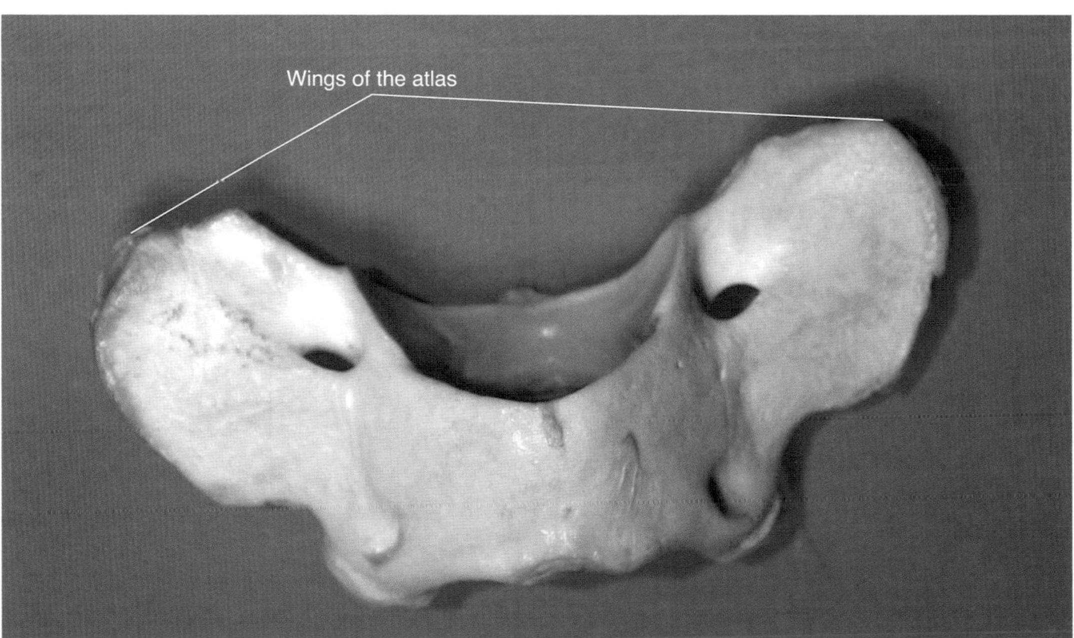

• **Fig. 6.27** Wings of the atlas (first cervical) vertebra.

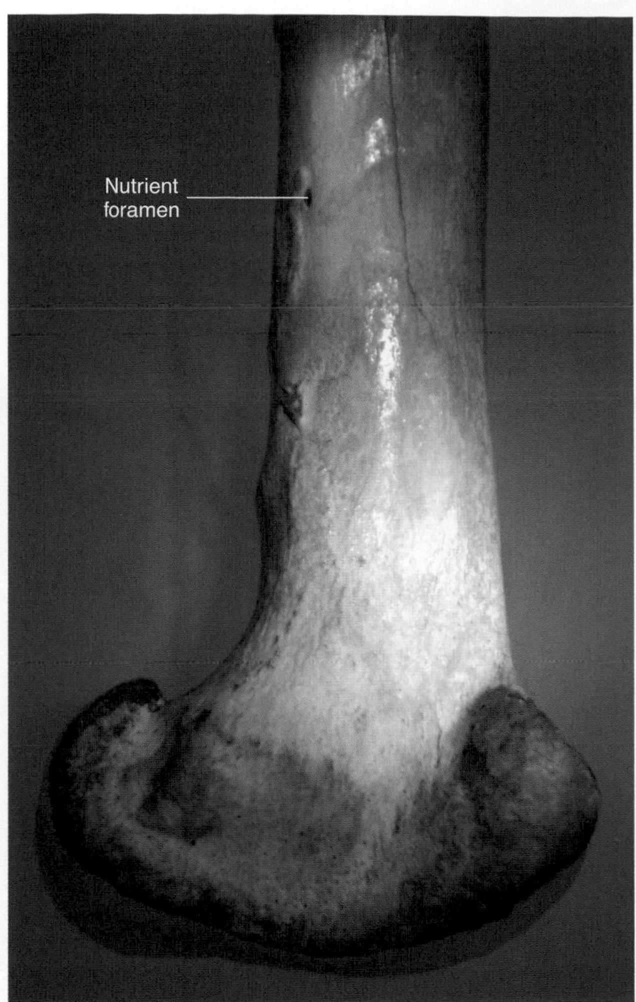

• **Fig. 6.28** Nutrient foramen in an equine femur. Blood vessels supplying the interior of the bone enter and leave the femur through this hole.

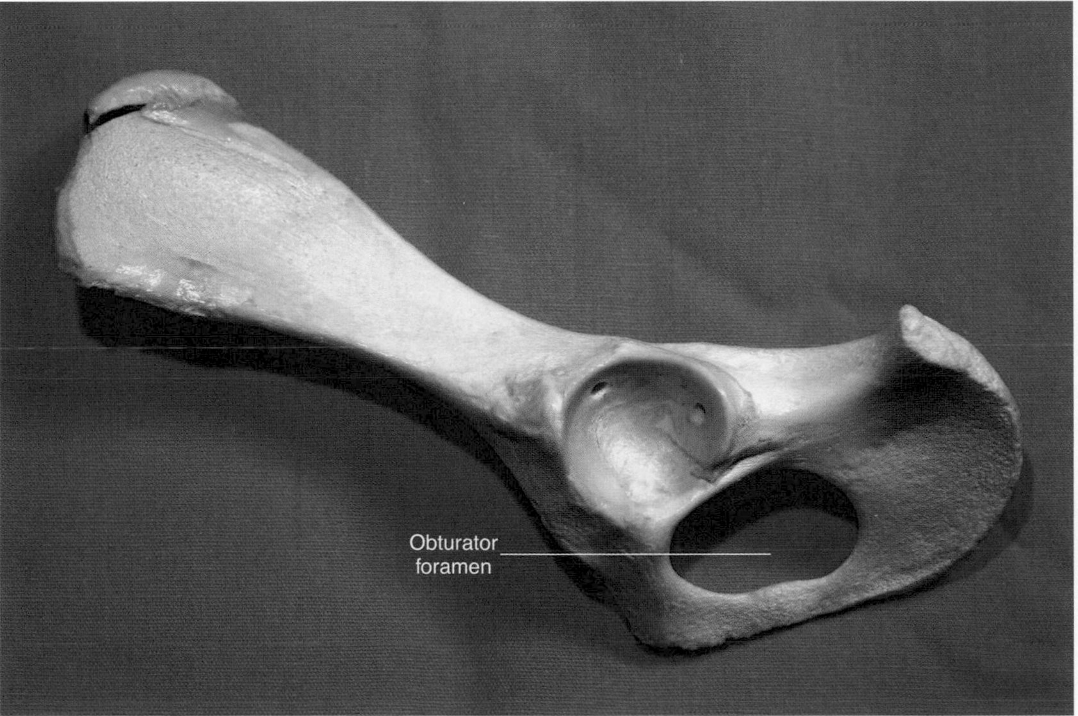

• **Fig. 6.29** Obturator foramen in a canine pelvic bone (lateral view). This foramen doesn't have anything large passing through it. It is there to make the pelvic bones lighter.

The Skeleton

Even though an animal has only one complete skeleton, we are going to divide it into two main parts (skeletons) for the purpose of studying the bones. The **axial skeleton** is made up of the bones located on or near the central cranial-caudal axis of the body—the skull, hyoid bone, spinal column, ribs, and sternum. The **appendicular skeleton** is made up of the main "appendages" of the body: the thoracic limbs and the pelvic limbs.

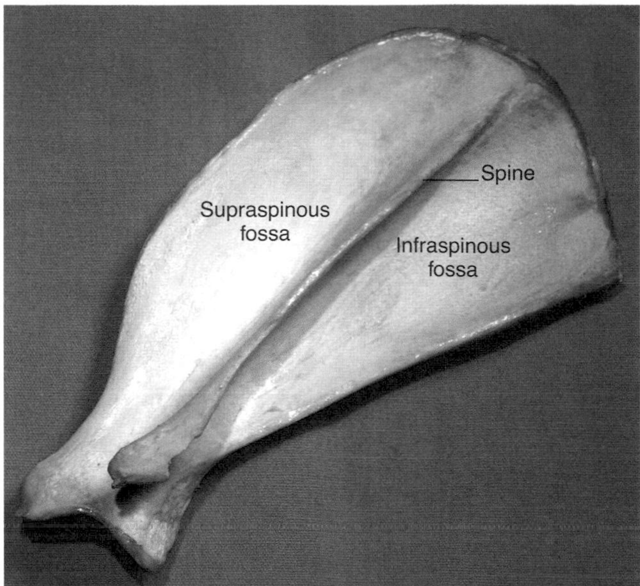

• **Fig. 6.30** Fossae on canine scapula (lateral view). The supraspinous and infraspinous fossae on either side of the scapular spine are attachment sites for two shoulder muscles—the infraspinatus and supraspinatus muscles.

Axial Skeleton

The axial skeleton is made up of the skull, hyoid bone, spinal column, ribs, and sternum. All the bones of the axial skeleton are located at or near the median plane of the animal's body (Box 6.1 and Fig. 6.32).

Skull

The **skull** is the most complex part of the skeleton. It is made up of bones that, with one exception, are united by jagged, immovable, fibrous joints called sutures. The only freely movable joint is the one between the mandible and the temporal bone. This joint is called the temporomandibular joint or TMJ.

The bones of the skull can be conveniently grouped into the bones of the cranium, which surround the brain, and the bones of the face. We will restrict our examinations to the external bones in each group, which are at least partly visible on the outside of the skull (Box 6.2). The names of these external skull bones are often used to describe locations on

• BOX 6.1 The Axial Skeleton

Skull
Hyoid bone
Spinal column
- Cervical vertebrae
- Thoracic vertebrae
- Lumbar vertebrae
- Sacral vertebrae
- Coccygeal vertebrae

Ribs
Sternum

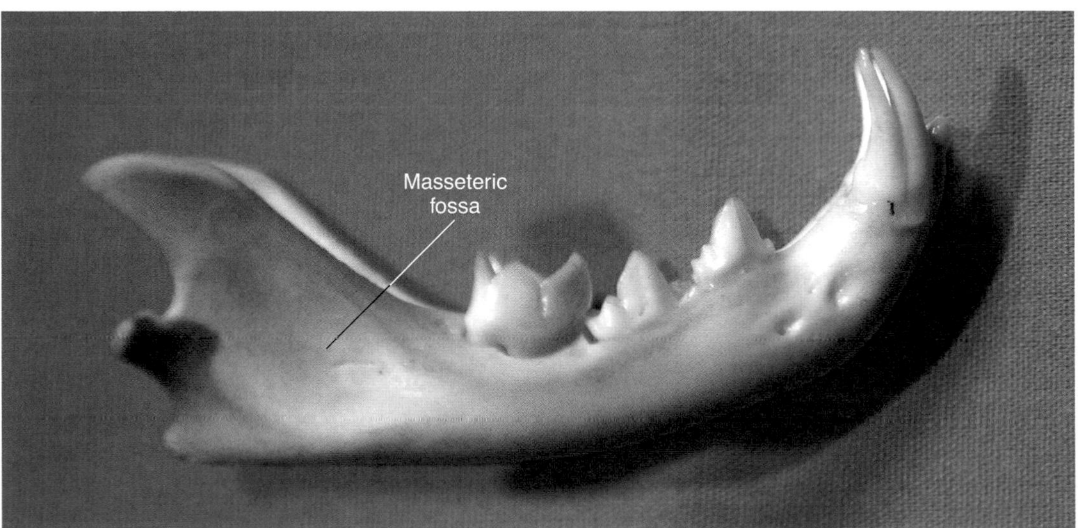

• **Fig. 6.31** Fossa on feline mandible (lateral view). The masseteric fossa on the lateral surface of the mandible is an attachment site for the large masseter jaw muscle.

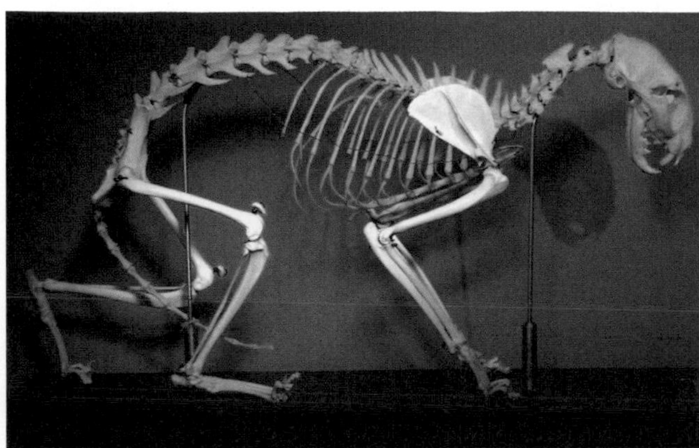

• **Fig. 6.32** Feline skeleton with the bones of the axial skeleton shaded red.

• BOX 6.2 External Skull Bones

Bones of the Cranium

Frontal bones (2)
Interparietal bones (2)
Occipital bone (1)
Parietal bones (2)
Temporal bones (2)

Bones of the Face

Incisive bones (2)
Lacrimal bones (2)
Mandible (1 or 2)
Maxillary bones (2)
Nasal bones (2)
Zygomatic bones (2)

animals' heads (e.g., left parietal region, right maxillary area) in medical records. The internal skull bones are hidden within the skull. The only internal bones we will cover are the nasal turbinates, which play important roles in the conditioning of inhaled air on its way to the lungs (Figs. 6.33–6.38).

External Bones of the Cranium

Occipital Bone

- Single bone that forms the "base" (caudoventral portion) of the skull
- The **foramen magnum** is the large opening where the spinal cord exits the skull
- **Occipital condyles** form a joint with the atlas (first cervical vertebra)

Interparietal Bones

- Two small bones on the dorsal midline between the occipital bone and the parietal bones

Parietal Bones

- Two bones that form the dorsolateral portion of the cranium

Temporal Bones

- Two bones that form the ventrolateral portion of the cranium
- Contain the middle and inner ear structures
- Form a portion of the zygomatic arch
- Form the temporomandibular joint with the mandible
- The **external acoustic meatus** opening leads to the middle and inner ear cavities
- The **tympanic bullae**, "egg-shaped" swellings on the ventral surface, contain the middle ear structures

Frontal Bones

- Two bones that form the "forehead" part of the skull
- Form the rostrolateral part of the cranium and part of the orbit of the eye
- Contain the large frontal sinuses
- In horned animals, the horn develops around the **cornual process** of the frontal bone

External Bones of the Face

Incisive Bones

- Two bones that are the most rostral skull bones
- House the upper incisor teeth (most animals) or dental pad (ruminants)

Nasal Bones

- Two bones that form the "bridge" of the nose—the dorsal part of the nasal cavity

Maxillary Bones

- Two bones that make up most of the upper jaw
- House upper canine teeth (if present) and upper premolar and molar teeth
- Contain the maxillary sinuses
- Form a portion of the hard palate

Lacrimal Bones

- Two small bones that form part of the orbit of the eye
- Contain the lacrimal sacs—part of the tear drainage system

Zygomatic Bones

- "Cheekbones"
- Two bones that form a portion of the orbit of the eye and a portion of the zygomatic arch

Note: The zygomatic arches can easily be palpated on each side of an animal's head just below and behind the eyes. They form the widest part of dog and cat skulls.

Mandible

- Lower jaw
- Two bones united rostrally by the mandibular symphysis in dogs, cats, and cattle
- One solid bone in adult horses and swine
- The **shaft** is the horizontal part that houses all the lower teeth

Text continued on page 118

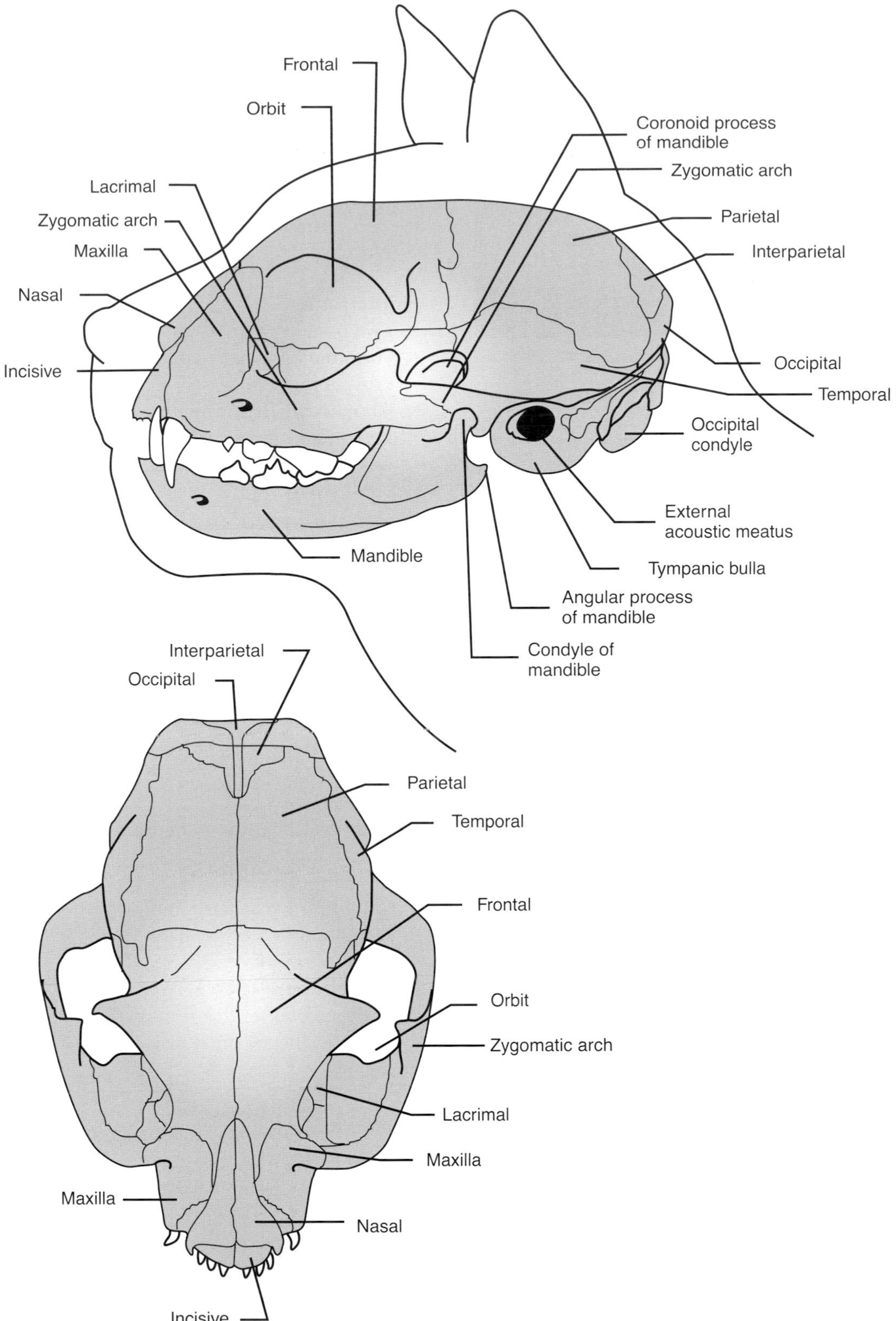

• **Fig. 6.33** The skull of a cat.

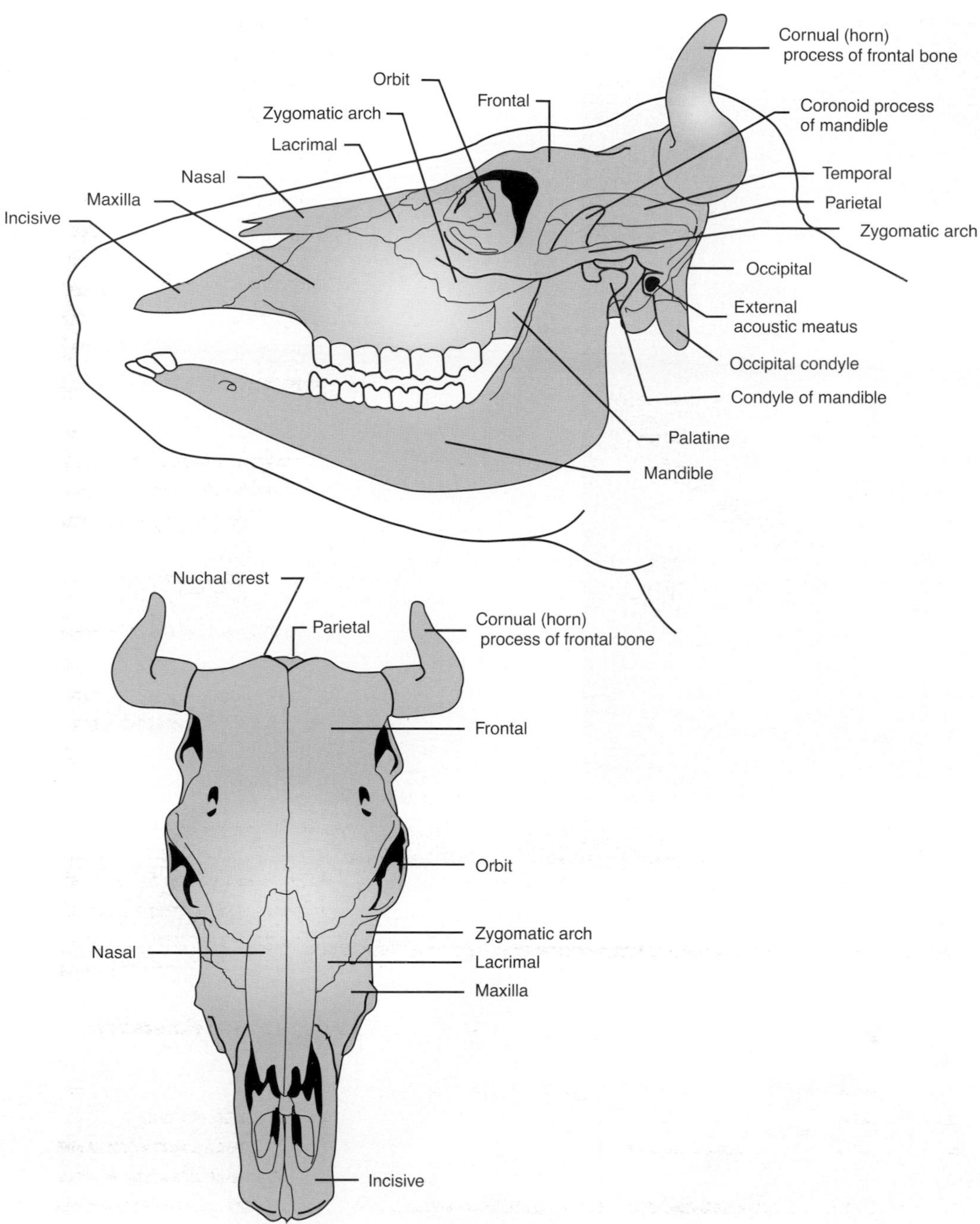

• **Fig. 6.34** Bovine skull.

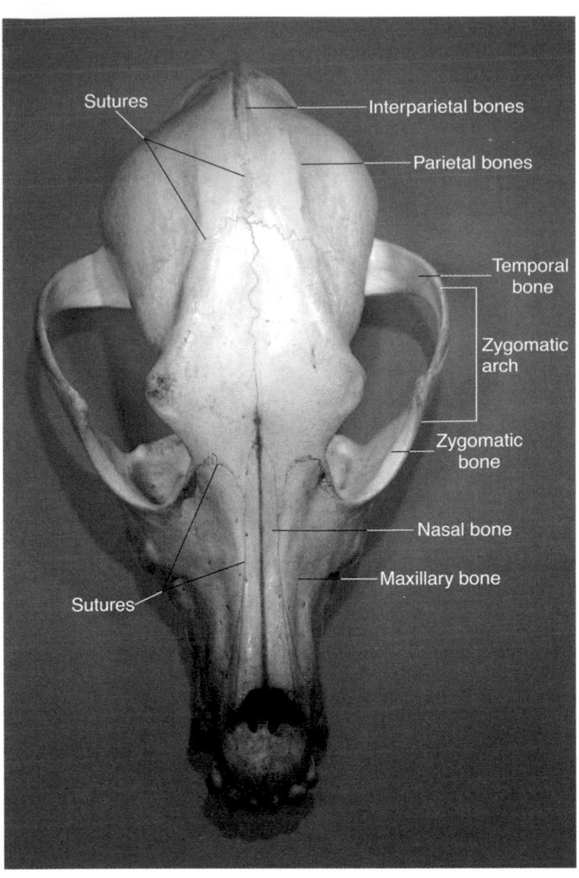

• **Fig. 6.35** Dorsal view of a canine skull.

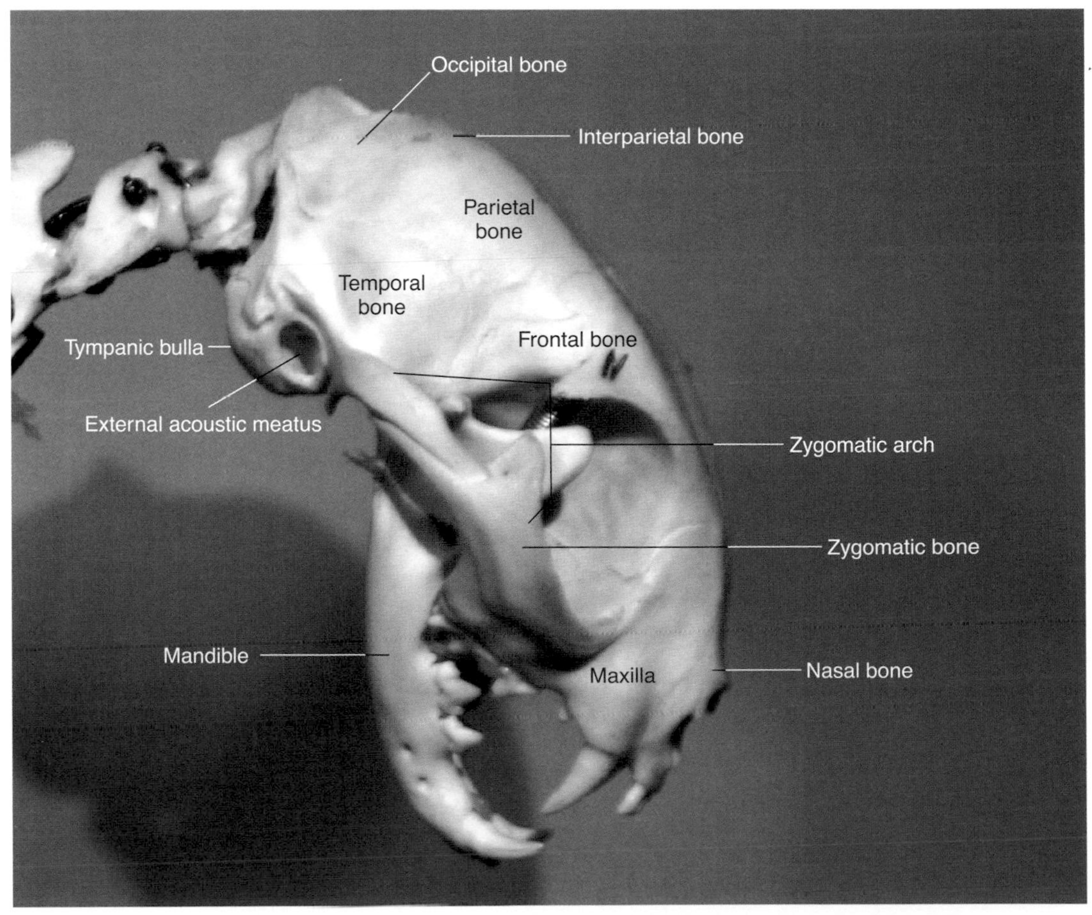

• **Fig. 6.36** Lateral view of a feline skull.

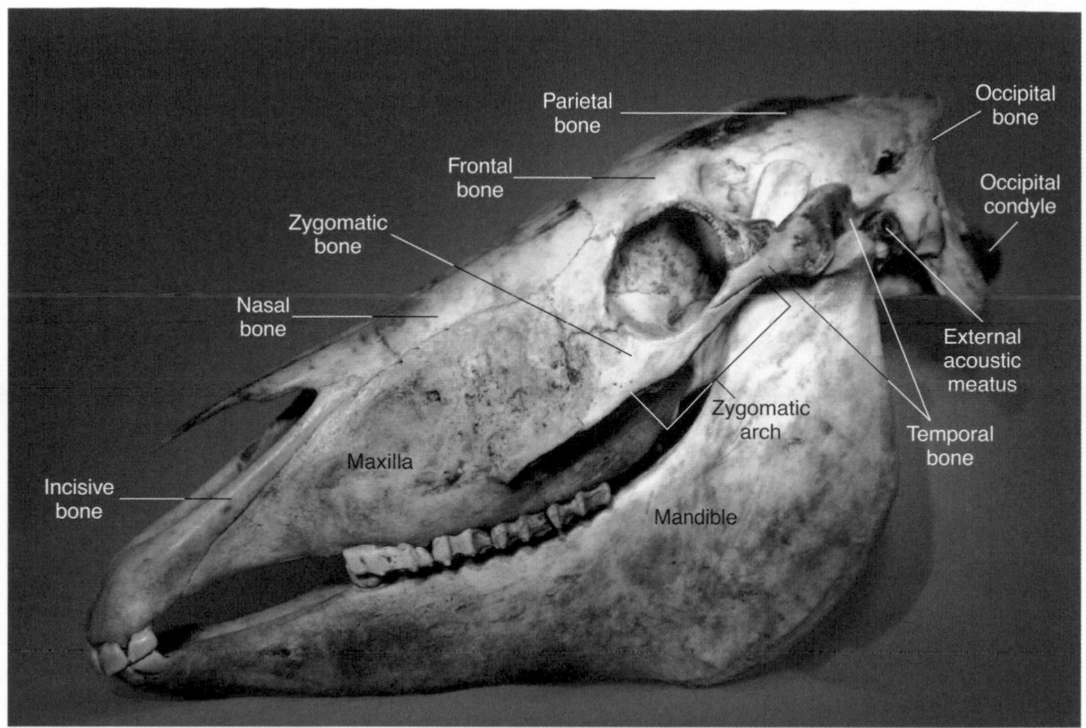

• **Fig. 6.37** Lateral view of an equine skull.

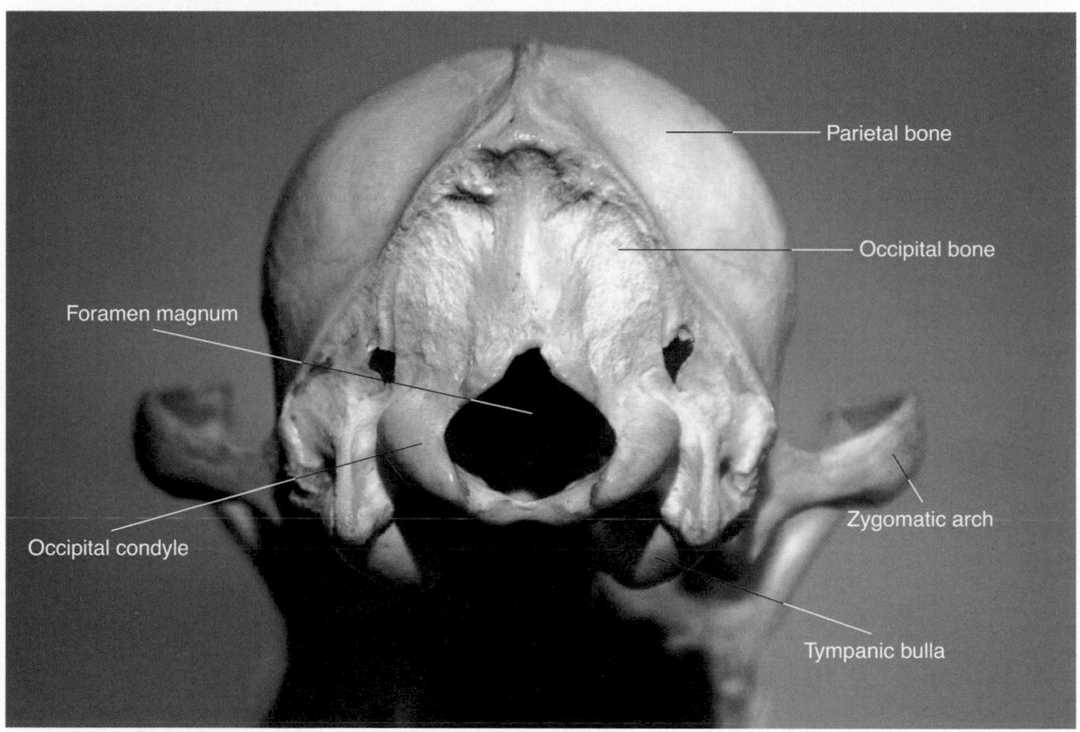

• **Fig. 6.38** Canine skull caudal view.

- The **ramus** is the vertical part at the caudal end that forms the temporomandibular joint with the temporal bone. This is also where the powerful jaw muscles attach

Internal Bones of the Face

Turbinates

- Thin scroll-like bones that fill most of the space in the nasal cavities
- Play important roles in "conditioning" inhaled air

Hyoid Bone

The hyoid bone (also known as the hyoid apparatus) attaches to the temporal bones and supports the base of the tongue, the pharynx, and the larynx. It consists of several individual parts united by cartilage but is usually referred to as a single bone (Fig. 6.39).

Spinal Column

The spinal column, also known as the vertebral column, consists of a series of irregular bones called **vertebrae** that extend from the skull to the tip of the tail. A typical vertebra consists of a ventral **body**, a dorsal **arch**, and a group of **processes**. The body is the heaviest, most dense part of the bone. The bodies of adjacent vertebrae are separated by cartilaginous intervertebral discs. The arch dorsal to the vertebral body houses the spinal cord in the living animal. Three kinds of process are commonly found on vertebrae: a single **spinous process** that projects dorsally, two **transverse processes** that project laterally, and **articular processes** on the cranial and caudal ends of the vertebra (Fig. 6.40).

Vertebrae are grouped into five regions—**cervical** (neck region, abbreviated "C"), **thoracic** (chest region, abbreviated "T"), **lumbar** (abdominal region, abbreviated "L"), **sacral** (pelvic region, abbreviated "S"), and **coccygeal** (tail region, abbreviated "Cy"). Most vertebrae do not have specific names but are identified by numbers within each region from cranial to caudal. A shorthand method of identifying

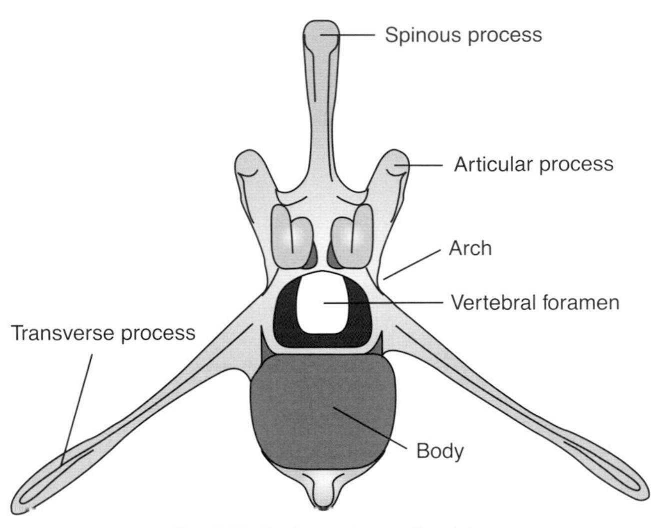

• **Fig. 6.40** Basic anatomy of vertebra.

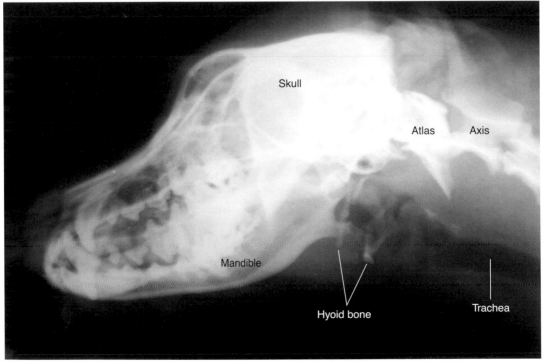

• **Fig. 6.39** Skull radiograph showing hyoid bone.

• BOX 6.3 Regions of the Spinal Column

Cervical (C) vertebrae—neck region
Thoracic (T) vertebrae—chest (thoracic) region
Lumbar (L) vertebrae—abdominal region
Sacral (S) vertebrae—pelvic region
Coccygeal (Cy) vertebrae—tail

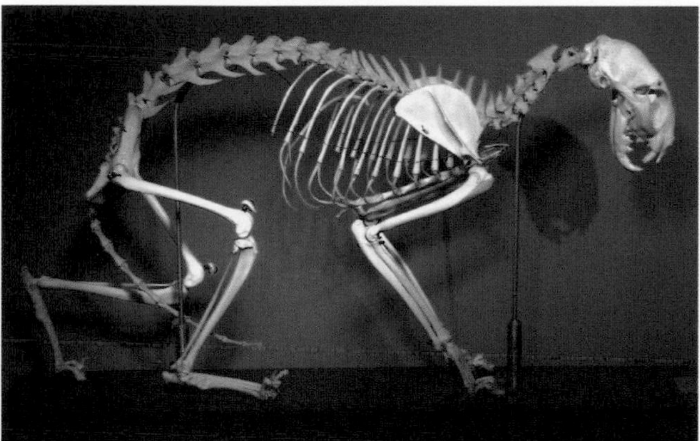

• **Fig. 6.41** Feline vertebral column. The five sections of the vertebral column are shaded red. The sacral region is located primarily between the two halves of the pelvis and is only partially visible.

vertebrae uses the abbreviation for the vertebral group followed by the number of the particular vertebra. For example, vertebra C5 is the fifth cervical vertebra and T10 is the tenth thoracic vertebra (Box 6.3 and Fig. 6.41).

The first two cervical vertebrae are unusual in shape compared with the rest of the vertebrae, and they have specific names. The first cervical vertebra (C1) is called the **atlas**. It does not have a vertebral body but consists of a bony ring that the spinal cord passes through, and two large transverse processes called the "wings" of the atlas. The occipital bone of the skull forms a joint with the atlas—the atlantooccipital joint. The second cervical vertebra (C2) is called the **axis**. Its main characteristics are a large, bladelike spinous process and the peglike dens on its cranial end that tucks into the caudal end of the atlas to help form and stabilize the atlantoaxial (C1–C2) joint. The rest of the cervical vertebrae are fairly normal in appearance and are just identified by number, like the rest of the vertebrae (Fig. 6.42).

The number of thoracic vertebrae is usually equal to the numbers of pairs of ribs the animal has. The main characteristics of thoracic vertebrae are their tall spinous processes and their lateral articular facets, which form joints with the heads of the ribs.

The lumbar vertebrae are the most massive-looking vertebrae of the spinal column. They have to support the

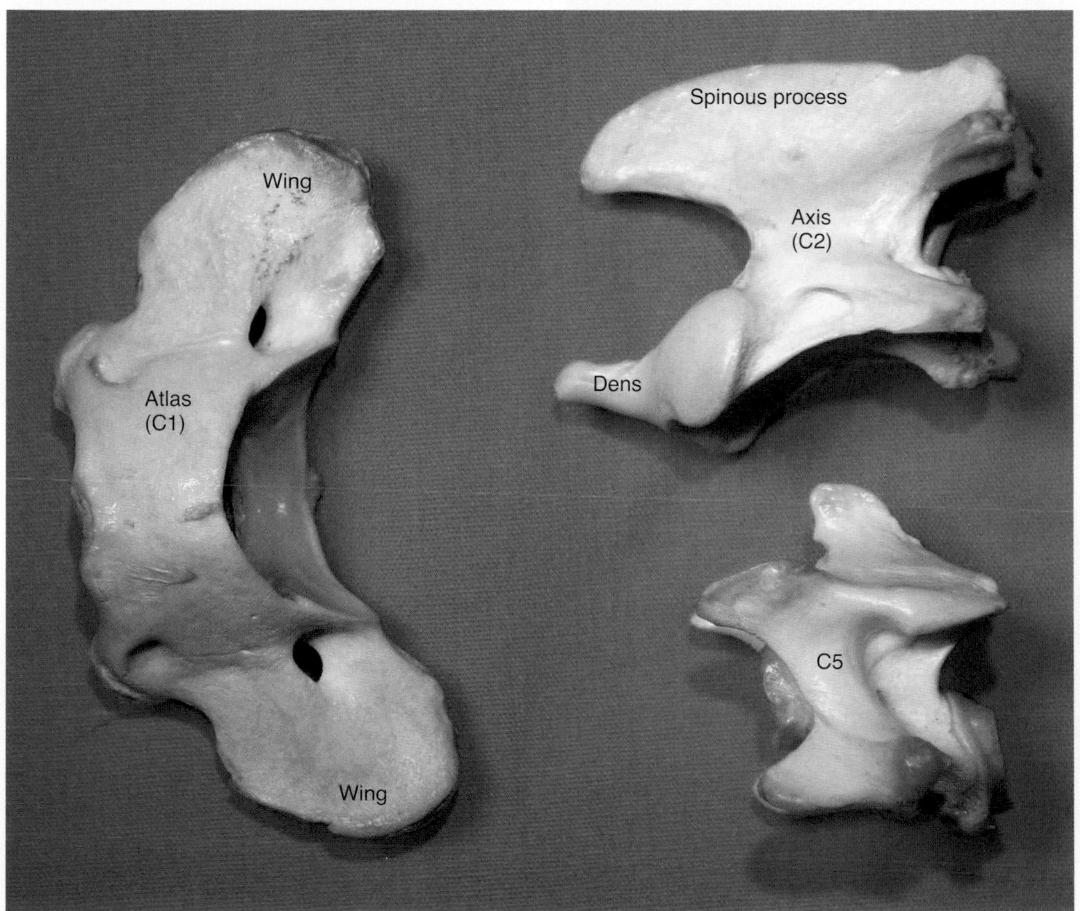

• **Fig. 6.42** Canine cervical vertebrae.

weight of the abdominal organs without the aid of the ribs, which help support the organs in the chest.

The sacral vertebrae are fused into a single solid structure called the sacrum. The sacrum forms a joint with the ilium of the pelvis—the sacroiliac joint.

The coccygeal vertebrae are the bones of the tail. At the cranial end, the first few coccygeal vertebrae look like small versions of normal vertebrae. They have bodies, arches, and processes. Further caudally, however, they gradually turn into simple little rods of bone.

Ribs

Ribs are flat bones that form the lateral sides of the thorax. They articulate with the thoracic vertebrae dorsally. The ventral part of a rib is composed of **costal (rib) cartilage**. Where the cartilaginous part meets the bony part is the **costochondral junction**. The costal cartilages join either the sternum or the costal cartilage of the ribs ahead of them (Figs. 6.43–6.46).

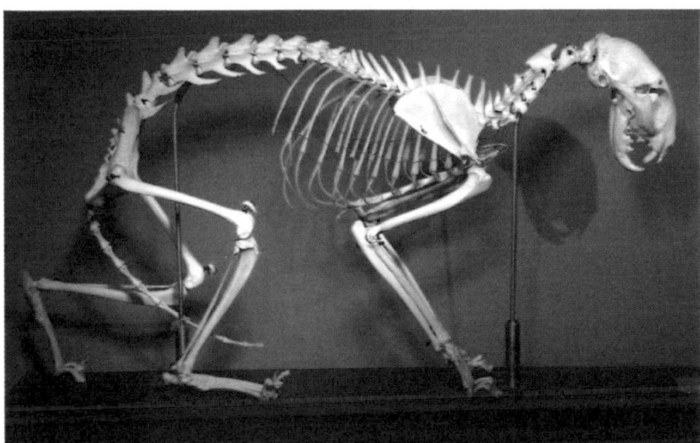

• **Fig. 6.43** Feline skeleton with the ribs shaded red.

Sternum

The **sternum** (breastbone) is made up of bones called sternebrae. The first sternebra is named the **manubrium** (full name manubrium sterni). The last sternebra is named the **xiphoid** (full name xiphoid process). A piece of cartilage that extends off the caudal end of the xiphoid process is the xiphoid cartilage, which can be palpated at the caudal end of the sternum in most animals (Fig. 6.47).

Appendicular Skeleton

The **appendicular skeleton** is made up of the thoracic (front) and pelvic (hind) limb bones of the animal. They make up the main appendages of the body, hence the name (Box 6.4 and Fig. 6.48).

Thoracic Limb

The **thoracic limb** is the front leg. In most domestic animals, it has no bony connection to the axial skeleton. Instead, the weight of the front part of the body is supported by a sluglike arrangement of muscles and tendons. From proximal to distal, the bones of the thoracic limb are the **scapula**, **humerus**, radius and ulna, carpal bones, metacarpal bones, and phalanges.

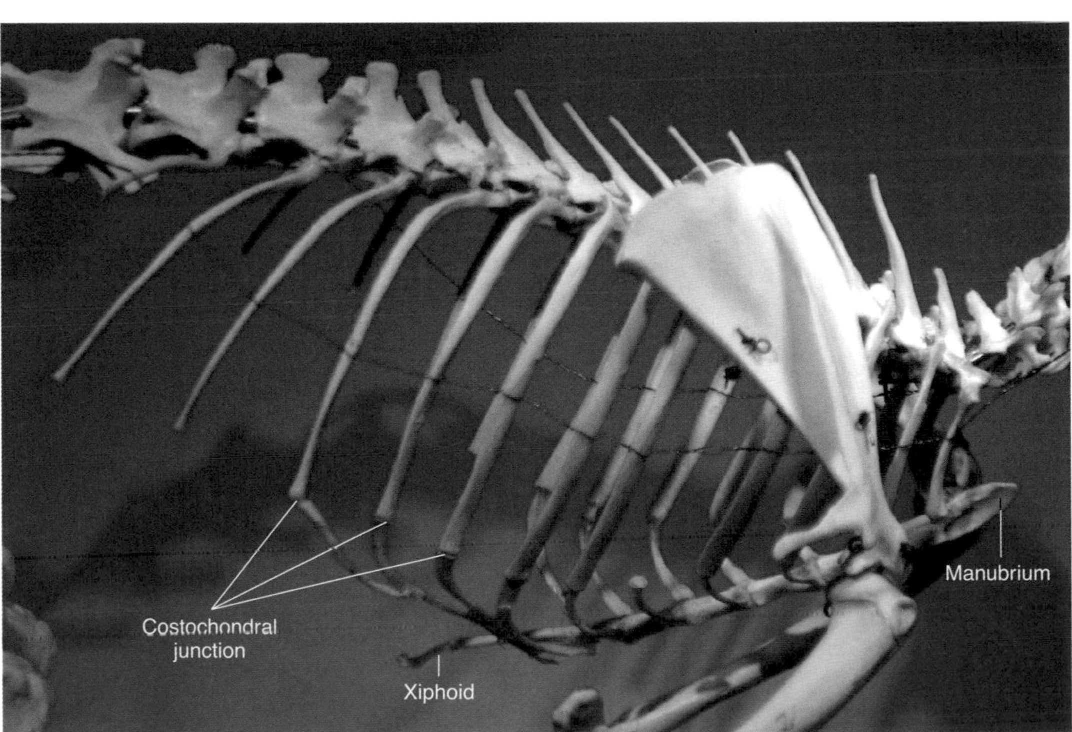

• **Fig. 6.44** Rabbit rib cage, sternum, and thoracic vertebrae. The point at which the bony part of the rib meets the cartilaginous part of the rib is the costochondral junction. Some of the costal cartilages join the sternum, and other costal cartilages attach to the costal cartilage of the rib in front.

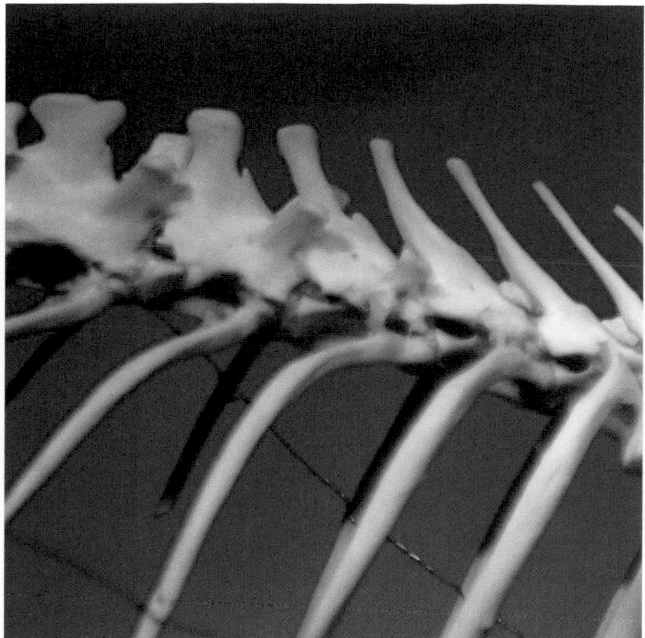

• **Fig. 6.45** Rabbit ribs articulating dorsally with thoracic vertebrae.

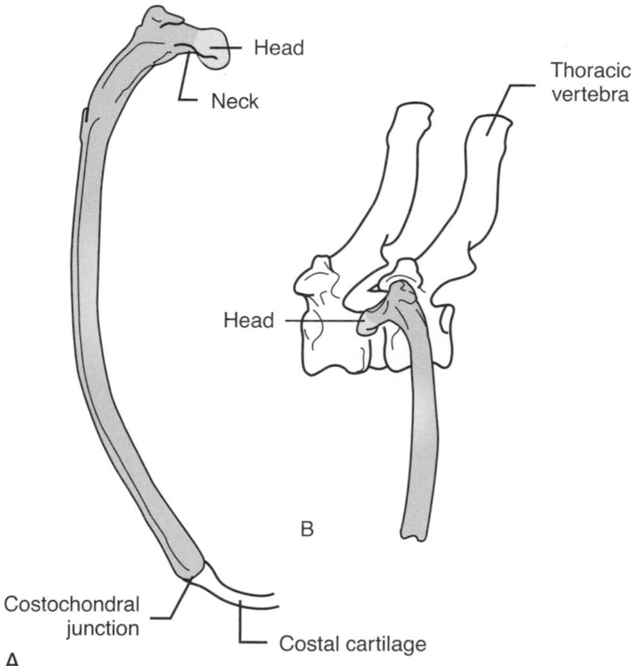

• **Fig. 6.46** Canine rib. (A) Caudal view of rib. (B) Lateral view of rib articulating with vertebrae.

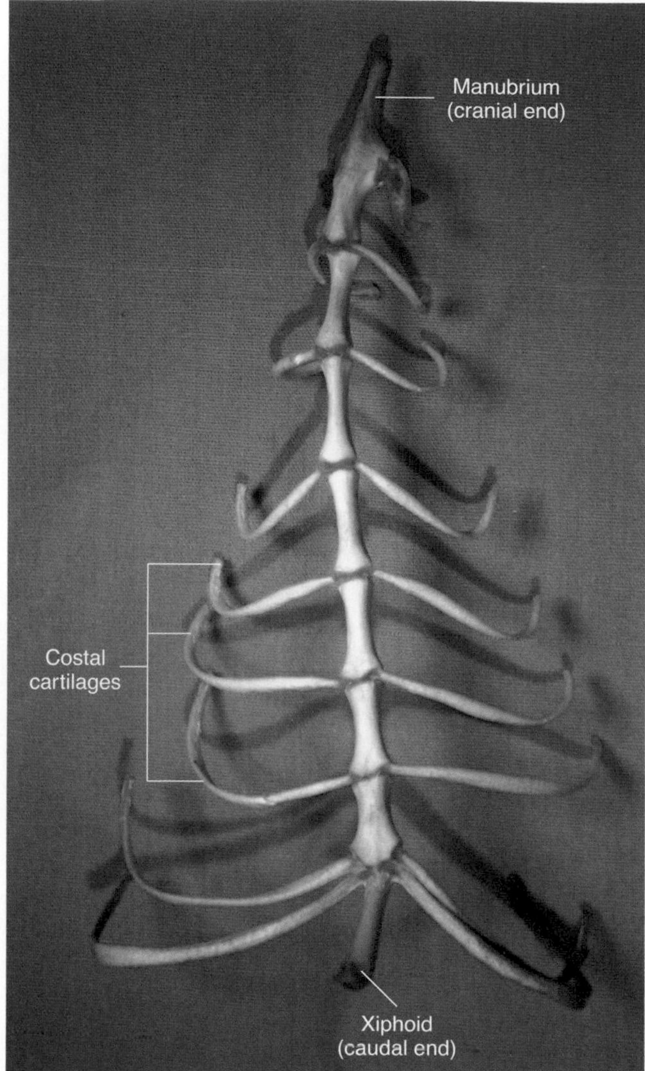

• **Fig. 6.47** Canine sternum and costal cartilages.

• BOX 6.4 Bones of the Appendicular Skeleton

Thoracic Limb

Scapula
Humerus
Radius
Ulna
Carpal bones
Metacarpal bones
Phalanges

Pelvic Limb

Pelvis
Femur
Patella
Tibia
Fibula
Tarsal bones
Metatarsal bones
Phalanges

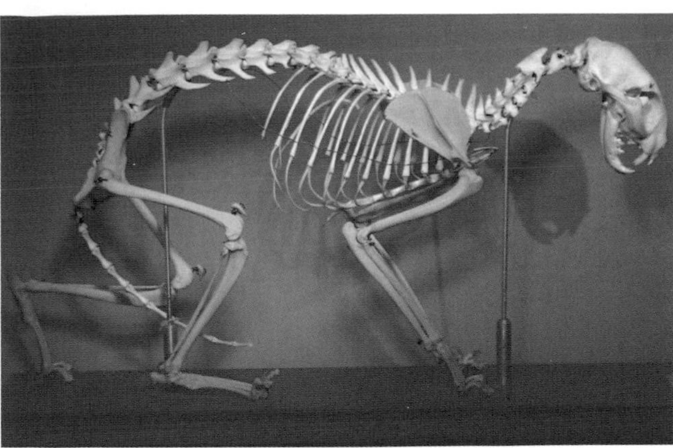

• **Fig. 6.48** Feline skeleton with the bones of the appendicular skeleton shaded red.

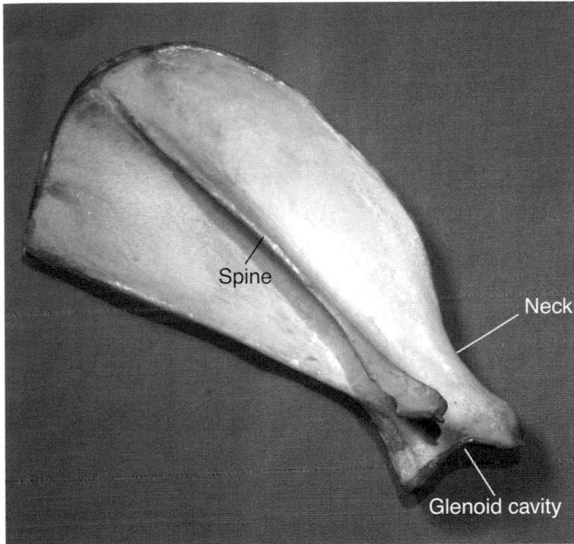

• **Fig. 6.49** Canine scapula. (Lateral view.)

Scapula

- Commonly called the shoulder blade
- Flat and somewhat triangular in shape (Fig. 6.49)
- The scapular **spine** is a ridge that projects laterally
- The concave **glenoid cavity** is the socket part of the ball-and-socket shoulder joint
- The **neck** joins the glenoid cavity to the main part of the bone

Humerus

- Long bone of the brachium ("upper arm") (Fig. 6.50)
- The rounded **head** on proximal end is the ball part of the ball-and-socket shoulder joint
- The **neck** joins the head to the shaft (not as obvious as the neck of the femur)
- The **greater tubercle** on proximal end is a large process to which shoulder muscles attach
- The distal articular surface is collectively called the **condyle** (the medial part is the trochlea, and the lateral part is the capitulum)
- Medial and lateral **epicondyles** are the "knobs" on the medial and lateral sides of the condyle
- The **olecranon fossa** is the indentation on the caudal surface just proximal to the condyle, which the anconeal process of the ulna tucks into when the elbow is extended

Ulna

- Long bone of the antebrachium ("forearm") (Fig. 6.51)
- Along with the radius, forms the elbow joint with the humerus
- The large **olecranon process** on the proximal end is the attachment site for the triceps brachii muscle
- The **trochlear notch** is a half-moon-shaped, concave articular surface that wraps around the trochlea of the humeral condyle to help make the elbow joint a very tight and secure joint
- The **anconeal process** is a beak-shaped process at the proximal end of the trochlear notch
- Medial and lateral **coronoid processes** on distal end of trochlear notch are located on the ends of the horizontal, concave **radial notch** where the proximal end of the radius articulates with the ulna
- The shaft of the ulna extends down to the carpus in all common domestic species except the horse
- The equine ulna consists only of the proximal structures and joins the radius about midshaft
- The **styloid process** on distal end articulates with the carpus

Radius

- Main weight-bearing bone of the antebrachium ("forearm") (Fig. 6.52)
- The **head** on the proximal end has a large, concave articular surface that articulates with the capitulum of the humeral condyle to form part of the elbow joint
- The **neck** on the proximal end connects the head with the shaft of the bone
- The **styloid process** on the distal end articulates with the carpus

Carpal Bones (Carpus)

- Located immediately distal to the radius and ulna (Figs. 6.53–6.55)
- Equivalent to the human wrist
- Consist of two parallel rows of short bones
- Bones in the proximal row are named the radial carpal, ulnar carpal, **accessory carpal**, and, in some species, an intermediate carpal
- The accessory carpal bone protrudes backward on the lateral side of the carpus (useful landmark for radiography)
- Bones in the distal row are numbered starting at the medial side

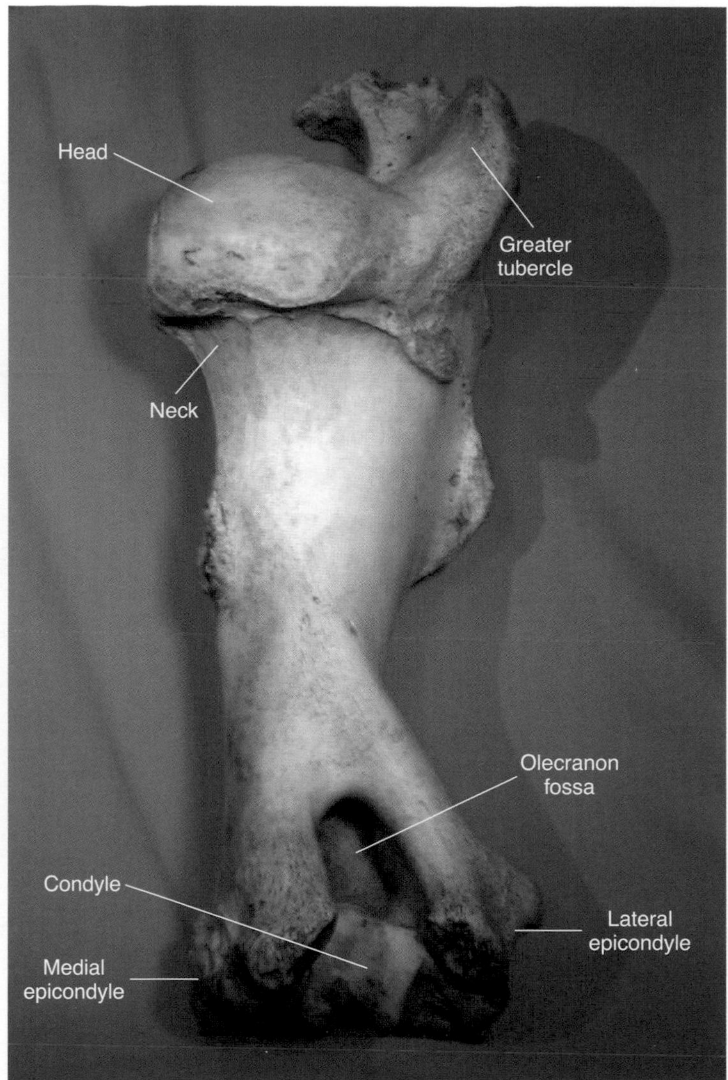

• **Fig. 6.50** Bovine right humerus. (Caudal view.)

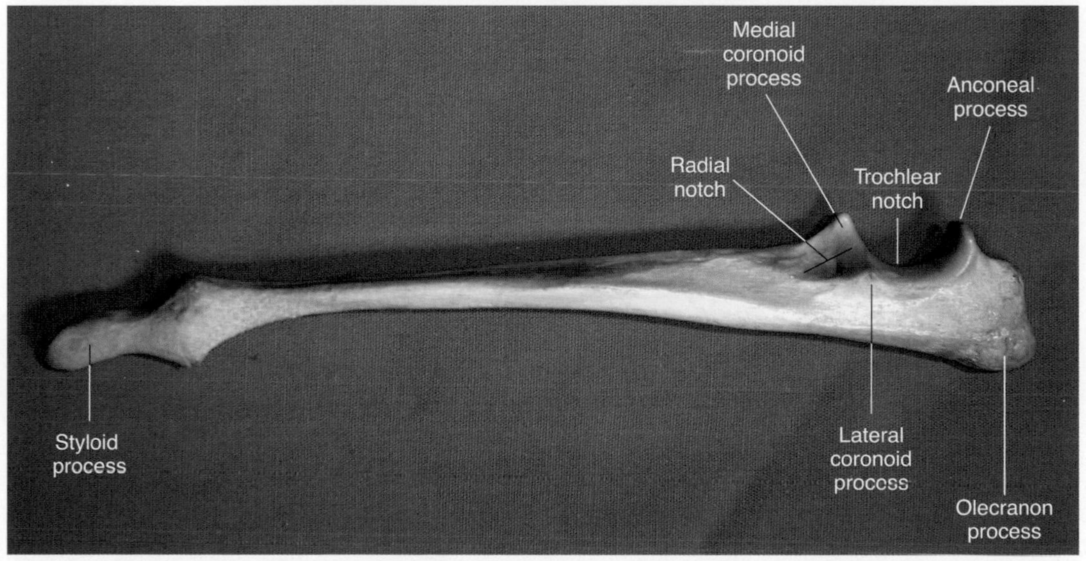

• **Fig. 6.51** Canine left ulna. (Lateral view.)

• **Fig. 6.52** Canine left radius. (Cranial view.)

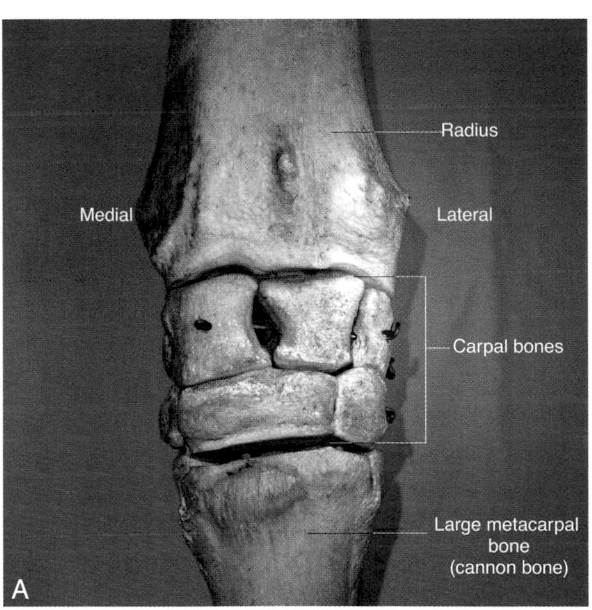

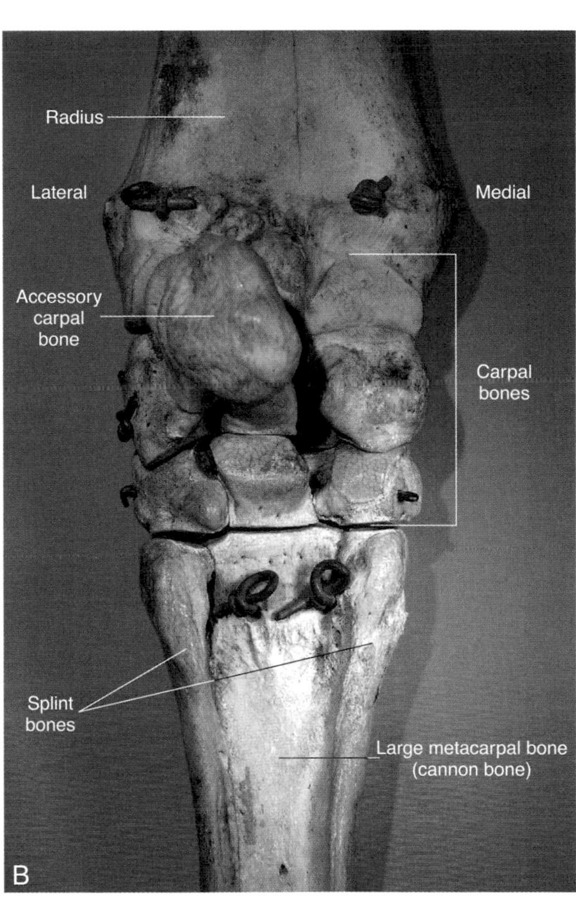

• **Fig. 6.53** Equine carpus. (A) Cranial view. (B) Caudal view.

Metacarpal Bones

- Extend distally from distal row of carpal bones to the proximal phalanges of the digit
- Dogs and cats typically have five metacarpal bones, numbered from medial (I) to lateral (V)
- Ruminants have a large metacarpal bone (commonly called the **cannon bone**) formed from two fused bones—metacarpals III and IV. A longitudinal groove shows its two-bone origin
- Horses have a single large metacarpal bone (metacarpal III, commonly called the cannon bone) with two small, incomplete metacarpal bones on either side (metacarpals II and IV, commonly called the **splint bones**)

Phalanges

- Phalanges (singular: phalanx) are the individual bones that make up the digits (toes)

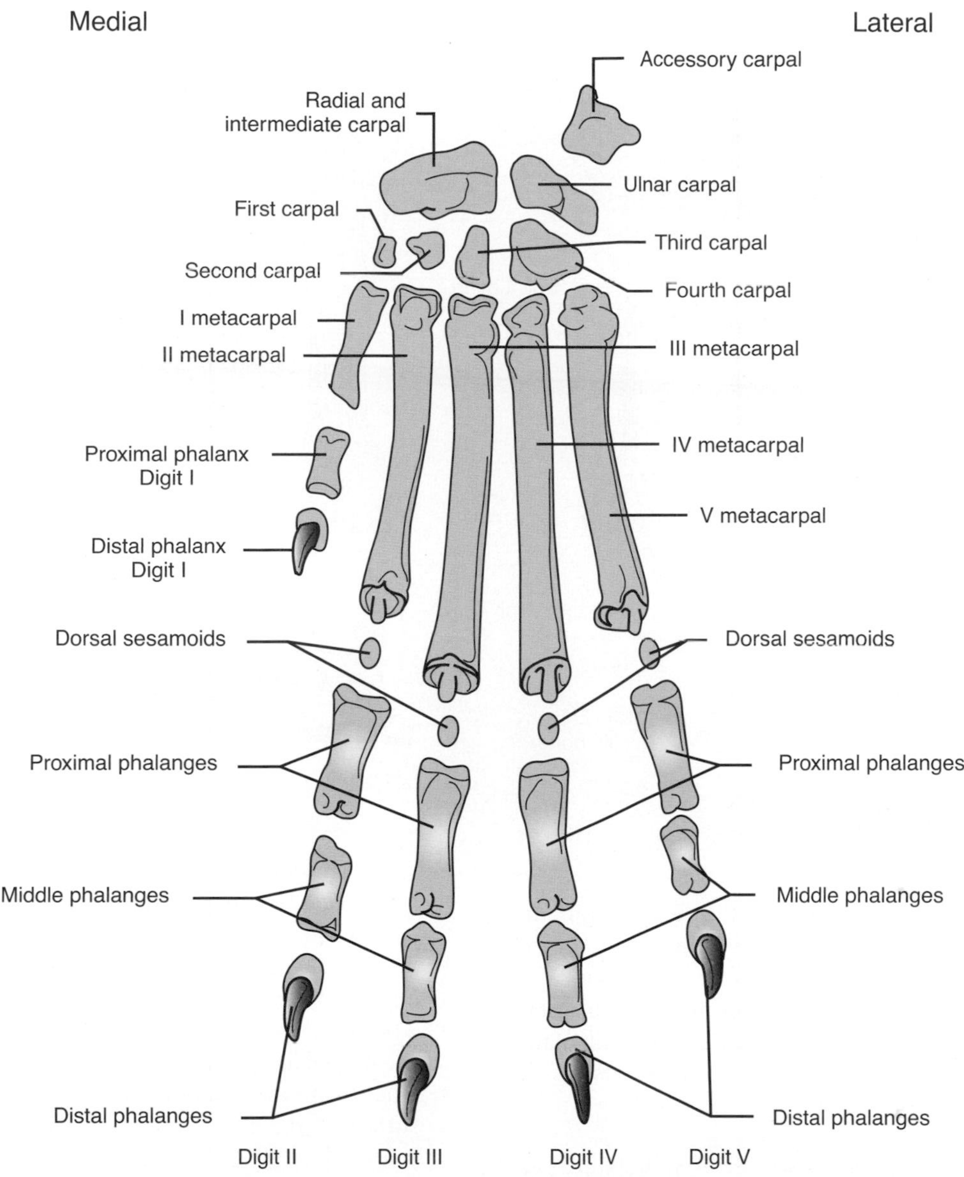

• **Fig. 6.54** Distal limb bones of canine front leg.

- Dog and cat forepaws typically have four or five digits numbered from medial to lateral:
  - Digit I, if present, is commonly called the dewclaw and has two phalanges—proximal and distal.
  - Digits II–V each contain three phalanges—proximal, middle, and distal.
  - The distal phalanx contains the ungual process that is surrounded by the claw.
- Ruminants have four digits on each limb:
  - Two support weight (III and IV).
  - Two are smaller non–weight-bearing "dewclaws" (II and V).
  - Weight-bearing digits each contain three phalanges—proximal, middle, and distal.
  - Weight-bearing digits each contain two proximal sesamoid bones on the palmar surface of the joint between the metacarpal and the proximal phalanx, and one distal sesamoid bone on the palmar surface of the joint between the middle and distal phalanges.
- Horses have one digit on each limb, composed of three phalanges and three sesamoid bones:
  - The phalanges are the proximal phalanx (common name: long pastern bone), middle phalanx (common name: short pastern bone), and distal phalanx (common name: coffin bone).
  - Two **proximal sesamoid bones** are located on the palmar surface of the joint between the metacarpal and the proximal phalanx.
  - The single **distal sesamoid bone** (common name: navicular bone) is located on the palmar surface of the joint between the middle and distal phalanges.

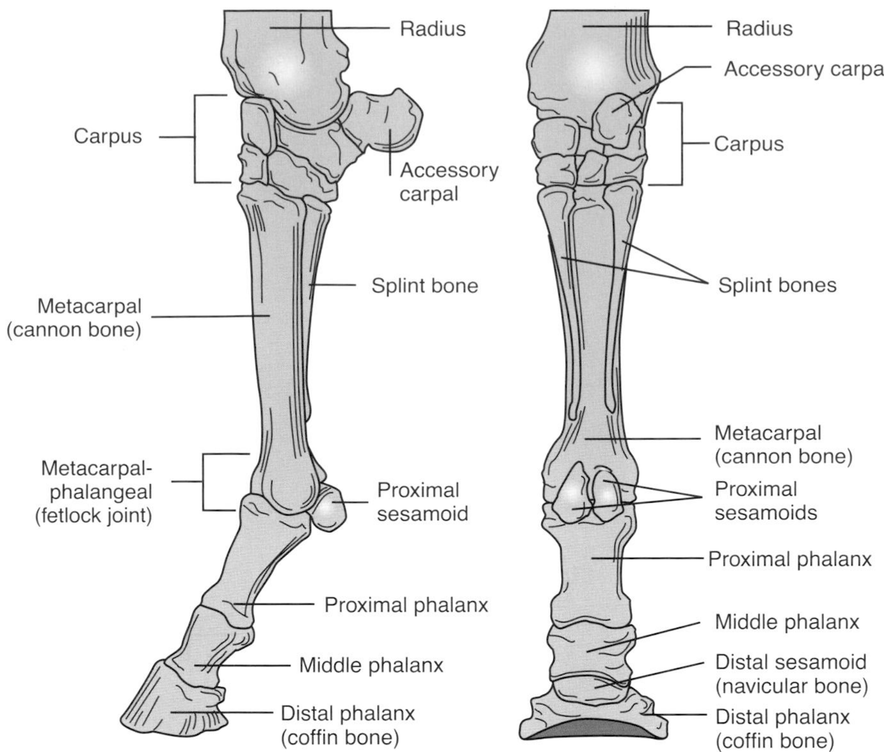

• **Fig. 6.55** Distal limb bones of equine front leg.

Pelvic Limb

The **pelvic limb** is the hind leg. Unlike the thoracic limb, the pelvic limb is connected to the axial skeleton through the sacroiliac joint that unites the ilium of the pelvis with the sacrum of the spinal column. From proximal to distal, the bones of the pelvic limb are the pelvis, femur, tibia and fibula, tarsal bones, metatarsal bones, and phalanges.

Pelvis

- Develops from three separate bones (ilium, ischium, and pubis) on each side that eventually fuse into a solid structure (Fig. 6.56)
- The names of the separate bones are used to indicate the main regions of the pelvis
- The **ilium** is the cranial-most area of the pelvis
- The **ischium** is the caudal-most area of the pelvis
- The **pubis** is located medially and forms the cranial part of the pelvic floor (the ischium forms the caudal part)
- The concave **acetabulum** on the lateral surface receives the head of the femur to form the hip joint
- The two halves of the pelvis are joined ventrally by a cartilaginous joint—the pelvic symphysis
- The **obturator foramina** are two large holes on either side of the pelvic symphysis that serve to reduce the weight of the pelvis

Femur

- Long bone of the "thigh" (Fig. 6.57)
- The rounded **head** on proximal end is the ball part of the ball-and-socket hip joint
- The **neck** joins the head to the shaft
- The **greater trochanter** on proximal end is the large process to which the gluteal muscles attach
- The distal articular surfaces are rounded medial and lateral **condyles**
- The medial and lateral **epicondyles** are the "knobs" on the medial and lateral sides of the condyles
- The trochlea is a smooth articular surface on the cranial surface of the distal end in which the patella (kneecap) rides

Patella

- "Kneecap"
- Largest sesamoid bone in the body
- Located in the distal tendon of the large quadriceps femoris muscle and helps protect it as it passes down over the trochlea of the femur to insert on the tibial crest (Fig. 6.58)

Fabellae

- The medial and lateral fabellae (see Fig. 6.58) are two small sesamoid bones in the proximal gastrocnemius (calf) muscle tendons of dogs and cats
- Located just proximal to (above) and caudal to (behind) the femoral condyles

Tibia

- Main weight-bearing bone of the lower leg
- The proximal end forms the stifle joint with the femur and the distal end forms the hock joint with the tarsus

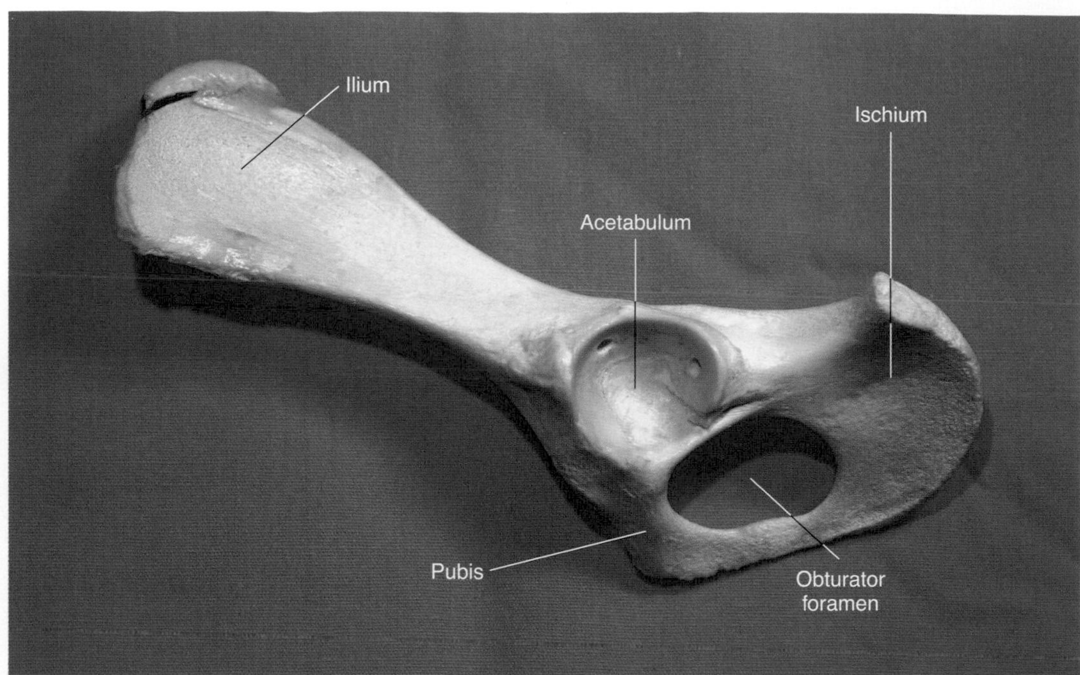

• **Fig. 6.56** Canine pelvis. (Left lateral view.)

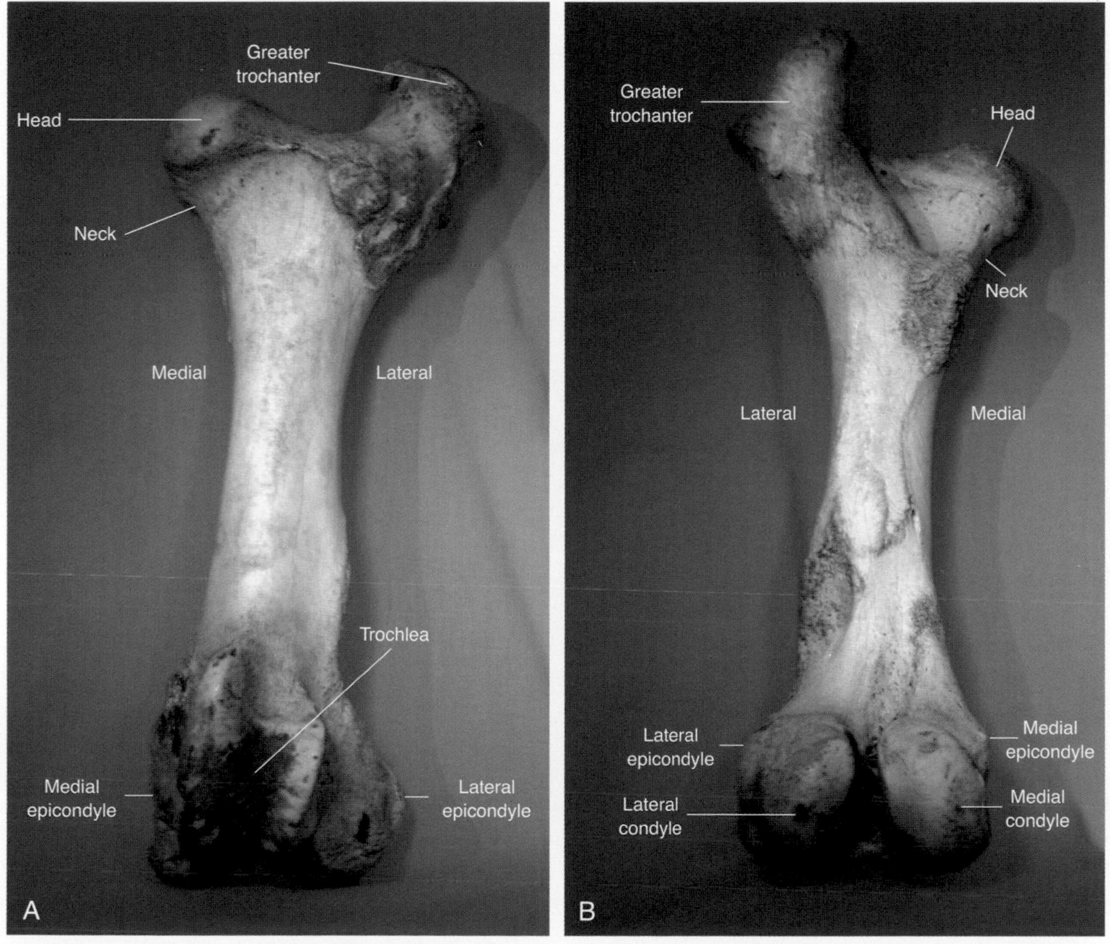

• **Fig. 6.57** Bovine left femur. (A) Cranial view. (B) Caudal view.

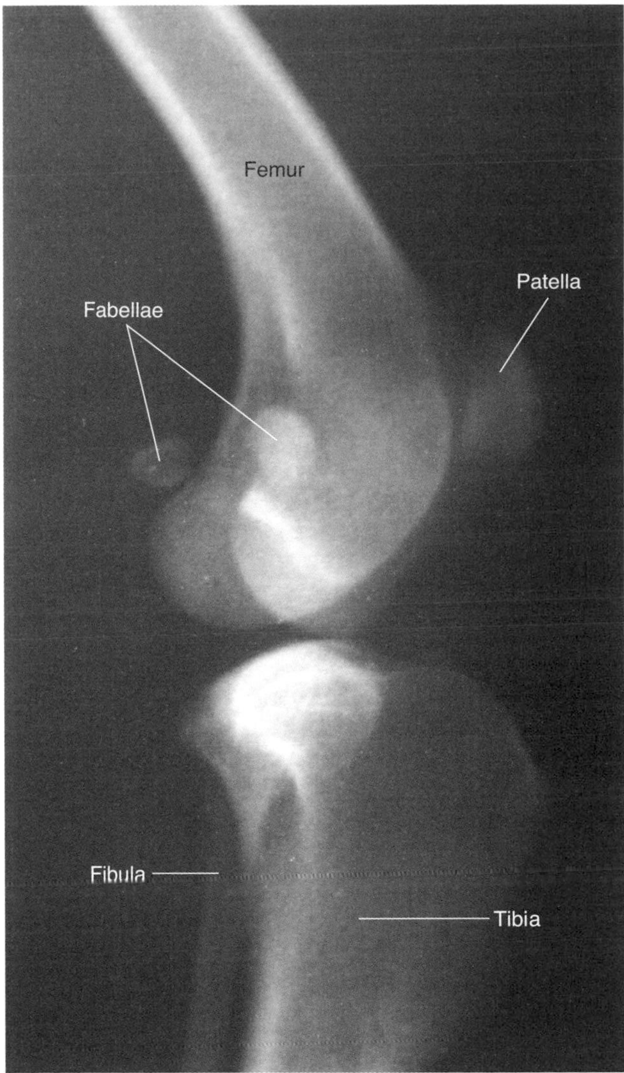

• **Fig. 6.58** Patella and fabellae. Radiograph of canine stifle.

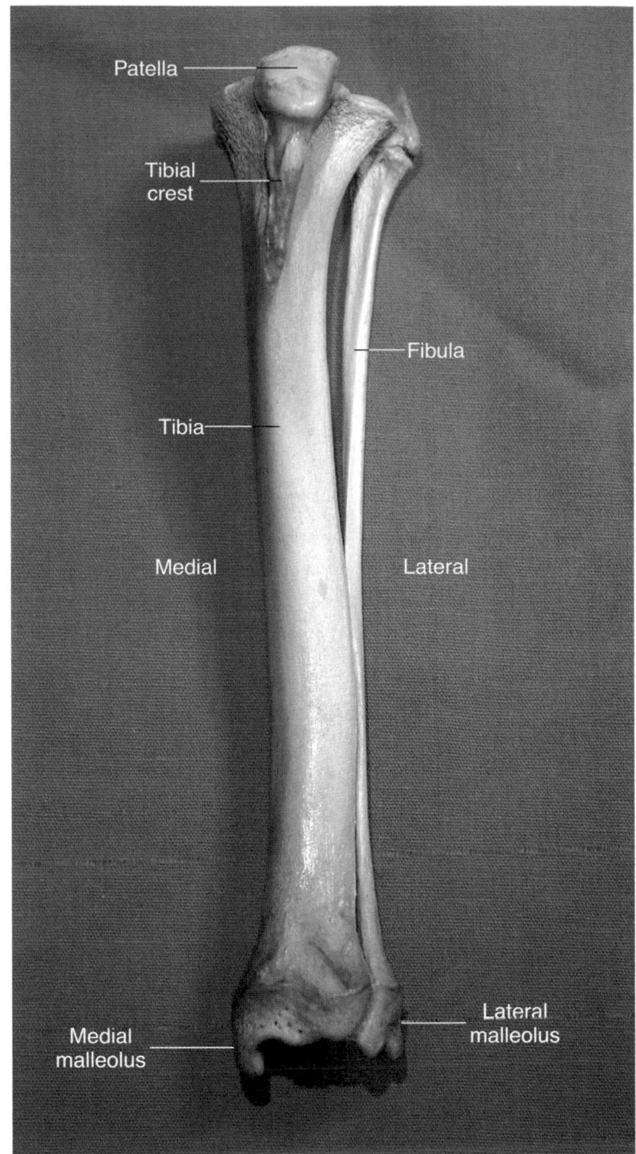

• **Fig. 6.59** Canine left tibia and fibula. (Cranial view.)

- Concave tibial **condyles** on the proximal end articulate with the condyles of the femur
- Proximal end looks triangular when viewed from above, with the apex, the tibial tuberosity, pointed forward; the patellar tendon attaches to the tibial tuberosity
- The **tibial crest** is a ridge of bone that continues distally from the **tibial tuberosity**
- The **medial malleolus** is a medially facing rounded process on the distal end of the tibia (the "knob" on the medial side of our ankle is our medial malleolus)

Fibula

- Thin but complete bone in dog and cat (Fig. 6.59)
- Incomplete in horses and cattle—only the proximal and distal ends are present
- Does not support significant weight
- Serves as muscle attachment site and helps form a stable joint distally with tarsus
- The **lateral malleolus** is the laterally facing rounded process on the distal end of the fibula (the lateral "knob" on our ankle is our lateral malleolus)

Tarsal Bones (Tarsus, Hock)

- Located immediately distal to the tibia and fibula
- Equivalent to the human ankle
- Consist of two rows of short bones
- Bones in the proximal row are named—large tibial tarsal and fibular tarsal, and small central tarsal
- The tibial tarsal bone has a large, rounded trochlea that articulates with the distal end of the tibia to form the most movable part of the hock joint
- The large **calcaneus** (calcaneal tuberosity) projects upward and backward to form the point of the hock; this is

the attachment site for the tendon of the large gastrocnemius muscle and corresponds to our heel
- Bones in the distal row are numbered from medial to lateral, in a similar fashion to the distal row of carpal bones

Metatarsal Bones
- Similar to metacarpal bones
- Extend distally from the distal row of tarsal bones to the proximal phalanges of the digits
- Dogs and cats typically have four metatarsal bones, numbered from medial (II) to lateral (V)
- Ruminants have a large metatarsal bone (commonly called the **cannon bone**) formed from two fused bones—metatarsals III and IV. A longitudinal groove shows its two-bone origin
- Horses have a single large metatarsal bone (metatarsal III, commonly called the cannon bone) with two small, incomplete metatarsal bones on either side (metatarsals II and IV, commonly called the **splint bones**)

Phalanges
- Similar to the phalanges of the thoracic limb (Figs. 6.60 and 6.61)
- Dog and cat hind paws typically have four digits, numbered from medial to lateral

  If digit I is present, it is commonly called the dewclaw and has two phalanges—proximal and distal.

  Digits II–V each contain three phalanges—proximal, middle, and distal.

  The distal phalanx contains the ungual process that is surrounded by the claw.

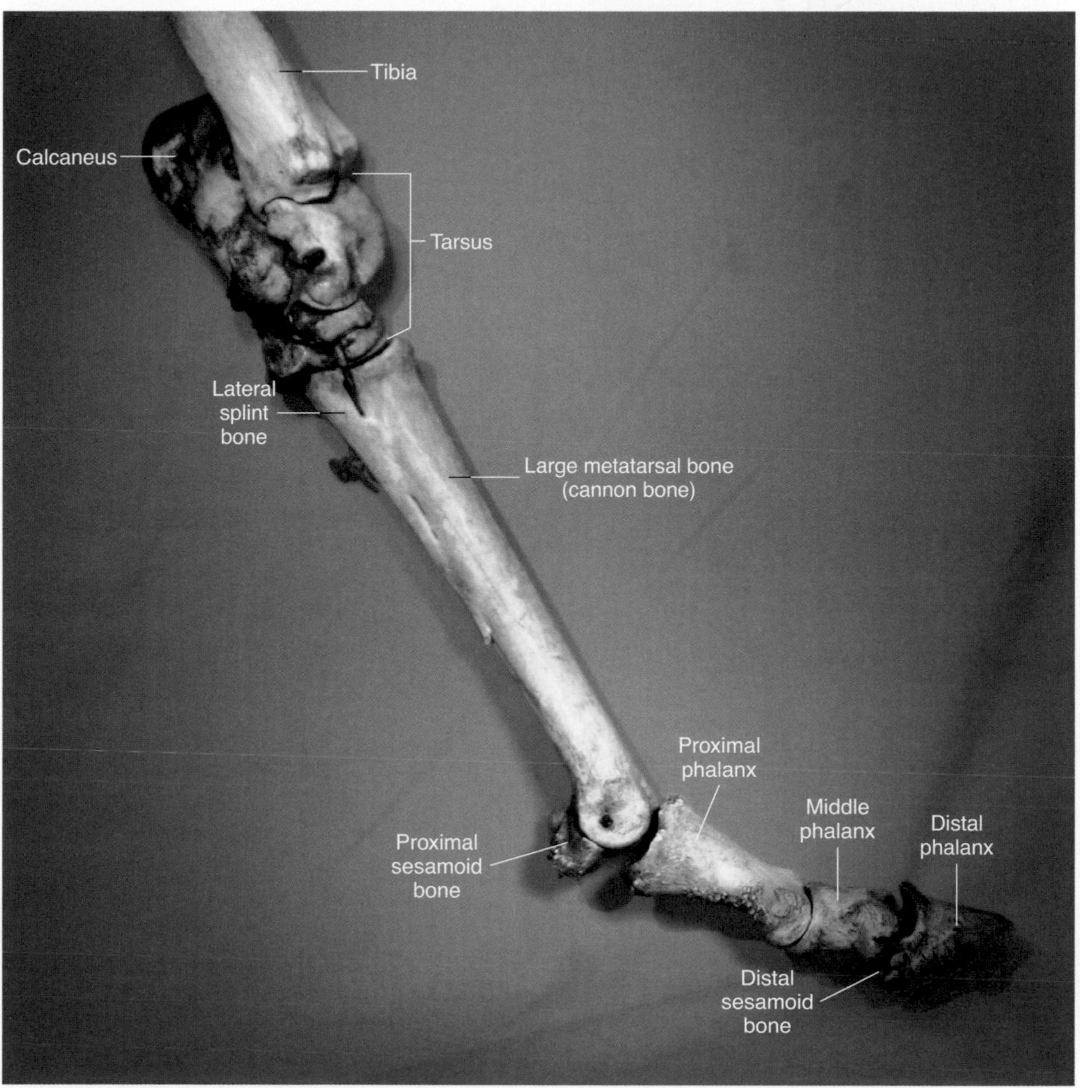

• **Fig. 6.60** Equine left hind leg. This is the distal portion of the hind leg of a horse, from the distal part of the tibia to the distal phalanx.

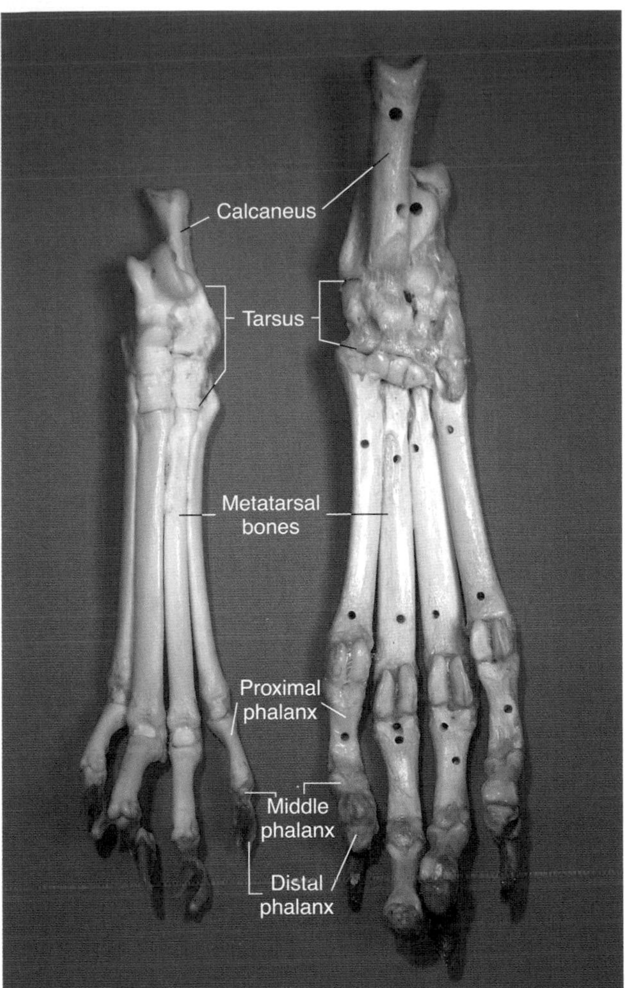

• **Fig. 6.61** Feline (dorsal view) and canine (plantar view) hind feet.

- Ruminants have four digits on each limb
  Two support weight (III and IV).
  Two are smaller non–weight-bearing "dewclaws" (II and V).
  Weight-bearing digits each contain three phalanges—proximal, middle, and distal.
  Weight-bearing digits each contain two proximal sesamoid bones on the plantar surface of the joint between the metatarsal and the proximal phalanx, and one distal sesamoid bone on the plantar surface of the joint between the middle and distal phalanges.
- Horses have one digit on each limb, composed of three phalanges and three sesamoid bones
  The phalanges are the proximal phalanx (common name: long pastern bone), middle phalanx (common name: short pastern bone), and distal phalanx (common name: coffin bone).
  Two **proximal sesamoid bones** are located on the plantar surface of the joint between the metatarsal and the proximal phalanx.
  A single **distal sesamoid bone** (common name: navicular bone) is located on the plantar surface of the joint between the middle and distal phalanges.

Joints

Joints are where bones connect with each other. The three types of joints in the animal body are immovable **fibrous** joints, slightly movable **cartilaginous** joints, and freely movable **synovial** joints.

Fibrous Joints

- Also known as synarthroses
- Bones are firmly united by fibrous tissue
- Allow no movement
- Examples: sutures uniting most of the skull bones (Fig. 6.62)

Cartilaginous Joints

- Also known as amphiarthroses
- Bones are united by fibrocartilage
- Allow slight rocking movement
- Examples: pelvic symphysis, mandibular symphysis (Fig. 6.63)

Synovial Joints

- Also known as diarthroses
- Allow free movement
- Characteristics:
  Smooth articular surfaces covered with smooth articular cartilage
  Joint capsule surrounds joint cavity that contains synovial fluid
  Ligaments (fibrous connective tissue) may connect the bones together
  (Note: ligaments connect bones to other bones; tendons connect muscles to bones)
- Types:
  Hinge joint—e.g., elbow, joints of digits (Fig. 6.64)
  Gliding joint—e.g., carpus (Fig. 6.65)
  Pivot joint—e.g., atlantoaxial joint (joint between C1 and C2 vertebrae) (Fig. 6.66)
  Ball-and-socket joint—e.g., shoulder and hip (Fig. 6.67)
- Movements possible:
  Flexion—decreased angle between the bones
  Extension—increased angle between the bones
  Adduction—movement of an extremity toward the median plane (inward)
  Abduction—movement of an extremity away from the median plane (outward)
  Rotation—twisting (rotational) movement
  Circumduction—movement of an extremity so the distal end moves in a circle

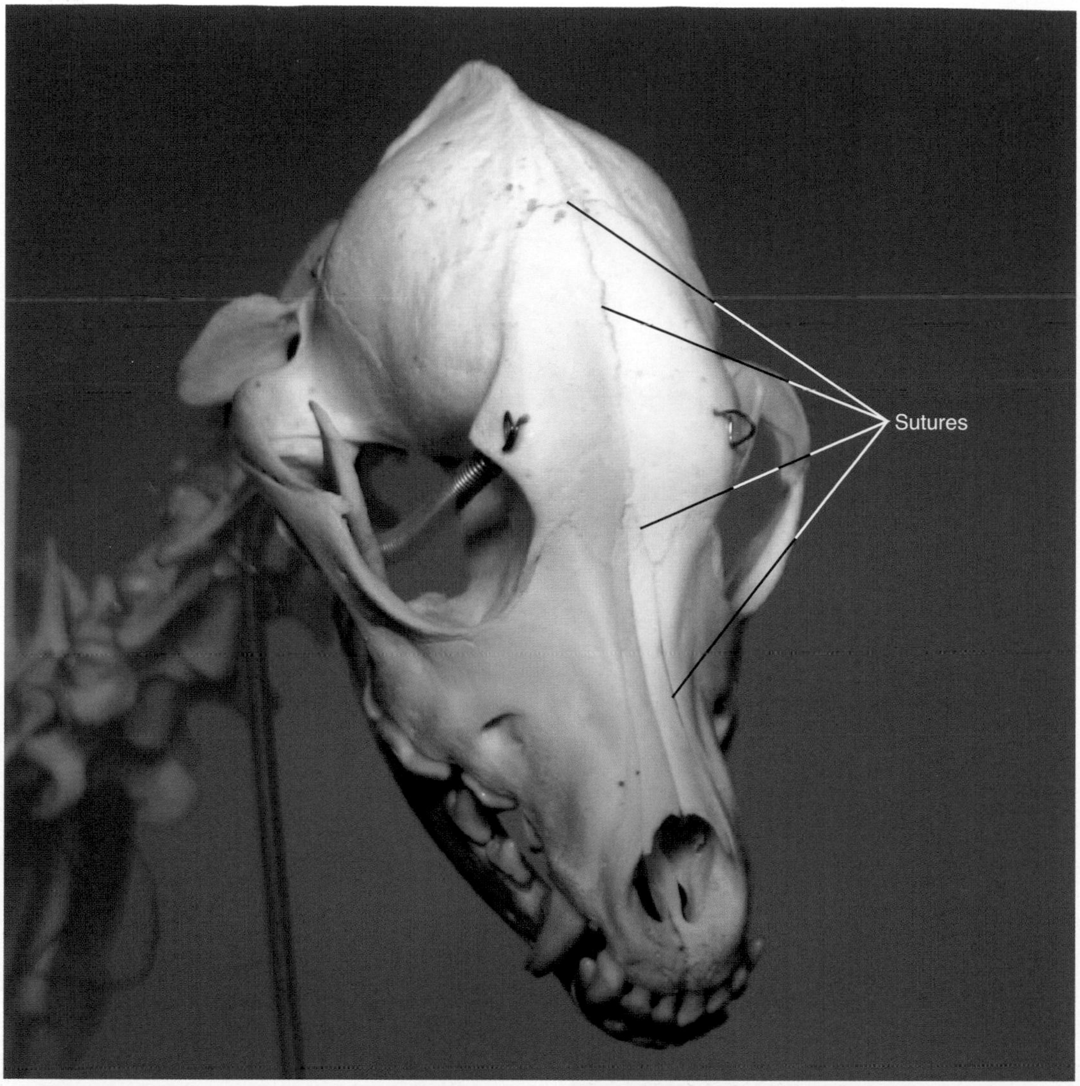

• **Fig. 6.62** Canine skull. The sutures that hold most of the skull bones together are examples of fibrous joints.

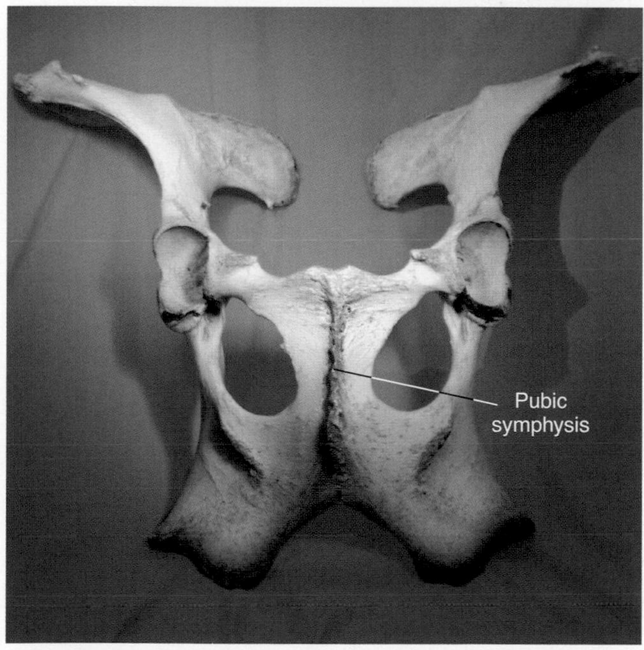

• **Fig. 6.63** Bovine pelvis. The two halves of the pelvis are joined together by the pelvic symphysis, a cartilaginous joint (ventral view).

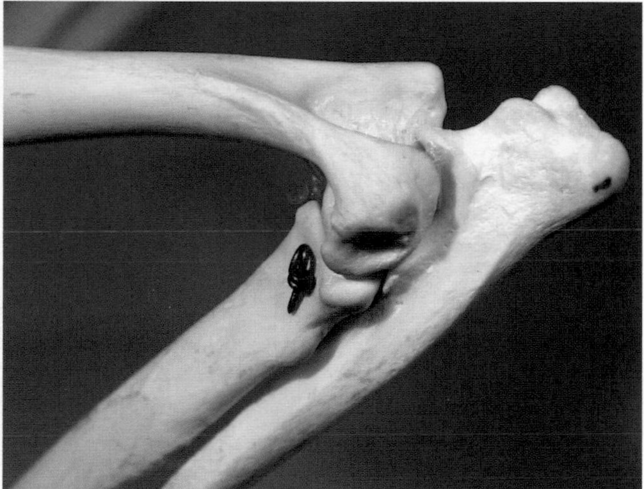

• **Fig. 6.64** Canine elbow joint. This is an example of a hinge joint.

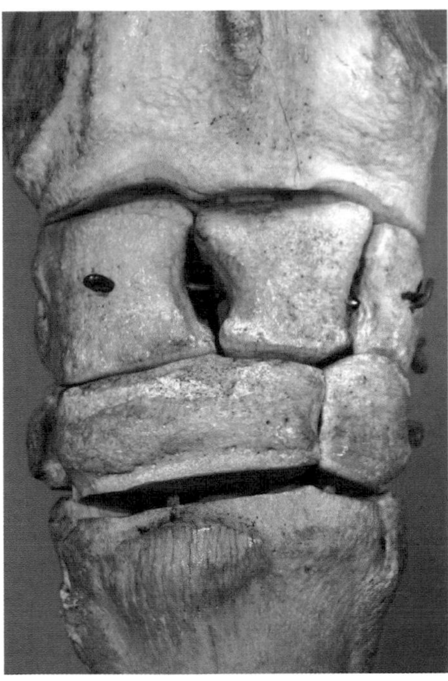

• **Fig. 6.65** Equine carpus. This is an example of a gliding joint.

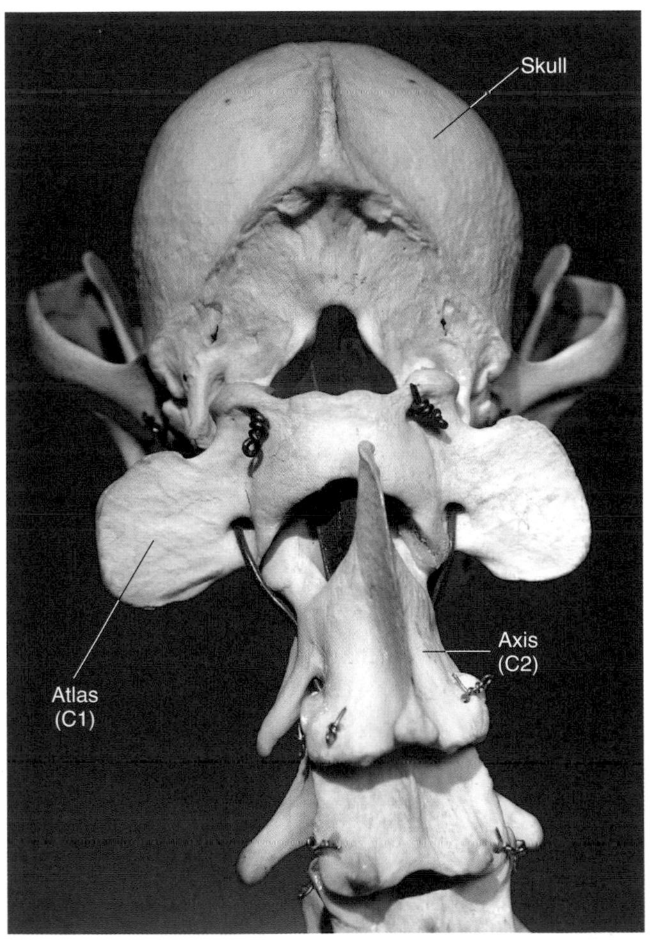

• **Fig. 6.66** Canine skull and first two cervical vertebrae. The joint between the atlas (C1) and axis (C2) cervical vertebrae is the only true pivot joint in the animal's body.

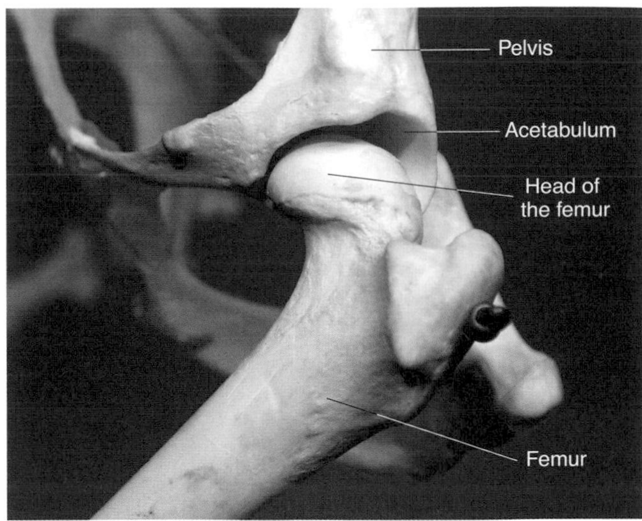

• **Fig. 6.67** Canine hip joint. This is an example of a ball-and-socket joint. The ball is the head of the femur, and the socket is the acetabulum in the pelvic bone.

SUGGESTED IN-CLASS ACTIVITIES

Bone Shapes and Features

Bone Shape and Feature Identification

Find bones that represent the various types of bone and the processes on them.

Supplies needed: disarticulated bones

Bone Shape and Feature Hunt

Students draw a shape or feature name out of a hat. They then must locate a bone on a skeleton that represents that shape or contains that feature. The student must also identify the bone.

OR

Students draw the name of a bone out of a hat. They must then locate the bone on the skeleton and identify the shape and what features the bone may possess.

Supplies needed: articulated skeleton

The Axial Skeleton

Skull Bone Identification

Students examine various skulls from different species of animal, identifying the bones of the skull.

Supplies needed: various skulls

Live Animal Palpation

Students palpate and identify the bones of the skull on live animals.

Supplies needed: live animals

Skull Bone Hunt

Students draw the name of a skull bone out of a hat. They then must locate that bone on a live animal.

Supplies needed: live animals

Vertebral Process Identification

Various vertebrae are set out. Students are to identify each vertebra by identifying the specific process types.

Supplies needed: vertebrae

Axial Assembly

Students assemble the bones of the axial skeleton in order.

Supplies needed: disarticulated skeleton

Radiographic Identification

Students identify bones of the axial skeleton on radiographs.

Supplies needed: radiographs

Live Animal Palpation

Students palpate the bones of the axial skeleton on live animals.

Supplies needed: live animals

The Appendicular Skeleton

Appendicular Limb Assembly

Students assemble, in order, both the thoracic and pelvic limbs.

Supplies needed: disarticulated skeleton

Radiographic Identification

Students identify bones of the appendicular skeleton on radiographs.

Supplies needed: radiographs

Live Animal Palpation

Students palpate the bones of the appendicular skeleton on live animals.

Supplies needed: live animals

Animals in Motion

Each student is given a laminated drawing or photograph of an animal in motion. The student is to draw the location of the bones of the animal's skeleton on the picture with an erasable marker. It is helpful to have live animals in the room for the students to position similar to their picture, then palpate for the bone locations and directions.

Supplies needed: laminated drawings and photographs of animals, erasable markers, and live animals

Appendicular Bone Hunt

Students draw the name of a bone out of a hat. They then must locate that bone on an animal skeleton and/or a live animal.

Supplies needed: various animal skeletons and live animals

EXERCISES

The Skeletal System

Exercise 1

Identify Structures of Compact and Cancellous Bone

Identify each of the compact and cancellous bone structures by labeling where indicated.

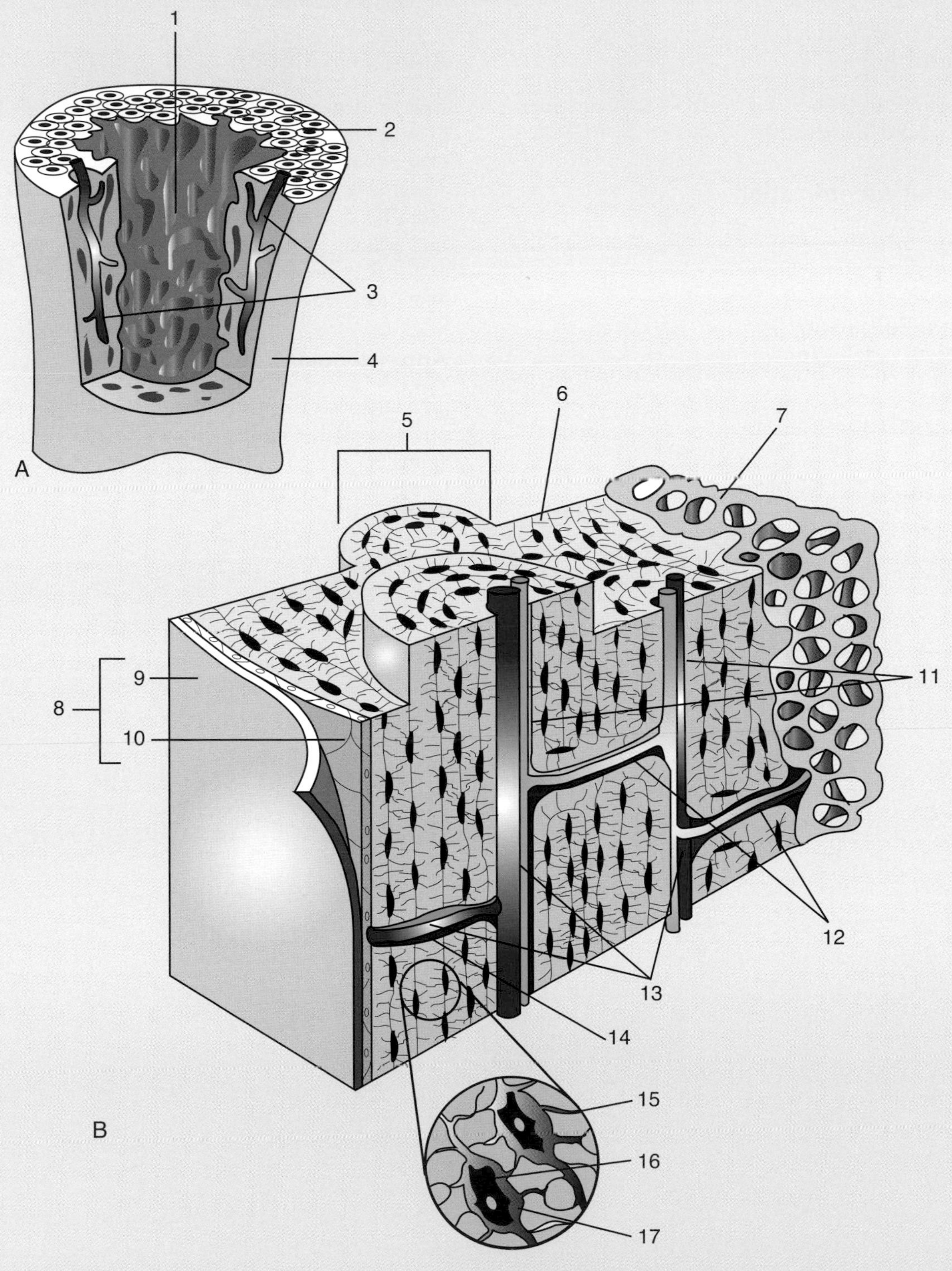

Exercise 1—cont'd

Identify Structures of Compact and Cancellous Bone

1. ______
2. ______
3. ______
4. ______
5. ______
6. ______
7. ______
8. ______
9. ______
10. ______
11. ______
12. ______
13. ______
14. ______
15. ______
16. ______
17. ______

Exercise 2

Identify Structures of Long Bone

______ 1. (What area of the bone)
______ 2. (What area of the bone)
______ 3. (What area of the bone)
______ 4. (What type of bone)
______ 5. (What normally fills this cavity)
______ 6. (What type of bone)
______ 7. (What is this line called)
______ 8. (What type of cartilage)

Exercise 3

Identify Bone Shape

For each of the bones pictured, identify the shape of the bone.

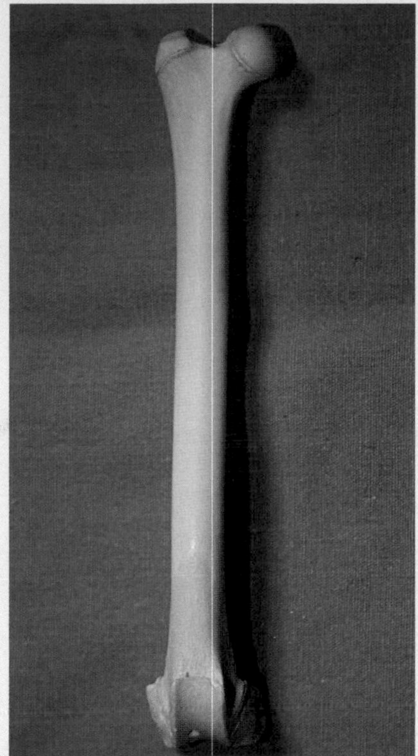

1. ______________________________

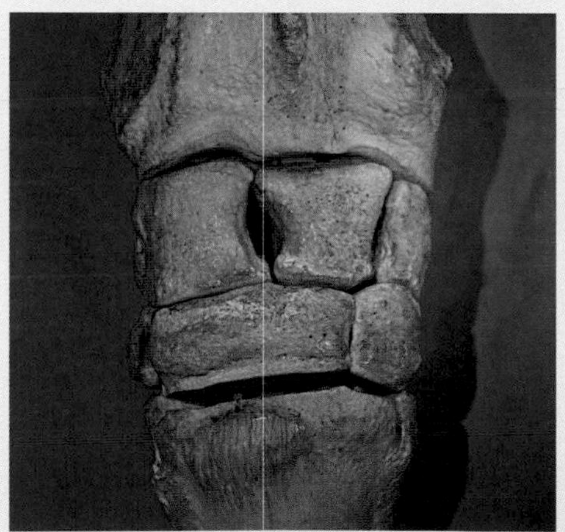

2. ______________________________

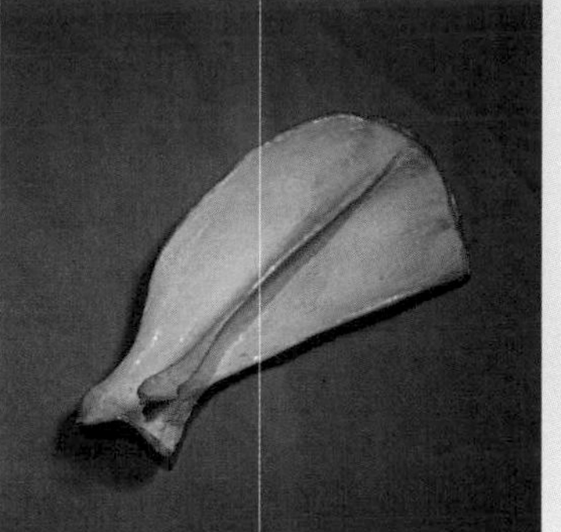

3. ______________________________

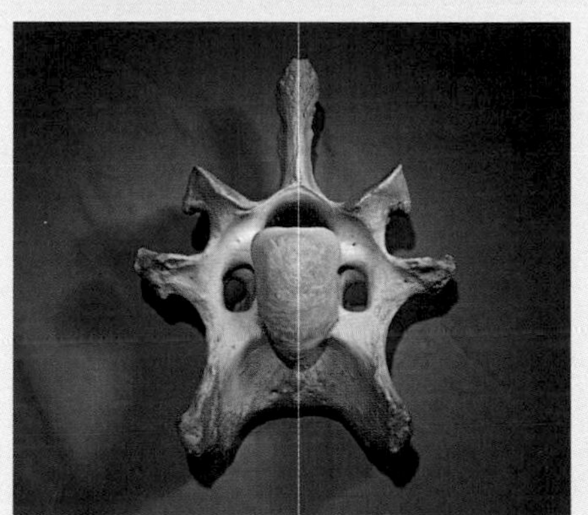

4. ______________________________

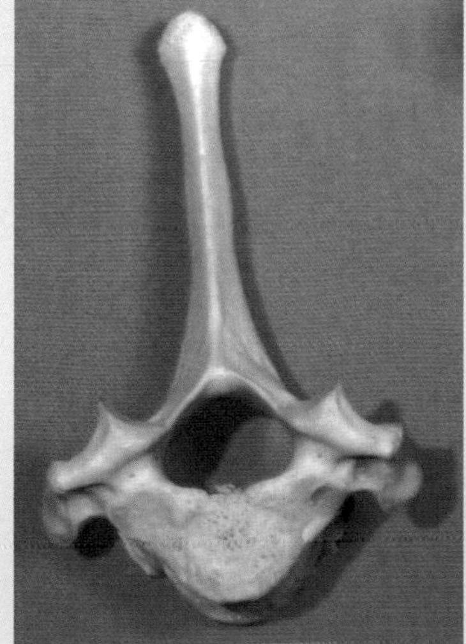

5. ______________________________

The Skeleton

Exercise 4

Identify Rabbit Skeletal Structures

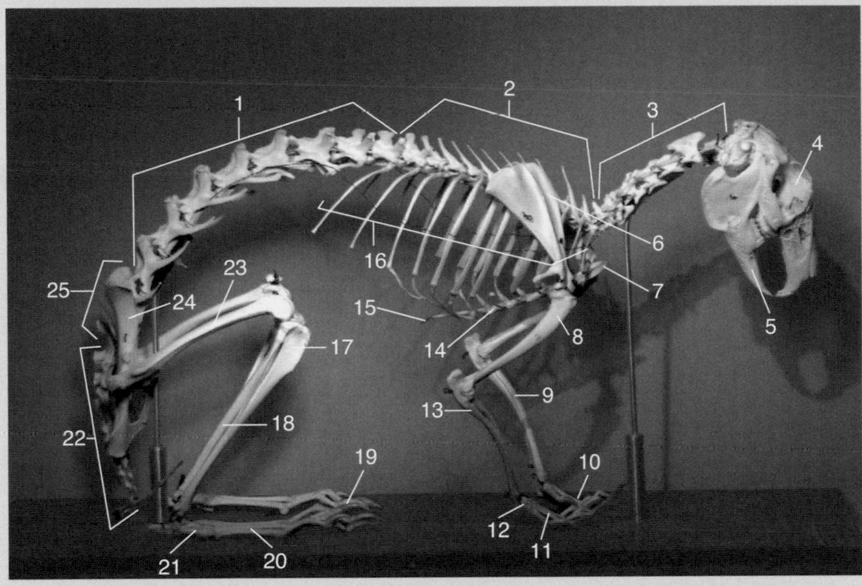

1. ______
2. ______
3. ______
4. ______
5. ______
6. ______
7. ______
8. ______
9. ______
10. ______
11. ______
12. ______
13. ______
14. ______
15. ______
16. ______
17. ______
18. ______
19. ______
20. ______
21. ______
22. ______
23. ______
24. ______
25. ______

Exercise 5

Identify Rat Skeletal Structures

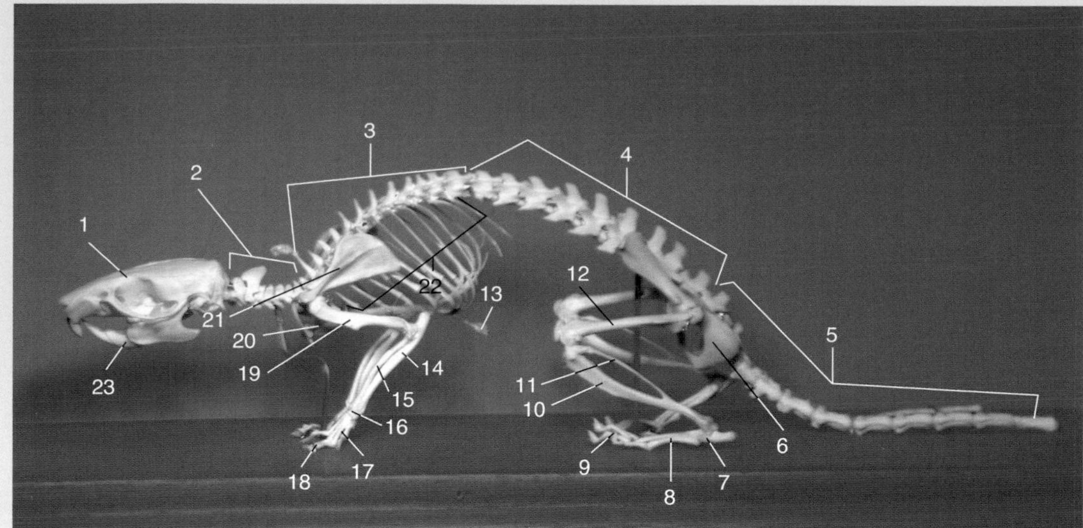

1. ______________________
2. ______________________
3. ______________________
4. ______________________
5. ______________________
6. ______________________
7. ______________________
8. ______________________
9. ______________________
10. ______________________
11. ______________________
12. ______________________
13. ______________________
14. ______________________
15. ______________________
16. ______________________
17. ______________________
18. ______________________
19. ______________________
20. ______________________
21. ______________________
22. ______________________
23. ______________________

Exercise 6

Identify Skeletal Features of the Cat Skull

Label the bones of the skull using the following terms:

External auditory meatus
Incisive
Interparietal
Lacrimal
Mandible
Maxilla
Nasal
Occipital
Occipital condyle
Parietal
Temporal
Tympanic bulla
Zygomatic
Zygomatic arch

Label the bones of the skull using the following terms:

Frontal
Incisal
Interparietal
Lacrimal
Maxilla
Nasal
Occipital
Orbit
Parietal
Temporal
Zygomatic arch

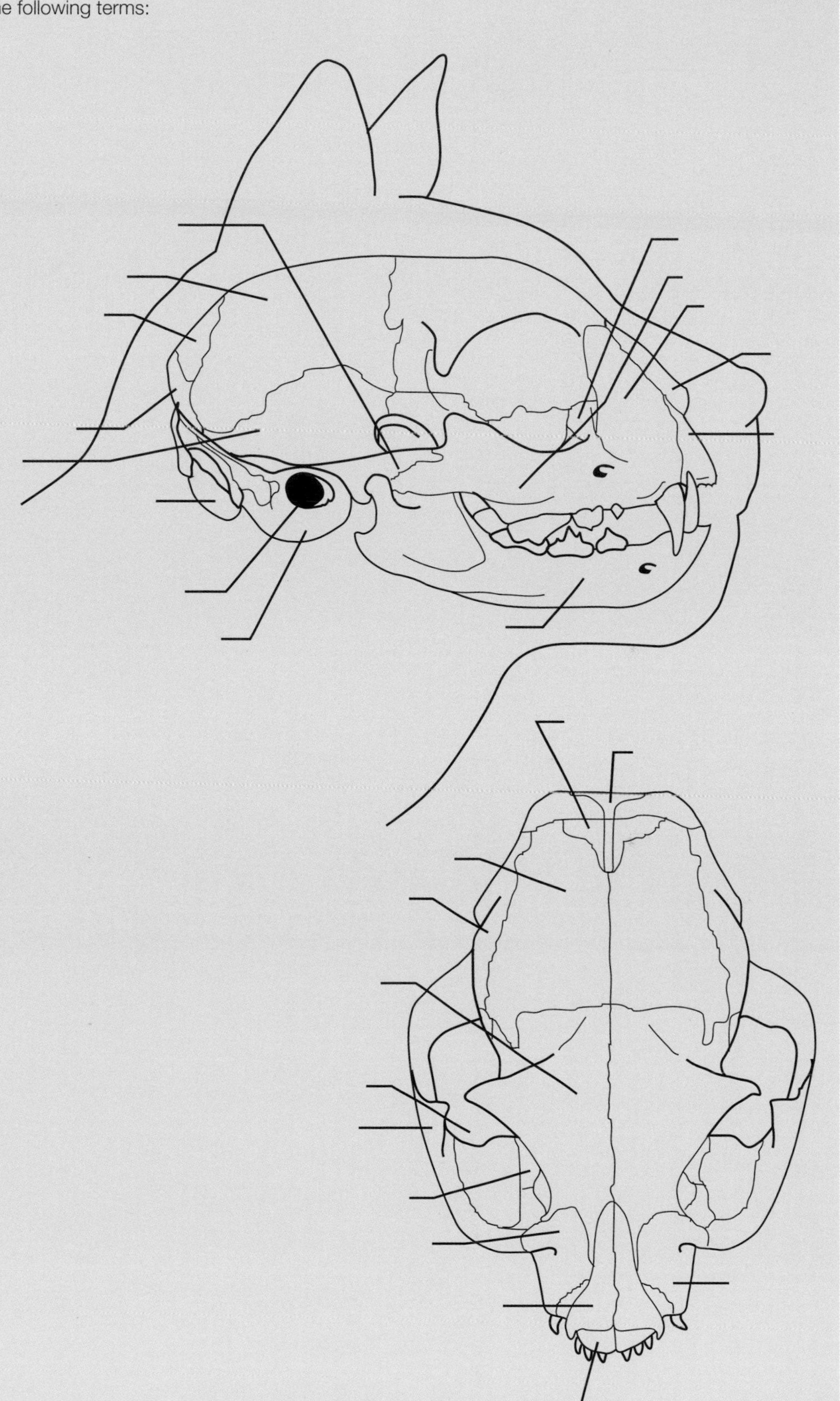

Exercise 7

Identify Bones and Processes of the Equine Thoracic Limb

__________________ 1.
__________________ 2.
__________________ 3. (Name the process)
__________________ 4. (Name the bone)
__________________ 5.
__________________ 6. (Name the bone—be specific)
__________________ 7. (Name the joint)
__________________ 8.
__________________ 9.
__________________ 10.
__________________ 11.
__________________ 12.
__________________ 13.
__________________ 14.

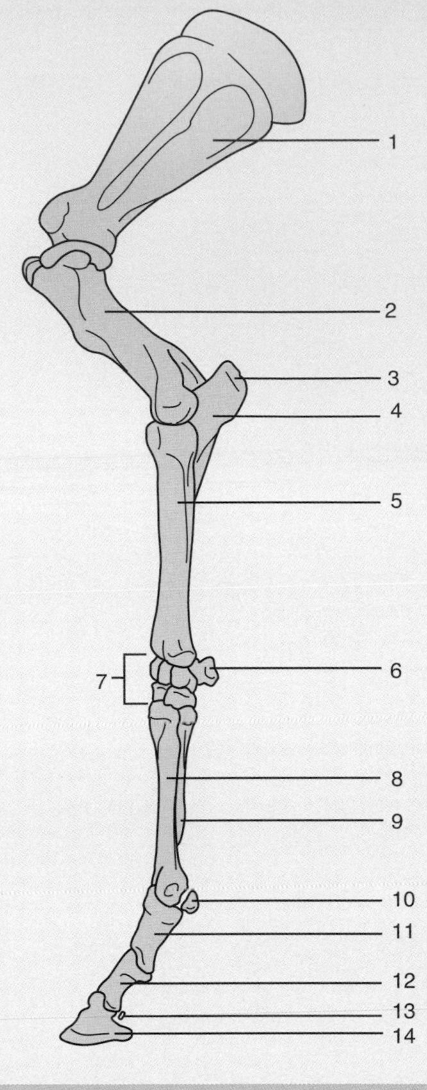

Exercise 8

Identify Bones, Joints, and Processes of the Equine Pelvic Limb

_______________ 1.
_______________ 2.
_______________ 3.
_______________ 4.
_______________ 5.
_______________ 6.
_______________ 7.
_______________ 8. (Name the process)
_______________ 9. (Name the joint)
_______________ 10.
_______________ 11.
_______________ 12.
_______________ 13.
_______________ 14.
_______________ 15.
_______________ 16.

Exercise 9

Label the Bones of the Horse Foot From Proximal to Distal

______________________ 1.
______________________ 2.
______________________ 3.
______________________ 4.
______________________ 5.

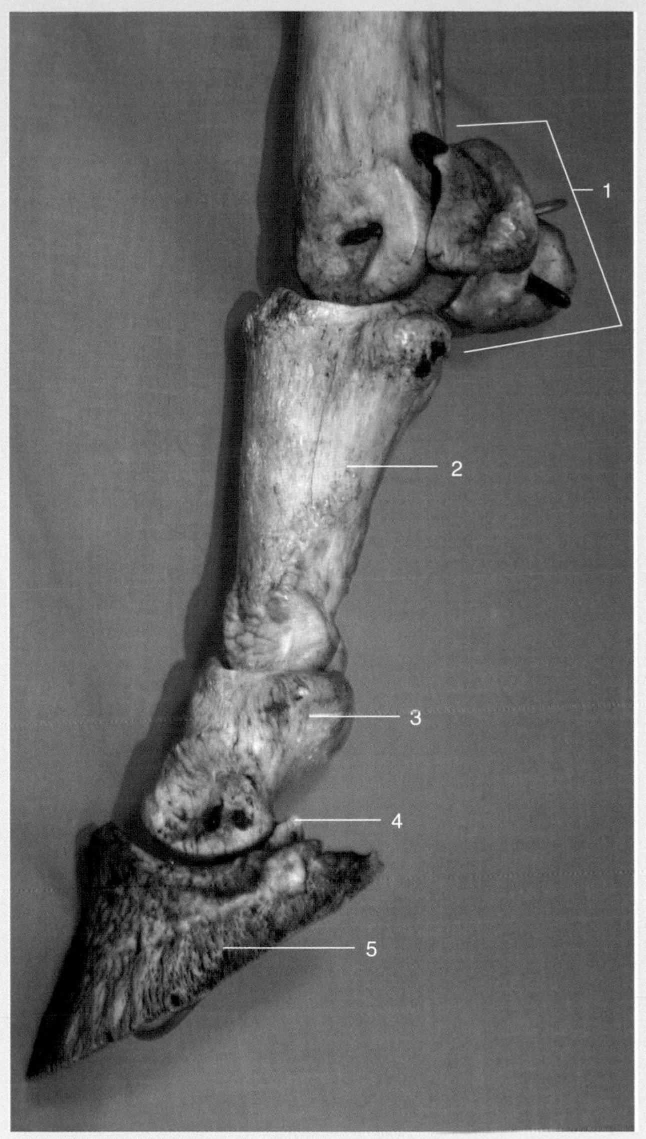

Joints

Exercise 10

Identify Joint Type

Identify each of the joint types represented here.

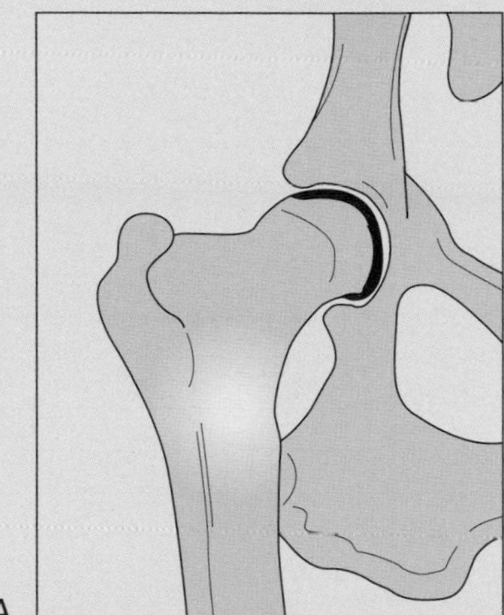

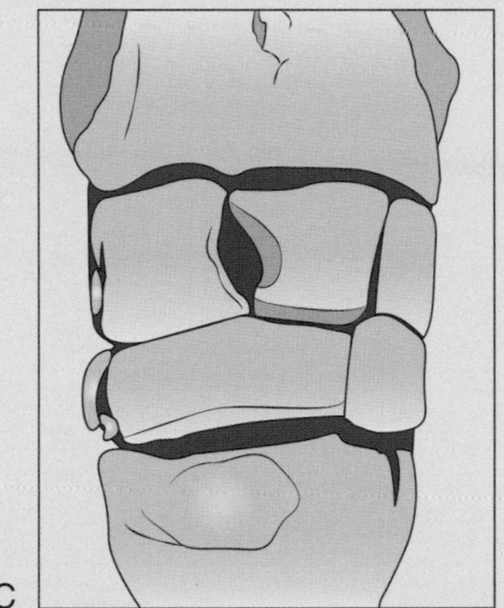

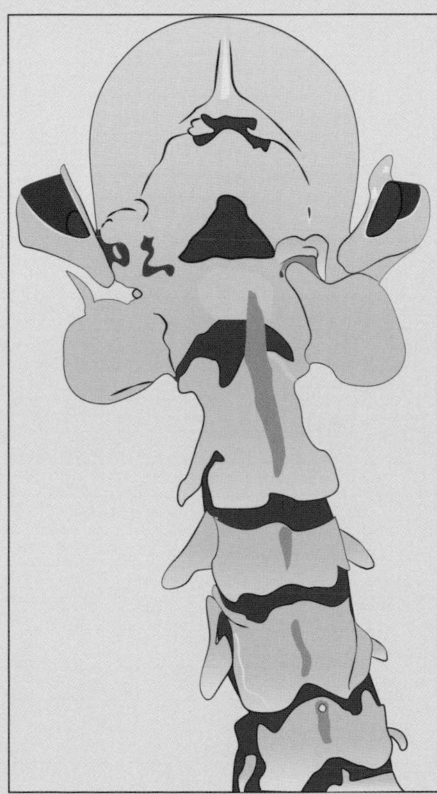

Critical and Clinical Thinking

Exercise 11

Defining Clinical Terms

Write the definition for each term.

1. Acetabulum ______
2. Articular process ______
3. Articular surface ______
4. Atlas ______
5. Axis ______
6. Calcaneus ______
7. Cancellous bone ______
8. Cannon bone ______
9. Carpus ______
10. Cartilaginous joint ______
11. Cervical vertebrae ______
12. Coccygeal vertebrae ______
13. Compact bone ______
14. Condyle ______
15. Costal cartilage ______
16. Costochondral junction ______
17. Fibrous joint ______
18. Flat bones ______
19. Foramen ______
20. Foramen magnum ______
21. Fossa ______
22. Irregular bones ______
23. Joint ______
24. Long bones ______

Exercise 11—cont'd

Defining Clinical Terms

25. Lumbar vertebrae ______________________________
26. Manubrium sterni ______________________________
27. Metacarpals ______________________________
28. Metatarsals ______________________________
29. Obturator foramina ______________________________
30. Olecranon ______________________________
31. Patella ______________________________
32. Pelvis ______________________________
33. Phalanges ______________________________
34. Process ______________________________
35. Sacral vertebrae ______________________________
36. Sesamoid bones ______________________________
37. Short bones ______________________________
38. Spinous process ______________________________
39. Splint bones ______________________________
40. Synovial joint ______________________________
41. Tarsus ______________________________
42. Thoracic vertebrae ______________________________
43. Transverse process ______________________________
44. Xiphoid process ______________________________

Exercise 12

Clinical Thinking Challenge

1. Name the four functions of bone.
   1. ______________________________
   2. ______________________________
   3. ______________________________
   4. ______________________________
2. ____________________ The ulna is an example of a/an _______ bone.
3. ____________________ A vertebra is an example of a/an _______ bone.
4. ____________________ The carpal bones are examples of _______ bones.
5. ____________________ The parietal bone in the skull is an example of a/an _______ bone.
6. ____________________ Name an example of a flat bone.
7. ____________________ Name an example of an irregular bone not found in the axial skeleton.
8. What bones make up the axial skeleton?

   ____

   ____
9. ____________________ The appendicular skeleton is made up of the _____ and ______.
10. ____________________ The bones of the front leg make up the _____ limb.
11. ____________________ The bones of the back leg make up the _____ limb.
12. ____________________ What attaches skeletal muscles to bones?
13. Explain where the epiphyseal plates are located in a long bone.

    ____

    ____
14. ____________________ What does the epiphyseal plate allow the bone to do?
15. ____________________ Another name for the epiphyseal plate is _______.
16. ____________________ The bones of the cranium and the bones of the face make up the _______.
17. ____________________ Skull bones that make up most of the upper jaw.
18. ____________________ Lower jaw.
19. ____________________ Skull bones that form the dorsolateral portion of the cranium.
20. ____________________ Bones of the "temple" area of the skull that also contain middle and inner ear structures.
21. ____________________ Bones of the "forehead" region of the skull.
22. ____________________ Bone that forms the "base" of the skull and articulates with the first cervical vertebra.
23. ____________________ Skull bones that form the "bridge of the nose."
24. ____________________ Thin, scroll-like bones found inside the nasal cavity of the skull.
25. ____________________ "Cheek bones" of the skull, made up of processes from the zygomatic and temporal bones.
26. ____________________ The tail vertebrae.
27. ____________________ The second cervical vertebra.
28. ____________________ Vertebrae that are the largest in size and also support the abdominal region.
29. ____________________ Fused vertebrae of the pelvic region.
30. ____________________ The first cervical vertebra articulates with the skull.
31. ____________________ Vertebrae that articulate with the ribs.
32. ____________________ Vertebrae in the neck.
33. ____________________ What distinguishing processes does the atlas possess?
34. ____________________ What distinguishing process does the axis possess?
35. ____________________ The _______ joins the ribs to the sternum.

Exercise 12—cont'd

Clinical Thinking Challenge

36. Name all the bones of the thoracic limb in order from proximal to distal.

____

____

37. ____________ The socket portion of the shoulder joint.
38. ____________ The main weight-bearing bone of the "lower arm."
39. ____________ These bones make up the joint that is the equivalent of our "wrist."
40. ____________ "Finger" or digit bones.
41. ____________ The long bone of the "forearm" that has a proximal process that is the point of the elbow.
42. ____________ Shoulder blade.
43. ____________ The "hand" bones.
44. ____________ The long bone in the "upper arm."
45. ____________ The point of the elbow.
46. ____________ What bone is partly or completely removed during feline declaw surgery?
47. Name all the bones of the pelvic limb from proximal to distal.

____

____

48. ____________ The socket portion of the hip joint.
49. ____________ The small, long bone of the "lower leg."
50. ____________ These bones make up the "ankle" or "hock."
51. ____________ "Toe" or digit bones.
52. ____________ The large, long bone of the "lower leg."
53. ____________ Part of the pelvic limb. Made up of three pairs of bones that are fused together.
54. ____________ The "foot" bones.
55. ____________ The long bone in the upper "thigh" region.
56. What three fused pairs of bones make up the pelvis?

____

____

57. What is the purpose of the obturator foramen?

____

____

58. ____________ and ____________ What are the anatomic names of the two splint bones in the thoracic limb of a horse?
59. ____________ The equivalent of our "heel" bone, the large process that forms the point of the hock.
60. ____________ The name for a joint that allows free movement.
61. ____________ The name for a joint that allows only a slight rocking movement.
62. ____________ The name for a joint that does not allow any movement.

7 The Muscular System[a]

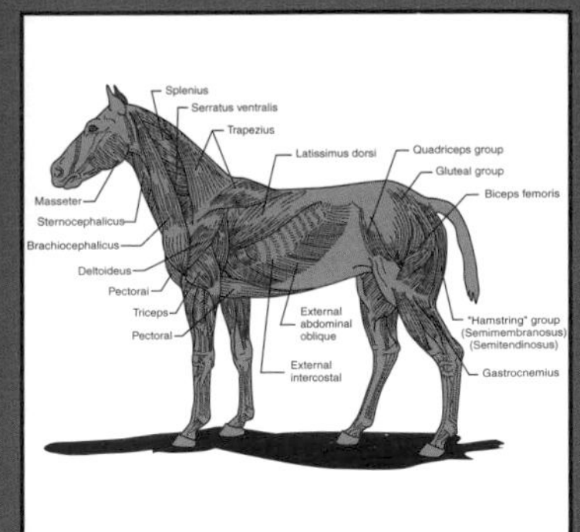

OVERVIEW AT A GLANCE

Laboratory I 149

Extrinsic Muscles of the Thoracic Limb and Related Areas 149

Extrinsic Muscles of the Thoracic Limb 152

Muscles of the Neck and Head 155

Muscles of Mastication 157

Suggested In-Class Activity 158

Laboratory II 159

Intrinsic Muscles of the Thoracic Limb 159

Suggested In-Class Activity 173

Laboratory III 173

Muscles of the Pelvic Limb 173

Muscles of the Abdominal Wall 189

Exercises 192–203

Laboratory I: Extrinsic Muscles of the Thoracic Limb and Related Areas 192–194

1. *Identify and Color Muscles in the Cat 192*
2. *Identify Muscle Name, Origin, Insertion, and Action 194*

Laboratory II: Intrinsic Muscles of the Thoracic Limb 194–198

3. *Identify and Color Intrinsic Muscles 194*
4. *Identify and Describe Muscles and Terms 196*
5. *Identify Muscle Name, Origin, Insertion, and Action 198*

Laboratory III: Muscles of the Pelvic Limb and Abdominal Wall 199–202

6. *Identify and Color Muscles of the Pelvic Limb 199*
7. *Identify Muscle Name, Origin, Insertion, and Action 202*

Critical and Clinical Thinking 203

8. *Clinical Thinking Challenge 203*

LEARNING OBJECTIVES

On completion of this lab series, the student will be able to:

- Identify the muscles used for locomotion and support in the preserved cat.
- Compare those muscles noted on the preserved cat to the live animal.
- Describe the action of the muscles studied.
- Determine what muscles are involved when giving an intramuscular injection.
- Locate nerves that must be avoided when giving intramuscular injections.

CLINICAL SIGNIFICANCE

Survival of any being, human or animal, depends on the ability to maintain a relatively constant internal environment, an ability that often relies on body movement. Muscles supply energy, and that energy turns into motion. The architecture of the body is supplied by the skeletal system; working together with the muscular system, the bones and joints provide the flexibility, agility, and necessary movements to sustain life. Understanding the muscular system can provide cues and clues to determining health and disease, whether chronic or acute, and movement is one of the most easily observed physical characteristics.

INTRODUCTION

When we hear the word *muscle* we usually think of large muscles, like the biceps or gluteal muscles. Actually, three different types of muscle make up the muscular system: *skeletal muscle* (the most familiar kind), *cardiac muscle,* and *smooth muscle.* Read Chapter 8 in *Clinical Anatomy and Physiology for Veterinary Technicians* for a description of the muscle types.

A general knowledge of muscles is important to have when performing clinical exams and administering drugs by injection.

[a]The authors and publisher wish to acknowledge Ronald J. Epps for previous contributions to this chapter.

INTRODUCTION—cont'd

Skeletal muscles can be divided into two major groups: those that attach a limb to the body (called extrinsic muscles) and those that attach to bones within the limb itself (called intrinsic muscles).

During the dissection of the cat, the student will systematically examine the muscles of the head, neck, forelimb, pelvic limb, thorax, and abdomen. Where appropriate, these areas will be compared to those of other species of animals that are routinely seen in practice.

- In Laboratory I, extrinsic muscles of the thoracic limb and muscles of the head and neck will be discussed.
- Laboratory II covers intrinsic muscles of the thoracic limb.
- In Laboratory III, intrinsic and extrinsic muscles of the pelvic limb and abdominal muscles are addressed.

MATERIALS NEEDED

Cat in preservation fluid
Exam gloves and lab coat
Dissection kit consisting minimally of:
- Scalpel handle and disposable scalpel blade
- Large dressing or thumb forceps
- Large Mayo scissors
- Blunt probes are also useful, but not required

Dissection tray
Map colors or colored pencils
A medical dictionary

LABORATORY I

Extrinsic Muscles of the Thoracic Limb and Related Areas

Items to Be Identified

The following is a list of muscles the student must be able to identify on dissected cat specimens and on anatomic drawings or photographs. The student should be careful to learn the correct spelling of each muscle. In addition, the student is responsible for being able to define the list of terms summarized as follows.

Muscles

Subcutaneous Muscle

1. Cutaneous trunci

Extrinsic Muscles

1. Superficial pectoral
2. Deep pectoral
3. Brachiocephalicus
   a. Cleidobrachialis
   b. Cleidomastoideus
   c. Cleidocervicalis
4. Omotransversarius
5. Trapezius
6. Rhomboideus
7. Latissimus dorsi
8. Serratus ventralis

Muscles of the Head and Neck

1. Sternocephalicus
2. Platysma

Muscles of Mastication

1. Temporalis
2. Masseter
3. Digastricus
4. Mylohyoideus

Terms

1. Attachments
   a. Tendon
   b. Aponeurosis
   c. Fleshy
2. Origin
3. Insertion
4. Action
5. Umbilicus
6. Mammary papilla (or teats)
7. Costal arch
8. Clavicular intersection
9. Jugular groove
10. Superficial cervical lymph node
11. Raphae

Getting Started

As each muscle is examined it is important to have an understanding of the following terms:

- **Attachment**—the junction of a skeletal muscle to bone
  - **Tendon**—an extension of the epimysium that consists of dense connective cordlike tissue
  - **Aponeurosis**—dense fibrous connective tissue much like the tendon but organized into a thin sheet of tissue
  - **Fleshy**—an apparent direct attachment of muscle to the bone; in reality, the muscle attaches to the periosteum of the bone by very short tendons

- **Origin**—the attachment at the less movable end of the muscle or usually the more proximal end
- **Insertion**—the attachment at the more movable end of the muscle; in the limbs, this is usually the most distal end
- **Action**—the body movement that a contraction of the muscle will produce

As each muscle is studied, refer to the anatomy of the skeleton to determine accurately the sites of origin and insertion for each muscle (Table 7.1). This is also an excellent way to review the skeletal anatomy of the animal.

As each muscle is isolated, concentrate on the name of the muscle, the origin and insertion of the muscle, and the action. Be sure to read the information in the lab manual before you begin dissection. Never cut into or remove any part of a muscle until instructed to do so. At the end of the lab session, wrap the cat in wet or formalin-soaked towels. Paper towels work well, but inexpensive surgical hand towels work even better because they are more absorbent and durable. Be sure your name is on the bag.

Following dissection, use the map colors to color in each muscle on the line drawings provided. Use a different color for each muscle, but color each muscle the same color in all of the drawings. For example, in every drawing you see the triceps muscle, color it purple. This will help you to learn the name and location of the muscles, their orientation in the body, and their origin and insertion.

The name of the muscle often contains descriptive information about the muscle. For example, the sternocephalicus muscle runs from the sternum (sterno-) to the head (cephalo-). If the attachments of the muscle are known, the action can usually be determined. During dissection, clean the fat and fascia off the muscle, particularly the origin and insertion, and free it from the underlying structures. Look for changes in muscle fiber orientation and the faint white lines of connective tissue that indicate the borders of the muscle. Visualize how the muscle lies within the body, what joint the muscle will affect when it contracts, and what other muscles surround it.

Before beginning the dissection, observe the following structures on the ventral aspect of the cat.

- **Umbilicus**—a small scar that will either be flat or slightly raised on the ventral midline of the abdomen about one-third of the distance from the xiphoid cartilage to the penis or vulva; the umbilicus serves as a landmark when abdominal surgery is performed.
- **Teats**—mammary papillae or mammae; the number of mammae varies. Tomcats usually have two, queens have eight, and dogs have eight to 12. They are positioned in two rows on either side of the abdomen and are usually divided into thoracic, abdominal, and inguinal.
- **Costal arch**—caudal ventral border of the rib cage formed by the costal cartilages of the 10th, 11th, and 12th ribs; the 13th rib does not attach to the costal arch.

TABLE 7.1 Name, Origin, Insertion, and Action of Extrinsic Muscles and Those of the Head and Neck

Muscle	Origin	Insertion	Action
Superficial pectoral	Cranial sternum	Greater tubercle of humerus	Adducts thoracic limb
Deep pectoral	Sternum	Greater tubercle of humerus	Adducts and pulls limb caudally
Brachiocephalicus	Clavicular intersection	Ulna, mastoid, dorsal neck	Pulls limb forward, extends shoulder
Omotransversarius	Wing of atlas	Spine and acromion of scapula	Advances leg
Trapezius muscle	Dorsal aspect of neck	Spine of scapula	Elevates and abducts limb
Rhomboideus	Occipital bone of head	Dorsal border of scapula	Elevates forelimb
Latissimus dorsi	Last 7 thoracic vertebrae and spinous process of lumbar vertebrae	Teres major tuberosity of humerus	Draws limb caudally Flexes shoulder joint
Serratus ventralis	Cervical vertebrae and ribs	Dorsomedial scapula	Supports trunk
Sternocephalicus	Sternum	Occipital bone	Draws head to side
Platysma	Tendinous raphe on dorsal midline	Attaches to muscles surrounding lips	Draws commissures of lips caudally
Temporalis	Parietal bone of skull	Coronoid process of mandible	Closes mouth when chewing
Masseter	Zygomatic arch	Lateral side of the mandible	Elevates the mandible to close the mouth when chewing
Digastricus	Occipital and temporal bones	Ventral mandible	Opens mouth
Mylohyoideus	Medial mandible	Median raphe between mandibles	Raises floor of mouth

Dissection of the Musculature

To begin the dissection, lay the cat on its right side with the head on your left. **Make the following incision through the skin only.** Incise the midline of the ventral aspect of the body, extending from the umbilicus to the most cranial aspect of the neck. Make a transverse incision from the umbilicus extending to the dorsal midline. Incise from the cranial aspect of the ventral incision dorsally, stopping at the midline. This incision should pass just caudal to the ear. Make an additional transverse incision medial to the left foreleg, extending from the midline incision transversely up the foreleg to the elbow. Make a circular incision around the elbow (Fig. 7.1).

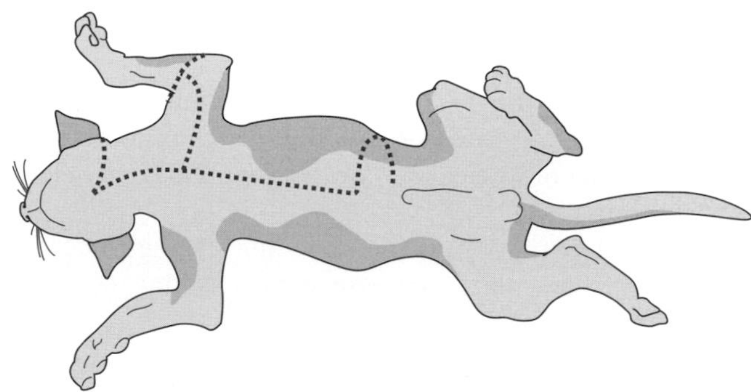

• **Fig. 7.1** Position of animal and initial skin incisions.

Reflect the flap of skin created from the left cervical, thoracic, and abdominal regions to the dorsal midline. While doing this, you will encounter the thin **cutaneous trunci** muscle (Fig. 7.2). This muscle covers the dorsal, lateral, and ventral walls of the thorax and abdomen, is tightly adherent and is not easily separated from the skin. The action of the muscle is to twitch the skin, as when an animal twitches the skin to remove flies. Use steady tension on the skin flap while using your fingers or scalpel handle to separate it bluntly from the underlying fascia.

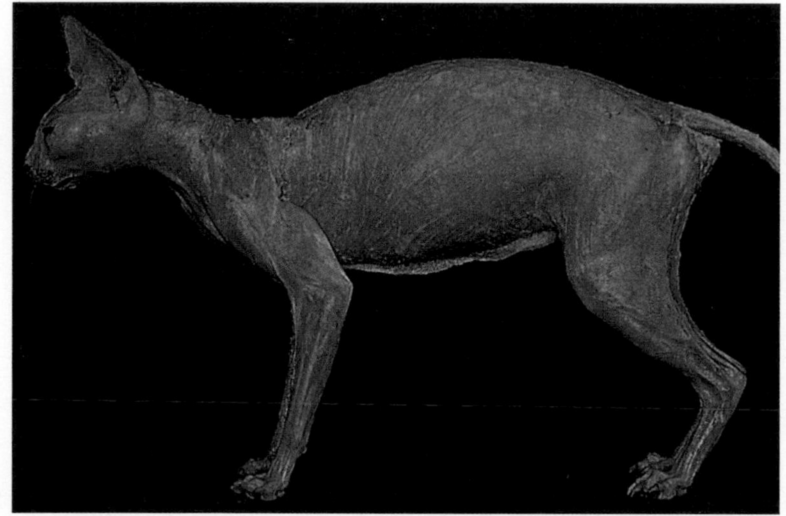

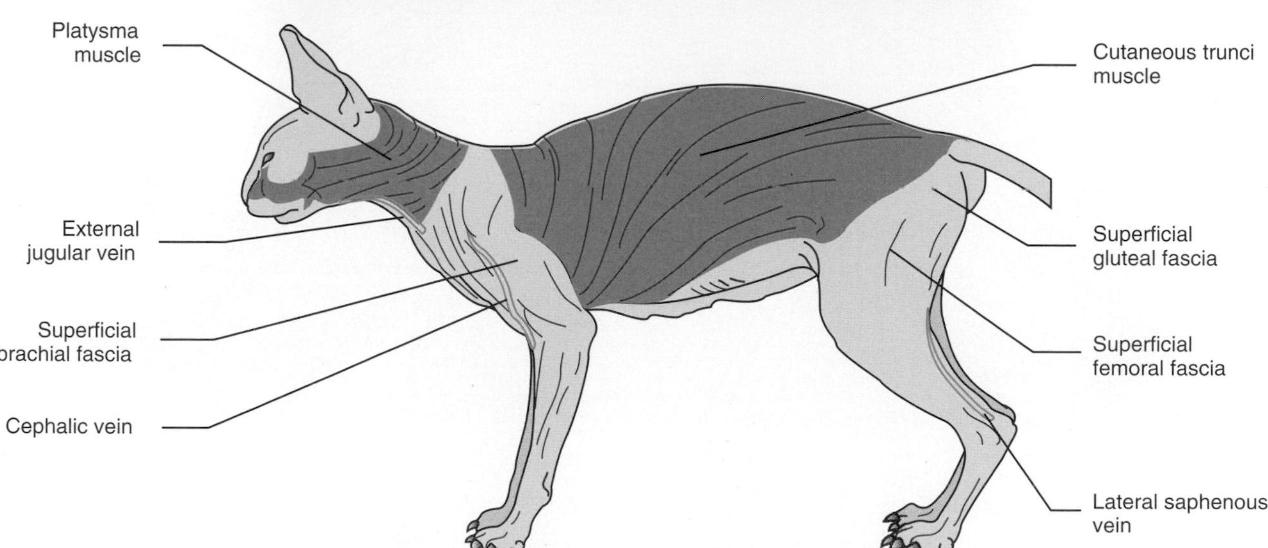

• **Fig. 7.2** Superficial muscles of the cat. (From Done SH et al: Color atlas of veterinary anatomy, vol 3, The dog and cat, London, 1996, Mosby Ltd.)

Extrinsic Muscles of the Thoracic Limb

Extrinsic muscles are those that attach the limb to the body. These muscles originate in the neck and thorax and extend to the shoulder or foreleg. All domestic mammals have eight extrinsic muscles.

The eight extrinsic muscles of the thoracic limb are:

- Superficial pectoral (transverse and descending)
- Deep pectoral
- Brachiocephalicus
- Omotransversarius
- Trapezius
- Rhomboideus
- Latissimus dorsi
- Serratus ventralis

Carefully clean the fat from the region between the forelegs on the ventral aspect of the cat. The two parts of the superficial pectoral muscle lie immediately under the skin at the cranial end of the sternum. It may be divided into a superficial descending portion and a broader transverse part.

Superficial Pectoral Muscle

It is sometimes difficult to make out both parts of this muscle (Fig. 7.3). The key is to remember that the smaller descending superficial portion arises from the first two

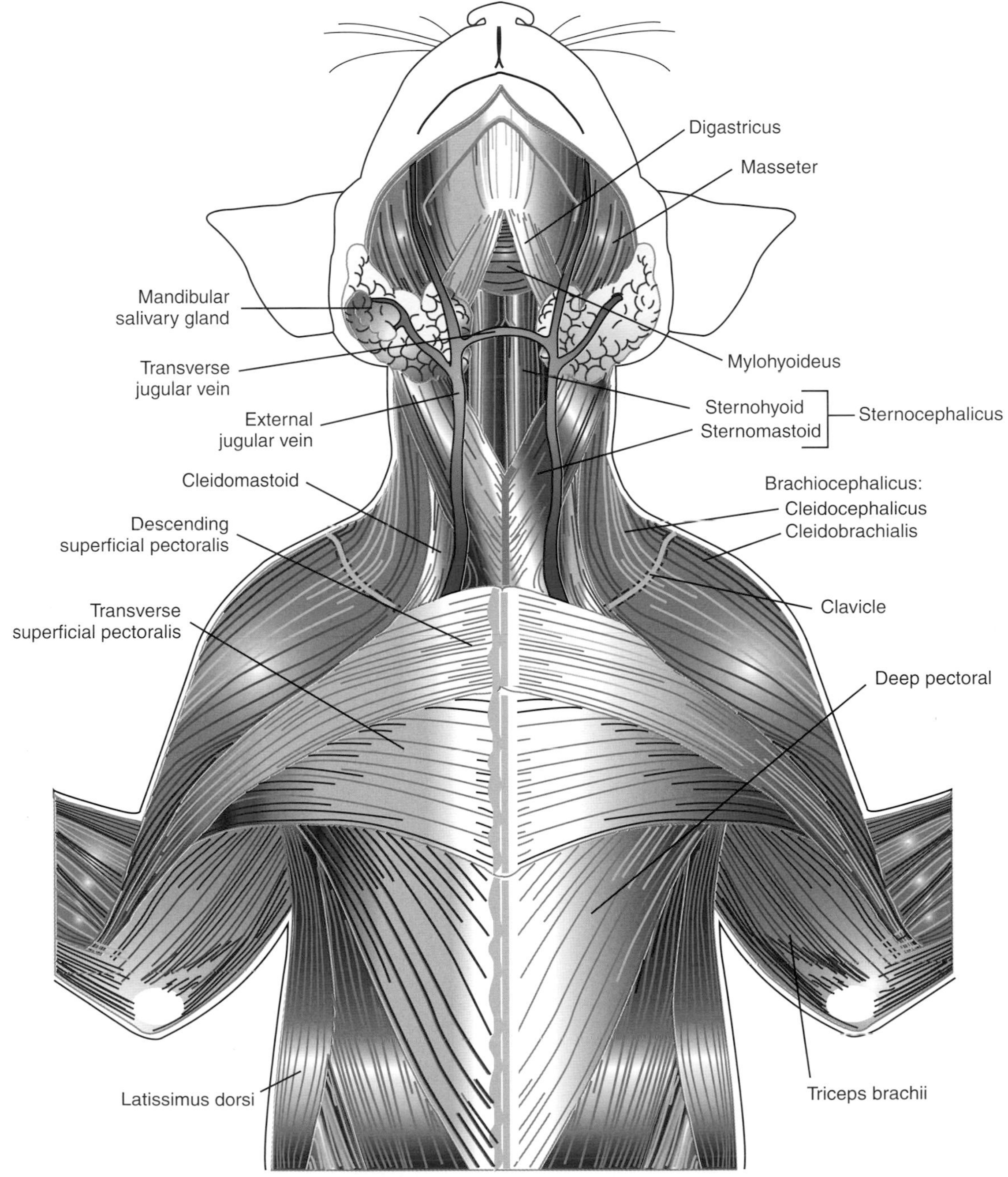

• **Fig. 7.3** Ventral aspect of thoracic and neck regions.

sternebrae, and its fibers run in a craniolateral direction, whereas the wider transverse portion of the muscle usually originates from the first three sternebrae and its fibers run more transversely.

Origin—cranial sternum; the smaller descending pectoral originates on the first two sternebrae. The larger transverse portion originates on the first two or three sternebrae

Insertion—the descending portion and the transverse portion insert on the greater tubercle of the humerus

Action—adducts the thoracic limb

Transect the superficial pectoral muscle approximately 1 to 2 cm from the sternum and reflect the cut end toward the humerus, paying particular attention to the insertion on the humerus. The insertion of the superficial pectoral muscle may be difficult to ascertain because it lies between the brachiocephalicus and the biceps brachii muscles.

Deep Pectoral Muscle

The deep pectoral muscle (see Fig. 7.3) is covered cranially by the superficial pectoral but is larger and wider than the superficial pectoral so that only the cranial portion of this muscle is covered. The deep pectoral muscle extends farther caudally where it lies immediately subcutaneously.

Origin—sternum

Insertion—crest of the greater tubercle in the cat but primarily the lesser tubercle of the humerus in the dog with some attachment to the greater tubercle

Action—adducts the limb and pulls the limb caudally

Transect the deep pectoral muscle approximately 3 cm from and parallel to the sternum and reflect the cut ends of the muscle to get a better view of the insertion.

Brachiocephalicus Muscle

Even though this muscle may appear as one muscle, it is actually a compound Y-shaped muscle with three parts (Figs. 7.3–7.5). As the name implies, this muscle runs from the foreleg (the brachium) to the head. This muscle has two major subdivisions, which are separated by a tendinous insertion in all domestic animals. This tendinous region, which is considered the origin of the brachiocephalicus muscle, is a vestige of the clavicle found in humans. The region from the clavicle to the foreleg is the cleidobrachialis,

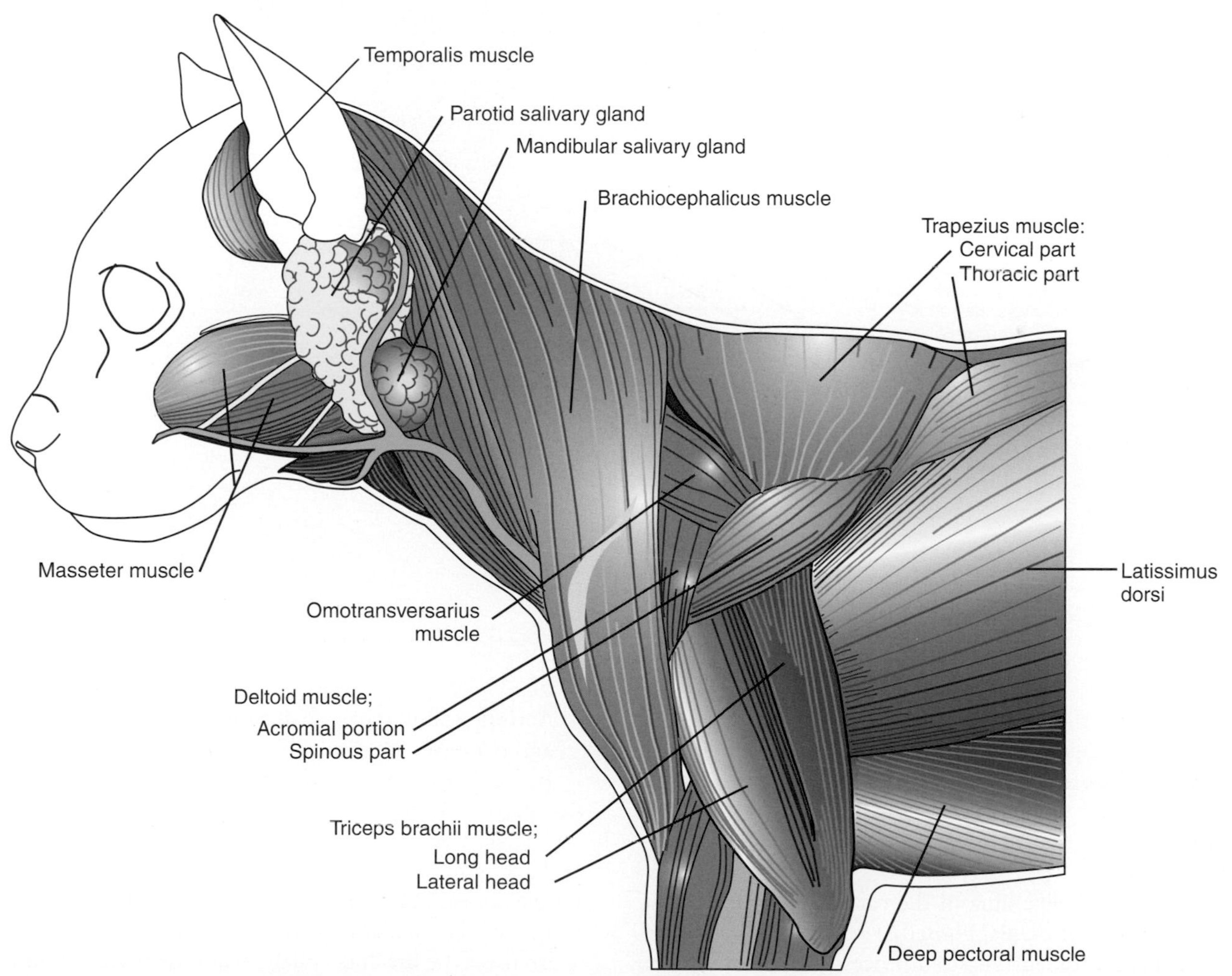

• **Fig. 7.4** Superficial muscles of the lateral thorax and proximal aspect of forelimb.

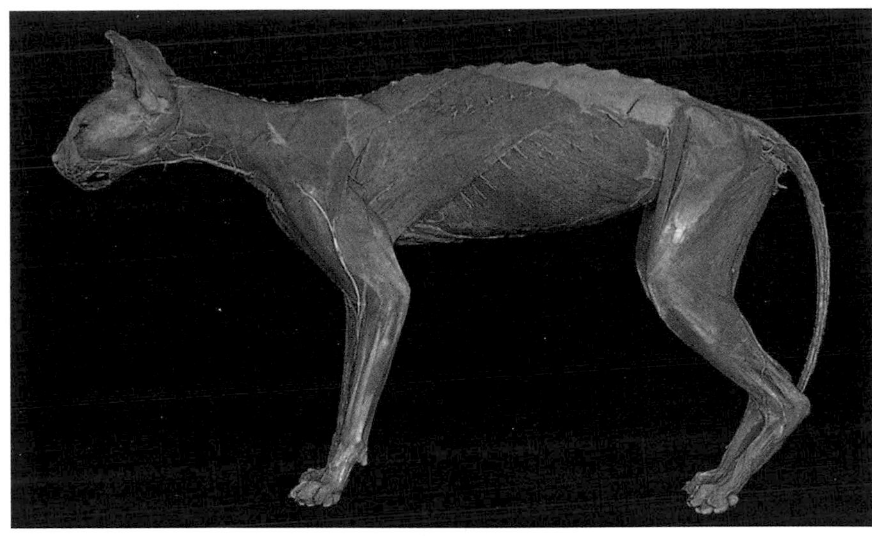

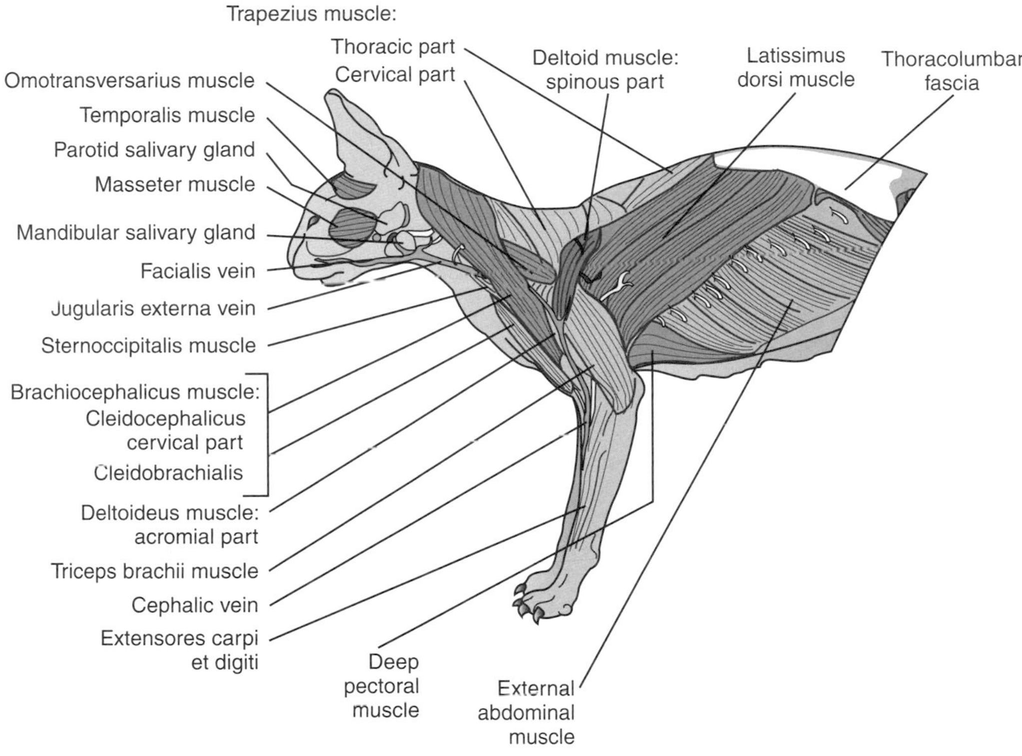

• **Fig. 7.5** Superficial muscles of the shoulder and thorax. (From Done SH et al: Color atlas of veterinary anatomy, vol 3, The dog and cat, London, 1996, Mosby Ltd.)

and that from the clavicle to the head is the cleidocephalicus. The cleidocephalicus can further be subdivided into two additional parts—the cleidomastoideus and the cleidocervicalis.

- **Origin**—clavicular intersection
- **Insertion**
  - Cleidobrachialis: ulna in the cat (in other animals it inserts on the cranial humerus)
  - Cleidomastoideus: mastoid process of temporal bone
  - Cleidocervicalis: dorsal neck
- **Action**—pulls the limb forward, extends the shoulder, and depresses and pulls the head and neck laterally

In the horse, the cleidocephalicus does not branch into two parts as it does in carnivores, ruminants, and pigs. In the horse, the clavicular intersection divides the brachiocephalicus into only two parts: the cleidomastoideus and the cleidobrachialis. The brachiocephalicus forms the upper margin of the jugular groove in animals.

Transect the brachiocephalicus approximately 2 cm from the tendinous intersection.

Omotransversarius Muscle

This straplike muscle is partially covered by the brachiocephalicus as the muscle leaves its insertion in the spine of the scapula (see Figs. 7.3–7.5).
Origin—wing of the atlas
Insertion—spine and acromion of scapula
Action—advances the limb and/or pulls the head and neck to the side

In the horse and ruminants, the omotransversarius ends in the lateral fascia of the shoulder and attaches indirectly to the spine of the scapula. The omotransversarius is intimately joined to the brachiocephalicus in the neck of the horse.

Transect the omotransversarius muscle through its middle and observe the **superficial cervical lymph node** in the fascia medial to this muscle and cranial to the scapula. This is one of the lymph nodes that are routinely palpated during physical exams.

Trapezius Muscle

This thin triangular muscle lies over the dorsal part of the scapula (see Figs. 7.4 and 7.5). The muscle can be divided into the cervical portion, which lies cranial to the scapular spine, and the thoracic portion, which lies caudal to the scapular spine.
Origin—dorsal aspect of neck and thorax
Insertion—spine of scapula
Action—elevates and abducts the forelimb

Transect the trapezius muscle by making a curving cut, beginning in the middle of the cervical portion, extending over the dorsum of the scapula, and continuing down through the middle of the thoracic portion.

Rhomboideus Muscle

The rhomboideus muscle lies beneath the trapezius muscle and holds the dorsal border of the scapula close to the body. This muscle can further be divided into three parts: capital, cervical, and thoracic.
Origin
- Rhomboideus capitis: nuchal crest of the occipital bone
- Rhomboideus cervicis: median fibrous tissue on the dorsal aspect of the neck
- Rhomboideus thoracis: spinous process of the first seven thoracic vertebrae
- **Insertion**—dorsal border of the scapula and/or its cartilage

Action—elevates forelimb

In the horse and cow, the rhomboideus muscle consists of only two parts: thoracic and cervical.

Transect the rhomboideus near its insertion on the scapula.

Latissimus Dorsi Muscle

This large triangle-shaped muscle lies caudal to the scapula and covers much of the thoracic wall (see Figs. 7.3–7.5).
Origin—spinous process of the lumbar and last seven or eight thoracic vertebrae
Insertion—teres major tuberosity of the humerus and the teres major tendon
Action—draws limb caudally; flexes the shoulder joint

Transect the latissimus dorsi muscle several centimeters from its insertion on the humerus.

Serratus Ventralis Muscle

This large muscle can be divided into two parts, based on its origin (Figs. 7.6 and 7.7). The cervical portion originates on the cervical vertebrae, and the thoracic portion originates on the ribs. The name *serratus* comes from the serrated appearance of the muscle on the ventral aspect of the thoracic portion. This muscle acts like a sling to support the body between the forelegs.
Origin—cervical part, cervical vertebrae; thoracic part, ribs
Insertion—serrated face on the dorsomedial aspect of the scapula
Action—supports the trunk and depresses the scapula

Abduct the limb and note the axillary artery and vein and the nerves of the brachial plexus. Using your scalpel, sever these structures along with the accompanying fascia. Notice the axillary lymph node in the fascia caudal to the shoulder joint. The serratus ventralis muscle can be detached from its insertion on the scapula by using forceful abduction of the limb. This will separate the forelimb from the body. Wrap the limb in wet paper towels as we continue our dissection of the muscles of the head.

Question

Injections in large animals are frequently given in the neck region cranial to the scapula and ventral to the cervical vertebrae. What muscles will the needle encounter after it has penetrated the skin?

Muscles of the Neck and Head

There are several muscles of the neck and head that are clinically significant. Some of these are involved in mastication or as landmarks when drawing blood from the jugular vein.

Remove the skin covering the head. Carefully make an incision through the skin, leaving a thin strip around the eyes and the lips. Remove the skin from the entire head but only to the base of the ear. Carefully remove any subcutaneous fat from the head to assist in viewing the muscles.

Sternocephalicus Muscle

The major importance of this muscle is that it forms, along with the brachiocephalicus, the jugular groove. The paired sternocephalicus muscle attaches the sternum to the head (see Fig. 7.3). In carnivores and ruminants, it is divided into two subparts, which are named for their attachments (mastoid and occipital). In the horse, the muscle is undivided.
Origin—sternum
Insertion
- Sternomastoideus—mastoid part of the occipital bone
- Sterno-occipitalis—nuchal crest of the occipital bone

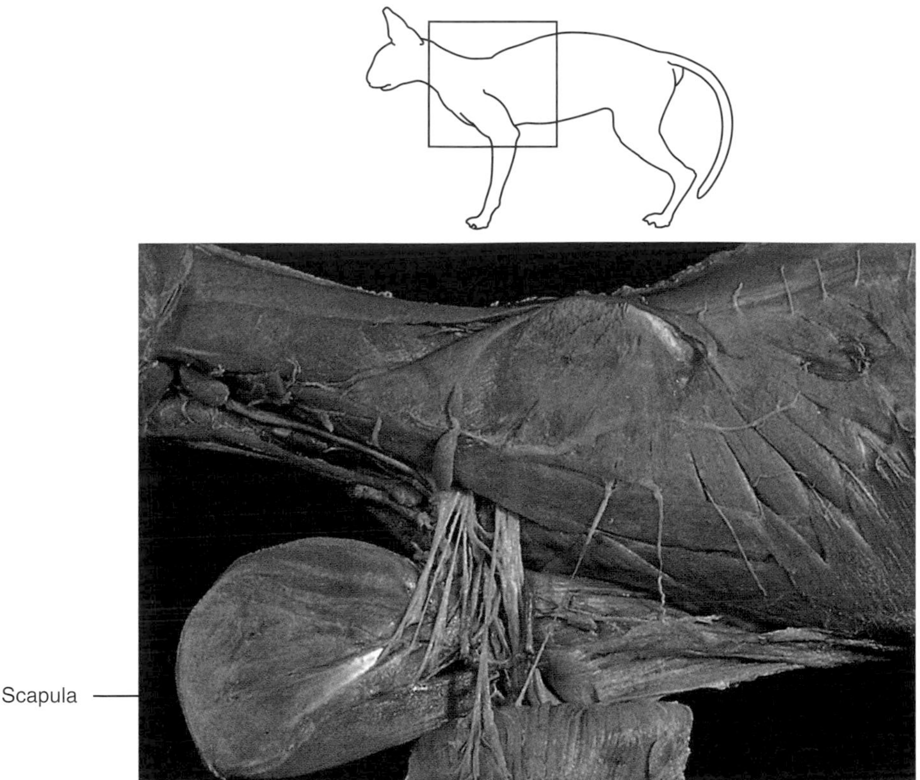

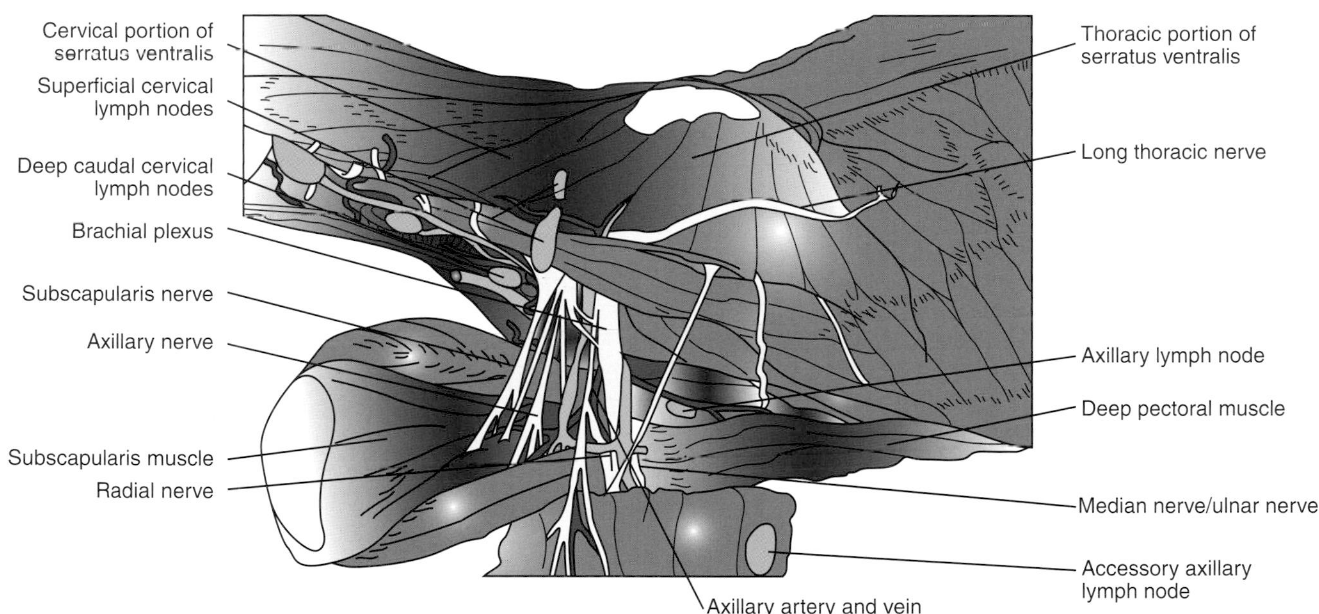

• **Fig. 7.6** Medial scapula showing the nerves of the brachial plexus and accompanying arteries and veins. (From Done SH et al: Color atlas of veterinary anatomy, vol 3, The dog and cat, London, 1996, Mosby Ltd.)

- **Action**—depresses the head and neck and/or draws the head and neck to the side

Platysma Muscle

This well-developed sheet-like muscle is one of the major cutaneous muscles of the neck and head (see Fig. 7.2). It is usually tightly adherent to the skin and may be reflected when the skin is removed from the neck and head region.

Origin—dorsal tendinous raphe at the dorsal midline

Insertion—fibers of this muscle attach to the muscles surrounding the lips

Action—draws the commissures of the lips caudally

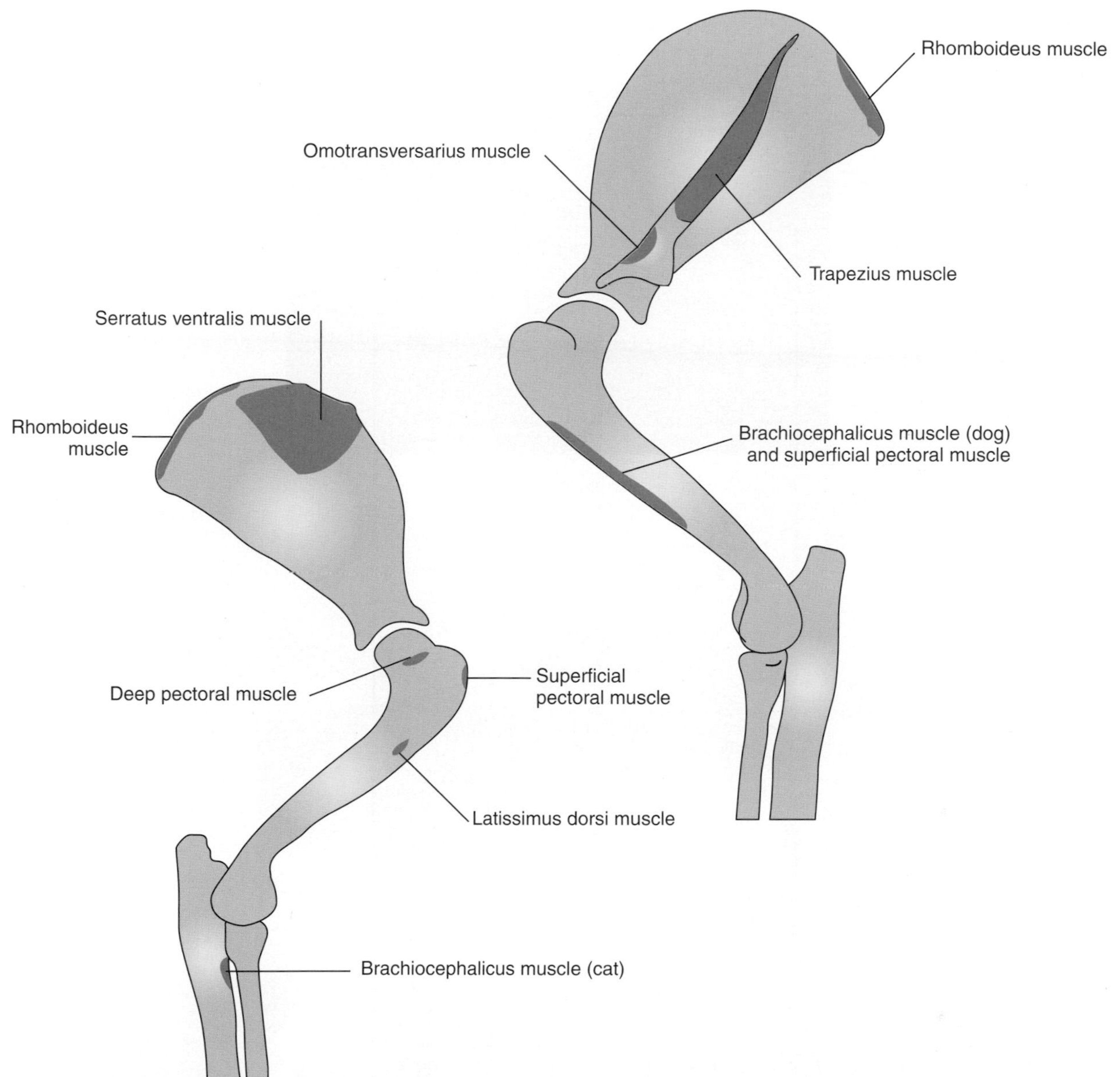

• **Fig. 7.7** Lateral and medial aspects of the foreleg showing the insertion of the extrinsic muscles of the thoracic limb.

Muscles of Mastication

Temporalis Muscle

This muscle is the largest muscle on the head and is found on the lateral and dorsal aspects of the skull (Fig. 7.8). It is prominent between the ears and extends down into the temporal fossa region of the skull.

Origin—the majority of muscle arises from the parietal bone, but the muscle also arises from the temporal, frontal, and occipital bones

Insertion—coronoid process of the mandible

Action—elevates the mandible to close the mouth when chewing; moves the mandible laterally

Masseter Muscle

This large muscle is found ventral to the zygomatic arch and lies on the lateral surface of the ramus of the mandible (see Fig. 7.8). It makes up the cheek region of the cat and is covered by an aponeurosis. The muscle consists of three layers whose fibers run in three different directions.

Origin—zygomatic arch

Insertion—lateral side of the mandible

Action—elevates the mandible to close the mouth when chewing

Digastricus Muscle

This thin, superficial, straplike muscle can be found along the ventral caudal edge of the mandible (see Fig. 7.3).

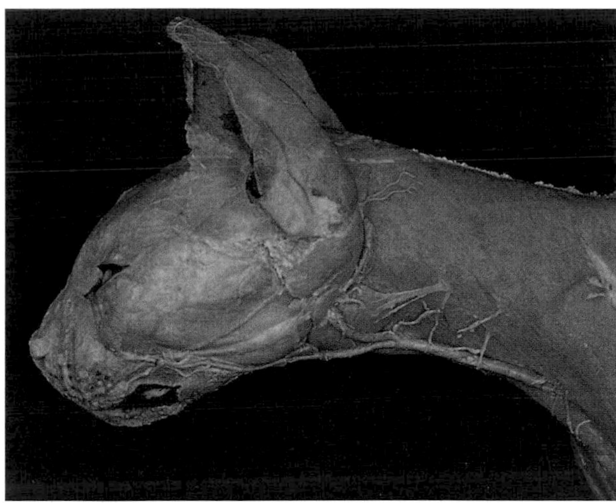

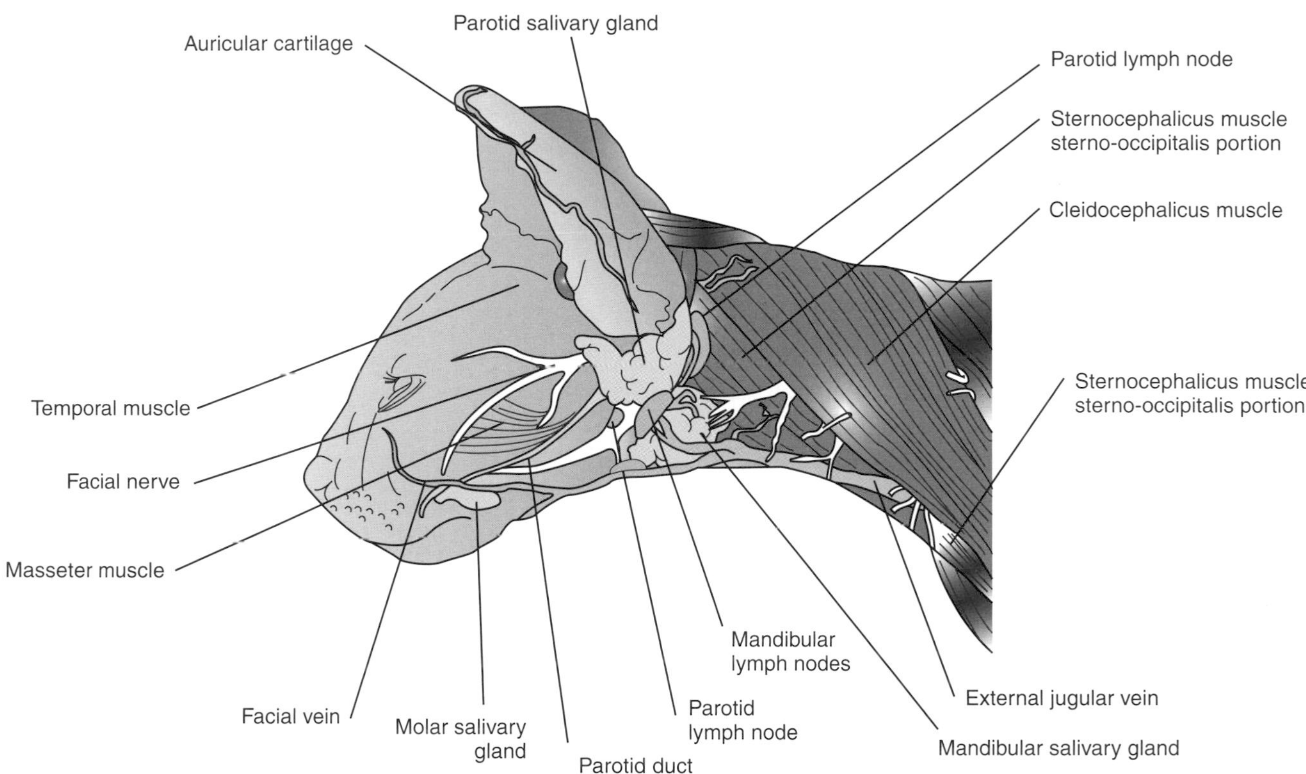

• **Fig. 7.8** Superficial muscles and structures of the head and neck. (From Done SH et al: Color atlas of veterinary anatomy, vol 3, The dog and cat, London, 1996, Mosby Ltd.)

Origin—occipital and temporal bones caudal to the external acoustic meatus
Insertion—ventral mandible
Action—opens the mouth

Mylohyoideus Muscle

This thin muscular sheet has fibers that run in a transverse direction. The muscle forms a sling for the tongue (see Fig. 7.3).
Origin—medial surface of the mandible
Insertion—ventral median raphe between the bones of the mandible
Action—raises the floor of the mouth

Suggested In-Class Activity

Live Animal

Visualize where the muscles are that you have studied today by palpating the live animal. Flex and extend the joints of the thoracic limb and visualize what muscles would cause this action. Palpate the jugular groove and visualize how the sternocephalicus and the brachiocephalicus muscles form this furrow. Palpate the dorsal and lateral aspects of the head and note how the temporal muscle makes feeling the occipital crest more difficult in some animals.

CLINICAL APPLICATION

Masticatory Myositis

Masticatory myositis is an inflammatory disease in the dog that affects the muscles of mastication. The exact cause is unknown, but it is thought to be immune mediated. This disease can occur in any breed of dog, but young or middle-aged German Shepherds, Dobermans, and retriever breeds are most commonly affected.

The clinical signs include fever, swelling of the muscles of mastication, and, in the acute form, submandibular lymphadenopathy. The chronic form is seen more commonly; the dog presents with very prominent bony features of the skull. Dogs with masticatory myositis usually have difficulty opening their mouths to eat but otherwise are very normal. Treatment typically involves the use of steroids.

LABORATORY II

Intrinsic Muscles of the Thoracic Limb

Intrinsic muscles attach only to the bones within the limb itself. For ease of learning, these muscles can be broken down into six groups based on their position on the foreleg (Table 7.2). Remove the skin from the shoulder, foreleg, and paw. As you are doing this, observe the **cephalic vein** located cranially on the leg (Fig. 7.9). This is an important structure because it is frequently used for intravenous injection in small animals. Visualizing its position on the leg will assist you when giving intravenous injections to the live animal. The major muscles we will study within each group are listed in the following categories:

- Lateral muscles of the scapula and shoulder
  - Deltoideus
  - Infraspinatus
  - Supraspinatus
- Medial muscles of scapula and shoulder
  - Subscapularis
  - Teres major

TABLE 7.2 Intrinsic Muscles of the Foreleg, with Origin, Insertion, and Action

Muscle	Origin	Insertion	Action
Deltoideus	Spine/acromion of scapula	Deltoid tuberosity of humerus	Flexes shoulder
Infraspinatus	Infraspinous fossa of scapula	Greater tubercle of humerus	Flexes shoulder/abducts limb
Supraspinatus	Supraspinous fossa of scapula	Greater tubercle of humerus	Extends shoulder
Subscapularis	Subscapular fossa of scapula	Lesser tubercle of humerus	Adducts limb/rotates forearm
Teres major	Caudal border of scapula	Teres major tuberosity of humerus	Flexes shoulder
Triceps brachii	Caudal border of scapula/ proximal border of humerus	Olecranon of ulna	Extends elbow/flexes shoulder
Biceps brachii	Supraglenoid tubercle of scapula	Ulna and radial tuberosities	Flexes elbow/extends shoulder
Brachialis	Caudolateral aspect of proximal humerus	Ulna and radial tuberosities	Flexes elbow
Brachioradialis	Lateral aspect of distal humerus	Distal radius	Rotates forearm (supination)
Extensor carpi radialis	Lateral supracondylar crest of humerus	Proximal aspect of second and third metacarpal bones	Extends carpus
Common digital extensor	Lateral epicondyle of humerus	Dorsal surface of distal phalanges of digits II, III, IV, V	Extends carpus and digits
Lateral digital extensor	Lateral epicondyle of humerus	Proximal ends of digits II, III, IV, V	Extends digital joints
Extensor carpi ulnaris	Lateral epicondyle of humerus	Lateral aspect of metacarpal V and accessory carpal bone	Flexes carpal joint
Abductor pollicis longus	Lateral border of ulna	Proximal end of metacarpals I and II	Extends carpal joint abducts digit
Flexor carpi radialis	Medial epicondyle of humerus	Palmar aspect of metacarpals II and III	Flexes carpal joint
Flexor carpi ulnaris	Medial epicondyle and olecranon	Accessory carpal bone	Flexes carpal joint
Superficial digital flexor	Medial epicondyle of humerus	Palmar aspect of phalanges of digits II, III, IV, V	Flexes carpus and digits
Deep digital flexor	Medial epicondyle/proximal ulna	Palmar aspect of distal phalanges	Flexes carpus and digits
	Medial radius		

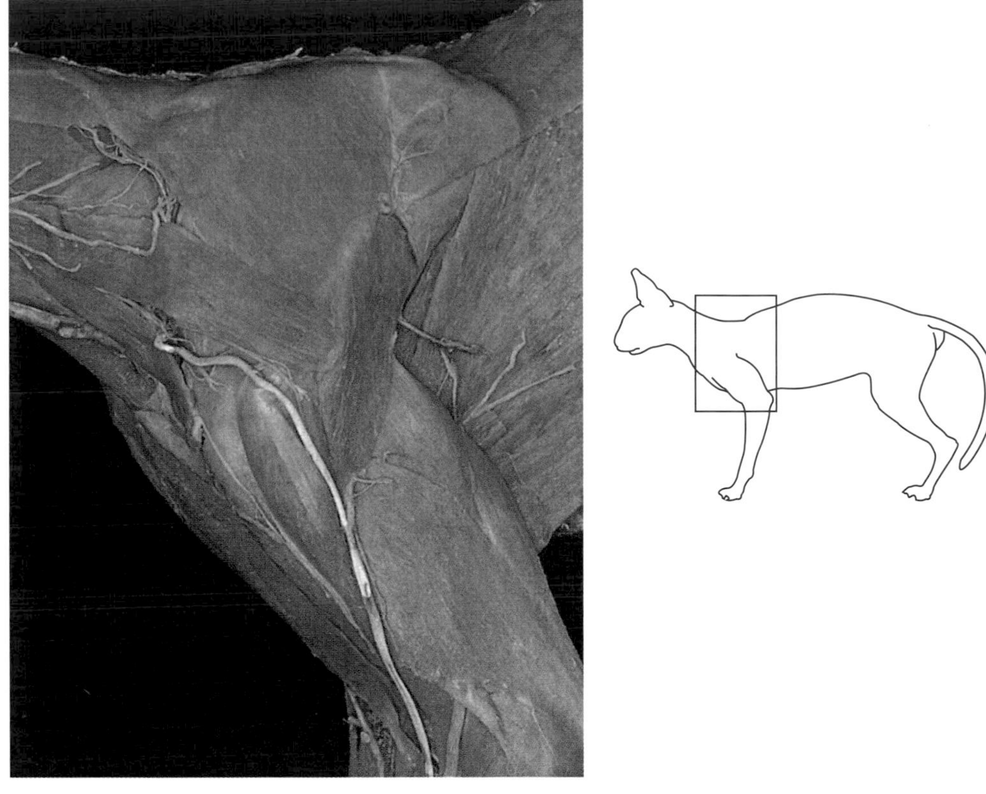

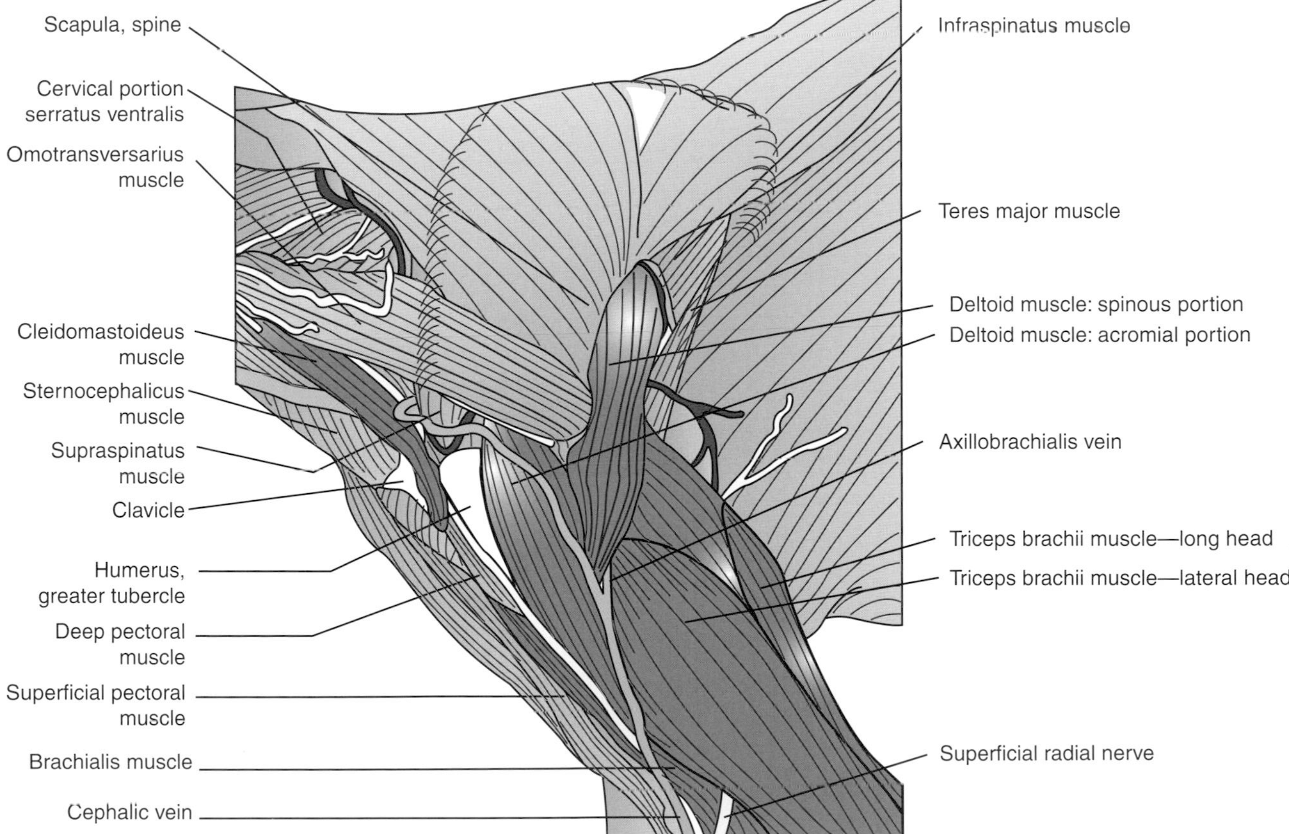

• **Fig. 7.9** Lateral aspect of foreleg and shoulder of cat. (From Done SH et al: Color atlas of veterinary anatomy, vol 3, The dog and cat, London, 1996, Mosby Ltd.)

- Caudal muscles of the foreleg
  - Triceps brachii
- Cranial muscles of the foreleg
  - Biceps brachii
  - Brachialis
- Craniolateral muscles of the foreleg
  - Extensor carpi radialis
  - Common digital extensor
  - Lateral digital extensor
  - Extensor carpi ulnaris
  - Abductor pollicis longus
- Caudomedial muscles of the foreleg
  - Flexor carpi radialis
  - Flexor carpi ulnaris
  - Superficial digital flexor
  - Deep digital flexor

Lateral Muscles of the Scapula and Shoulder

Except for the supraspinatus muscle, the lateral muscles of the scapula and shoulder are primarily flexors of the shoulder joint.

Deltoideus Muscle

The deltoideus muscle consists of two parts (scapular and acromion) that join and act in common (see Fig. 7.9). The scapular portion covers the majority of the infraspinatus muscle located below it. The two parts of the muscle fuse before they insert into the deltoid tuberosity of the humerus.
Origin—spine and acromion of scapula
Insertion—deltoid tuberosity of the humerus
Action—flexes the shoulder joint

In the pig and the horse, the deltoideus does not appear to be divided into two parts. Transect the deltoideus muscle approximately 2.5 cm distal to the acromion of the scapula and reflect the stumps.

Infraspinatus Muscle

This muscle fills the infraspinous fossa caudal to the spine of the scapula (Fig. 7.10). Transect the infraspinatus approximately halfway down from the dorsal portion of the scapula. Use your scalpel handle to scrape away the fibers where the muscle inserts on the infraspinous fossa of the scapula and reflect the freed portion of the muscle to the insertion

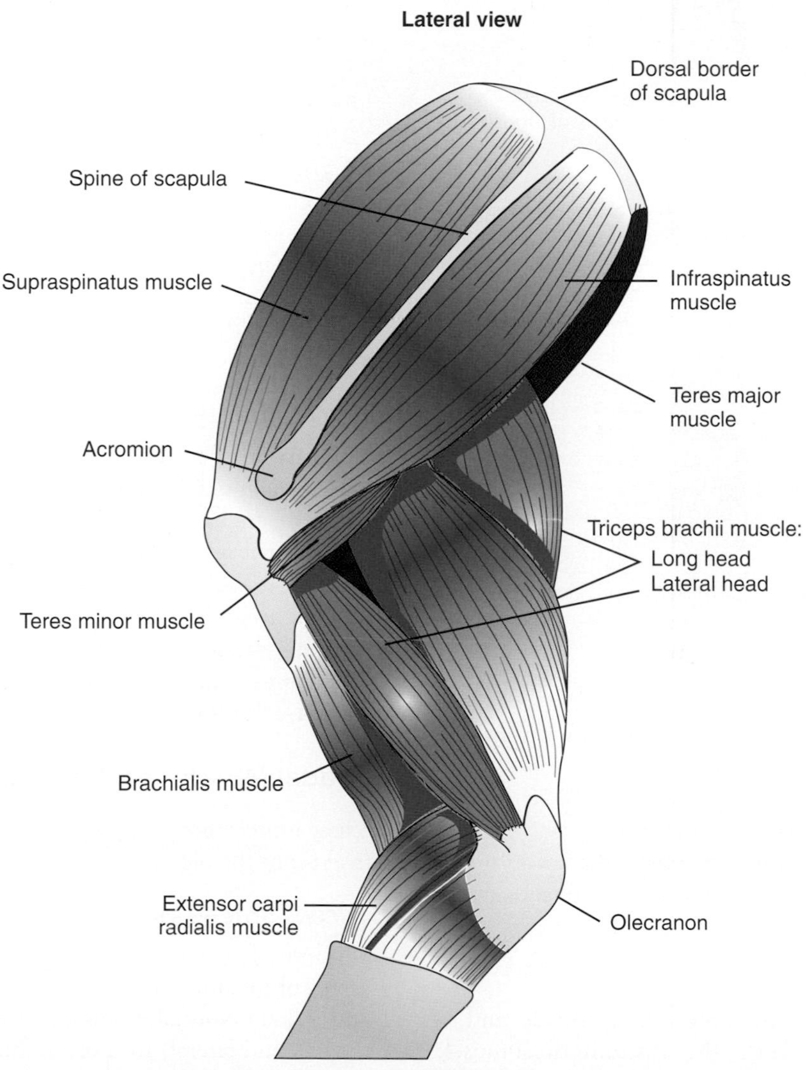

• **Fig. 7.10** Lateral aspect of the left foreleg of the cat.

on the greater tubercle of the humerus. Notice the small teres minor muscle on the caudal aspect of the scapula, deep to the infraspinatus. This muscle will not be studied because it plays only a minor role in support of the shoulder in our animals but a major role in people, being involved in the various movements of the shoulder.

Origin—infraspinous fossa of the scapula
Insertion—lateral side of the greater tubercle of the humerus
Action—flexes the shoulder joint and abducts the limb at the shoulder

The horse and cow have a cranial and caudal part to the greater tubercle of the humerus. The infraspinatus muscle attaches to both parts. In the pig, it attaches to a depression distal to the greater tubercle.

Supraspinatus Muscle

This muscle fills the supraspinous fossa cranial to the spine of the scapula and is wider and longer than the infraspinatus muscle (see Figs. 7.3 and 7.10). A large part of the supraspinatus is covered by the trapezius and omotransversarius muscles.

Origin—supraspinous fossa
Insertion—greater tubercle of the humerus
Action—extends the shoulder joint

Medial Muscles of the Shoulder

The muscles in this group are primarily flexors of the shoulder joint.

CLINICAL APPLICATION

Shoulder Slip

When animals of large mass, such as horses, are placed on their sides for extended periods of time, for example during a procedure requiring anesthesia, it is important to lay the animal down on soft soil or place pads under the animal's shoulder. If an animal of large mass is in this position for an extended length of time and is not padded well, damage to the nerves supplying the shoulder muscles can result. This nerve damage can lead to atrophy of the muscles of the shoulder and instability in the shoulder joint itself. Such atrophy and instability are commonly called shoulder slip or "Sweeney."

Subscapularis Muscle

This muscle occupies the subscapular fossa on the medial aspect of the scapula (see Figs. 7.6 and 7.11).

Origin—subscapular fossa of the scapula
Insertion—lesser tubercle of the humerus
Action—adducts limb at the shoulder and rotates foreleg medially; it also functions as a medial collateral ligament to the shoulder

Teres Major Muscle

This muscle lies caudal to the subscapularis muscle, and its tendon of insertion joins that of the latissimus dorsi muscle (see Figs. 7.9–7.12)

Origin—caudal border of scapula
Insertion—teres major tuberosity of the humerus
Action—flexes the shoulder

CLINICAL APPLICATION

Why Animals Don't Get Rotator Cuff Injuries

The support of the shoulder joint is primarily achieved by the muscles surrounding the joint as they attach distally to the foreleg. Animals do not have as much shoulder trouble as humans because the foreleg does not routinely make the same movements, such as throwing a baseball, rotation of the leg, or circumduction of the leg. Pain in the shoulder from a group of muscles called the rotator cuff is a frequent problem in humans and usually requires surgical correction. Four muscles make up the "rotator cuff": the supraspinatus, infraspinatus, subscapularis, and teres minor.

Cranial Muscles of the Foreleg

These muscles primarily flex the elbow.

Biceps Brachii Muscle

This muscle is located on the craniomedial aspect of the humerus (see Figs. 7.11 and 7.12; see also Figs. 7.18 and 7.19). It has only one head in animals.

Origin—supraglenoid tubercle of the scapula
Insertion—ulnar and radial tuberosities
Action—flexes the elbow and extends the shoulder

The tendon of the biceps brachii is bound into the intertubercular groove of the humerus by the transverse humeral ligament. This position of attachment gives additional support to the shoulder joint.

Brachialis Muscle

This muscle is located on the lateral side of the humerus (see Figs. 7.10 and 7.12; see also Figs. 7.18 and 7.19). After its origin on the lateral humerus, it courses distally, following the brachial groove of the humerus, twisting laterally and cranially toward its insertion on the medial side of the proximal radius and ulna.

Origin—caudolateral aspect of the proximal humerus
Insertion—ulnar and radial tuberosities
Action—flexes the elbow

Caudal Muscles of the Foreleg

These muscles are primarily extensors of the elbow joint and insert into the olecranon.

Triceps Brachii Muscle

This muscle makes up the large muscle mass on the caudal aspect of the humerus (see Figs. 7.9-7.11; see also Figs. 7.18 and 7.19). Normally this muscle has three heads (long, medial, and lateral) in most animals, but carnivores have a fourth head called the accessory head.

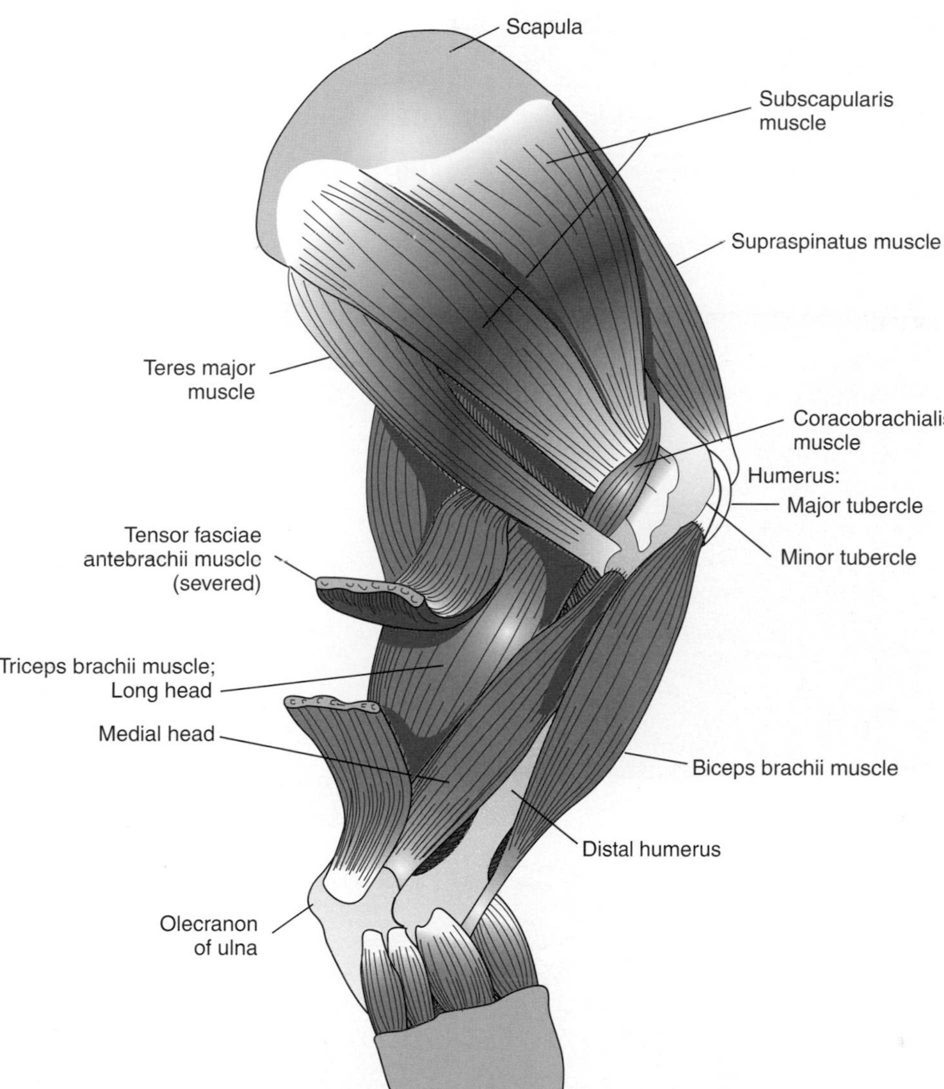

• **Fig. 7.11** The medial muscles of the shoulder and upper foreleg.

Origin—the long head originates from the caudal border of the scapula; the other heads originate from the proximal border of the humerus
Insertion—all four heads insert on the olecranon of the ulna
Action—extends the elbow and flexes the shoulder

CLINICAL APPLICATION

Avoiding Damage to the Radial Nerve

The triceps brachii is innervated by the radial nerve. If this nerve is damaged proximal to where it innervates the triceps brachii, it will lead to atrophy of the triceps and an inability to extend the elbow, or "dropped elbow," resulting in an inability to support the body weight on this limb. An awareness of the location of this nerve is important when giving intramuscular injections in the upper foreleg.

Craniolateral Muscles of the Foreleg

These muscles are primarily extensors of the carpal and digital joints and originate on or close to the lateral epicondyle of the humerus. Many of these muscles have a minor flexor action on the elbow joint because of their origin proximal to the joint. A thick fascial band, the extensor retinaculum, near the carpal joint holds the tendons of these muscles in place. Cut this fascial band when needed to follow the tendons of these muscles distally.

Brachioradialis Muscle

This is the most cranially located muscle in the forearm (see Figs. 7.12 and 7.14; see also Figs. 7.18 and 7.19). It may be confused with part of the extensor carpi radialis.
Origin—lateral aspect of the distal humerus

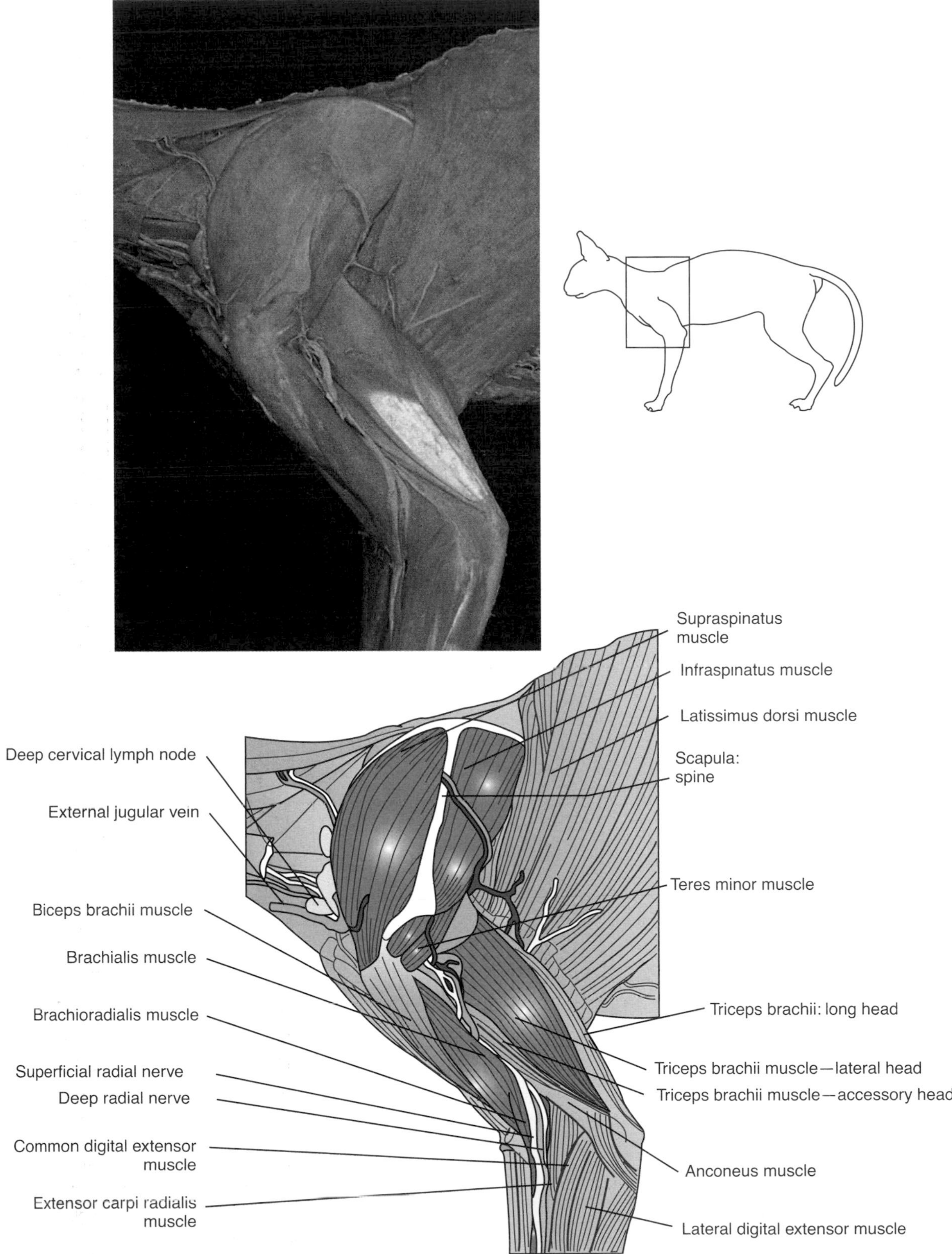

• **Fig. 7.12** Lateral aspect of the shoulder with the deltoideus muscle removed. (From Done SH et al: Color atlas of veterinary anatomy, vol 3, The dog and cat, London, 1996, Mosby Ltd.)

Insertion—distal radius
Action—rotates the forearm (supination of forearm)

The brachioradialis muscle is always present in the cat and usually in the dog. It is not present in the ungulates (cattle, horses, goats, pigs, and sheep).

The brachioradialis muscle runs beside the cephalic vein on the cranial aspect of the forearm. It is approximately the same size as the cephalic vein and may be mistaken for the vein during venipuncture.

Extensor Carpi Radialis Muscle

This is the largest of the craniolateral muscle group (see Figs. 7.12–7.14; see also Figs. 7.18 and 7.19). It lies on the cranial aspect of the radius and deep to the brachioradialis muscle as it courses distally. In the cat, it usually has two distinct heads. In the dog, the distinction between the two heads is not as evident. The tendon of insertion courses under the abductor pollicis longus muscle.
Origin—lateral supracondylar crest of the humerus

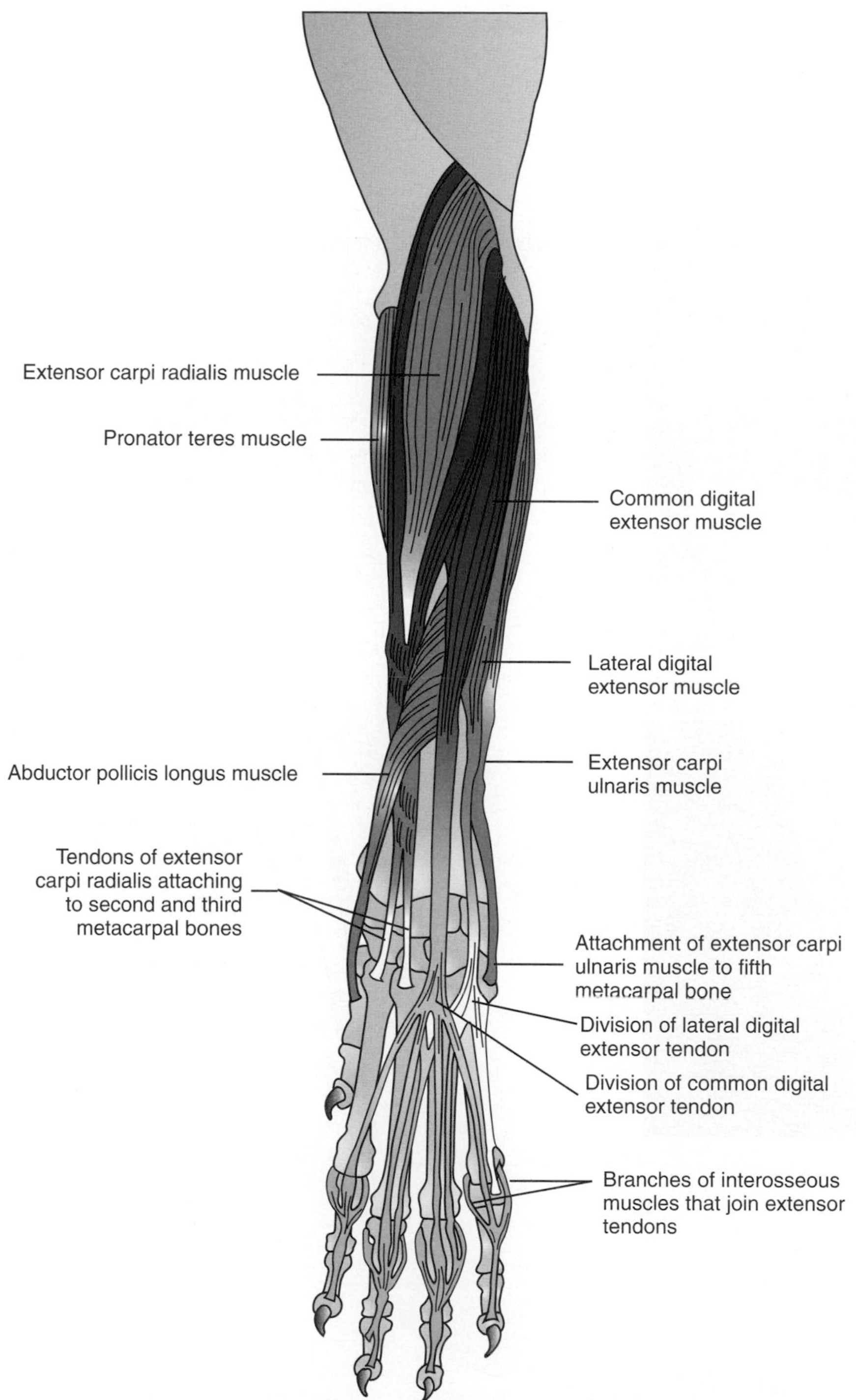

• **Fig. 7.13** The cranial muscles of the foreleg.

Insertion—proximal aspect of the second and third metacarpal bones
Action—extends the carpus

Common Digital Extensor Muscle

This muscle lies caudal to the extensor carpi radialis on the lateral side of the foreleg (see Figs. 7.12–7.14; see also Figs. 7.18 and 7.19). Its tendon of insertion branches into four separate branches and each branch inserts on the dorsal surface of the proximal phalanges of the major digits.
Origin—lateral epicondyle of humerus
Insertion—dorsal surface of distal phalanges of digits II, III, IV, and V
Action—extends the carpus and digits

In all domestic animals except the horse, the tendon is divided into parts that are distributed to each digit. In

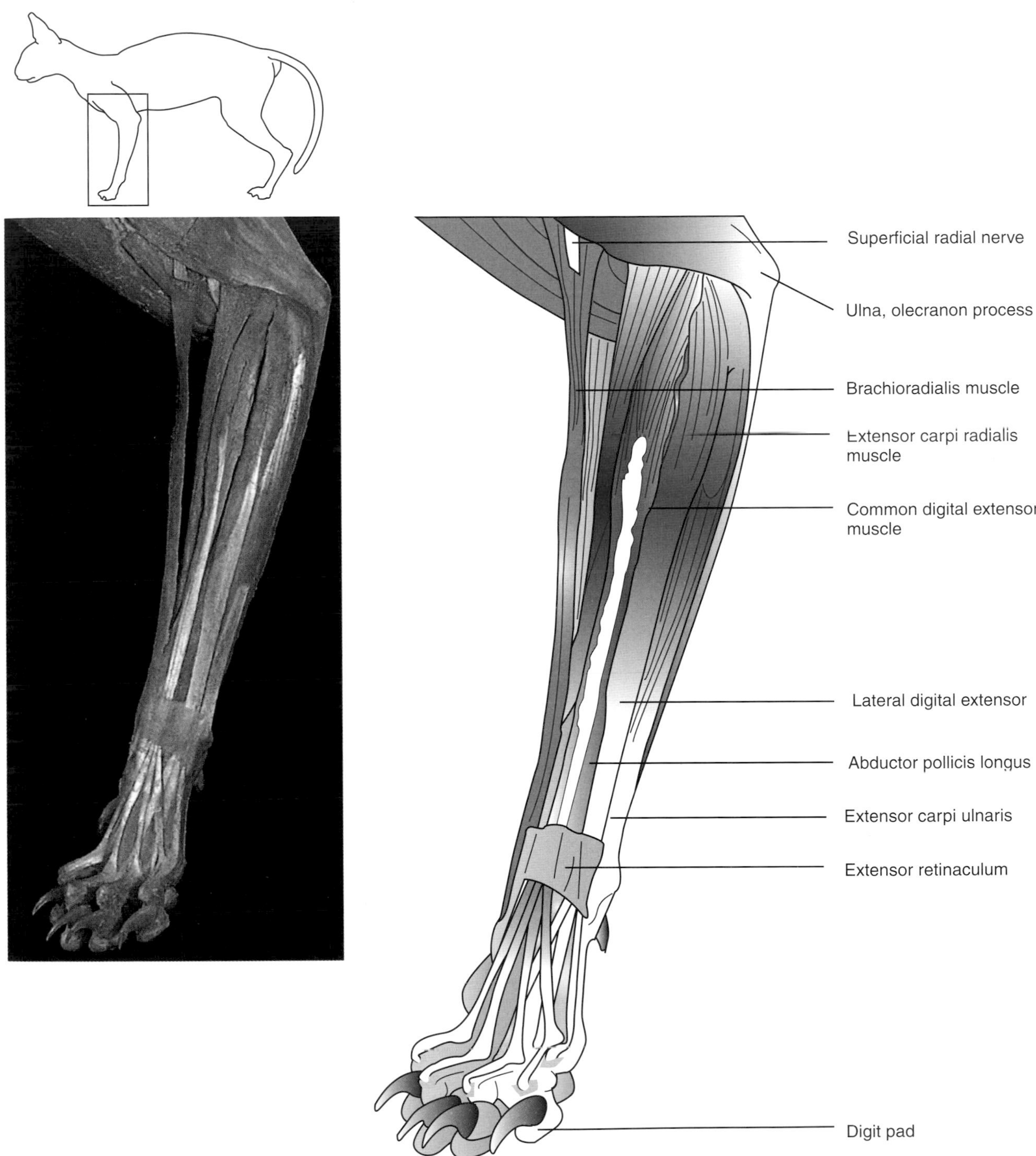

• **Fig. 7.14** Cranial muscles of the foreleg. (From Done SH et al: Color atlas of veterinary anatomy, vol 3, The dog and cat, London, 1996, Mosby Ltd.)

ruminants, the muscle is distinctly separated into a medial belly that attaches to the third digit and a lateral belly that attaches to digits III and IV.

Lateral Digital Extensor Muscle

This muscle is smaller than the common digital extensor and lies just caudolateral to it (Figs. 7.13 and 7.14; see also Figs. 7.18 and 7.19). The muscle splits into three tendons of insertion on the digits.

Origin—lateral epicondyle of humerus

Insertion—proximal ends of digits II, III, IV, and V in the cat (with the common digital extensor) or II, III, and IV in the dog

Action—extends the digital joints

In the horse, the lateral digital extensor attaches only as far distally as the proximal phalanx.

Extensor Carpi Ulnaris (Formerly Ulnaris Lateralis)

This muscle lies caudal and lateral to the lateral digital extensor (see Figs. 7.13 and 7.14; see also Figs. 7.18 and 7.19). This is the only flexor that arises on the lateral epicondyle.

Origin—lateral epicondyle

Insertion—lateral aspect of metacarpal V and the accessory carpal bone

Action—flexes the carpal joint

In horses and ruminants, this muscle attaches to the fourth metacarpal bone.

Abductor Pollicis Longus Muscle

This flat triangular muscle lies primarily in the groove between the radius and ulna (see Figs. 7.13 and 7.14). Its fibers run obliquely across the tendon of the extensor carpi radialis muscle.

Origin—lateral border of ulna

Insertion—proximal end of metacarpals I and II

Action—extends the carpal joint and abducts the digit

Caudomedial Muscles of the Foreleg

These muscles are primarily flexors of the carpal and digital joints. They originate in the medial epicondyle of the humerus.

Flexor Carpi Radialis Muscle

This muscle is the most cranial and medial of the caudomedial muscles (see Figs. 7.15 and 7.16). The thick fusiform belly of this muscle is partially attached to the deep digital flexor and extends only to the middle of the radius. Be careful not to confuse it with the small pronator teres muscle, which crosses the medial aspect of the humerus.

Origin—medial epicondyle of the humerus

Insertion—palmar aspect of metacarpals II and III

Action—flexes the carpal joint

Flexor Carpi Ulnaris Muscle

The flexor carpi ulnaris is the most caudal of this muscle group and lies next to the extensor carpi ulnaris (Figs. 7.15–7.19). It consists of two parts (the humeral head and ulnar head) that are distinct throughout their length but both parts attach to the accessory carpal bone.

Origin—medial epicondyle (humeral head) and olecranon (ulnar head)

Insertion—accessory carpal bone

Action—flexes the carpal joint

Superficial Digital Flexor Muscle

This muscle lies caudomedial to the ulna and covers the deep digital flexor (see Figs. 7.15–7.19). The tendon of insertion divides into four major branches and each branch inserts on one digit. Remove the flexor retinaculum, which is the fascia that binds it down at the carpus, and observe the division of this muscle into four parts.

Origin—medial epicondyle of the humerus

Insertion—palmar aspect of the middle phalanges of digits II, III, IV, and V

Action—flexes the carpal and digital joints

In the horse, the superficial digital flexor also attaches to the distal end of the proximal phalanx. A radial head consisting of a tendinous band from the radius joins this muscle. This band is termed the accessory ligament of the superficial digital flexor.

Deep Digital Flexor Muscle

This muscle has three heads of origin and makes up most of the remaining muscle mass on the caudal aspect of the foreleg (see Figs. 7.16, 7.18, and 7.19). The tendons of all three heads fuse at the carpus to form a single tendon and then subdivide to attach to the palmar aspect of each digit. The deep digital flexor lies deep to the superficial digit flexor muscle and the flexor carpi ulnaris. These two muscles can be transected for better observation of the deep digital flexor.

Origin—the humeral head arises from the medial epicondyle of the humerus; the ulnar head arises from the caudal aspect of the proximal ulna; the radial head arises from the middle of the medial radius.

Insertion—palmar aspect of the distal phalanges of each digit

Action—flexes the carpus and digits

In the horse, a strong tendinous band from the palmar carpal ligament joins this tendon distal to the carpus. This ligament is called the accessory ligament of the deep digital flexor. In the past, this ligament has been called the carpal or distal check ligament.

CLINICAL APPLICATION

Bowed Tendon

Bowed tendon, a condition most commonly seen in the superficial digital flexor in the foreleg of a horse, is actually a tear of the tendon usually resulting from stress placed on the tendons during racing.

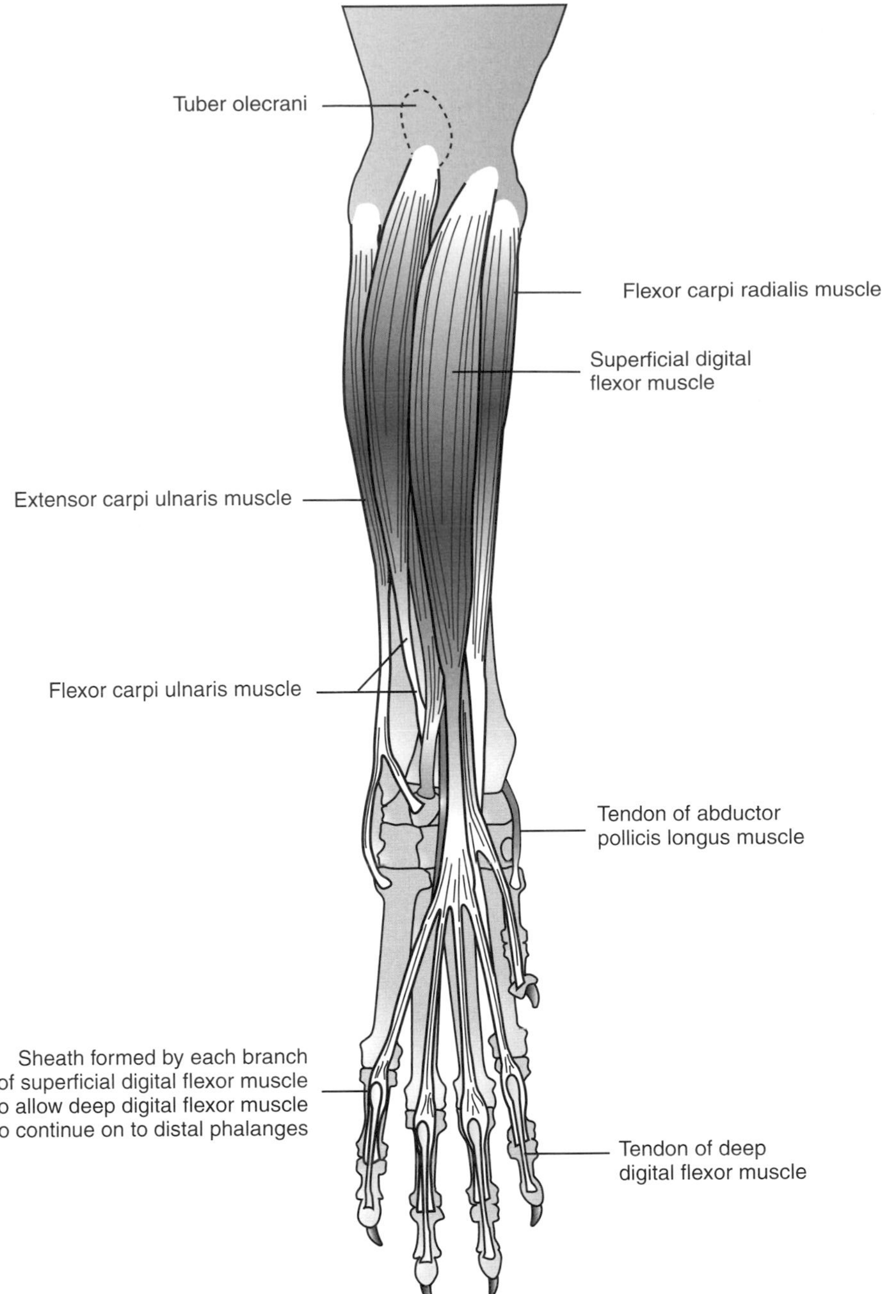

• **Fig. 7.15** Superficial muscles on the caudal aspect of the left foreleg.

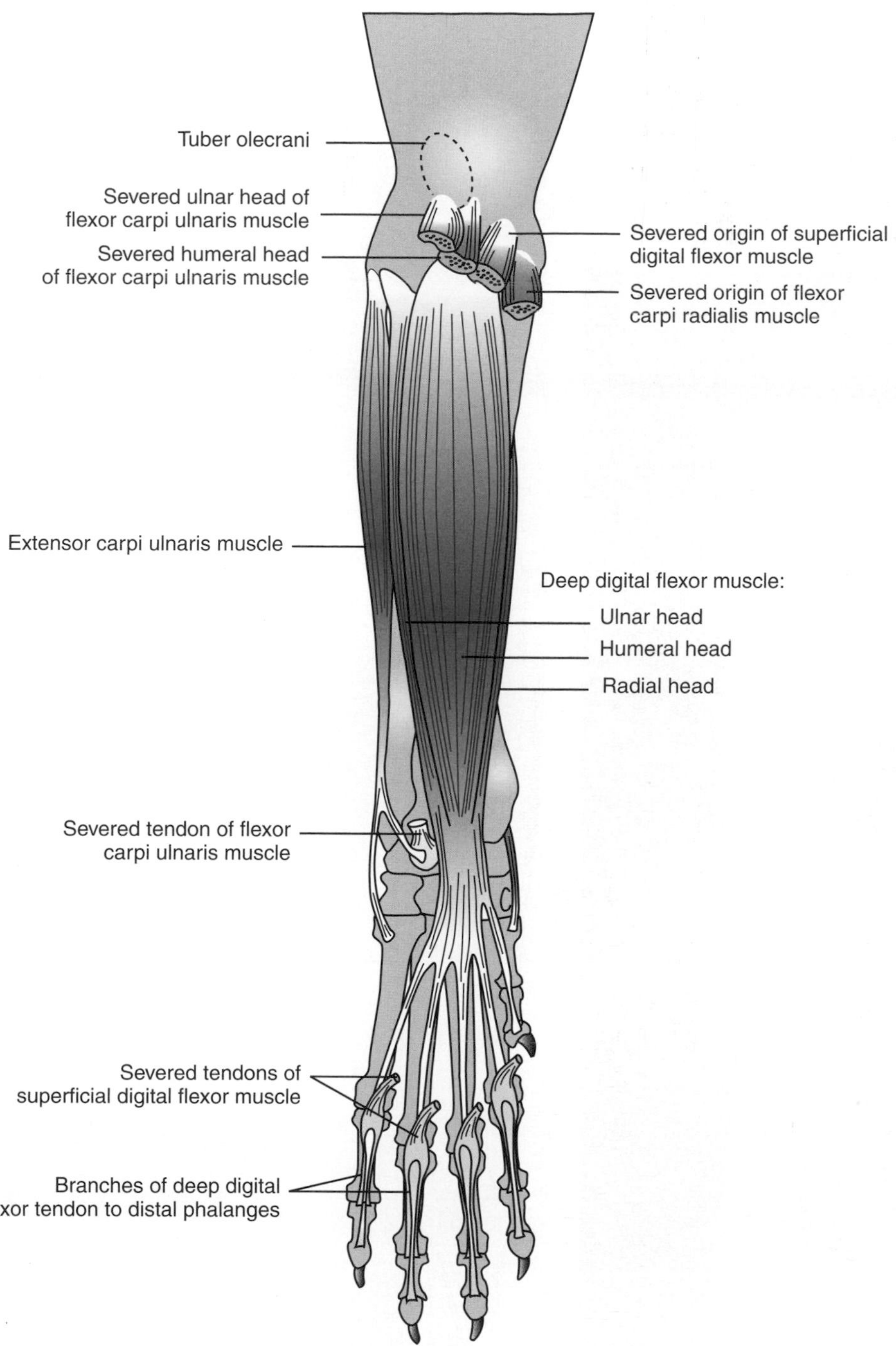

• **Fig. 7.16** Deep muscles on the caudal aspect of the left foreleg.

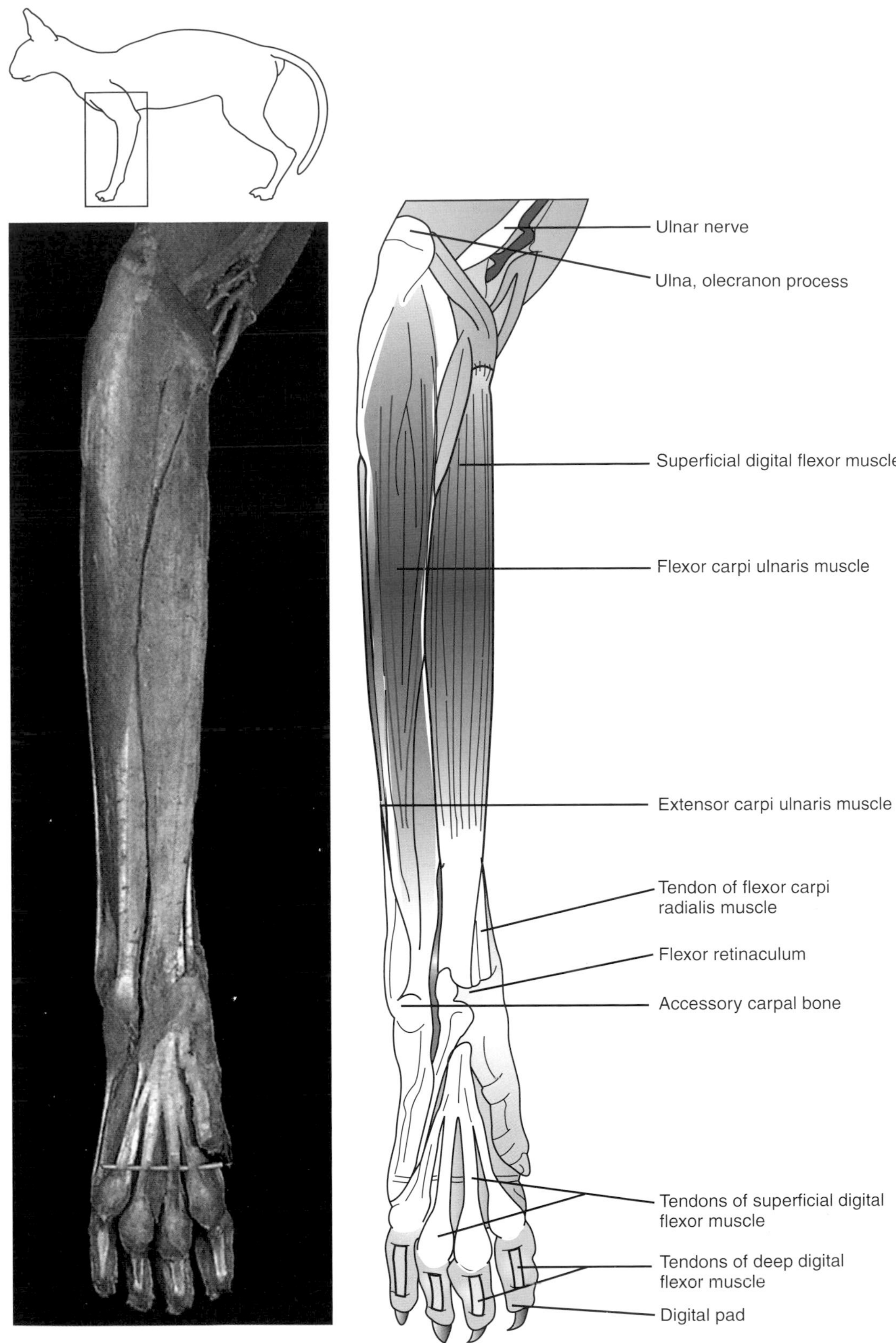

• **Fig. 7.17** Caudal aspect of the left foreleg of the cat. (From Done SH et al: Color atlas of veterinary anatomy, vol 3, The dog and cat, London, 1996, Mosby Ltd.)

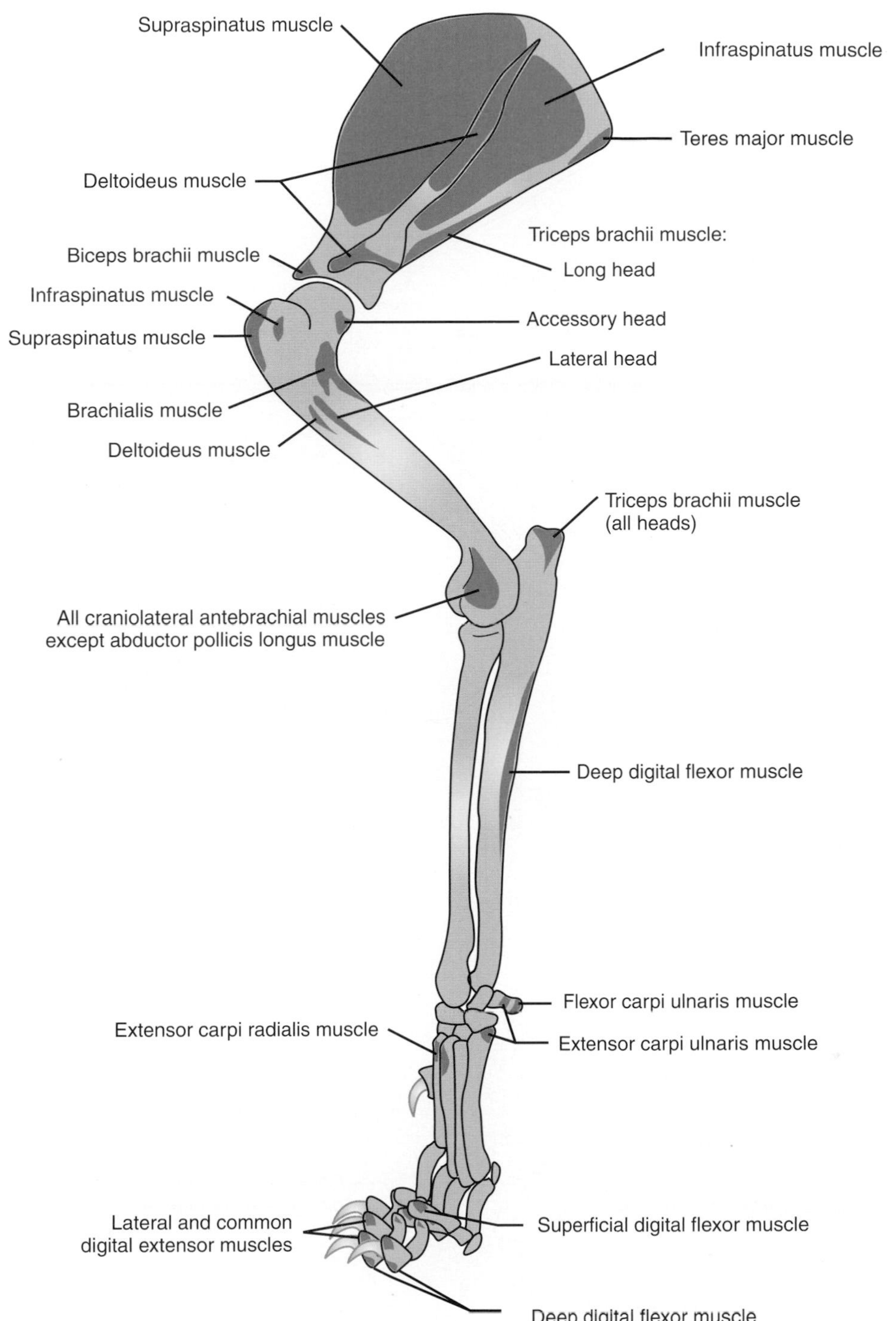

• **Fig. 7.18** Attachment of the muscles of the lateral aspect of the left forelimb.

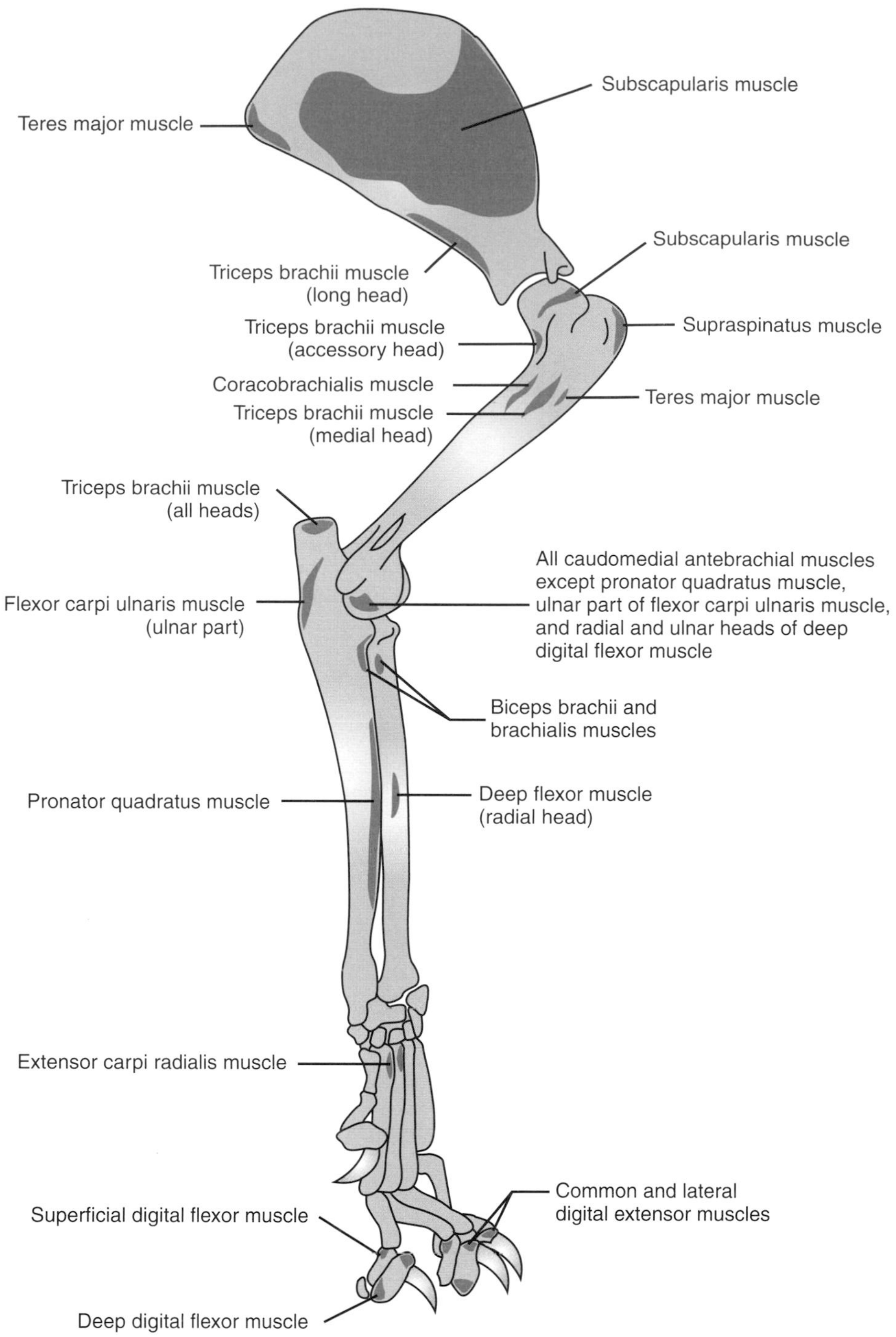

Teres major muscle
Subscapularis muscle
Triceps brachii muscle (long head)
Subscapularis muscle
Triceps brachii muscle (accessory head)
Supraspinatus muscle
Coracobrachialis muscle
Triceps brachii muscle (medial head)
Teres major muscle
Triceps brachii muscle (all heads)
Flexor carpi ulnaris muscle (ulnar part)
All caudomedial antebrachial muscles except pronator quadratus muscle, ulnar part of flexor carpi ulnaris muscle, and radial and ulnar heads of deep digital flexor muscle
Biceps brachii and brachialis muscles
Pronator quadratus muscle
Deep flexor muscle (radial head)
Extensor carpi radialis muscle
Superficial digital flexor muscle
Common and lateral digital extensor muscles
Deep digital flexor muscle

• **Fig. 7.19** Attachment of the muscles of the medial aspect of the left forelimb.

Muscles of the Forefoot (Manus)

There are a number of small rather insignificant muscles located in the front paw known as the interosseous muscles (Figs. 7.20 and 7.21). These four small muscles lie deep to the deep digital flexor on the palmar aspect of the four metacarpal bones. Each muscle originates from the base of the metacarpal bone and the carpal joint capsule. Its insertion is on the base of the proximal phalanx, via two tendons. Sesamoid bones are located in the tendons of insertion of these muscles. These muscles act as flexors of the metacarpophalangeal joint.

In the horse, the middle interosseous muscle is the only one of prominence and it is almost entirely tendinous. It is referred to as the suspensory ligament or proximal sesamoidean ligament. The suspensory ligament plays a role in the stay apparatus and in locomotion.

Suggested In-Class Activity

Live Animal

As you did in the last lab, visualize where the muscles are found in the live animal. Follow each muscle and visualize where the origin and insertion of the muscles would generally be. What muscles can you palpate easily? What are the actions of the muscles you palpate?

LABORATORY III

Muscles of the Pelvic Limb

The muscles of the rear limb are important in propelling the animal forward, for example when walking or jumping. The large muscle mass caudal to the femur is a common

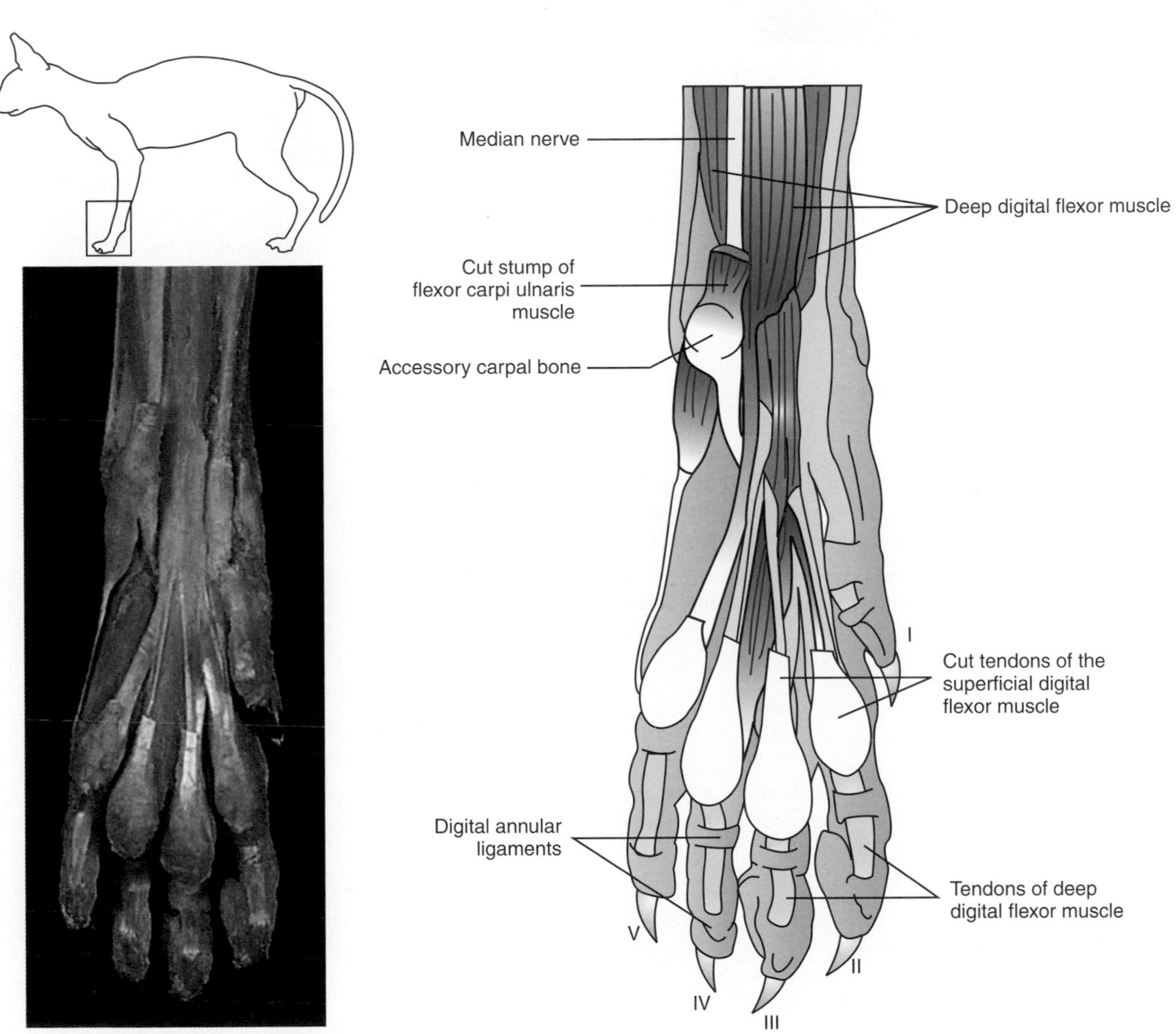

• **Fig. 7.20** Palmar aspect of the muscles of the paw of the left foreleg. (From Done SH et al: Color atlas of veterinary anatomy, vol 3, The dog and cat, London, 1996, Mosby Ltd.)

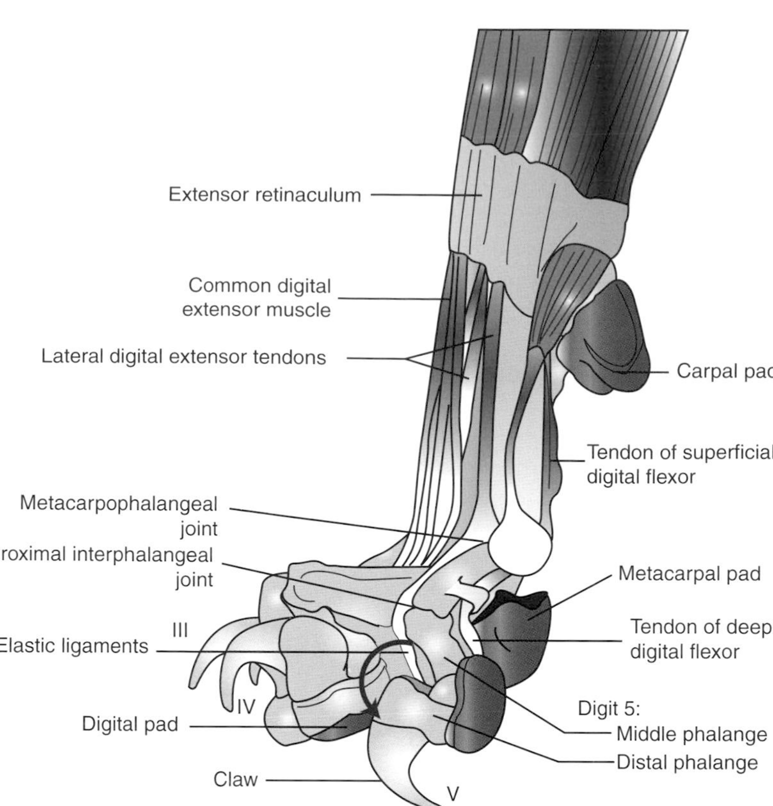

• **Fig. 7.21** Lateral aspects of the muscles of the paw of the left foreleg. (From Done SH et al: Color atlas of veterinary anatomy, vol 3, The dog and cat, London, 1996, Mosby Ltd.)

location for intramuscular (IM) injections. Knowledge of the location of the muscles and the major nerve that lies caudal to the femur (the sciatic nerve) is important when giving IM injections in this region. IM injection in the cranial aspect of the thigh, which includes the massive quadriceps, offers a greater degree of safety because the sciatic nerve cannot be reached via this route. Another common location for IM injection is in the caudal third of the narrow but deep epaxial muscles, which run parallel to the spine.

To Be Identified

The following is a list of the muscles and structures the student must be able to identify on the dissected cat specimens and on anatomic drawings and photos (Table 7.3). A list of terms that the student must be prepared to define is also given.

Muscles

Lateral Muscles of the Hip

1. Tensor fasciae latae muscle
2. Superficial gluteal muscle
3. Middle gluteal muscle
4. Deep gluteal muscle

Caudal Muscles of the Thigh

1. Biceps femoris muscle
2. Semitendinosus
3. Semimembranosus

Medial Muscles of the Thigh

1. Sartorius muscle
2. Gracilis muscle
3. Pectineus muscle
4. Adductor muscle

Cranial Muscles of the Thigh

Quadriceps femoris

1. Vastus lateralis
2. Vastus medialis
3. Vastus intermedius
4. Rectus femoris

Craniolateral Muscles of the Distal Hind Leg

1. Cranial tibial muscle
2. Long digital extensor muscle
3. Peroneus longus muscle

Caudal Muscles of the Distal Hind Leg

1. Gastrocnemius muscle
2. Superficial digital flexor
3. Deep digital flexor
4. Popliteus muscle

TABLE 7.3 Muscles of the Pelvic Limb and Abdomen, Showing Origin, Insertion, and Action

Muscle	Origin	Insertion	Action
Tensor fasciae latae muscle	Cranial wing of ilium	Lateral femoral fascia	Flexes hip/extends stifle
Superficial gluteal muscle	Sacrum and coccygeal vertebrae	Greater trochanter of femur	Abducts limb/extends hip
Middle gluteal muscle	Lateral ilium	Greater trochanter of femur	Abducts limb/extends hip
Deep gluteal muscle	Body of ilium and ischiatic spine	Cranial aspect of greater trochanter	Abducts and extends hip
Biceps femoris muscle	Ischiatic tuberosity of pelvis	Patella/proximal tibia/tuber calcanei	Extends hip/flexes stifle/extends tarsus
Semitendinosus	Ischiatic tuberosity of pelvis	Tibia and tuber calcanei	Extends hip/flexes stifle/extends tarsus
Semimembranosus	Ischiatic tuberosity of pelvis	Femur and tibia	Extends hip
Sartorius muscle	Crest of ilium	Patella/cranial part of tibia	Flexes hip/extends stifle
Gracilis muscle	Pelvic symphysis	Cranial border of tibia/tuber calcanei	Adducts limb/flexes stifle/ extends hip and hock
Pectineus muscle	Prepubic tendon/acetabulum	Caudal aspect of femur	Adducts limb
Adductor muscle	Pelvic symphysis	Caudal aspect of femur	Adducts limb and extends hip
Quadriceps femoris	Ilium/proximal femur	Tibial tuberosity	Extends stifle/flexes hip
Cranial tibial muscle	Cranial tibial border	Proximal metatarsus	Flexes tarsus
Long digital extensor muscle	Extensor fossa of femur	Extensor process of distal phalanges	Extends digits/flexes tarsus/ extends stifle
Peroneus longus muscle	Proximal tibia and fibula	Fourth tarsal bone/plantar aspect metatarsus	Flexes tarsus
Gastrocnemius muscle	Medial/lateral supracondylar tuberosities of femur	Proximal surface tuber calcanei	Extends tarsus/flexes stifle
Superficial digital flexor	Lateral supracondylar tuberosities of femur	Proximal surface of tuber calcanei and plantar surface of middle phalanges	Extends tarsus/flexes stifle and digital joints
Deep digital flexor	Caudal aspect of tibia and fibula	Plantar surface of distal phalanges	Extends tarsus/flexes digital joints
Popliteus muscle	Lateral condyle of femur	Caudal aspect of proximal tibia	Flexes stifle and rotates leg medially
External abdominal oblique	Thoracolumbar fascia of last rib	Linea alba	Flexes vertebral column/ abdominal press
Internal abdominal oblique	Thoracolumbar fascia	Linea alba	Flexes vertebral column/ abdominal press
Transversus abdominis	Last four to five ribs/transverse processes of lumbar vertebrae	Linea alba	Flexes vertebral column/ abdominal press

Muscles of the Abdominal Wall

1. External abdominal oblique
2. Internal abdominal oblique
3. Transversus abdominis
4. Rectus abdominis

Structures

1. Cunean tendon
2. Hamstrings
3. Common calcanean tendon
4. Crus
5. Femoral triangle
6. Popliteal lymph node
7. Extensor retinaculum
8. Sesamoid bone
9. Linea alba
10. Rectus sheath
11. Sciatic nerve

Terms

1. Bone spavin
2. Ankylosis
3. Rhabdomyolysis

Dissection of the Musculature

Remove the skin from the caudal half of the cat by extending the ventral incision from the umbilicus to the tail. Closely circle the external genitalia and the anus. Extend the incision on the medial aspect of the hind leg to the tarsus. Encircle the tarsus and remove the skin from the hind leg and caudal half of the body to the middorsal line. Observe the medial saphenous vein on the medial side between the stifle and the tarsus. This vein is frequently used for venipuncture in the cat, whereas the lateral saphenous is generally used in the dog.

Subcutaneous fat and fascia may need to be removed from the dorsal aspect lateral to the spine to enable you to visualize the proximal muscles of the pelvic limb.

Lateral Muscles of the Hip

This muscle group acts primarily on the hip joint, causing flexion, extension, and/or abduction.

Tensor Fasciae Latae

This triangle-shaped muscle can be divided into two portions (Figs. 7.22 through 7.24). The more cranial superficial portion radiates over the quadriceps in its insertion with the

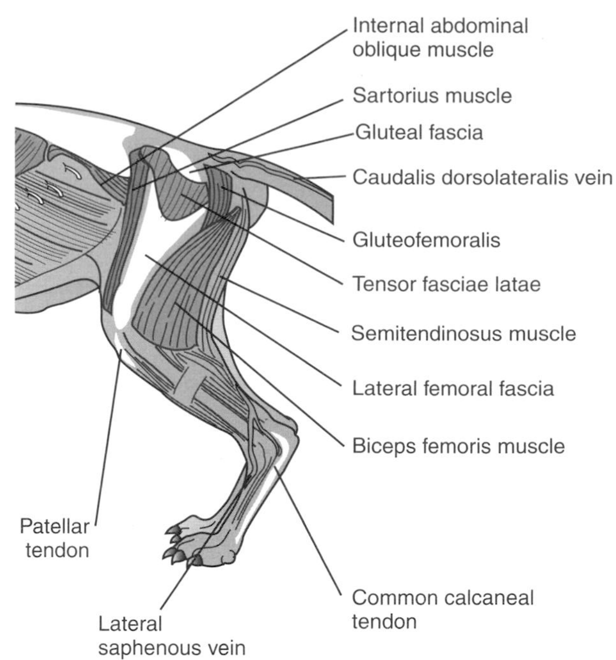

• **Fig. 7.22** Superficial muscles of the abdomen and pelvic limb.

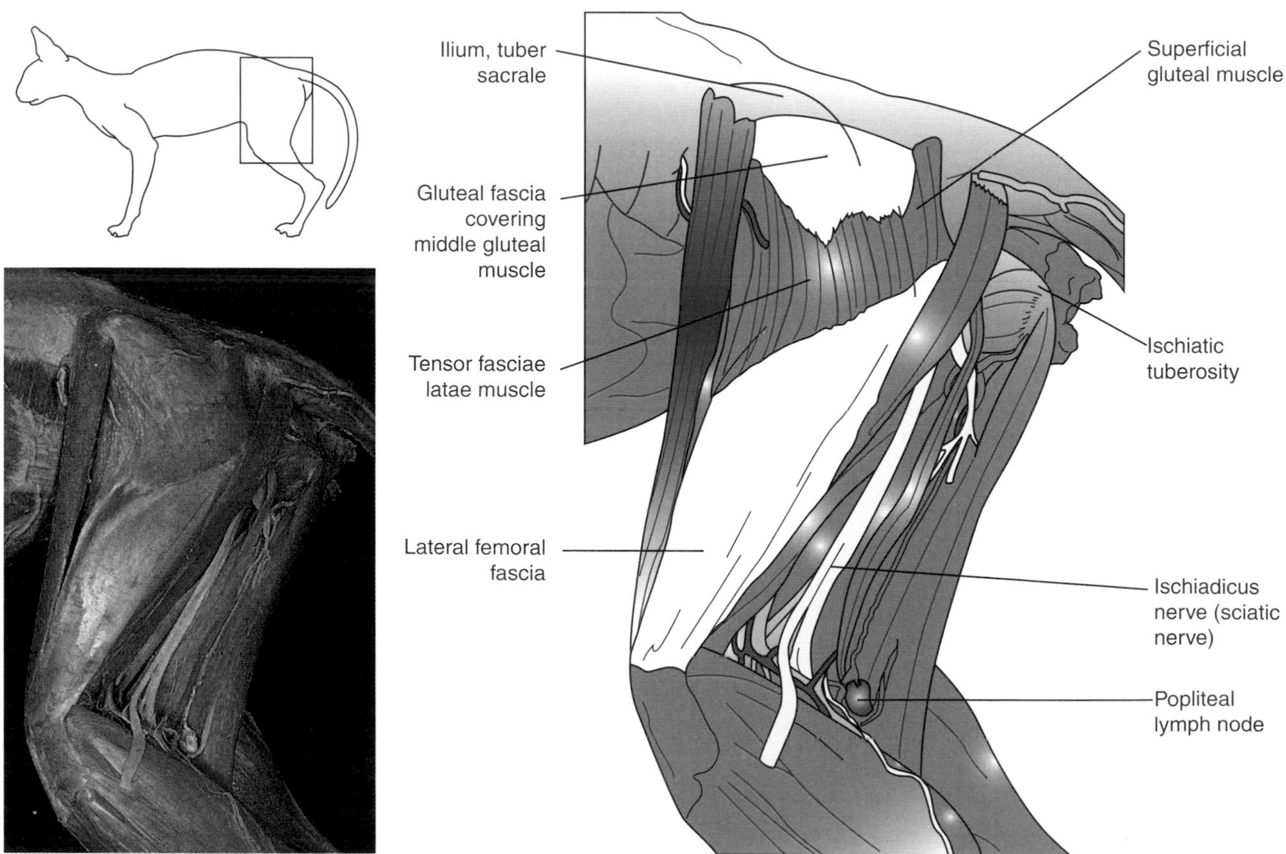

• **Fig. 7.23** Lateral muscle of the left hip and proximal rear leg. (From Done SH et al: Color atlas of veterinary anatomy, vol 3, The dog and cat, London, 1996, Mosby Ltd.)

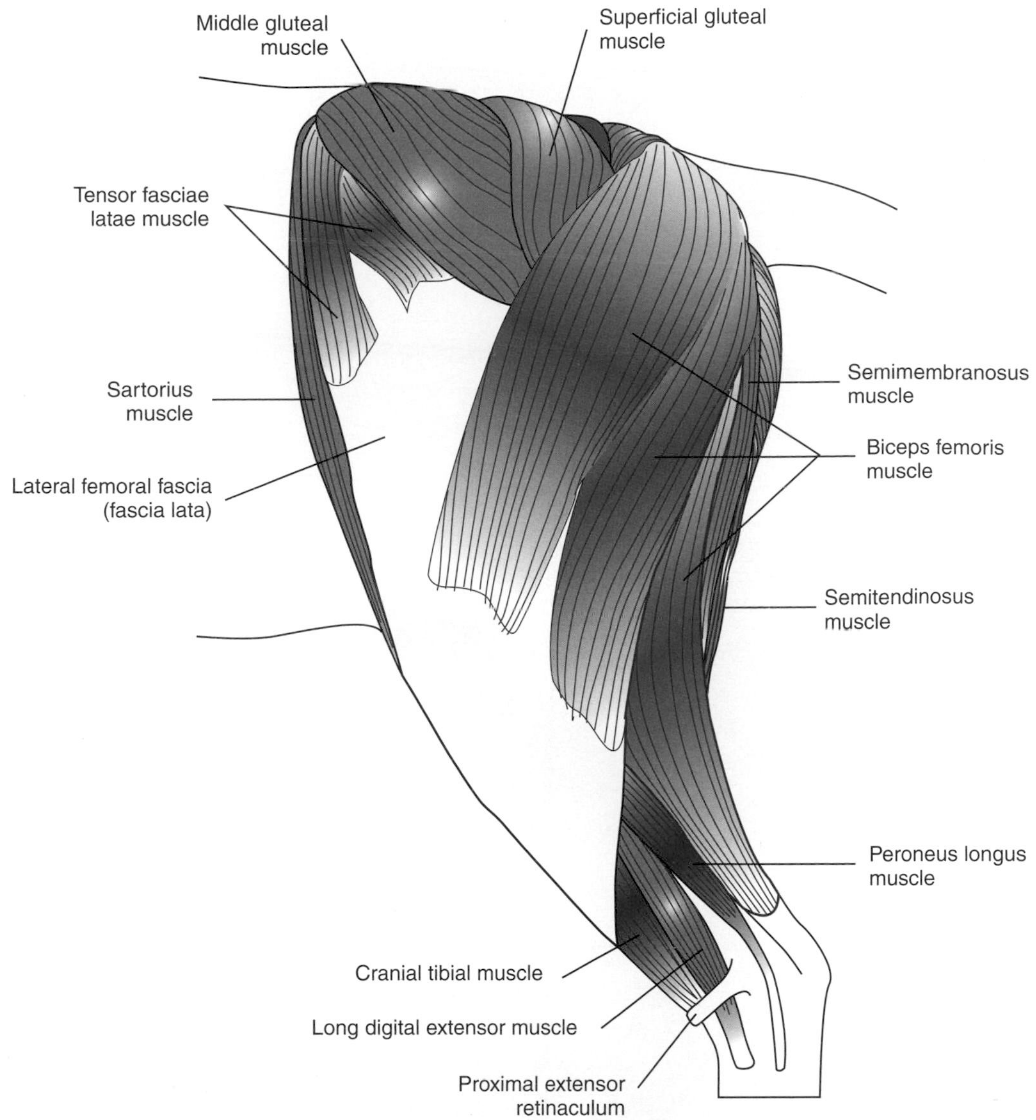

• **Fig. 7.24** Muscles of the left hip and proximal rear leg.

biceps femoris on the lateral femoral fascia. The deeper portion is inserted on the lateral femoral fascia that is deep to the biceps femoris.
Origin—cranial wing of the ilium
Insertion—lateral femoral fascia
Action—flexes the hip joint and extends the stifle

Superficial Gluteal Muscle

This small triangular muscle overlies the caudal part of the middle gluteal muscle (see Figs. 7.23 and 7.24). The fibers of the muscle extend laterally from its origin to the insertion on the femur.
Origin—sacrum and coccygeal vertebrae
Insertion—greater trochanter of femur
Action—abducts the limb and extends the hip

Transect the superficial gluteal muscle to better expose the middle gluteal. The middle gluteal muscle is covered by thick gluteal fascia. Transect the middle gluteal muscle to expose the deep gluteal.

Middle Gluteal Muscle

This large egg-shaped muscle lies cranial to the superficial gluteal and caudal to the tensor fasciae latae (see Fig. 7.24; see also Fig. 7.33). After its origin on the lateral ilium, the fibers are directed caudoventrally to their insertion on the femur.

CLINICAL APPLICATION

Rhabdomyolysis

Rhabdomyolysis, or "Monday morning disease," occurs in horses that are worked hard during the week and then given the weekend off. When Monday rolls around, the horses are again given their usual strenuous exercise, which can result in "tying up" or muscle stiffness and a stilted gait. In more severe cases the animal will exhibit azoturia, muscle fasciculations, muscle cramping, sweating, and myoglobin in the urine as a result of muscle breakdown. Kidney damage is occasionally a sequela.

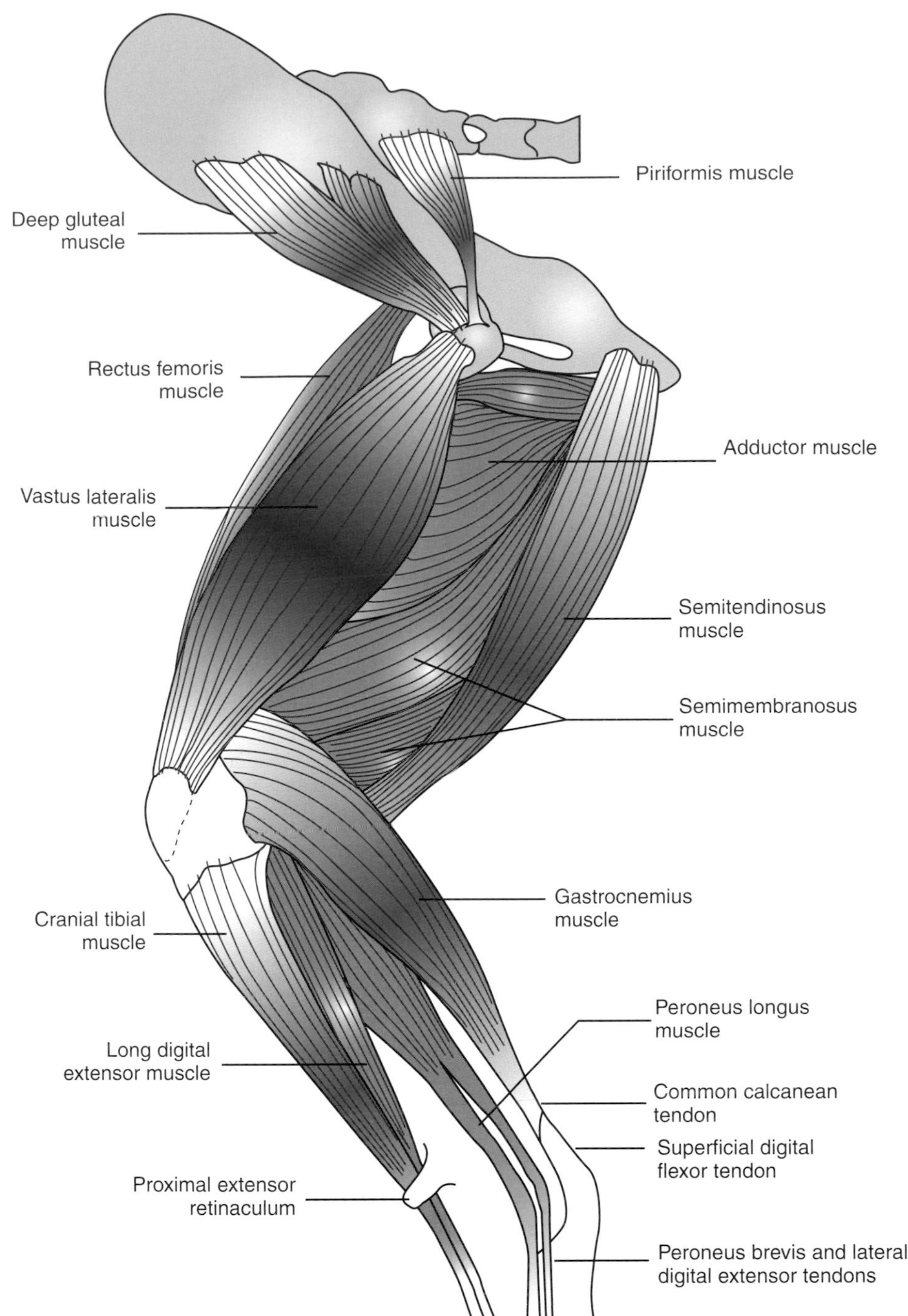

• **Fig. 7.25** Deep muscles of the lateral left leg after removal of the biceps femoris, semitendinosus, tensor fasciae latae, and superficial and middle gluteal muscles.

Origin—lateral ilium
Insertion—greater trochanter of femur
Action—abducts the limb and extends hip

Deep Gluteal Muscle

This fan-shaped muscle is totally covered by the middle gluteal (Figs. 7.25 and 7.33).
Origin—body of ilium and ischiatic spine
Insertion—cranial aspect of greater trochanter
Action—abducts and extends hip

Caudal Muscles of the Thigh

These muscles are informally referred to as the "hamstrings." The caudal thigh muscles from medial to lateral are the biceps femoris, the semitendinosus, and the semimembranosus.

Biceps Femoris Muscle

The biceps femoris is the longest and widest muscle of the thigh and covers its entire caudolateral aspect (see Figs. 7.22, 7.24, and 7.25; see also Fig. 7.34). This muscle spans three joints and can affect all three. The tendon of this muscle contributes to the formation of the common calcanean tendon (Achilles tendon) by a strand of heavy fascia. The biceps femoris exerts its action on the hip joint, stifle, and tarsus.

Origin—ischiatic tuberosity of the pelvis
Insertion—patella, proximal tibia, and tuber calcanei
Action—extends the hip joint, flexes the stifle joint, and extends the tarsal joints

Lying in the fat at the caudal border of the biceps femoris, directly opposite the stifle, is the popliteal lymph node. Transect the biceps femoris in the middle and reflect the cut ends. Notice the large sciatic nerve that runs on the caudal aspect of the femur beneath the biceps femoris. This nerve is to be avoided when giving intramuscular injections.

Semitendinosus Muscle

This straplike muscle lies medial to the biceps femoris and lateral to the semimembranosus (see Figs. 7.22 and 7.23–7.28; see also Figs. 7.33 and 7.34). The tendon of this muscle also contributes to the common calcanean tendon.

Origin—ischiatic tuberosity
Insertion—tibia and tuber calcanei
Action—extends the hip, flexes the stifle, and extends the tarsal joints

Semimembranosus Muscle

This muscle is not as long as the semitendinosus but is slightly larger in the transverse section (see Figs. 7.24, 7.27, and 7.28; see also Figs. 7.33 and 7.34). It is wedged between the biceps femoris laterally and the gracilis and adductor muscles medially. It consists of two bellies of equal size.

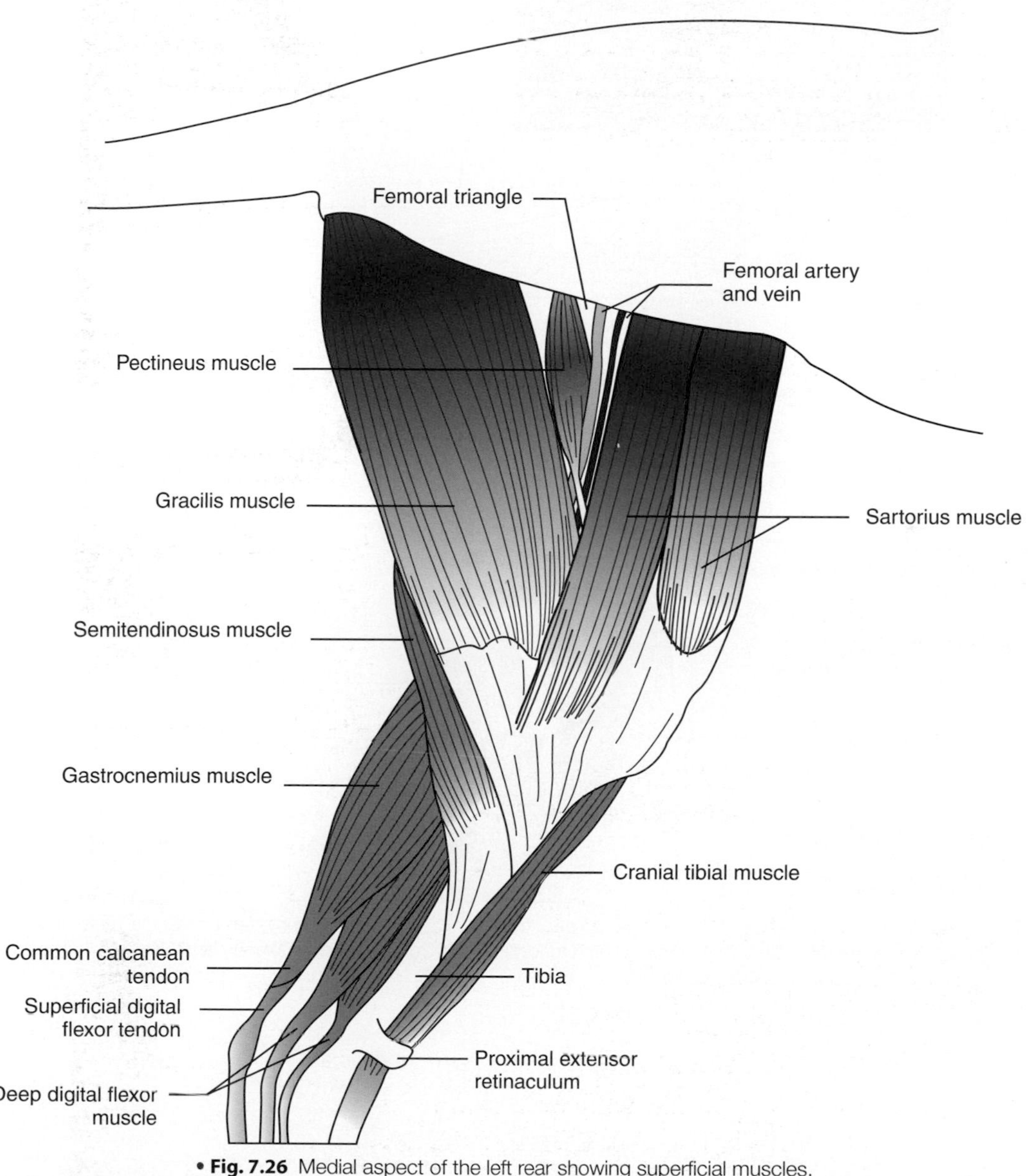

• **Fig. 7.26** Medial aspect of the left rear showing superficial muscles.

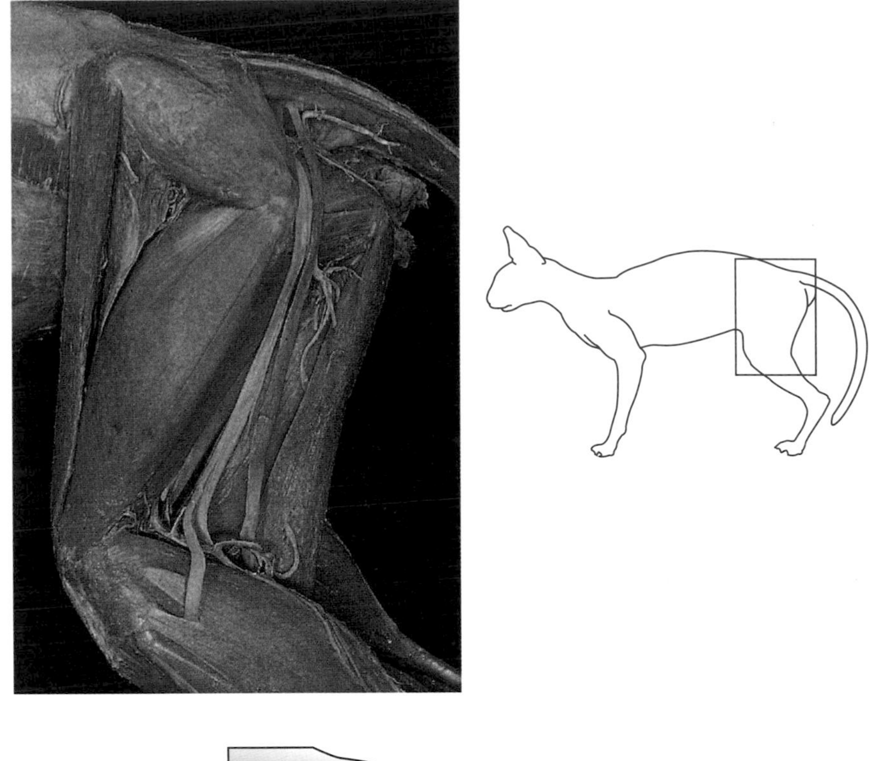

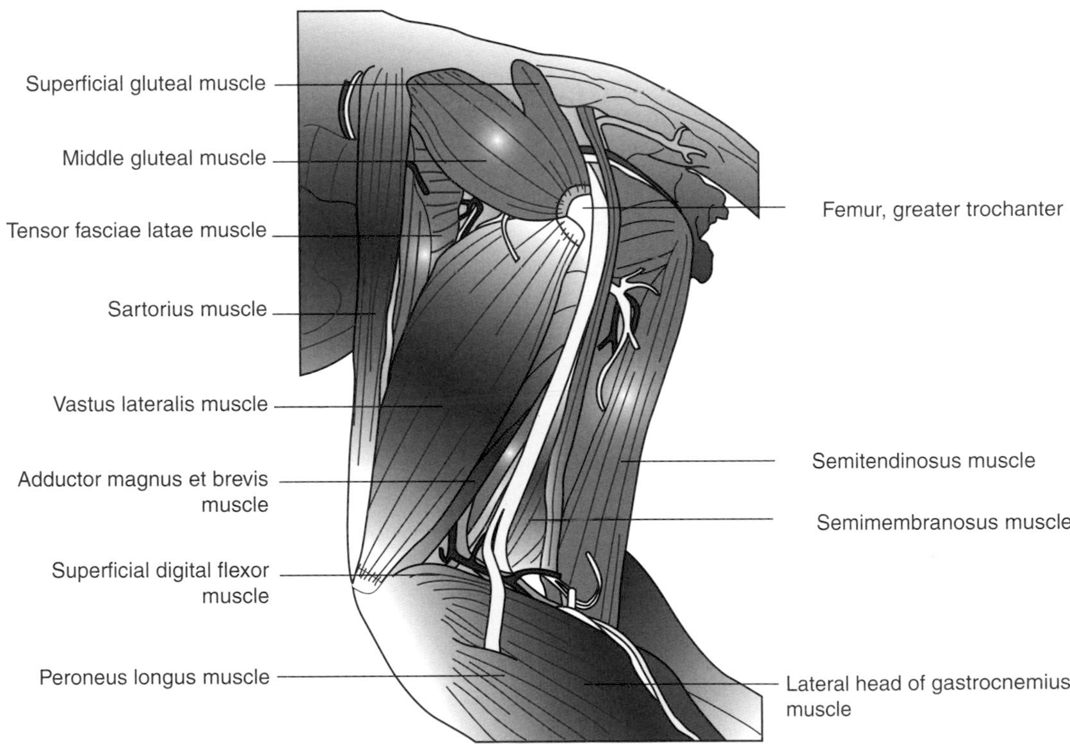

• **Fig. 7.27** Deep muscles of the left rear leg after the removal of biceps femoris, tensor fasciae latae, and the lateral femoral and gluteal fascia. (From Done SH et al: Color atlas of veterinary anatomy, vol 3, The dog and cat, London, 1996, Mosby Ltd.)

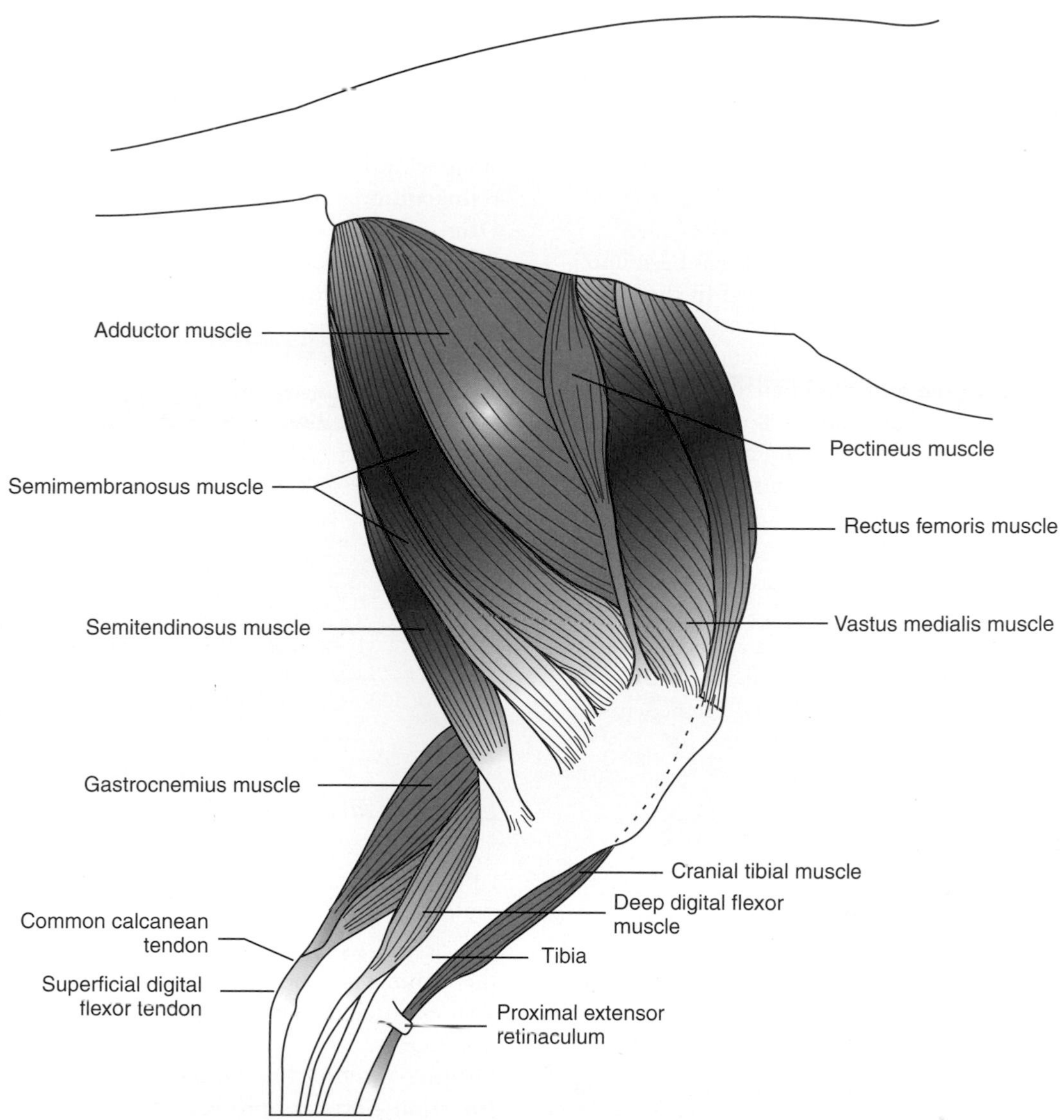

• **Fig. 7.28** Medial aspect of the left rear leg after removal of the gracilis and sartorius muscles and the fascial attachment of the semitendinosus muscle.

Origin—ischiatic tuberosity
Insertion—femur and tibia
Action—extends the hip and flexes the stifle

Medial Muscles of the Thigh

The four muscles in this group are primarily adductors of the rear leg. They also may have some action on the hip or stifle joints.

Sartorius Muscle

This muscle is made up of two straplike parts that lie on the cranial and craniomedial surfaces of the thigh (see Figs. 7.22 and 7.24 through 7.27; see also Figs. 7.33 and 7.34).
Origin—on or near the crest of the ilium
Insertion—the cranial part inserts on the patella along with the tendon of the quadriceps and the caudal part on the cranial border of the tibia
Action—flexes hip, extends stifle (cranial part), and flexes stifle (caudal part)

The sartorius has two distinct bellies in the dog but is undivided in the horse and cat. Transect the sartorius in the middle and reflect the ends toward its origin and insertion.

Gracilis Muscle

This large, wide, flat muscle covers the caudomedial surface of the medial thigh (Fig. 7.26; see also Figs. 7.33 and 7.34).
Origin—pelvic symphysis
Insertion—cranial border of tibia, and sends a small tendon down to insert on the tuber calcanei as well
Action—adducts the limb, flexes the stifle, and extends the hip and hock

Pectineus Muscle

This small spindle-shaped muscle is located on the medial aspect (see Fig. 7.26; see also Figs. 7.28, 7.33, and 7.34).

Origin—prepubic tendon and cranioventral to acetabulum on the pubis
Insertion—caudal aspect of distal femur
Action—adducts the limb

Surgical severing of the pectineus muscle has been implicated as an important procedure performed in the alleviation of pain associated with hip dysplasia.

The **femoral triangle** is the shallow triangular space created by the borders of the sartorius cranially, the pectineus and adductor muscles caudally, and the body wall medially. This triangular region contains the femoral artery and vein. The pulse is usually taken in this area in small animals.

Adductor Muscle

This large pyramid-shaped muscle consists of two muscles that are not easily divisible (se Fig. 7.25; see also Figs. 7.28 and 7.32). The larger portion is called the adductor magnus et brevis, whereas the smaller more cranial part is called the adductor longus. This muscle is found between the semitendinosus and the semimembranosus.

Origin—pelvic symphysis
Insertion—caudal aspect of femur
Action—adducts the limb and extends the hip

Cranial Muscles of the Thigh

These muscles primarily act to flex the hip joint and extend the stifle joint.

Quadriceps Femoris Muscle

This muscle consists of four heads (hence "quad") that fuse distally to form a common tendon (see Figs. 7.25, 7.27, and 7.28; see also Figs. 7.32 and 7.33). This muscle is the most powerful extensor of the stifle. The most cranial head of this muscle is termed the **rectus femoris.** The other three heads lie lateral, medial, and caudal to the rectus femoris, respectively. The **vastus lateralis** lies lateral, the **vastus medialis** medial, and the **vastus intermedius** caudal to the rectus femoris. The **patella** is a sesamoid bone in the tendon of insertion of the quadriceps and articulates with the trochlea of the femur.

Origin—rectus femoris on the ilium; the other three heads arise on the proximal femur
Insertion—tibial tuberosity
Action—extends the stifle joint and flexes the hip joint

In the horse, the patellar ligament is divided into three parts: the lateral patellar ligament, medial patellar ligament, and intermediate patellar ligament. The enlarged medial ridge of the femoral trochlea protrudes between the medial and intermediate patellar ligaments and is important in the stay apparatus.

Craniolateral Muscles of the Hind Leg

These muscles are primarily flexors of the tarsal joint and extensors of the digital joints.

Cranial Tibial Muscle

The cranial tibial is the most cranial muscle in this group (see Figs. 7.24–7.26 and 7.28–7.30; see also Figs. 7.33 and 7.34). Near the tarsal joint the muscle is held in position, along with the other muscles in this group, by the **extensor retinaculum**, a strong band of fascia.

Origin—lateral aspect of the cranial tibial border
Insertion—proximal metatarsus
Action—flexes the tarsal joint

CLINICAL APPLICATION

Bone Spavin

In the horse, the cranial tibial muscle is occasionally referred to as the "cunean" tendon. This muscle is occasionally resected to relieve "bone spavin." Bone spavin is osteoarthritis and periostitis usually of the distal intertarsal and tarsometatarsal joints of the hock. In severe cases, bone spavin can result in ankylosis of the hock.

Long Digital Extensor Muscle

This spindle-shaped muscle lies lateral to the cranial tibial muscle and is partly covered by it (see Figs. 7.24, 7.25, 7.29, and 7.30; see also Figs. 7.33 and 7.34). Expose the muscle and its tendon of origin from the extensor fossa of the femur. The tendons of this muscle run under the proximal extensor retinaculum and divide into four tendons of insertion.

Origin—extensor fossa of the femur
Insertion—extensor processes of the distal phalanges
Action—extends digital joints, flexes the tarsal joint, and extends the stifle joint

Peroneus Longus Muscle

This muscle lies caudal and lateral to the long digital extensor (see Figs. 7.24, 7.25, and 7.27; see also Figs. 7.32 and 7.33). Its tendon passes through a groove on the caudal aspect of the lateral malleolus to its insertion.

Origin—proximal end of tibia and fibula
Insertion—fourth tarsal bone and the plantar aspect of the base of the metatarsals
Action—flexes the tarsal joint

Caudal Muscles of the Hind Leg

These muscles primarily flex the digital joints and/or extend the tarsal joints (Fig. 7.31).

Gastrocnemius Muscle

This is the most superficial muscle of the caudal leg muscles and consists of two heads, each of which has a

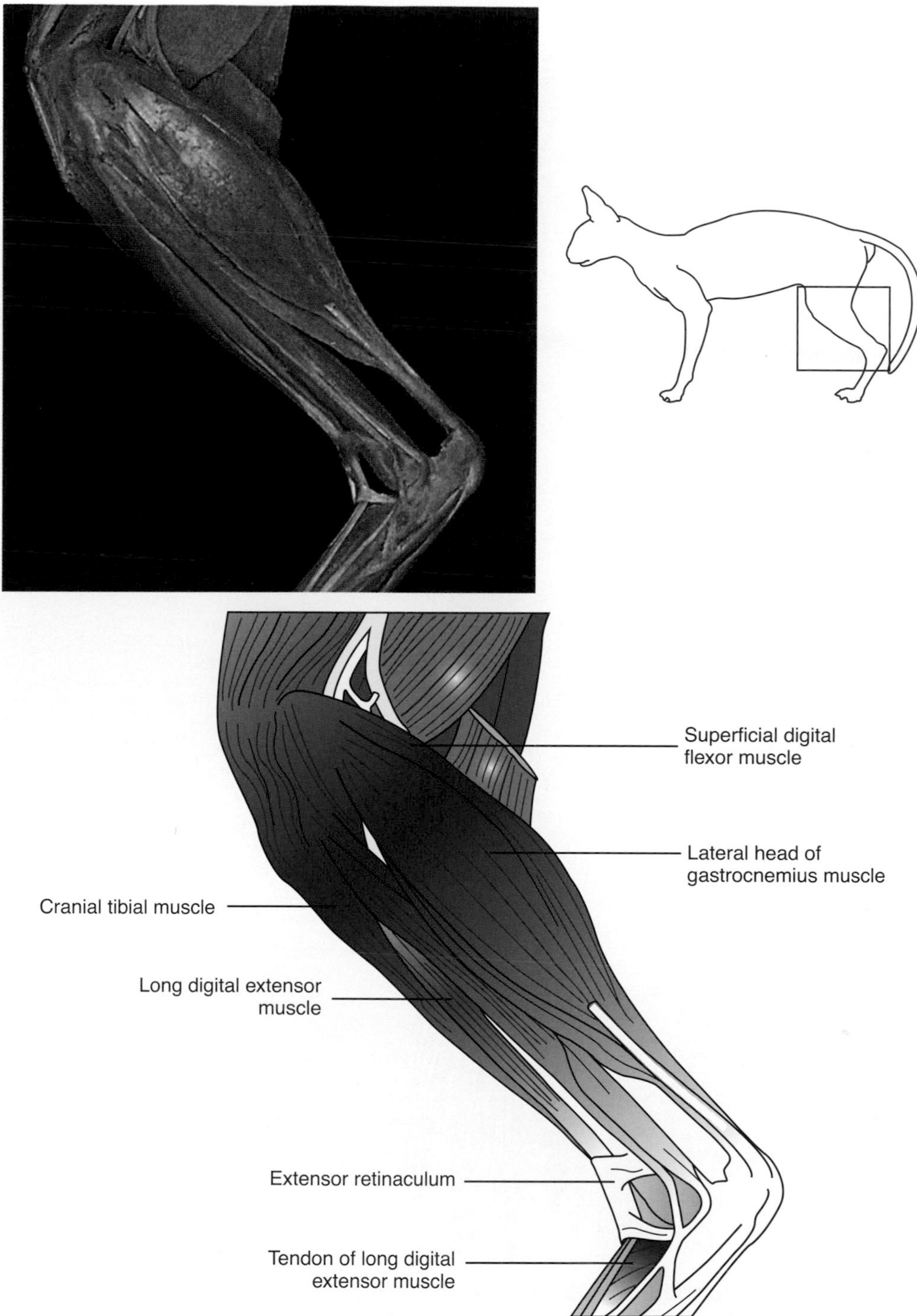

• **Fig. 7.29** Lateral aspect of the left rear leg distal to the stifle. The biceps femoris muscle has been removed. (From Done SH et al: Color atlas of veterinary anatomy, vol 3, The dog and cat, London, 1996, Mosby Ltd.)

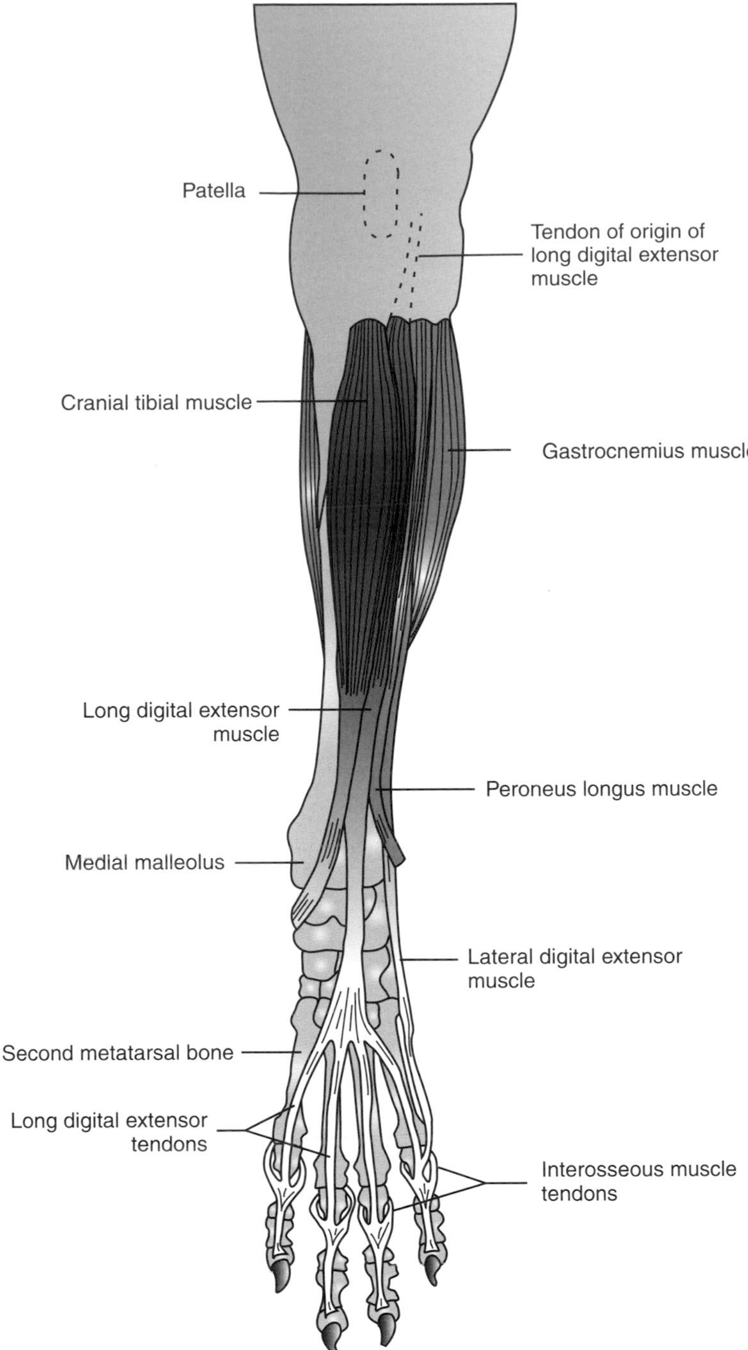

• **Fig. 7.30** Craniolateral muscles of the left rear leg distal to the stifle.

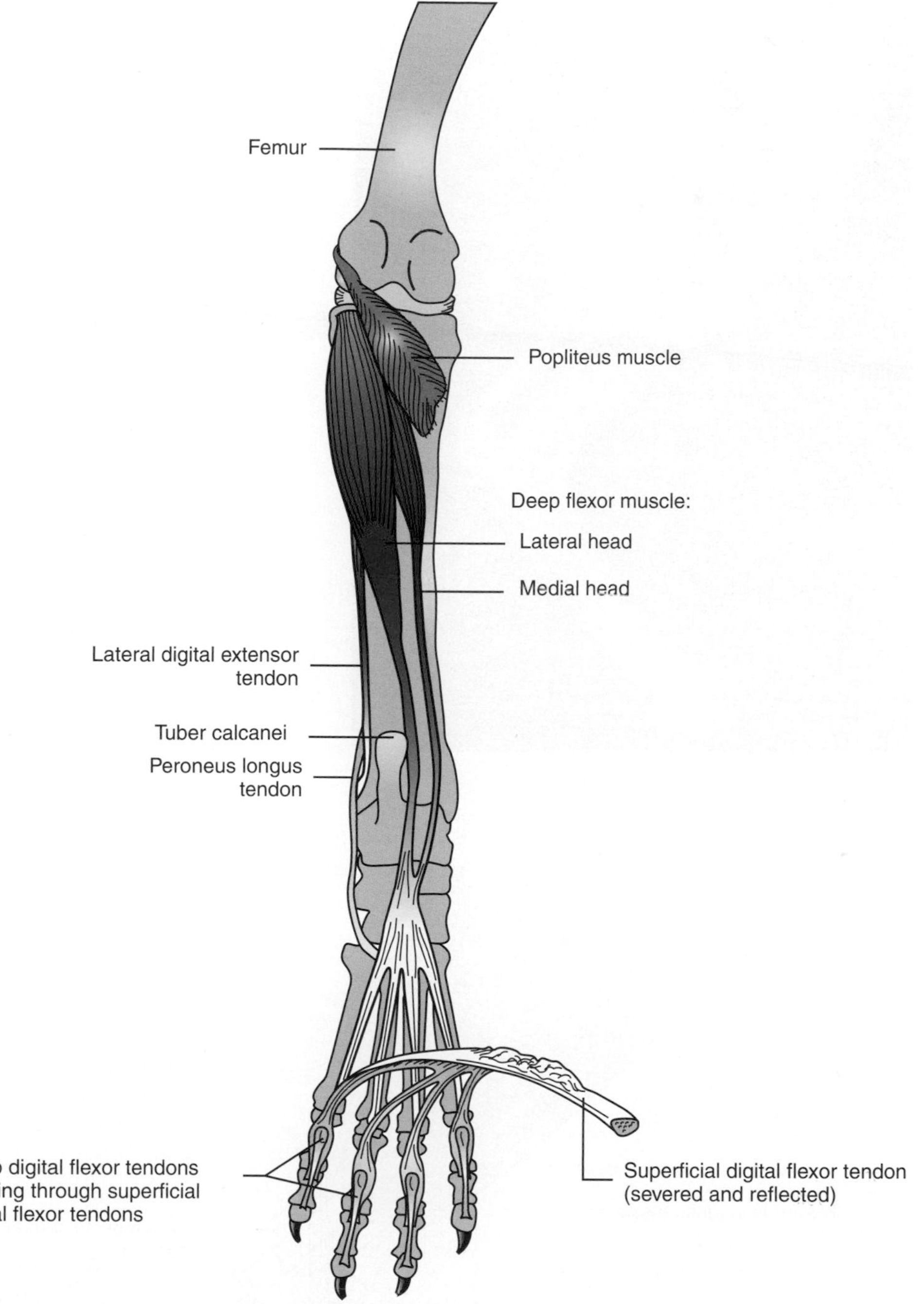

• **Fig. 7.31** Caudal muscles of the left rear leg distal to the stifle. The gastrocnemius muscle and the common calcanean tendon have been removed.

sesamoid bone embedded near its origin (see Figs. 7.25 to 7.30 and 7.32–7.34). This muscle is often called the calf muscle. The tendon of this muscle, along with that of the superficial digital flexor muscle, forms the bulk of the **common calcanean tendon** (Achilles tendon) (see Figs. 7.28 and 7.32).

Origin—medial and lateral supracondylar tuberosities of the femur

Insertion—proximal surface of the tuber calcanei

Action—extends the tarsus and flexes the stifle

Identify the two heads of the gastrocnemius muscle and follow it to its insertion on the tuber calcanei. Transect the gastrocnemius muscle and reflect to its attachments and note the two sesamoid bones in each head where it originates. Separate the gastrocnemius from the underlying superficial digital flexor muscle. (It is easiest to identify these tendons near the tuber calcanei and proceed proximally in your separation.) In the cat, a small muscle called the soleus is located next to the lateral head of the gastrocnemius. This muscle need not be studied.

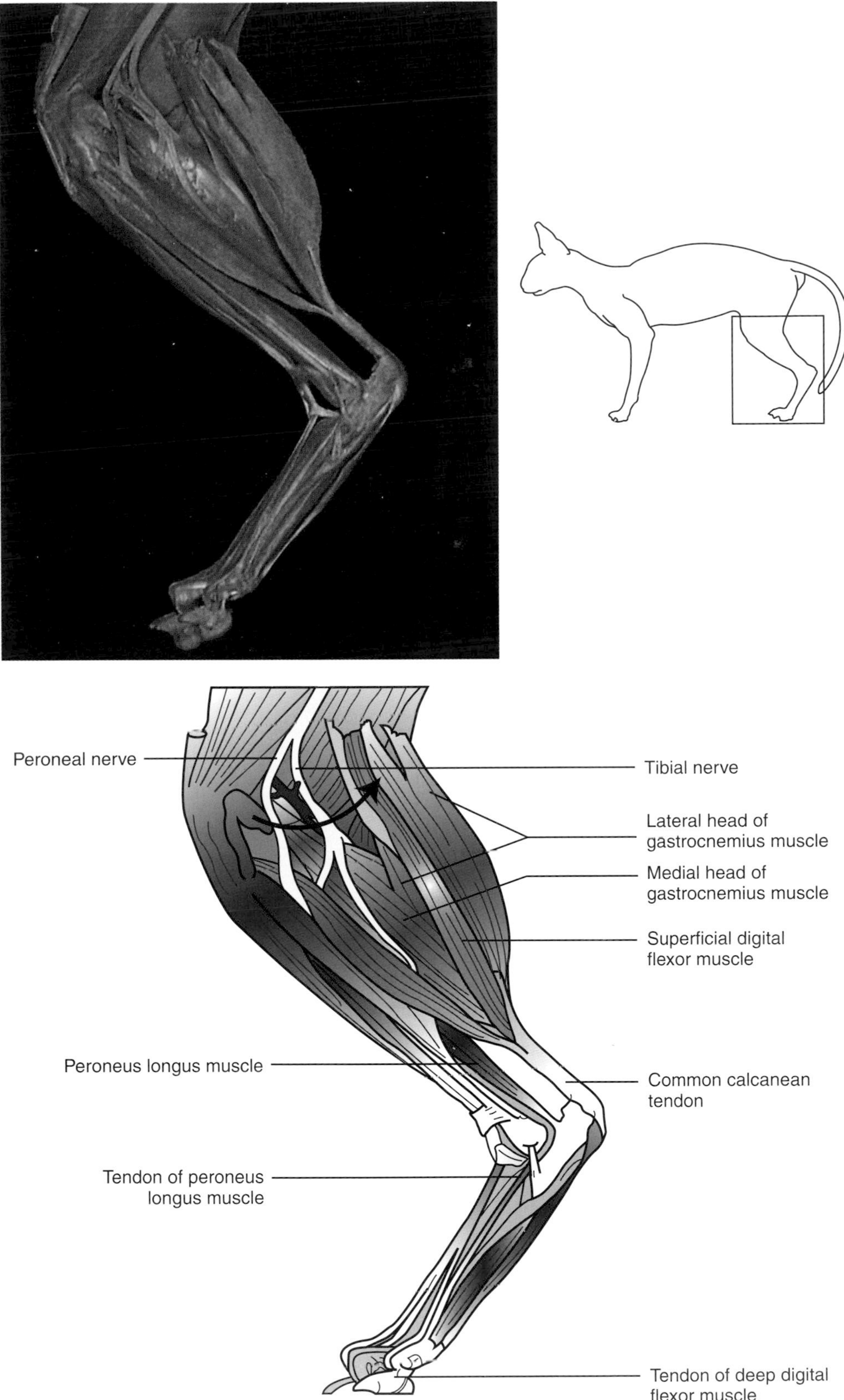

• **Fig. 7.32** Lateral aspect of the left rear leg distal to the stifle. A portion of the lateral head of the gastrocnemius muscle and the superficial digital flexor have been removed. (From Done SH et al: Color atlas of veterinary anatomy, vol 3, The dog and cat, London, 1996, Mosby Ltd.)

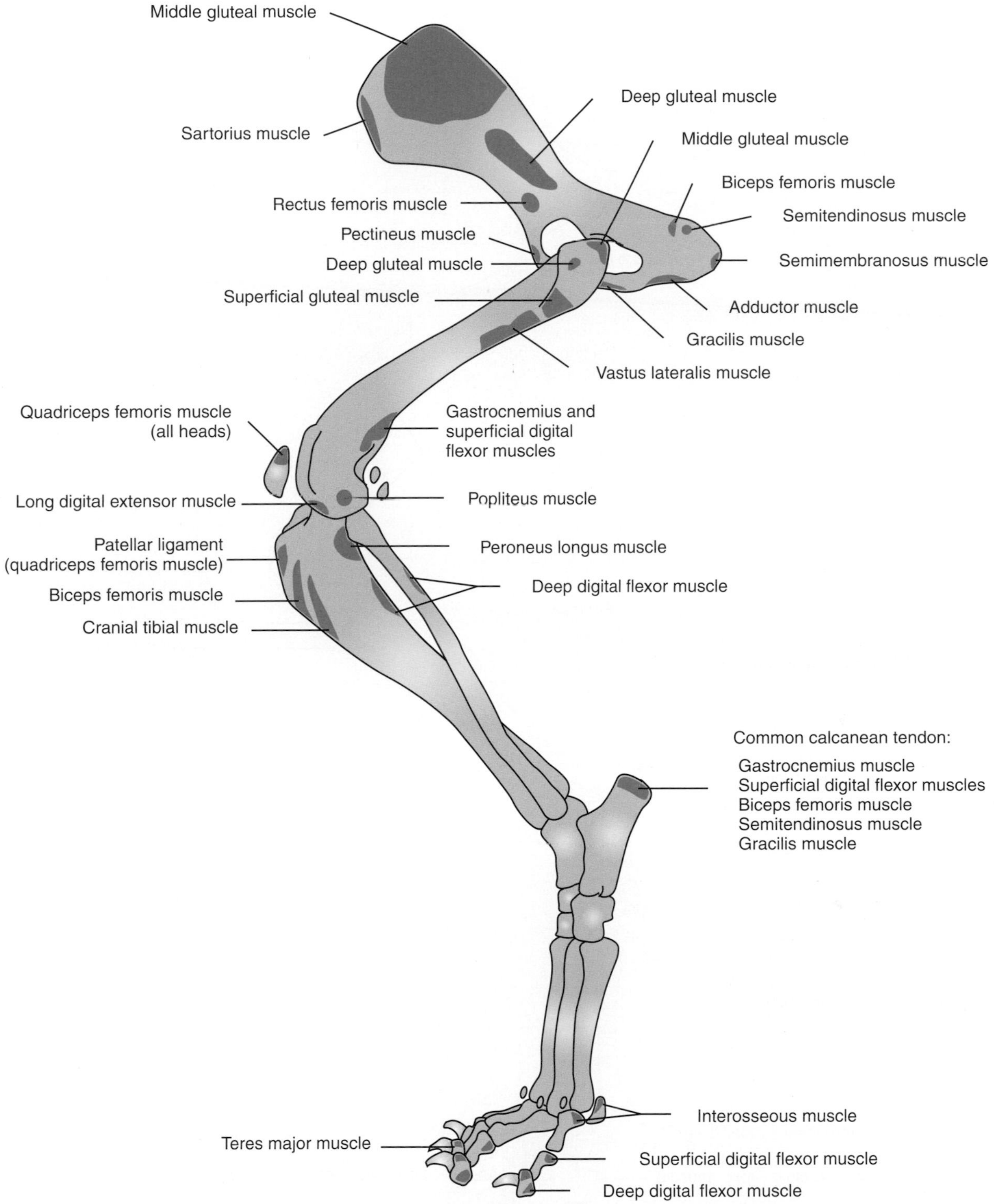

• **Fig. 7.33** Origins and insertions of the muscles on the lateral aspect of the left rear leg.

Superficial Digital Flexor Muscle

This spindle-shaped muscle arises from the lateral supracondylar tuberosity of the femur along with the lateral head of the gastrocnemius muscle (see Figs. 7.25, 7.26, 7.28, 7.29, 7.31, 7.33, and 7.34). The tendon of insertion twists medially around that of the gastrocnemius to insert on the sides of the tuber calcanei and phalanges.

Origin—lateral supracondylar tuberosity of the femur

Insertion—tuber calcanei and the plantar surface of phalanges II, III, IV, and V

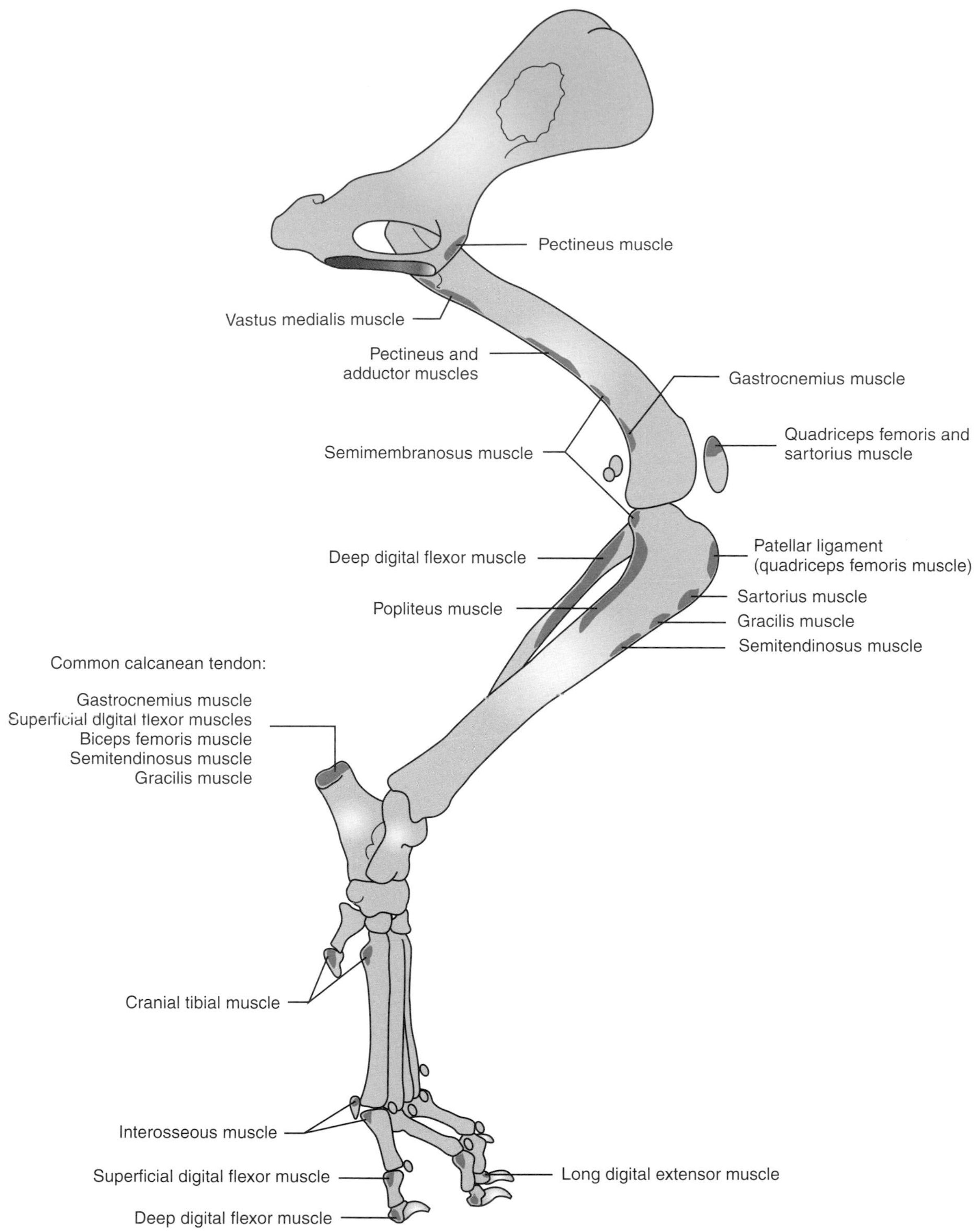

• Fig. 7.34 Origins and insertions of the muscles on the medial aspect of the left rear leg.

Action—flexes the stifle and digital joints and extends the tarsal joints

Deep Digital Flexor Muscle

This muscle originates on the proximal caudal aspect of the tibia and fibula and lies deep to the superficial digital flexor on the caudal aspect of the leg (see Figs. 7.26, 7.28, and 7.31 to 7.34). It consists of a lateral head and a much smaller medial head. The tendons from both heads join near the tarsus and then divide, sending a small tendon to insert into each of the four digits.

Origin—caudal aspect of proximal tibia and fibula

Insertion—plantar surfaces of the distal phalanges
Action—extends the tarsal joints and flexes the digital joints

Popliteus Muscle

This muscle is covered by the gastrocnemius and superficial digital flexor (see Figs. 7.31, 7.33, and 7.34). It lies on the caudal surface of the proximal tibia and medial to the proximal portion of the deep digital flexor. At the junction of the muscle belly with the tendon, there is a sesamoid bone that articulates with the caudal aspect of the lateral condyle of the tibia.
Origin—lateral condyle of femur
Insertion—caudal aspect of proximal tibia
Action—flexes the stifle and rotates the leg medially

Common Calcanean Tendon

The common calcanean tendon, or Achilles tendon, is a heavy band of connective tissue that inserts on the tuber calcanei (see Figs. 7.25, 7.26, and 7.28). It is made up of five different muscles. The muscles whose tendons of insertion make up this tendon are:

- Gastrocnemius
- Superficial digital flexor
- Semitendinosus
- Gracilis
- Biceps femoris

Muscles of the Rear Foot (PES)

These muscles are essentially the same as those in the forefoot (manus) and do not need to be dissected.

Muscles of the Abdominal Wall

The lateral and ventral abdominal wall is made up of four pairs of muscles (Figs. 7.35–7.38). These muscles, from superficial to deep, are the: **external abdominal oblique, internal abdominal oblique, transversus abdominis,** and **rectus**

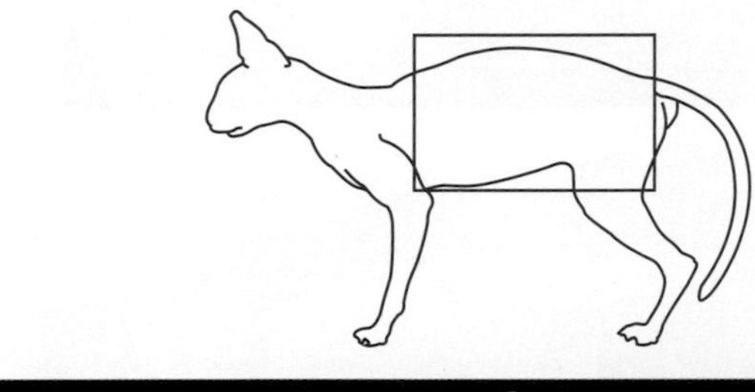

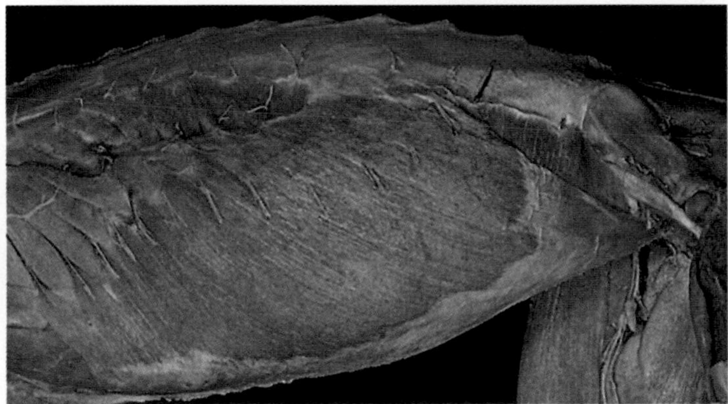

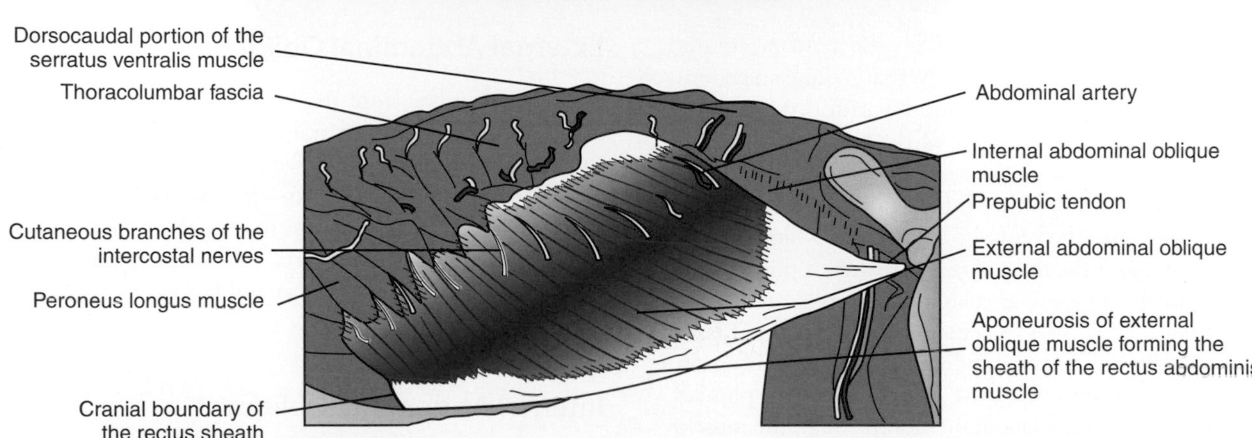

• **Fig. 7.35** Left lateral aspect of the muscles of the abdominal wall. (From Done SH et al: Color atlas of veterinary anatomy, vol 3, The dog and cat, London, 1996, Mosby Ltd.)

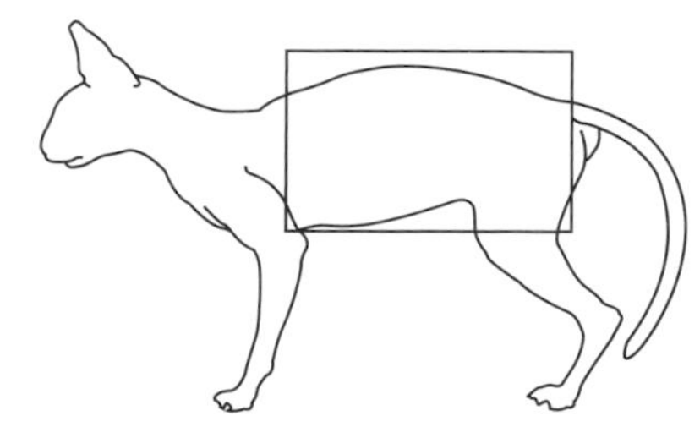

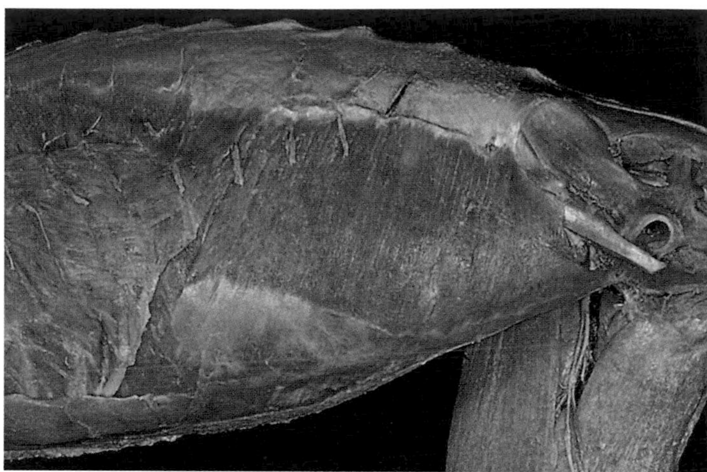

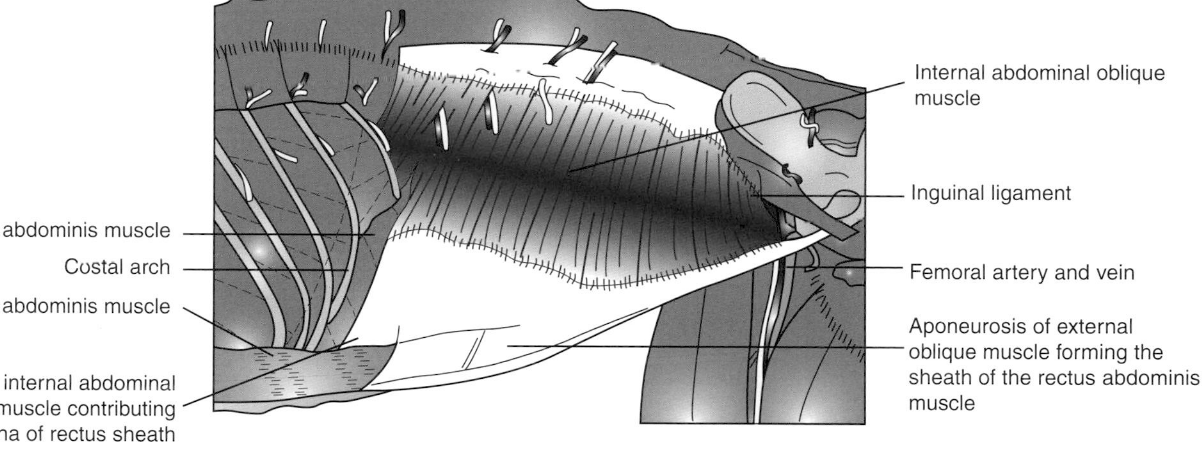

• **Fig. 7.36** Left lateral aspect of the muscles of the abdominal wall after removal of the external abdominal oblique muscle. (From Done SH et al: Color atlas of veterinary anatomy, vol 3, The dog and cat, London, 1996, Mosby Ltd.)

abdominis. These muscles work to flex the vertebral column and to assist in various body functions that require an abdominal press, such as urination, defecation, parturition, and vomiting. If these muscles on one side of the body contract, they cause the trunk to bend or twist toward the contracted side. Make an incision through the abdominal wall from the sternum to the pelvis on the ventral midline. The whitish line on the midline is called the linea alba. It is through this line that incisions into the abdominal cavity of domestic animals are routinely made. This "line" is actually a narrow strip of fascia that connects the two rectus abdominis muscles and is also made up of the insertions of the other abdominal muscles. At the umbilicus, make a lateral incision through the muscles dorsally to the lumbar area. Gently separate the muscles of the abdominal wall and note the orientation of their fibers.

External Abdominal Oblique

This muscle arises from the last rib and the thoracolumbar fascia and covers the ventral and lateral thoracic wall and the lateral abdominal wall (see Figs. 7.35, 7.36, and 7.38). The fibers of this muscle run caudoventrally. The belly of the muscle does not extend to the caudal midline but forms a wide aponeurosis that inserts on the linea alba.

Origin—thoracolumbar fascia and last rib

Insertion—linea alba

Internal Abdominal Oblique

This muscle is located medial to the external abdominal oblique and arises from the thoracolumbar fascia caudal to

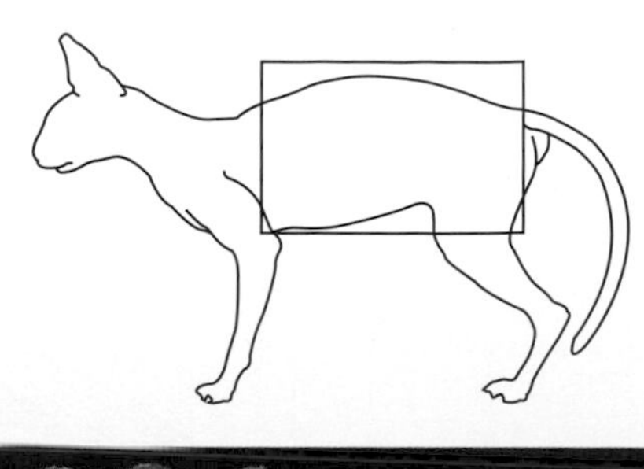

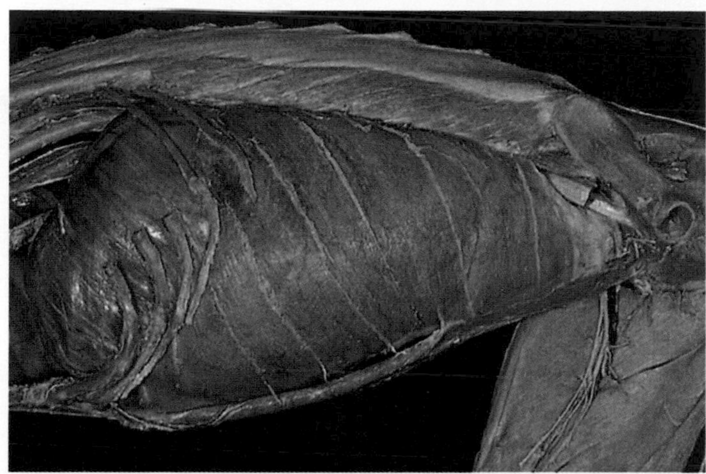

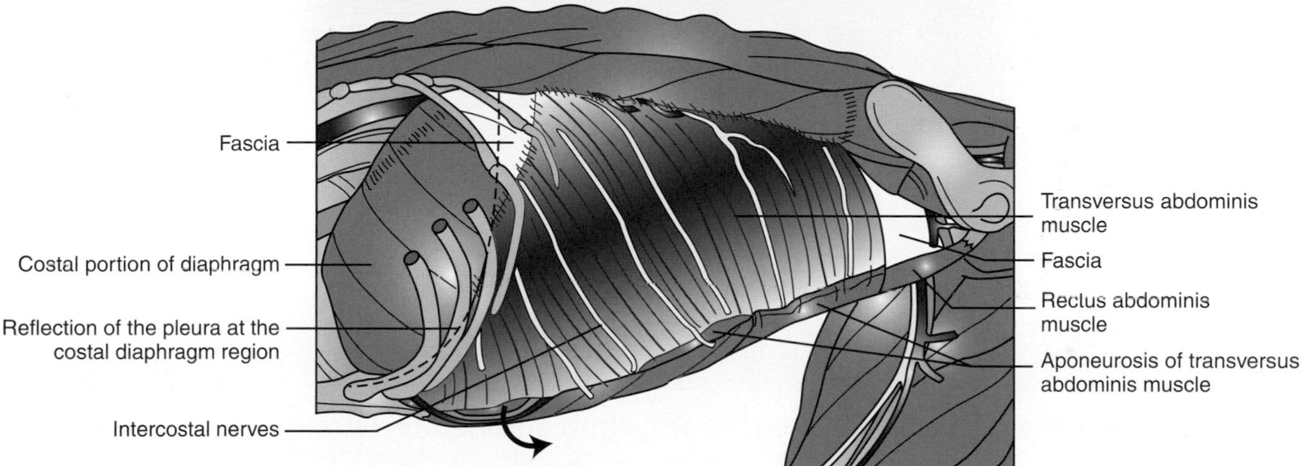

• Fig. 7.37 Left lateral aspect of the muscles of the abdominal wall after removal of the external abdominal oblique and internal abdominal oblique muscles. (From Done SH et al: Color atlas of veterinary anatomy, vol 3, The dog and cat, London, 1996, Mosby Ltd.)

the last rib (see Figs. 7.37 and 7.38). The fibers of this muscle run in a cranioventral direction.
Origin—thoracolumbar fascia
Insertion—linea alba

Transversus Abdominis

This muscle is medial to the internal abdominal oblique and the rectus abdominis and arises from the last four to five ribs and the transverse processes of the lumbar vertebrae (see Figs. 7.37 and 7.38). Its fibers run in a dorsoventral direction.
Origin—medial surface of last four to five ribs and transverse process of lumbar vertebrae
Insertion—linea alba

Rectus Abdominis

The rectus abdominis lies on either side of the ventral midline (see Figs. 7.35–7.37). This straplike muscle runs from the sternum to the pubis, lateral to the linea alba. This muscle is what forms the "six-pack" in physically fit individuals.
Origin—sternum
Insertion—pubis

The flat rectus abdominis muscle is encased in an aponeurosis known as the **rectus sheath.** The external rectus sheath, owing to its connective tissue, is the holding layer when the abdomen is closed during abdominal surgery.

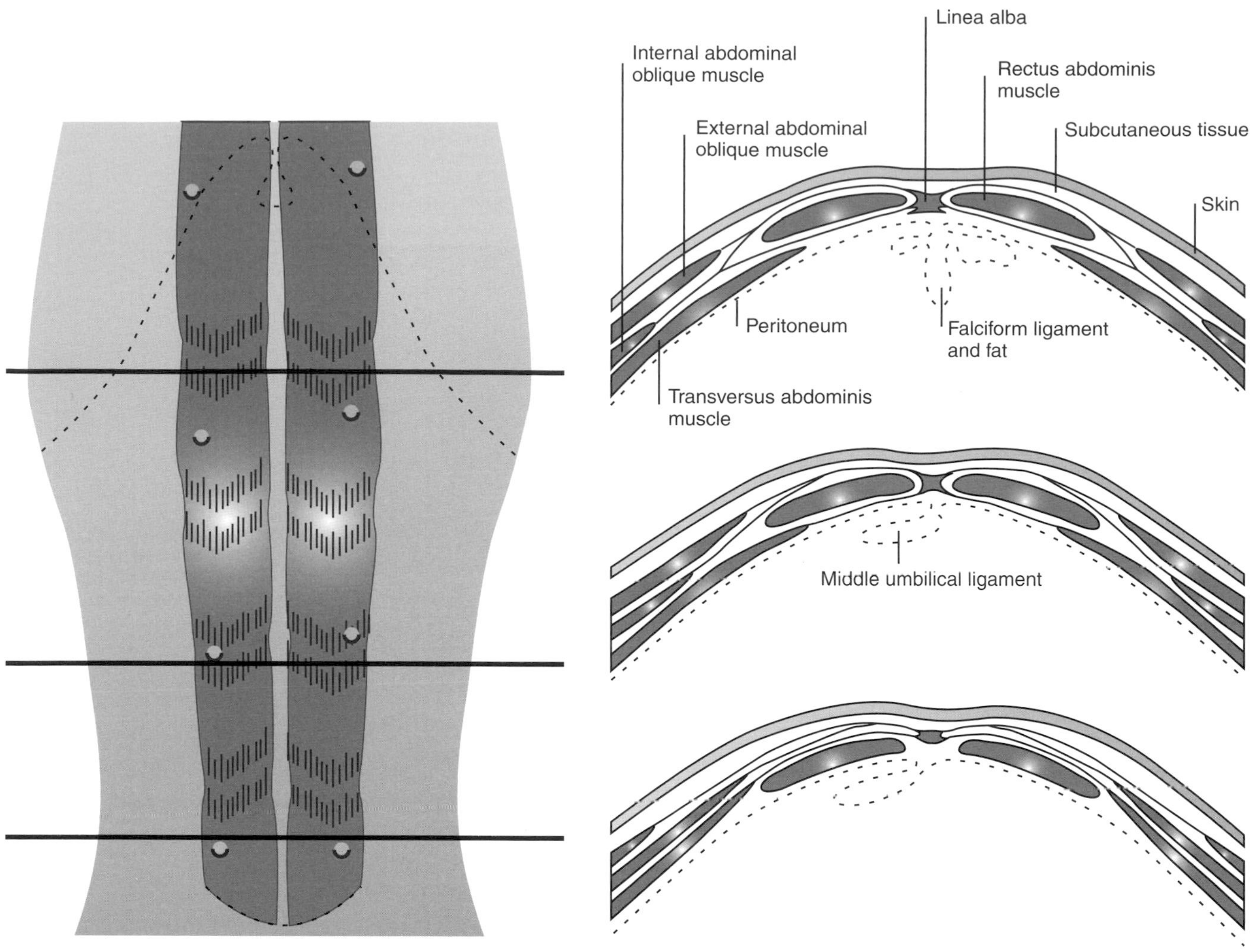

• **Fig. 7.38** Ventral aspect of the abdominal wall with the musculature sectioned at three different levels.

EXERCISES

Laboratory I: Extrinsic Muscles of the Thoracic Limb and Related Areas

Exercise 1

Identify and Color Muscles in the Cat

Color in the muscles in the following drawings. Use the same color for the same muscle in each. Then label the muscles.

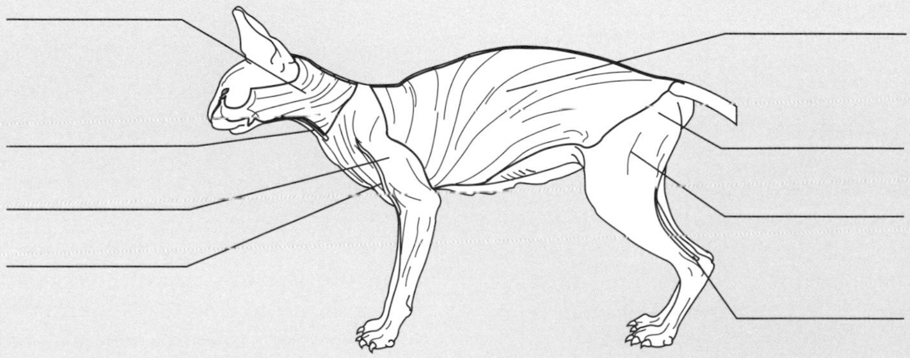

Exercise 1—cont'd

Identify and Color Muscles in the Cat

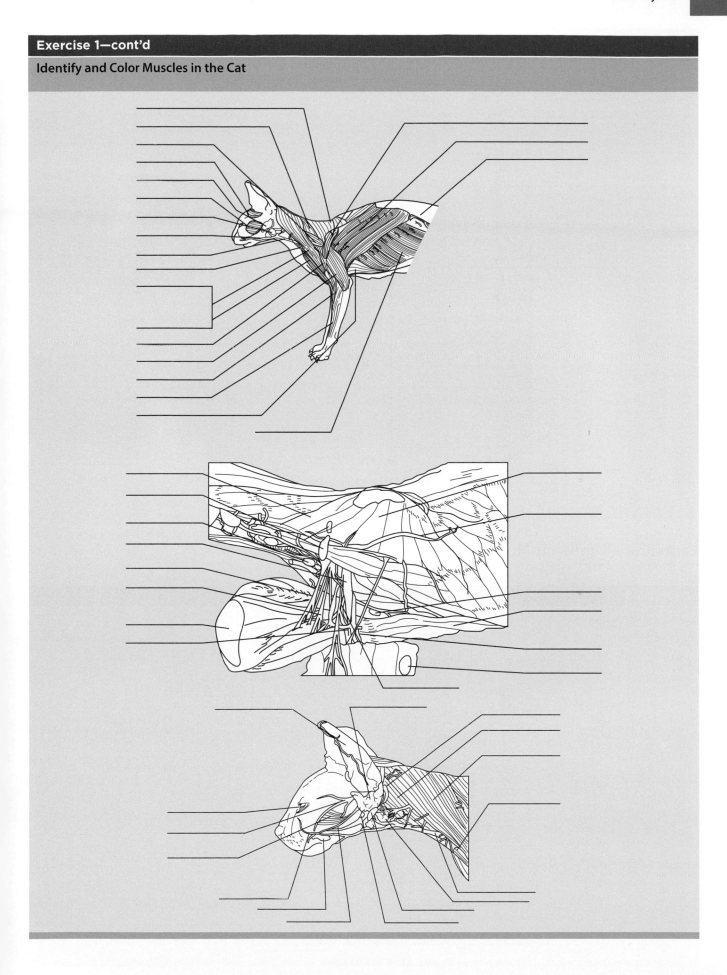

Exercise 2

Identify Muscle Name, Origin, Insertion, and Action

Fill in the blanks with the correct muscle name, origin, insertion, or action as needed. Then color the name of the muscle in the same color you colored the muscles in the drawings in Exercise 1.

Muscle	Origin	Insertion	Action
1. ______________	Cranial sternum	Greater tubercle of humerus	Adducts thoracic limb
Deep pectoral	Sternum	Greater tubercle of humerus	Adducts and pulls limb caudally
Brachiocephalicus	5. ______________	Ulna, mastoid, dorsal neck	Pulls limb forward, extends shoulder
Omotransversarius	Wing of atlas	Spine and acromion of scapula	Advances leg
Trapezius muscle	Dorsal aspect of neck	Spine of scapula	Elevates and abducts limb
Rhomboideus	Occipital bone of head	Dorsal border of scapula	Elevates forelimb
2. ______________	Last seven thoracic vertebrae and spinous process of lumbar vertebrae	Teres major tuberosity of humerus	Draws limb caudally Flexes shoulder joint
Serratus ventralis	Cervical vertebrae and ribs	Dorsomedial scapula	7. ______________
Sternocephalicus	Sternum	6. ______________	Draws head to side
3. ______________	Tendinous raphe on dorsal midline	Attaches to muscles surrounding lips	Draws commissures of lips caudally
Temporalis	Parietal bone of skull	Coronoid process of mandible	Closes mouth when chewing
Masseter	Zygomatic arch	Lateral side of mandible	8. ______________
Digastricus	Occipital and temporal bones	Ventral mandible	9. ______________
4. ______________	Medial mandible	Median raphe between mandible	Raises floor of mouth

Laboratory II: Intrinsic Muscles of the Thoracic Limb

Exercise 3

Identify and Color Intrinsic Muscles

Color in the muscles in the following drawings. Use the same color for the same muscle in each. Then label the muscles.

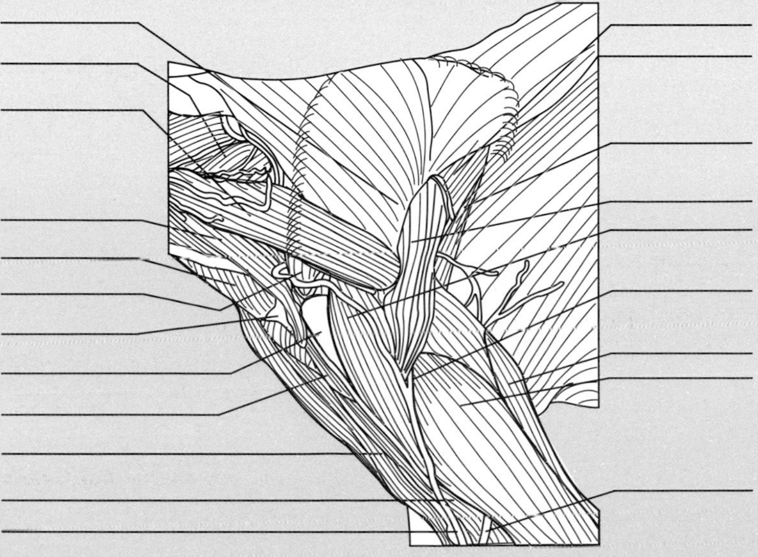

Exercise 3—cont'd

Identify and Color Intrinsic Muscles

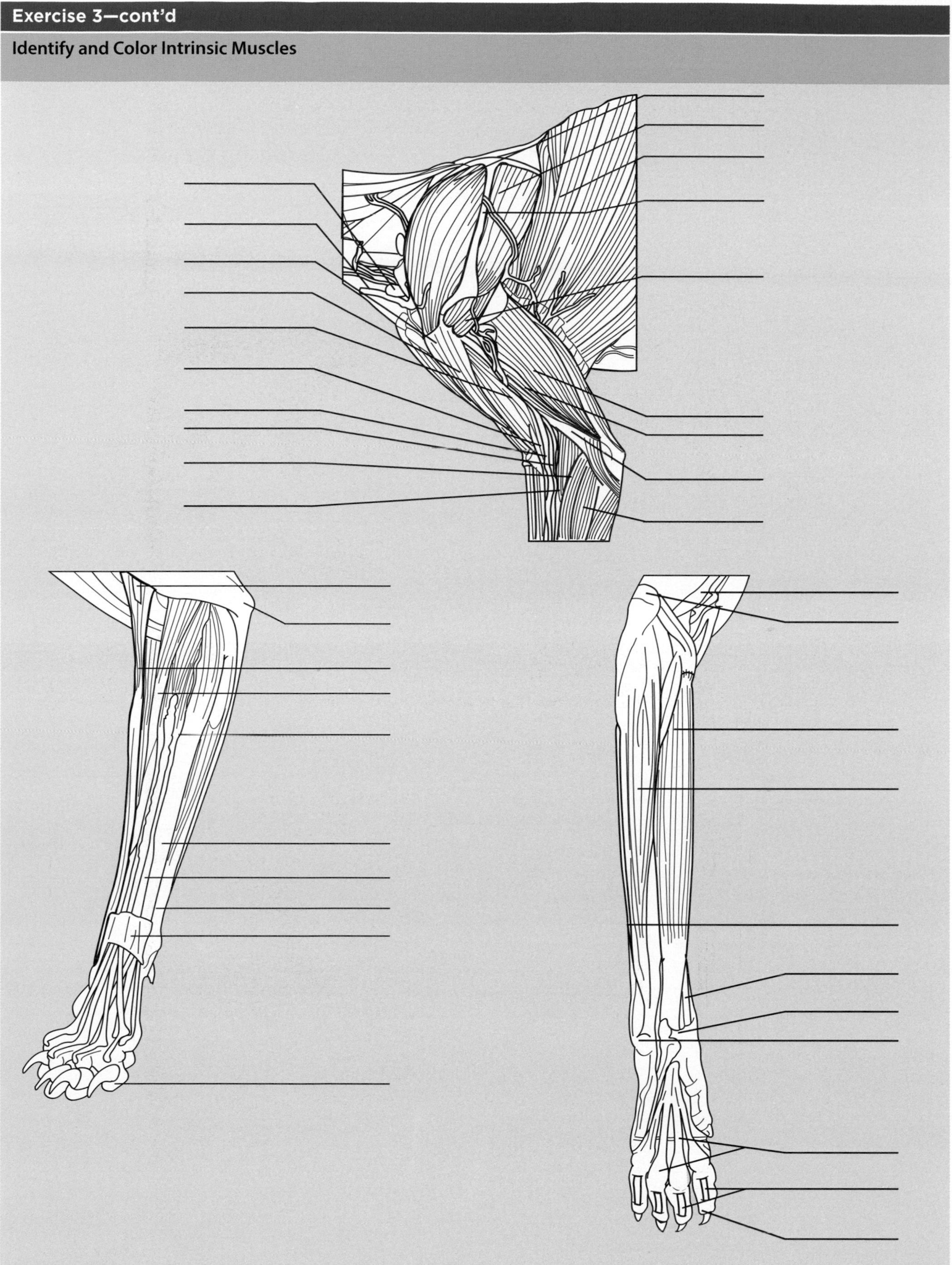

Continued

Exercise 3—cont'd

Identify and Color Intrinsic Muscles

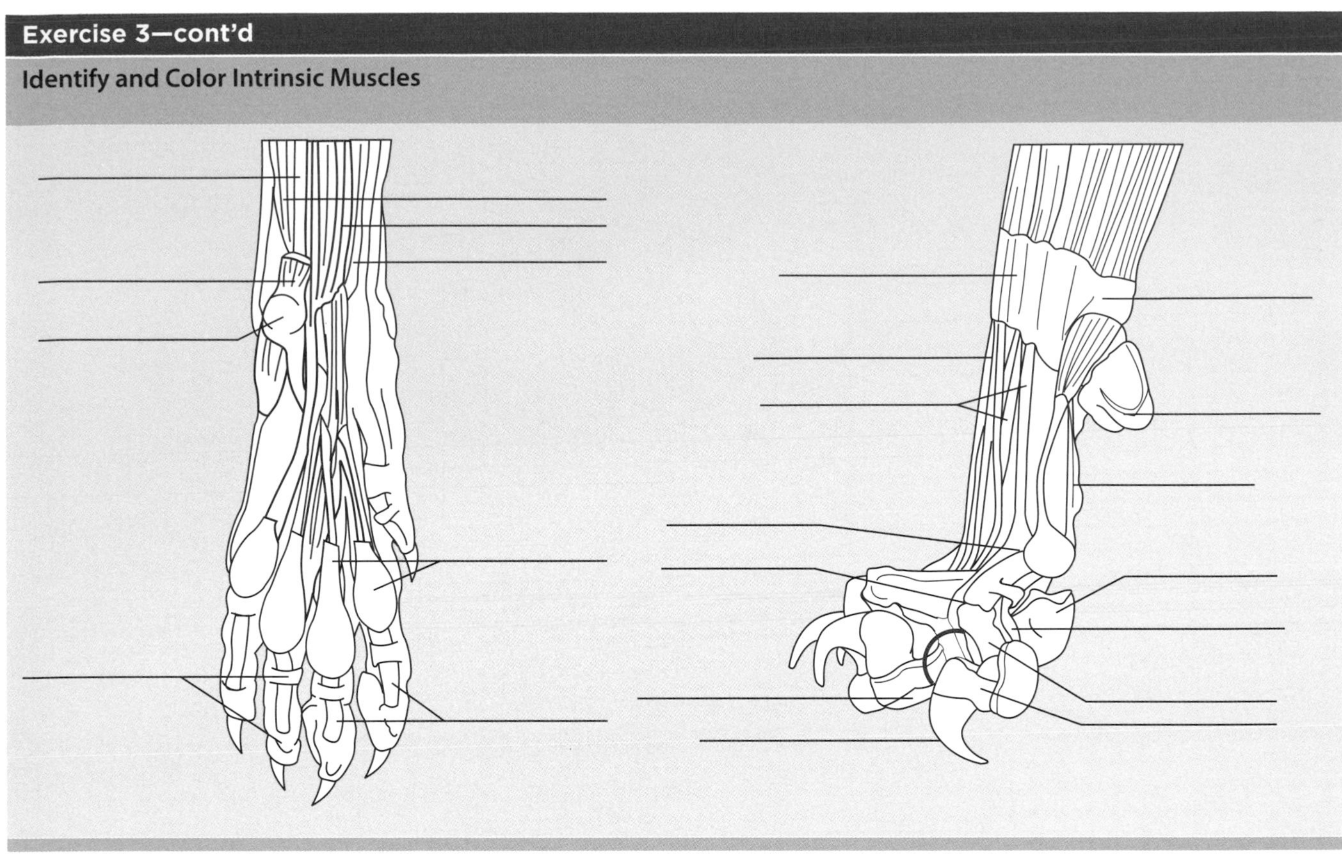

Exercise 4

Identify and Describe Muscles and Terms

The following is a list of the muscles and terms you must be able to identify on your cat specimen and describe their actions.

1. Deltoideus ______
2. Infraspinatus ______
3. Supraspinatus ______
4. Subscapularis ______
5. Teres major ______
6. Triceps brachii ______
7. Biceps brachii ______
8. Brachialis ______
9. Extensor carpi radialis ______
10. Lateral digital extensor ______

Exercise 4—cont'd

Identify and Describe Muscles and Terms

11. Extensor carpi ulnaris ______

12. Abductor pollicis longus ______

13. Flexor carpi ulnaris ______

14. Superficial digital flexor ______

15. Deep digital flexor ______

16. Cephalic vein ______

17. Radial nerve ______

18. Manus ______

19. Abduction ______

20. Adduction ______

21. Circumduction ______

22. Flexion ______

23. Extension ______

24. Extensor retinaculum ______

25. Fusiform ______

26. Ungulates ______

27. Flexor retinaculum ______

28. Phalanx ______

29. Interosseous muscle ______

30. Sesamoid bone ______

Exercise 5

Identify Muscle Name, Origin, Insertion, and Action

Fill in the blanks with the correct muscle name, origin, insertion, or action as needed. Then color the name of the muscle in the same color you colored the muscles in the drawings in Exercise 3.

Muscle	Origin	Insertion	Action
1. ________________	5. ________________	Deltoid tuberosity of humerus	Flexes shoulder
Infraspinatus	Infraspinous fossa of scapula	Greater tubercle of humerus	11. ________________
2. ________________	Supraspinous fossa of scapula	Greater tubercle of humerus	Extends shoulder
Subscapularis	Subscapular fossa of scapula	Lesser tubercle of humerus	Adducts limb/rotates forearm
Teres major	Caudal border of scapula	Teres major tuberosity of humerus	12. ________________
3. ________________	Caudal border of scapula/ proximal border of humerus	Olecranon of ulna	Extends elbow/flexes shoulder
Biceps brachii	6. ________________	Ulna and radial tuberosities	13. ________________
Brachialis	Humerus	Ulna and radial tuberosities	Flexes elbow
Brachioradialis	Lateral aspect distal humerus	Distal radius	Rotates forearm (supination)
Extensor carpi radialis	Lateral supracondylar crest of humerus	Proximal aspect of second and third metacarpal bone	Extends carpus
4. ________________	Lateral epicondyle of humerus	Dorsal surface of distal phalanges	Extends carpus and digits
		Digits II, III, IV, V	
Lateral digital extensor	Lateral epicondyle of humerus	10. ________________	Extends digital joints
Extensor carpi ulnaris	7. ________________	Lateral aspect metacarpal V and accessory carpal bone	Flexes carpal joint
Abductor pollicis longus	Lateral border of ulna	Proximal end of metacarpal I and II	14. ________________
Flexor carpi radialis	8. ________________	Palmar aspect of metacarpals II and III	Flexes carpal joint
Flexor carpi ulnaris	9.________________	Accessory carpal bone	Flexes carpal joint
Superficial digital flexor	Medial epicondyle of humerus	Palmar aspect of phalanges of digits II, III, IV, V	15. ________________
Deep digital flexor	Medial epicondyle/proximal ulna	Palmar aspect of distal phalanges	16. ________________
	Medial radius		

Laboratory III: Muscles of the Pelvic Limb and Abdominal Wall

Exercise 6

Identify and Color Muscles of the Pelvic Limb

Color in the muscles in the following drawings. Use the same color for the same muscle in each. Then label the muscles.

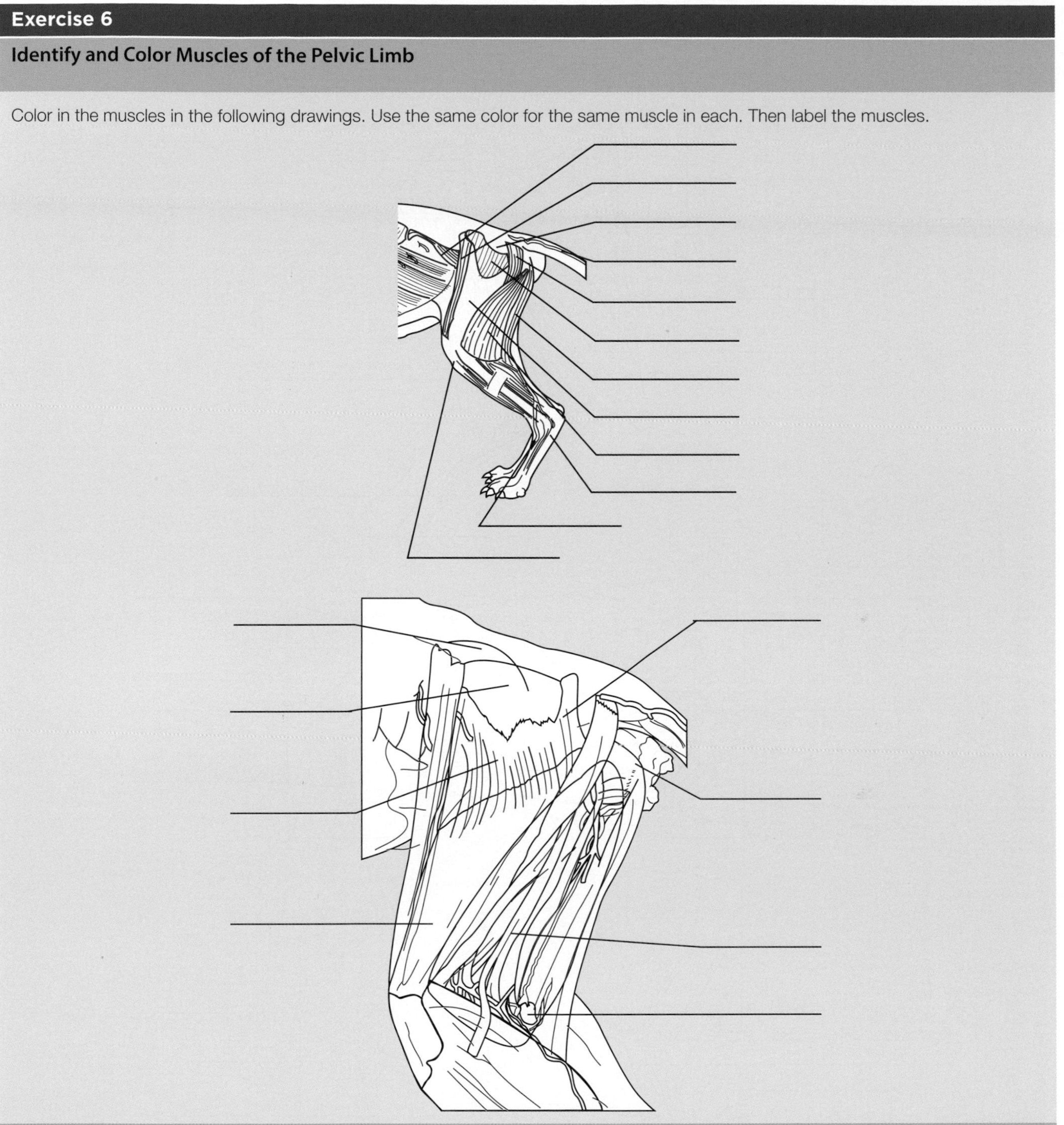

Continued

Exercise 6—cont'd

Identify and Color Muscles of the Pelvic Limb

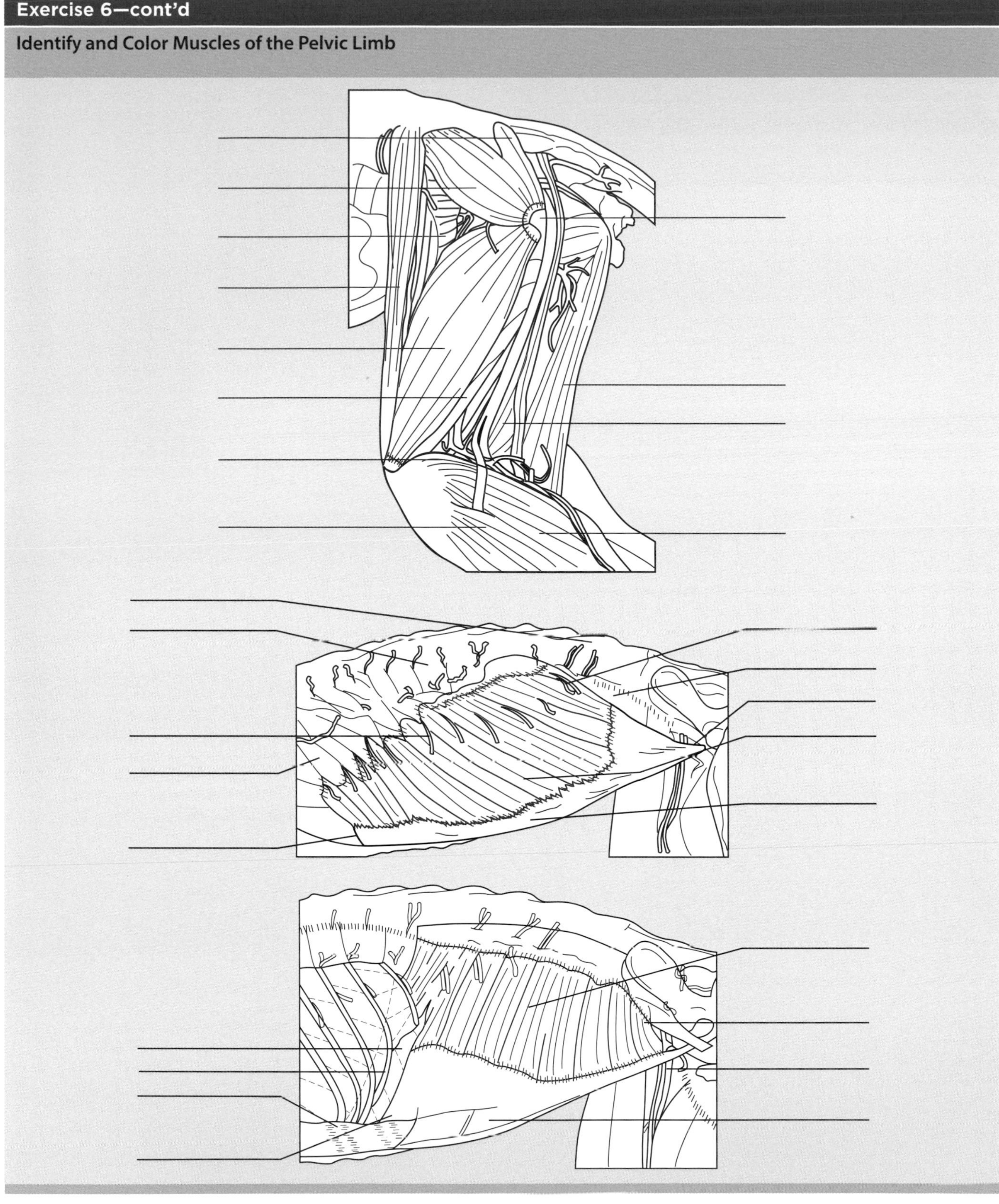

Exercise 6—cont'd

Identify and Color Muscles of the Pelvic Limb

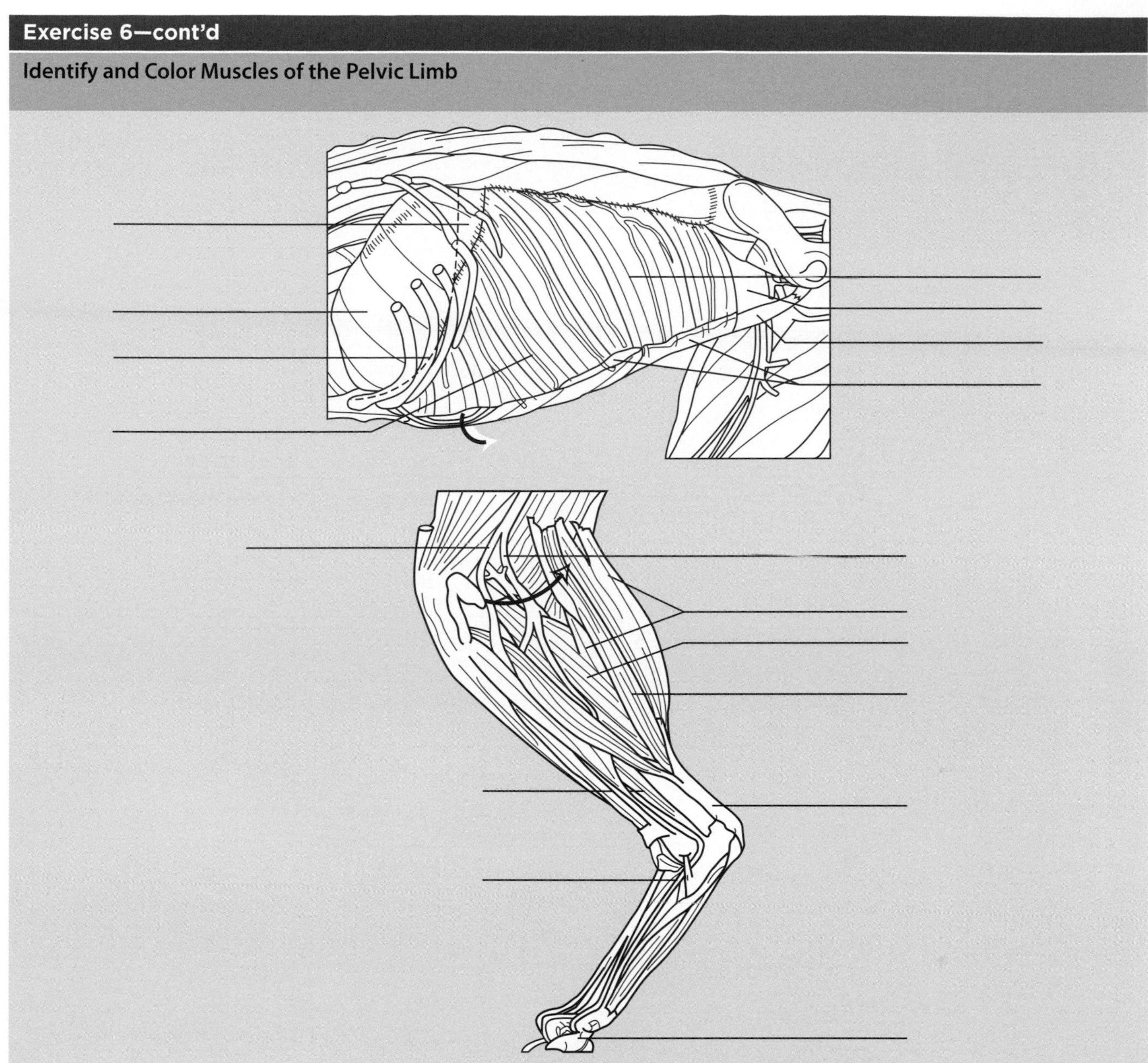

Exercise 7

Identify Muscle Name, Origin, Insertion, and Action

Fill in the blanks with the correct muscle name, origin, insertion, or action as needed. Then color the name of the muscle in the same color you colored the muscles in the drawings in Exercise 6.

Muscle	Origin	Insertion	Action
1. ________________	Cranial wing of ilium	Lateral femoral fascia	Flexes hip/extends stifle
Superficial gluteal muscle	Sacrum and coccygeal vertebrae	13. ________________	Abducts limb/extends hip
Middle gluteal muscle	Lateral ilium	Greater trochanter of femur	Abducts limb/extends hip
Deep gluteal muscle	Body of ilium and ischiatic spine	Cranial aspect of greater trochanter	18. ________________
Biceps femoris muscle	6.________________	Patella/proximal tibia/tuber calcanei	Extends hip/flexes stifle/ extends tarsus
2. ________________	Ischiatic tuberosity of pelvis	Tibia and tuber calcanei	Extends hip/flexes stifle/ extends tarsus
Semimembranosus	7. ________________	Femur and tibia	Extends hip
Sartorius muscle	Crest of ilium	Patella/cranial part of tibia	19. ________________
3. ________________	Pelvic symphysis	Cranial border of tibia/ tuber calcanei	20. ________________
Pectineus muscle	Prepubic tendon/ acetabulum	Caudal aspect of femur	Adducts limbs
Adductor muscle	Pelvic symphysis	14. ________________	Adducts limb and extends hip
4. ________________	Ilium/proximal femur	Tibial tuberosity	21.________________
Cranial tibial muscle	Cranial tibial border	15. ________________	Flexes tarsus
Long digital extensor muscle	8. ________________	Extensor process of distal phalanges	Extends digits/flexes tarsus/ extends stifle
5. ________________	Proximal tibia and fibula	Fourth tarsal bone plantar aspect metatarsus	Flexes tarsus
Gastrocnemius muscle	9. ________________	Proximal surface tuber calcanei	Extends tarsus/flexes stifle
Superficial digital flexor	Lateral supracondylar tuberosities of femur	Proximal surface of tuber calcanei and plantar surface middle phalanges	22. ________________
Deep digital flexor	Caudal aspect of tibia and fibula	Plantar surface distal phalanges	Extends tarsus/flexes digital joints
Popliteus muscle	Lateral condyle of femur	Caudal aspect of proximal tibia	Flexes stifle and rotates leg medially
External abdominal oblique	10. ________________	Linea alba	Flexes vertebral column/ abdominal press
Internal abdominal oblique	11. ________________	Linea alba	23. ________________
Transversus abdominis	Last four to five ribs/ transverse processes of lumbar vertebrae	16. ________________	Flexes vertebral column/ abdominal press
Rectus abdominis	12. ________________	17. ________________	Flexes vertebral column/ abdominal press

Critical and Clinical Thinking

Exercise 8

Clinical Thinking Challenge

Support each of the following correct statements with appropriate rationale, stating why or in what way each statement is correct.

1. A muscle has three primary functions: provide motion, maintain posture, and generate heat. To do so, it is made up of muscle cells with four common characteristics.
2. Three types of muscle make up the muscular system.
3. A skeletal muscle does only one thing but does it really well.
4. There is logic behind the names given to most muscles: they are often named for six physical characteristics.
5. Abdominal muscles, obviously, support the abdominal organs. But that is not all they do.
6. The most common abdominal incision site is the *ventral midline,* where the linea alba is located.
7. Abdominal surgery in cattle is often done while the animal is standing.
8. In theory, any skeletal muscle is appropriate to use for an intramuscular injection. In practice, not so.
9. A single muscle fiber contraction (a twitch contraction) can be divided into three phases.
10. The term rigor mortis, meaning "stiffness of death" in Latin, describes the stiffness of skeletal muscles shortly after death. It would seem more sensible for the muscles to go limp after death, but things at the cellular level go in another direction.
11. Cardiac and skeletal muscle cells are similar in that they contain many of the same organelles and intracellular structures, such as myofibrils. However, they are otherwise very different.
12. Smooth muscle cells can shorten to a greater extent than skeletal or cardiac muscle cells.
13. It is critically important that the smooth muscle in the pregnant uterus does not contract as the fetus grows.
14. Sympathetic stimulation results in different types of activity in cardiac and visceral smooth muscle.

8

The Nervous System[a]

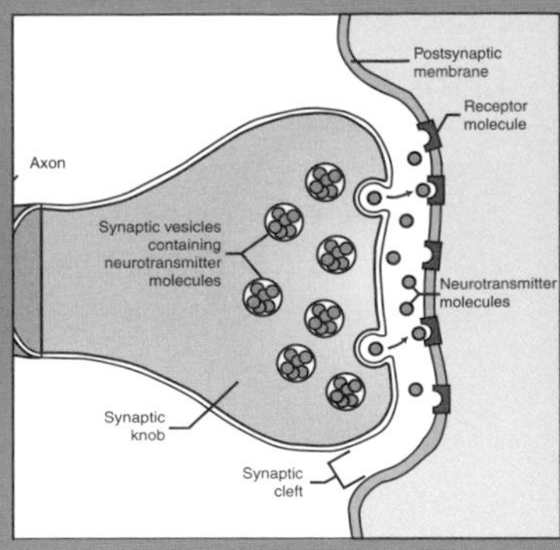

OVERVIEW AT A GLANCE

The Brain 205

The Spinal Cord 215

The Meninges 216

Peripheral Nerves of Clinical Importance 217

Exercises 222–230

The Brain 222–224

1. *Label the Indicated Divisions/Structures of the Sheep Brain 222*
2. *Label the Indicated Divisions/Structures of the Sheep Brain 222*
3. *Label the Indicated Structures of the Sheep Brain 223*
4. *Label the Indicated Divisions/Structures 223*
5. *Label the Indicated Structures 223*
6. *Label the Indicated Structures 224*
7. *Photo Quiz 224*

Peripheral Nerves of Clinical Importance 225–228

8. *Identify the Twelve Pairs of Cranial Nerves 225*
9. *Identify the Effect of the Sympathetic and Parasympathetic Nervous Systems 225*
10. *Identify the Nerve Indicated (Feline Groin Area) 226*
11. *Identify the Three Nerves Indicated (Medial Surface of a Cat Forelimb) 227*
12. *Identify the Nerve Indicated (Lateral View of Cat Thigh) 228*

Critical and Clinical Thinking 228–230

13. *Define Clinical Terms 228*
14. *Clinical Thinking Challenge #1 230*
15. *Clinical Thinking Challenge #2 230*

LEARNING OBJECTIVES

In this chapter, we will explore the anatomy of the brain and spinal cord. We will also locate clinically significant peripheral nerves. Read Chapter 9 in *Clinical Anatomy and Physiology for Veterinary Technicians* for detailed descriptions and locations of these structures.

CLINICAL SIGNIFICANCE

The nervous system controls, or at least influences, all other body systems. Therefore, nervous system diseases and injuries can have wide-reaching effects on the rest of the body. Knowledge of the nervous system is important in many situations and activities in the veterinary clinic. Local and general anesthesia, pain management, dealing with traumatic injuries that involve nervous system components, and communicating with clients are just some of these situations. We even have to keep the nervous system in mind when we do seemingly simple things, such as applying bandages and positioning animals for surgery, to help prevent damage to peripheral nerves.

INTRODUCTION

The nervous system is all about information and control. It receives, processes, and distributes information by way of nerve impulses, and it directly or indirectly controls nearly all body functions. At the microscopic level, the basic functional unit of the nervous system is the neuron (nerve cell). Neurons have long cellular processes called axons that are bundled together to make the cordlike structures we call nerves. It is the axons within the nerves that actually conduct the nerve impulses. Macroscopically (visible without magnification), the nervous system's two main divisions are the **central nervous system** (CNS) and the **peripheral nervous system** (PNS).

The central nervous system is made up of the brain and the spinal cord. The brain is located within the cranium of the skull. The spinal cord extends down the spinal canal formed by the dorsal arches of the vertebrae. The CNS is where the conscious mind resides along with the basic control centers that regulate

[a]The authors and publisher wish to acknowledge Joann Colville and Amy Ellwein for previous contributions to this chapter.

INTRODUCTION—cont'd

digestive, respiratory, and other body functions. It receives and processes sensory inputs from the peripheral nervous system and sends motor instructions back out to control body functions.

The peripheral nervous system is made up of cord-like nerves that either originate directly from the brain (cranial nerves) or originate from the spinal cord (spinal nerves). In either case, the nerves link the CNS with all parts of the body. Sensory fibers within nerves carry information inward to the spinal cord and brain. Motor fibers carry instructions outward to tell the body what to do.

TERMS TO BE IDENTIFIED

When you have completed this chapter, you will be able to identify the following structures/parts of the nervous system.

Central nervous system
- Brain
  - Spinal cord

Divisions of the brain
- Brainstem
- Cerebellum
- Cerebrum
- Diencephalon

Structures of the brain
- Corpus callosum
- Gray matter
- Gyri (singular ∇ gyrus)
- Hypothalamus
- Longitudinal fissure
- Medulla oblongata
- Midbrain
- Olfactory bulb
- Optic chiasm
- Optic nerve
- Pituitary gland
- Pons
- Sulci (singular ∇ sulcus)
- Thalamus
- White matter

Meninges
- Arachnoid
- Dura mater
- Pia mater

Peripheral nerves
- Facial nerve
- Femoral nerve
- Median nerve
- Radial nerve
- Sciatic nerve
- Ulnar nerve
- Vagus nerve

MEDICAL WORD PARTS

Encephal/o = brain (inside the head)
Meningi/o = meninges, the connective tissue covering the brain
Myel/o = spinal cord
Neur/o = nerve

The Brain

The **brain** has four divisions: the cerebrum, the cerebellum, the diencephalon, and the brainstem (Figs. 8.1–8.6). Each has its own particular functions.

- The **cerebrum** is the largest and most rostral part of the brain. It is responsible for learning and intelligence, for receiving and interpreting sensory information, and it is where the conscious mind resides.
- The **cerebellum** is caudal to the cerebrum. It coordinates movement, balance, posture, and complex reflexes.
- The **diencephalon** serves as a passageway between the brainstem and the cerebrum. This part of the brain is

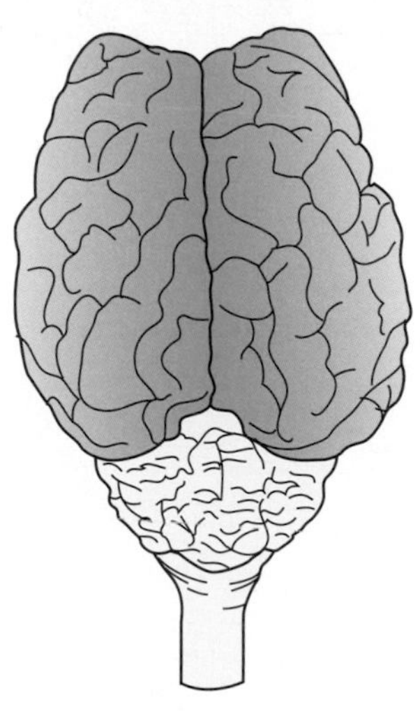

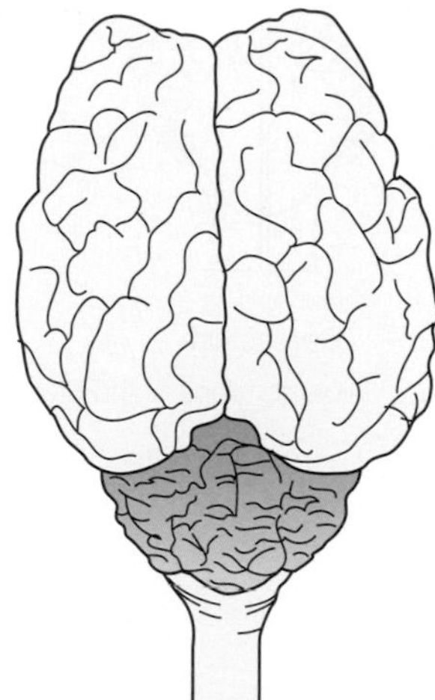

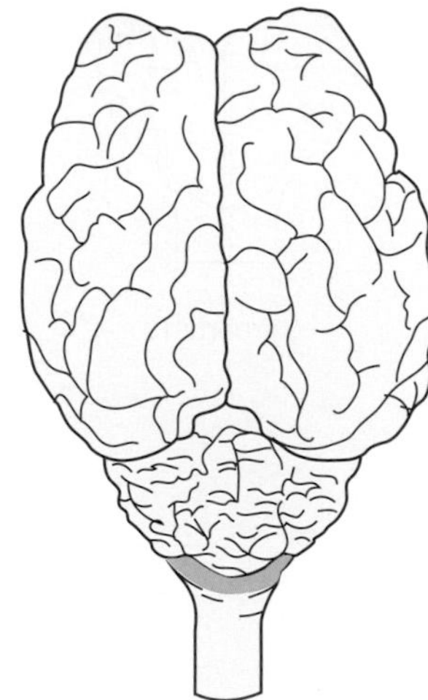

• **Fig. 8.1** Externally visible divisions of the brain. Dorsal view.

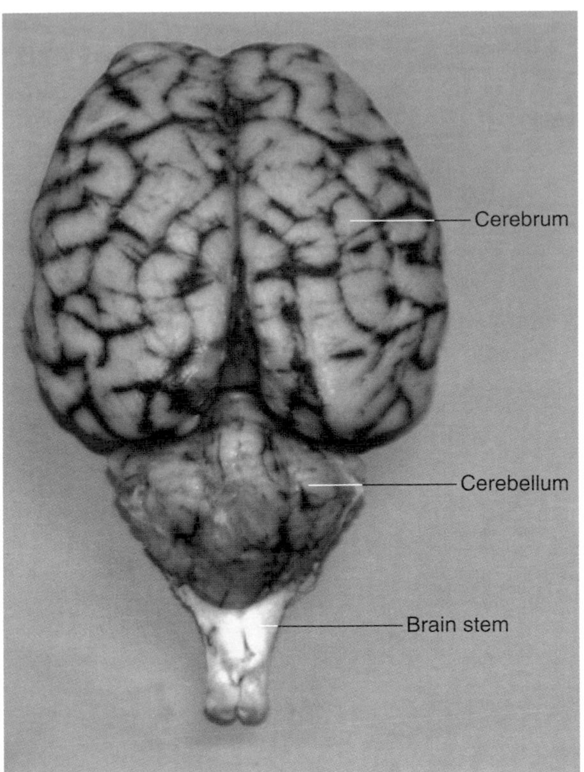

• **Fig. 8.2** Dorsal view of a sheep brain.

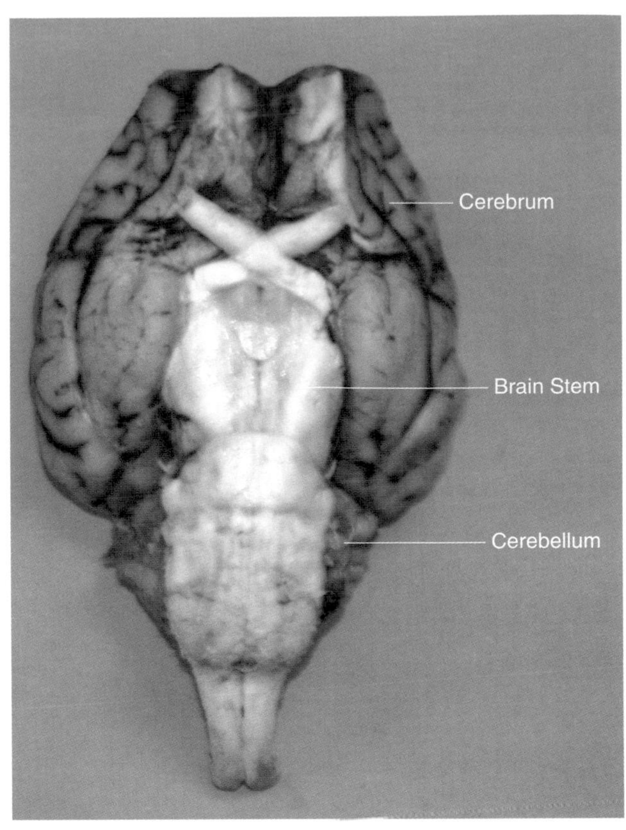

• **Fig. 8.4** Ventral view of a sheep brain.

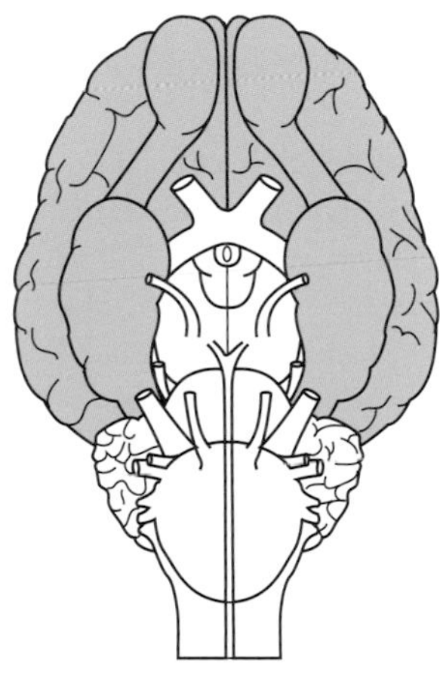

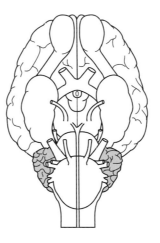

Cerebrum

Cerebellum

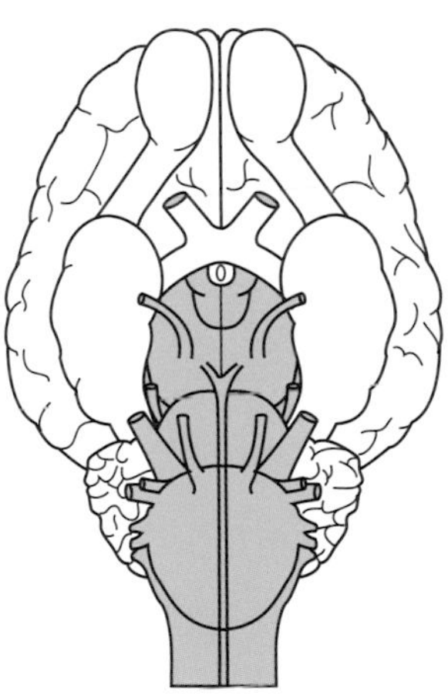

Brain stem

• **Fig. 8.3** Externally visible divisions of the brain. Ventral view.

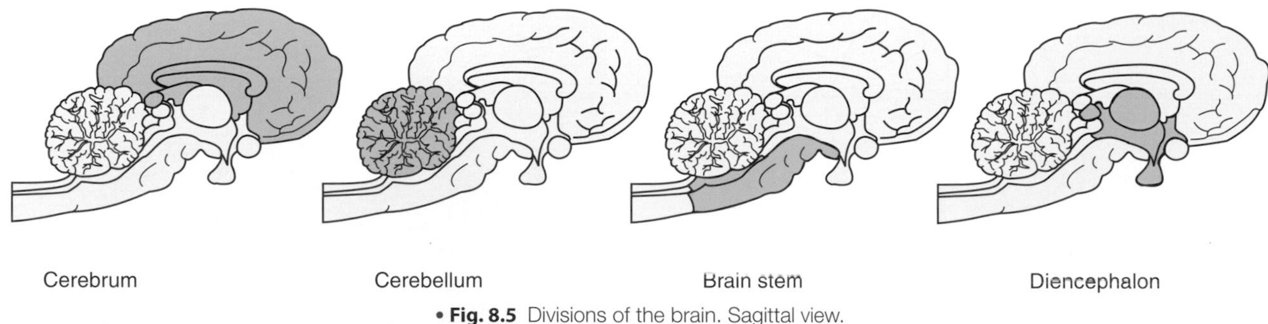

• **Fig. 8.5** Divisions of the brain. Sagittal view.

• **Fig. 8.6** Sagittal view of a sheep brain.

not as clearly defined as the others. It is more of an "area" than a distinctly visible "thing."

- The **brainstem** is the most primitive part of the brain. It contains centers that control basic body functions, such as breathing, cardiac function, and digestive tract function, and it connects the rest of the brain with the spinal cord.

External Structures of the Cerebrum

(Figures 8.7–8.10)

- The **longitudinal fissure** separates the cerebrum into right and left cerebral hemispheres.
- The **olfactory bulbs** receive information from the olfactory (sense of smell) nerves, then send the impulses to the cerebrum via the olfactory tracts.
- The **gyri** are the hills or ridges on the surface of the cerebrum.
- The **sulci** are the shallow depressions in the surface of the cerebrum between the gyri.

External Structures of the Cerebellum

(See Figures 8.7–8.10)

- There is no longitudinal fissure, but the right and left sides are described as the right and left cerebellar hemispheres.
- The gyri and sulci are small and tight, giving a "wrinkled" appearance to the surface of the cerebellum.

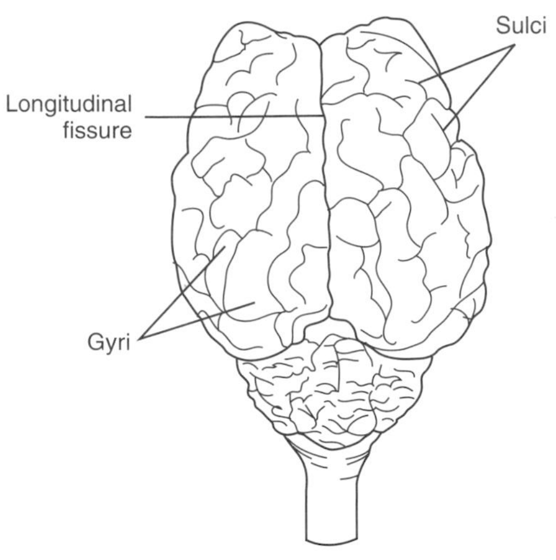

• **Fig. 8.7** Cerebrum and cerebellum. Dorsal view.

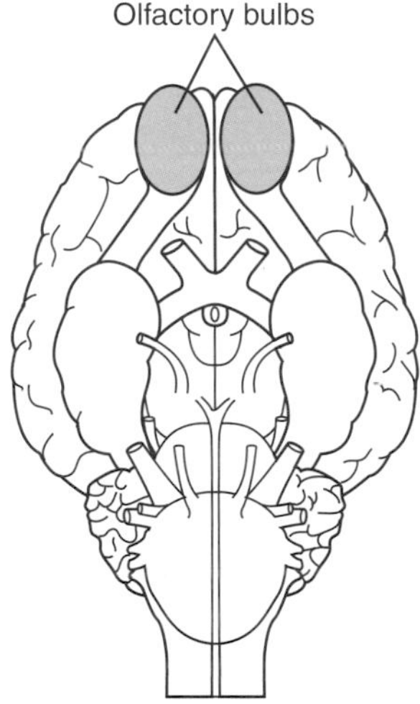

• **Fig. 8.8** Cerebrum and cerebellum. Ventral view.

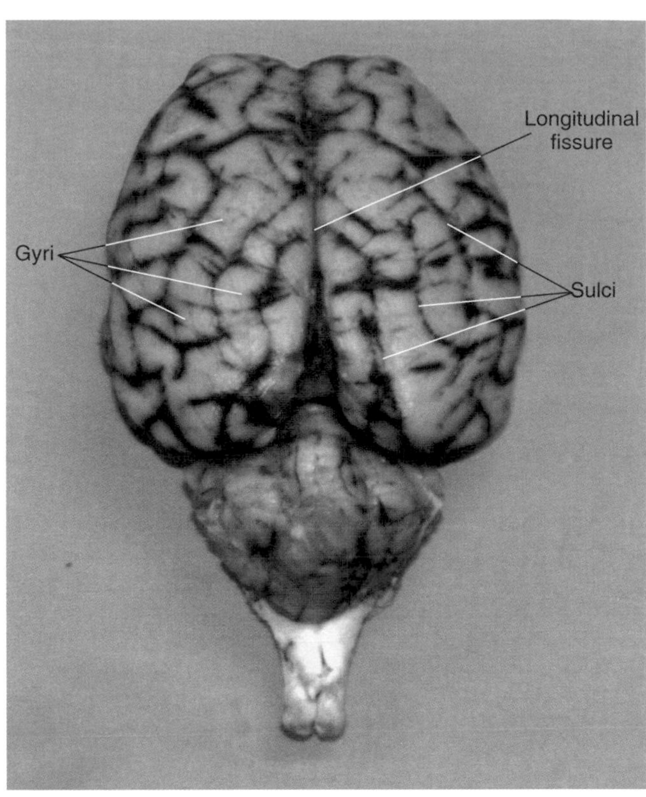

• **Fig. 8.9** Cerebrum and cerebellum. Sheep brain. Dorsal view.

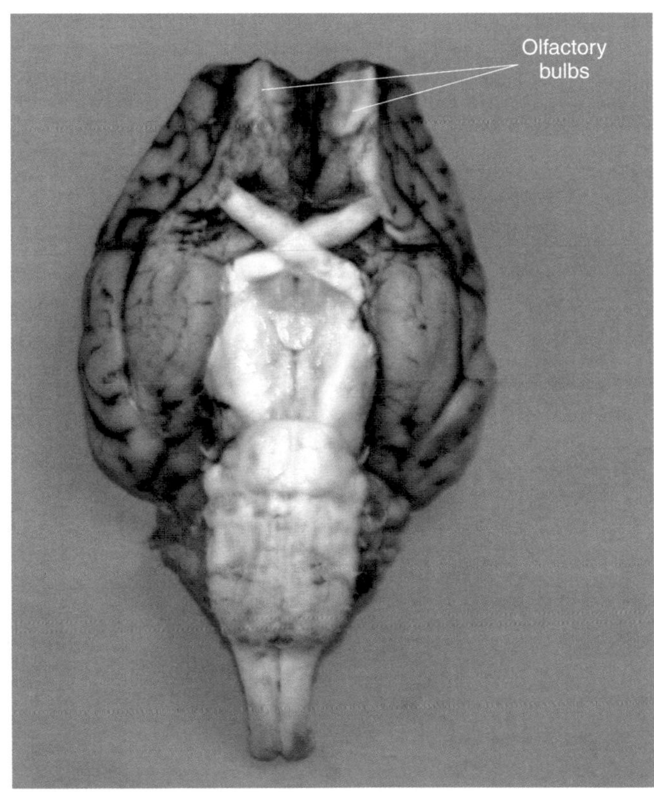

• **Fig. 8.10** Cerebrum and cerebellum. Sheep brain. Ventral view.

Cranial Nerves

The cranial nerves are 12 pairs of nerves that originate directly from the brain (Fig. 8.11). All other nerves are spinal nerves—they originate from the spinal cord. Cranial nerves are generally identified by the Roman numerals I through XII (1 through 12), although they have specific names as well. As you can see in Table 8.1, the cranial nerves have a variety of functions, some of which occur outside the head region.

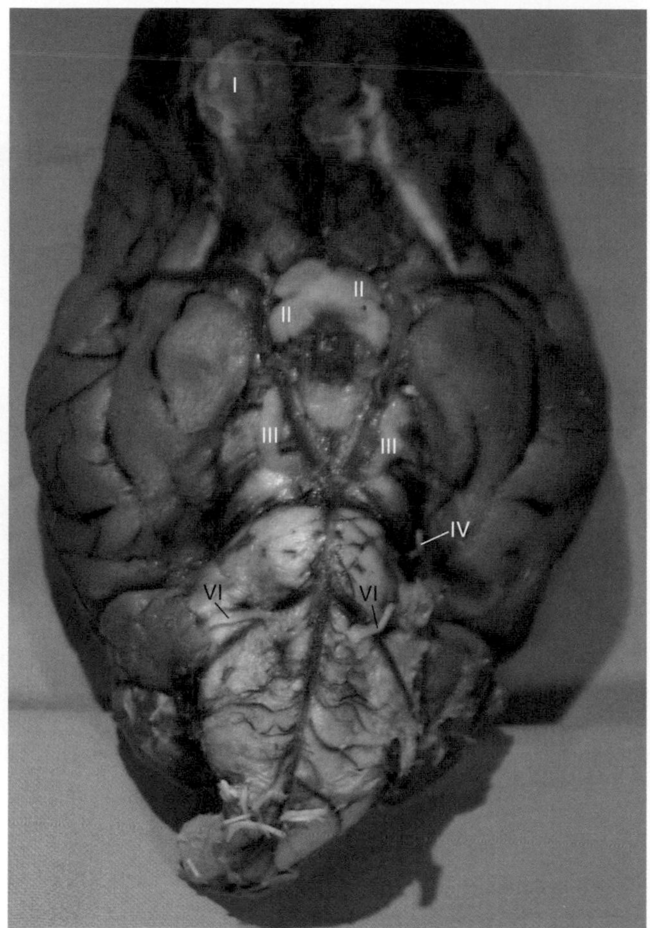

• **Fig. 8.11** Cranial nerves. Ventral view of sheep brain.

TABLE 8.1 Cranial Nerves

Number	Name	Sensory/Motor/Mixed	Sensation/Control
I	Olfactory	Sensory	Smell
II	Optic	Sensory	Vision
III	Oculomotor	Motor	External and internal eye muscles
IV	Trochlear	Motor	External eye muscles
V	Trigeminal	Mixed	Head and teeth sensations, chewing muscles
VI	Abducent	Motor	External eye muscles
VII	Facial	Mixed	Facial muscles, salivation, tear production, taste
VIII	Vestibulocochlear	Sensory	Balance, hearing
IX	Glossopharyngeal	Mixed	Tongue muscles, swallowing, salivation, taste
X	Vagus	Mixed	Sensory to respiratory tree and gastrointestinal tract. Motor to larynx, pharynx, abdominal and thoracic organs
XI	Accessory	Motor	Head movement. Partially joins with vagus nerve
XII	Hypoglossal	Motor	Tongue muscles

Internal Structures of the Cerebrum and Cerebellum

(Figs. 8.12 and 8.13.)

- The **corpus callosum** is made up of nerve fibers that connect the right and left cerebral hemispheres. It looks like a whitish "ear" inside the cerebrum.
- The locations of the gray and white matter in the cerebrum and cerebellum are obvious grossly (without magnification) when a cut surface is examined.

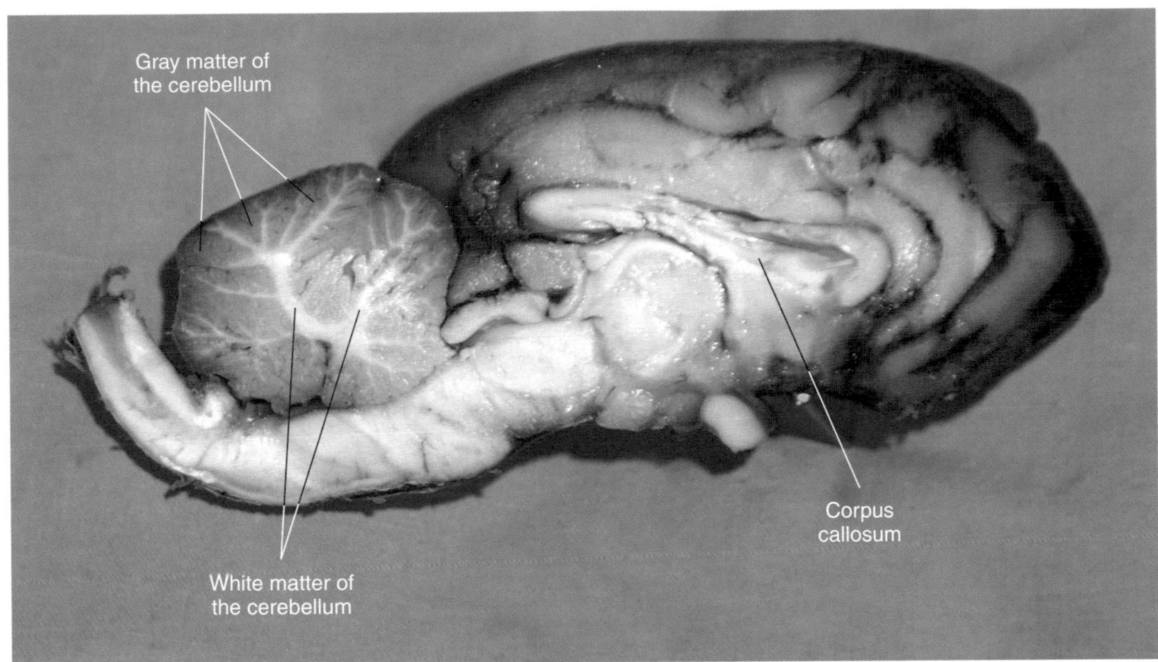

• **Fig. 8.12** Internal structures of the cerebrum and cerebellum. Sagittal view of the sheep brain.

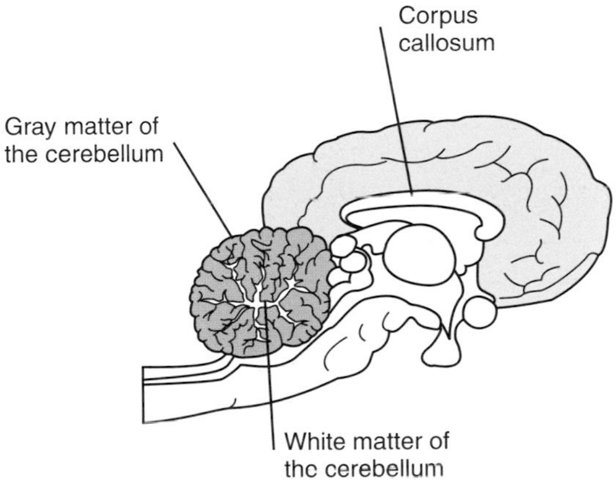

• **Fig. 8.13** Drawing of sagittal view of sheep brain.

External Structures of the Diencephalon

- The **pituitary gland** is the only externally visible part of the diencephalon (Fig. 8.14).
    - It is called the "master endocrine gland" because it regulates the production and release of other hormones throughout the body.
    - It resembles a brown "bean," protruding from the ventral surface of the brain just caudal to the **optic chiasm**.
    - It is often removed from preserved sheep brain specimens when the dura mater is removed.

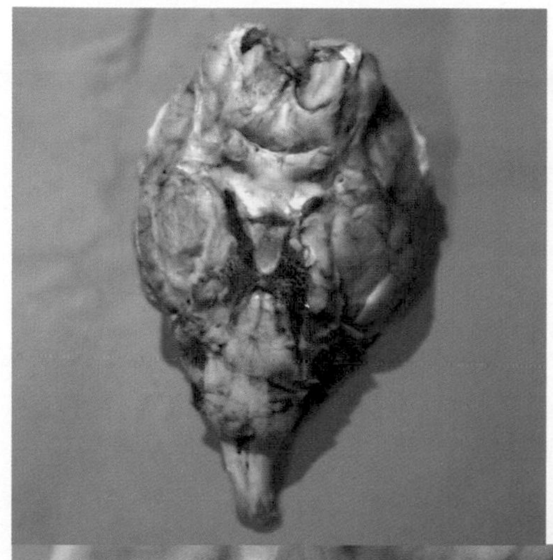

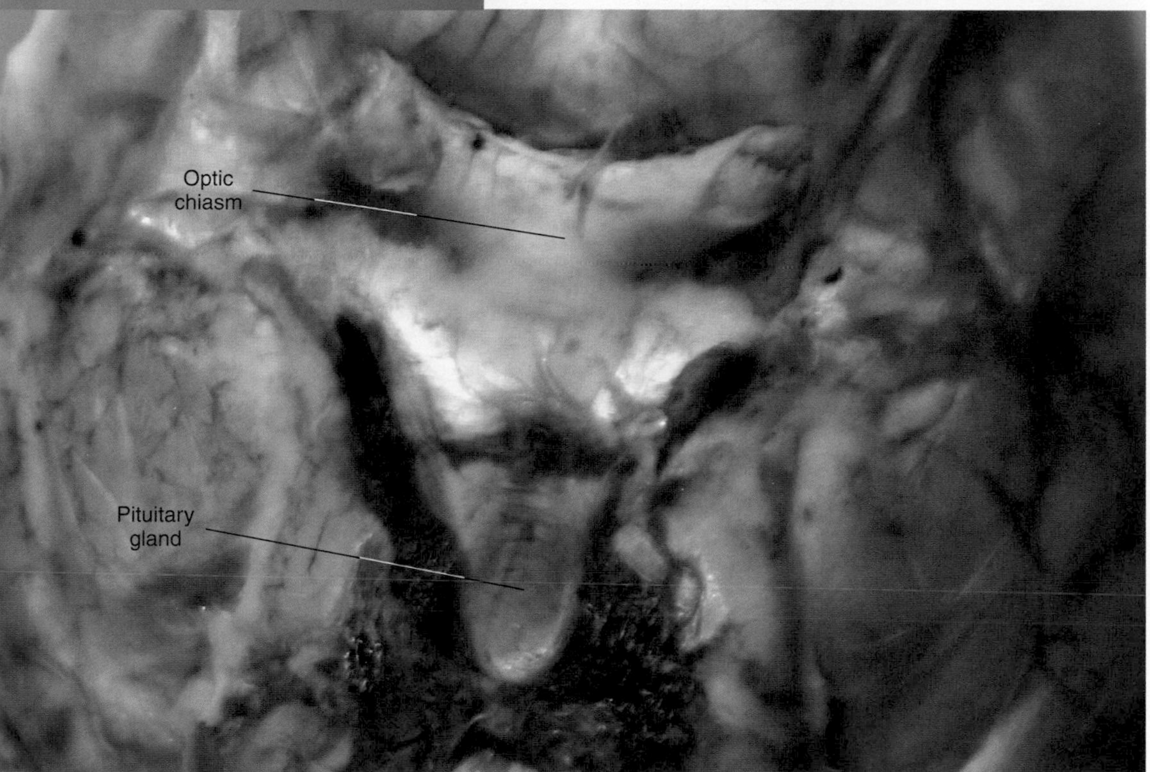

• **Fig. 8.14** Pituitary gland. Ventral view of a sheep brain. The dura mater is still attached to this brain.

Internal Structures of the Diencephalon

(Figs. 8.15 and 8.16.)

- The **thalamus** is a relay station for regulating sensory inputs to the cerebrum. It is a circular structure ventral to the corpus callosum.
- The **hypothalamus** is a bridge between the nervous system and the endocrine system. It is an area of the diencephalon rather than a distinct structure and is located between the thalamus and the pituitary gland.
- The pineal body is a small, bean-shaped structure located caudal to the thalamus.

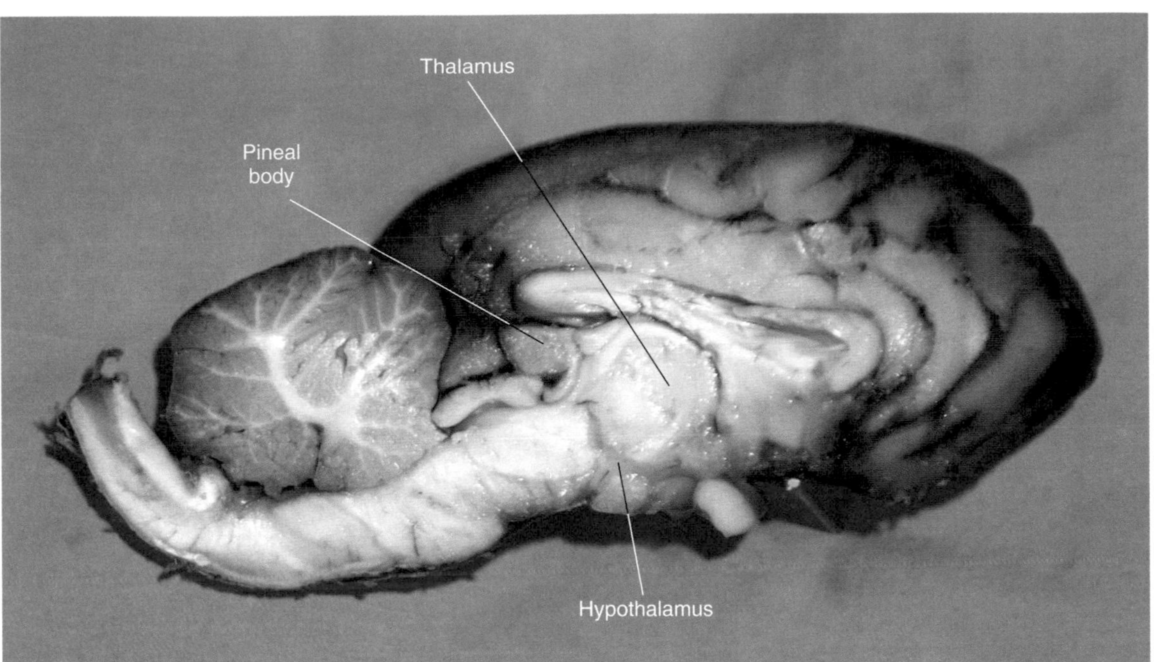

• **Fig. 8.15** Internal structures of the diencephalon. Sagittal view of a sheep brain.

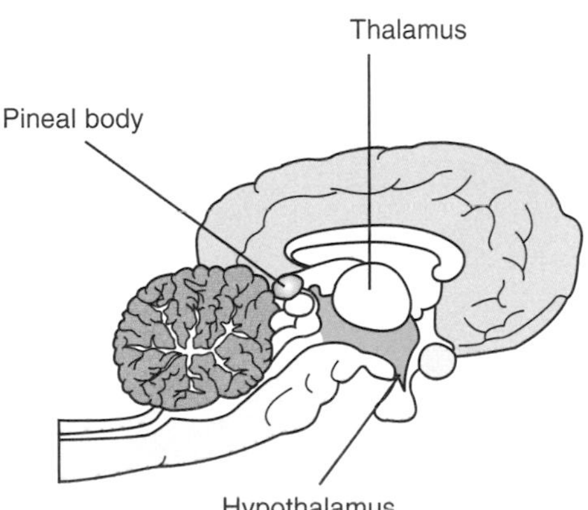

• **Fig. 8.16** Internal structures of the diencephalon.

External Structures of the Brainstem

(Figs. 8.17 and 8.18.)

- The **medulla oblongata** is the area of the brainstem that connects with the spinal cord.
- The **pons** is located just rostral to the medulla oblongata. It is separated from the medulla oblongata by a horizontal groove. Nerve fibers running transversely across the pons give it a rounded, plump look.
- The **midbrain** is located between the pons and the cerebrum.

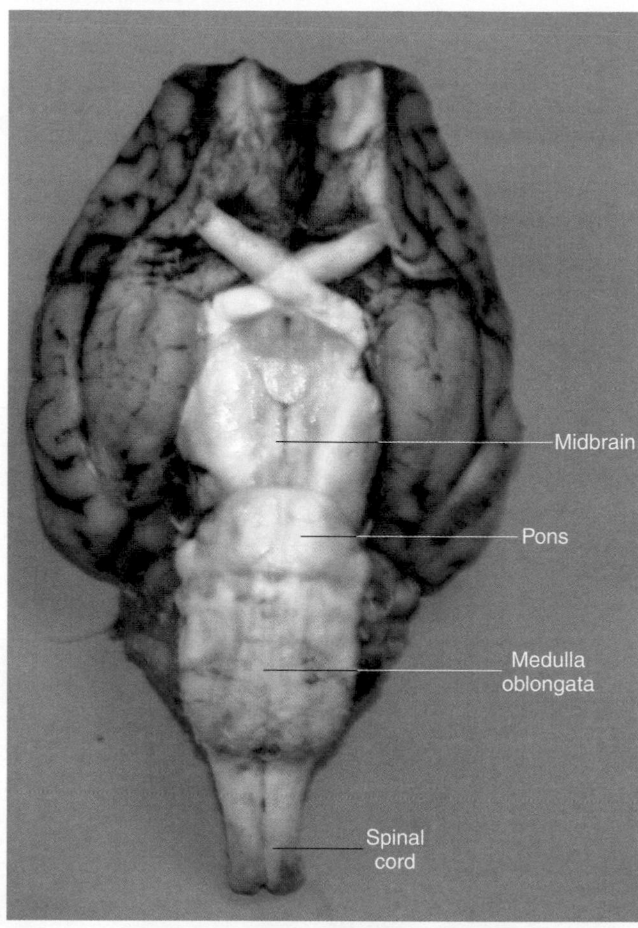

• **Fig. 8.17** External structures of the brainstem.

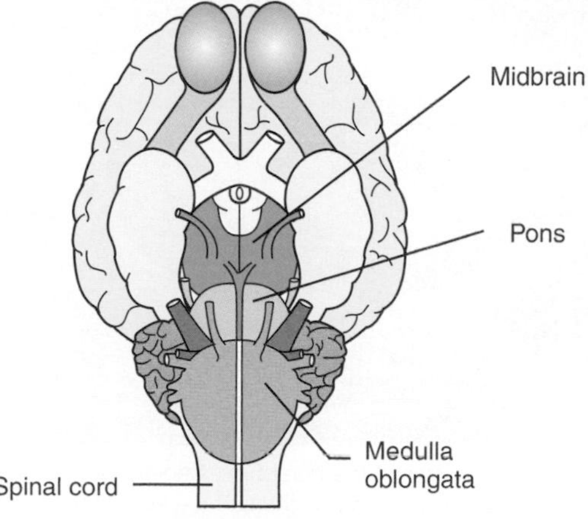

• **Fig. 8.18** Ventral view of a sheep brain.

Gray Matter and White Matter in the Brain

- Gray matter and white matter are named based on their gross appearance on cut sections of brain tissue (Figs. 8.19 and 8.20).
- **Gray matter** contains most of the neuron cell bodies and it is where many nerve impulses are initiated. Gray matter appears brownish gray grossly.
- **White matter** consists mainly of myelinated nerve fibers—it is the "wiring" that carries impulses in and out of the gray matter. The myelin sheath that covers the nerve fibers gives white matter a very pale whitish color grossly.
- Gray matter is found in the cortex (outer portion) of the cerebrum and cerebellum.
- White matter is found in the medulla (inner portion) of the cerebrum and cerebellum.
- The gyri and sulci on the outside of the cerebrum and cerebellum increase their surface areas, therefore allowing for more gray matter.
- In the diencephalon and brainstem, gray matter and white matter switch places from their positions in the cerebrum and cerebellum to their opposite positions in the spinal cord. When looking at a cut surface of the diencephalon or brainstem grossly (without magnification), there is no clear distinction between the gray and white matter.

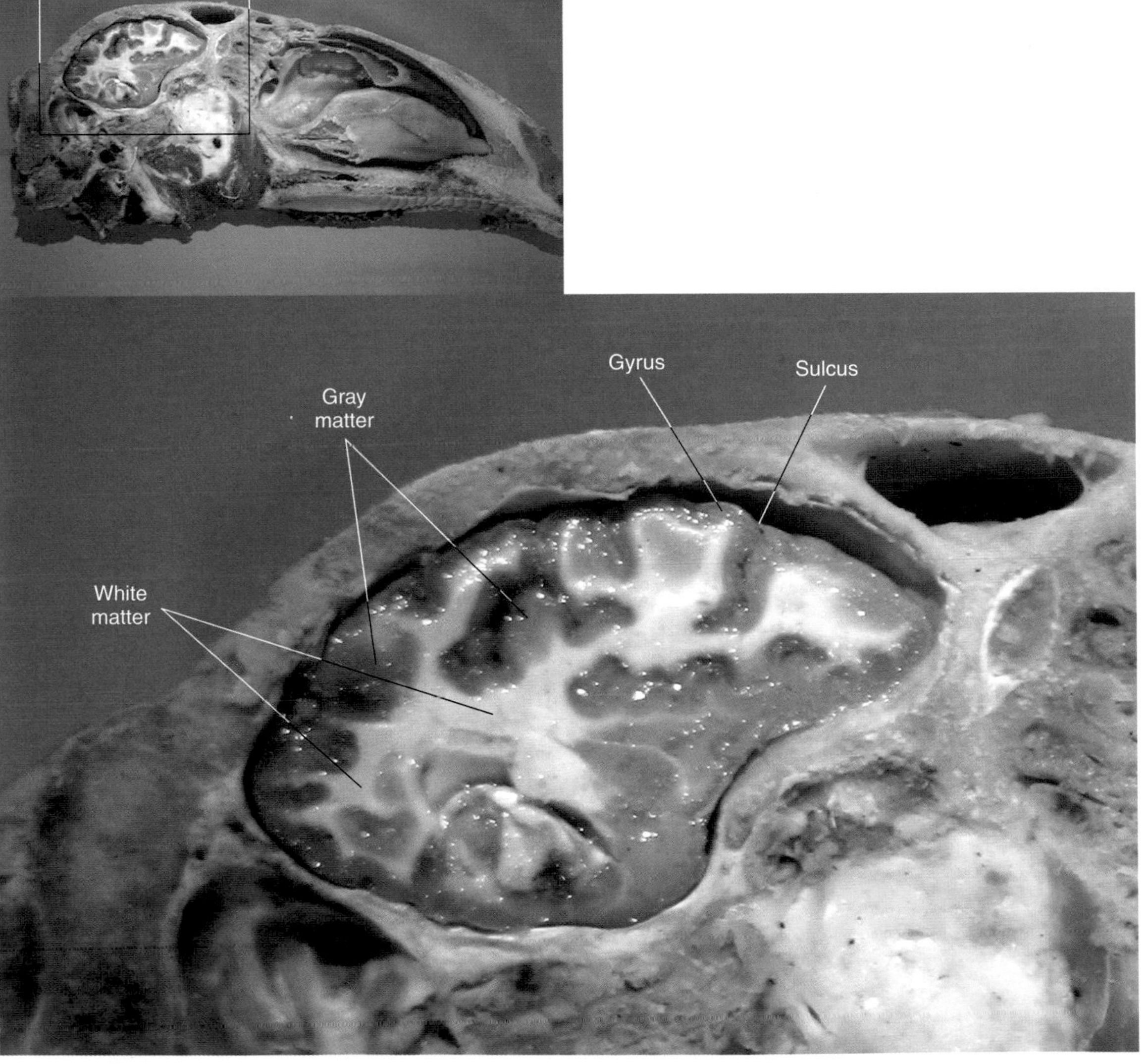

• **Fig. 8.19** Gray matter and white matter of the cerebrum. Sagittal view (longitudinal cross section) of a sheep skull. Notice how the gyri and sulci increase the surface area of the cerebrum, making more room for the gray matter.

The Spinal Cord

- In the **spinal cord**, the gray matter is in the medulla (inner portion) and white matter is in the cortex (outer portion) (Fig. 8.21).
- The gray matter in the spinal cord forms a butterfly shape. The dorsal horn of the butterfly carries sensory impulses up to the brain. The ventral horn carries motor impulses out to the rest of the body.
- The area occupied by the white matter is much larger in the spinal cord than in the brain.
- The central canal in the center of the spinal cord contains cerebrospinal fluid.

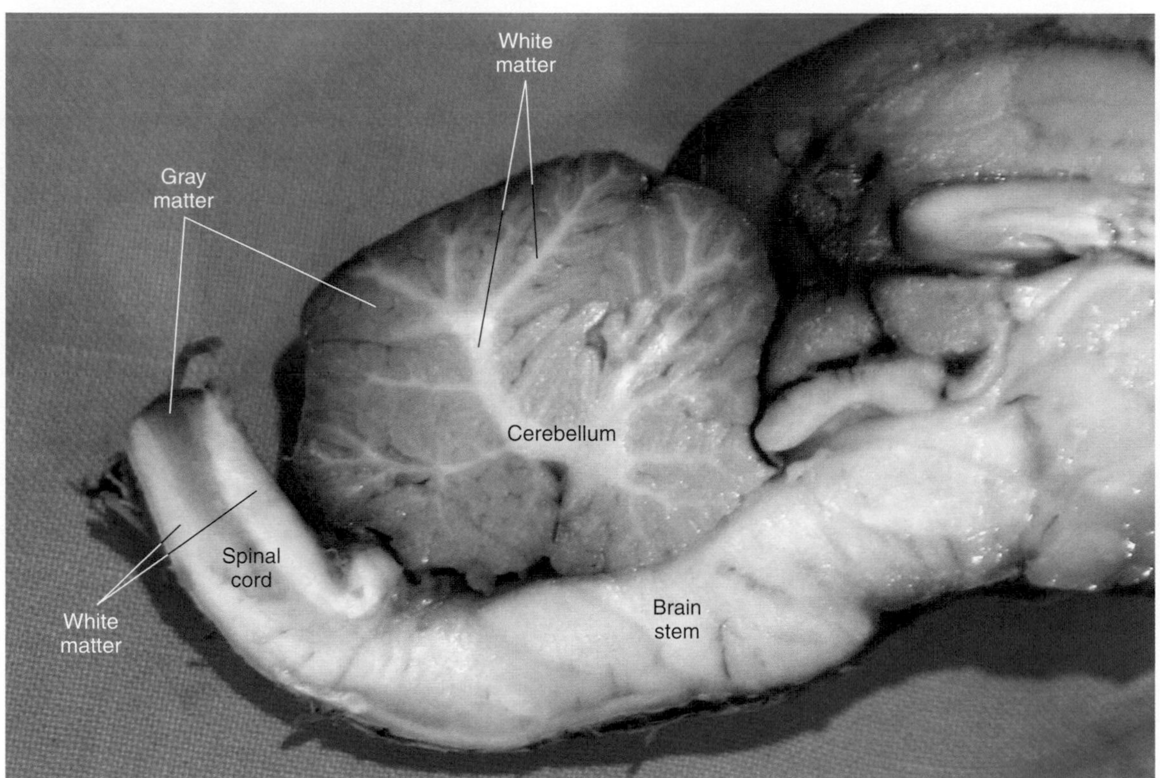

• **Fig. 8.20** Gray matter and white matter of the cerebellum. Sagittal view of a sheep brain. This view of the cerebellum shows the gray matter in the cortex and the white matter in the medulla. In the spinal cord, the gray matter is in the medulla (inside) and the white matter is in the cortex (outside). Notice that there is no clear distinction between gray and white matter in the brainstem.

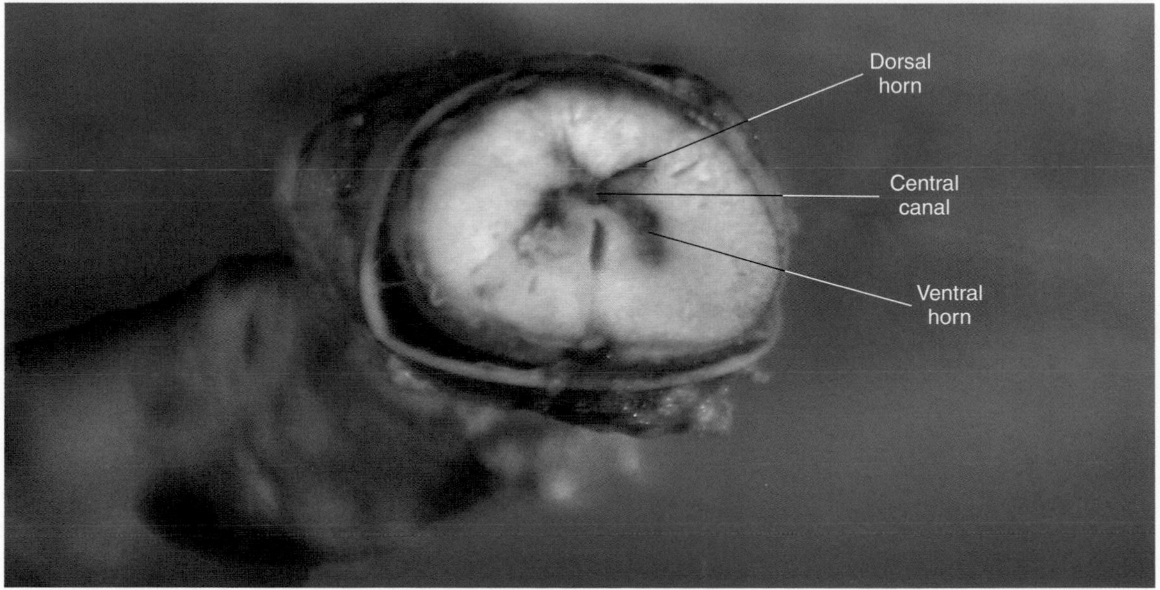

• **Fig. 8.21** Spinal cord cross section.

The Meninges

(Figs. 8.22–8.24.)

- The brain and spinal cord are covered and protected by three layers of connective tissue called the **meninges**.
- The outermost, thickest, and toughest layer is the **dura mater**. This layer is easily identified even on preserved brains if it has not been removed during processing.

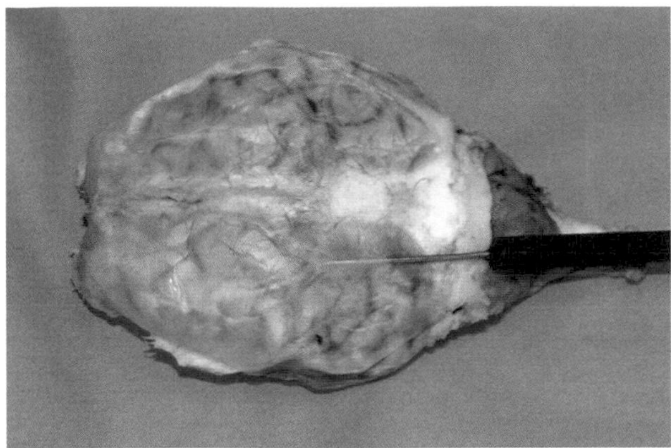

• **Fig. 8.22** Dura mater of a sheep brain. The dura mater is the cloudy-appearing membrane covering the cerebrum. The probe has been inserted through the dura mater.

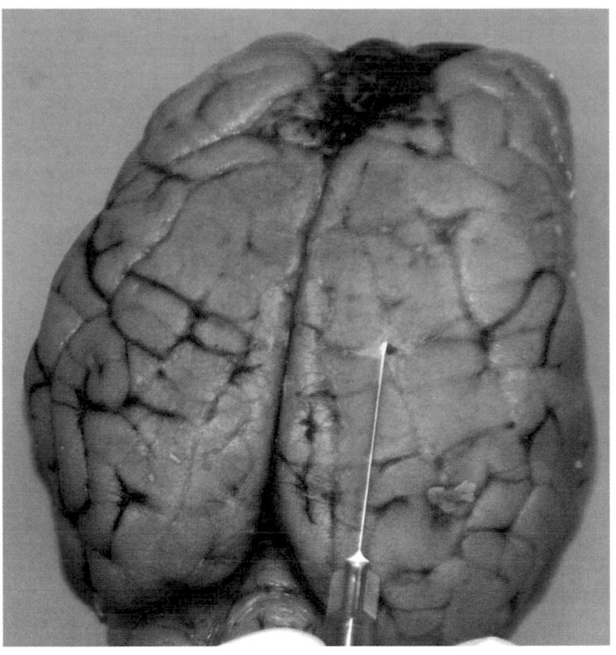

• **Fig. 8.24** Pia mater on a sheep brain. The pia mater is shown here being lifted from the surface of the cerebrum by the tip of a needle. It is a very thin, delicate layer that dries out very quickly on preserved specimens.

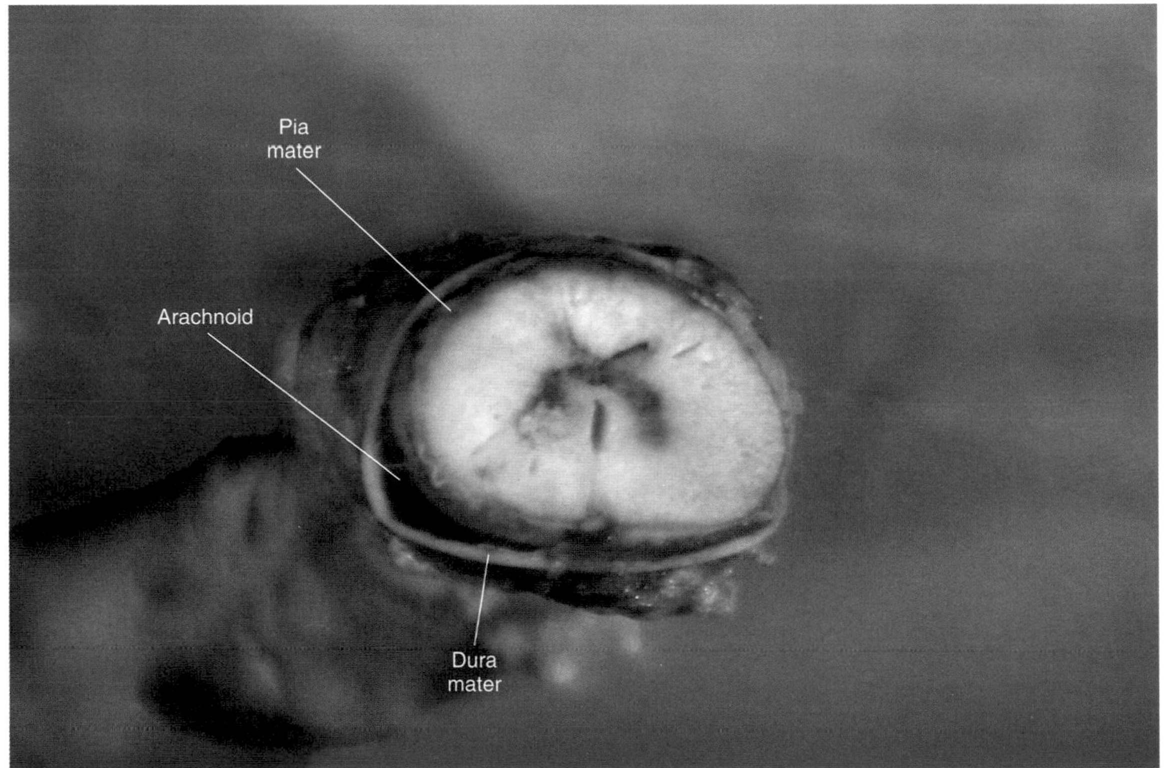

• **Fig. 8.23** Layers of the meninges. Sheep spinal cord. Note the fine fibers in the arachnoid space between the dura mater and the pia mater.

- The **arachnoid** is located between the dura mater and the pia mater. It is a cerebrospinal fluid-filled space that contains many filaments, like a spider's web.
- The innermost of the three meningeal layers is the **pia mater**. This is a very thin layer that tightly adheres to the surface of the brain and spinal cord.

Peripheral Nerves of Clinical Importance

Facial Nerve

The **facial nerve** is cranial nerve VII and is located very superficially on the lateral sides of the face (Fig. 8.25). Through its numerous branches, it controls many facial muscles and relays sensations from taste buds on the tongue. It also carries nerve fibers to the tear and salivary glands.

Damage to the facial nerve causes paralysis of facial muscles on the affected side. This is usually characterized by a drooping lip and nostril, although a drooping ear and a weak or absent palpebral reflex (touch the medial canthus of the eye and the eyelids blink) may also be seen. In large animals, facial nerve damage due to prolonged pressure can occur if they are in lateral recumbency for long periods of time without proper padding under the head. In horses, this can result if the animal's halter is not removed when the animal is anesthetized and placed in lateral recumbency. In small animals, facial nerve damage most often results from head trauma or facial surgery.

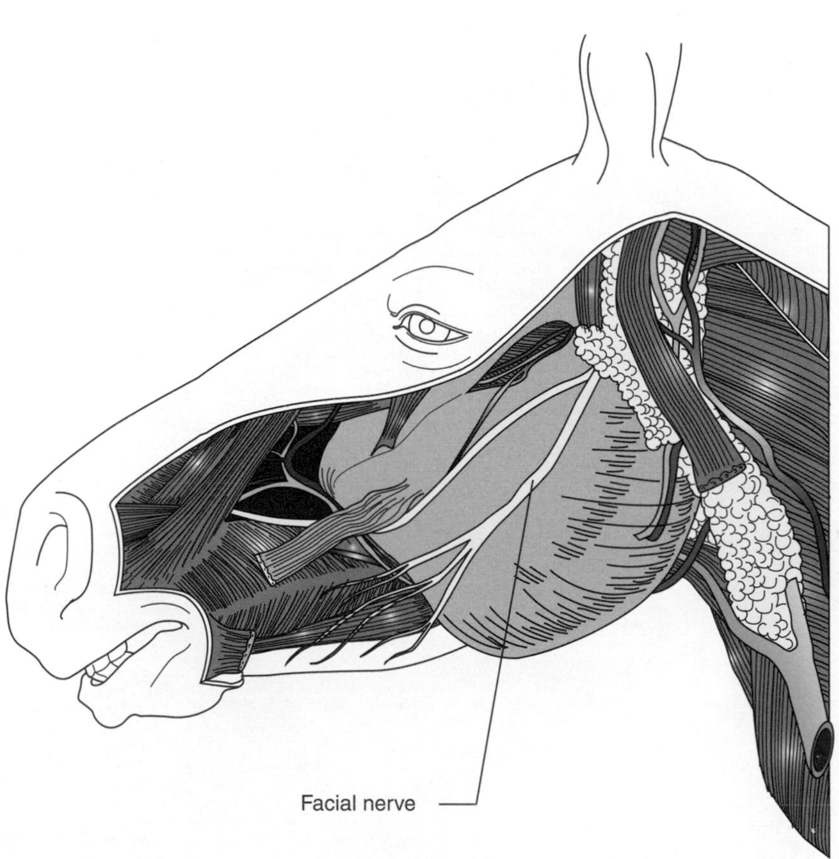

• **Fig. 8.25** Facial nerve.

Vagus Nerve

The **vagus nerve** is cranial nerve X, originating from the medulla oblongata (Fig. 8.26). It is the longest nerve in the body, traveling from the brainstem all the way to the colon. The vagus nerve supplies motor impulses to the pharynx, larynx, trachea, lungs, heart, esophagus, and rest of the digestive tract. It also brings sensory impulses from the ear, tongue, pharynx, and larynx back to the brain. It is found in the neck area, running next to the carotid artery and the jugular vein.

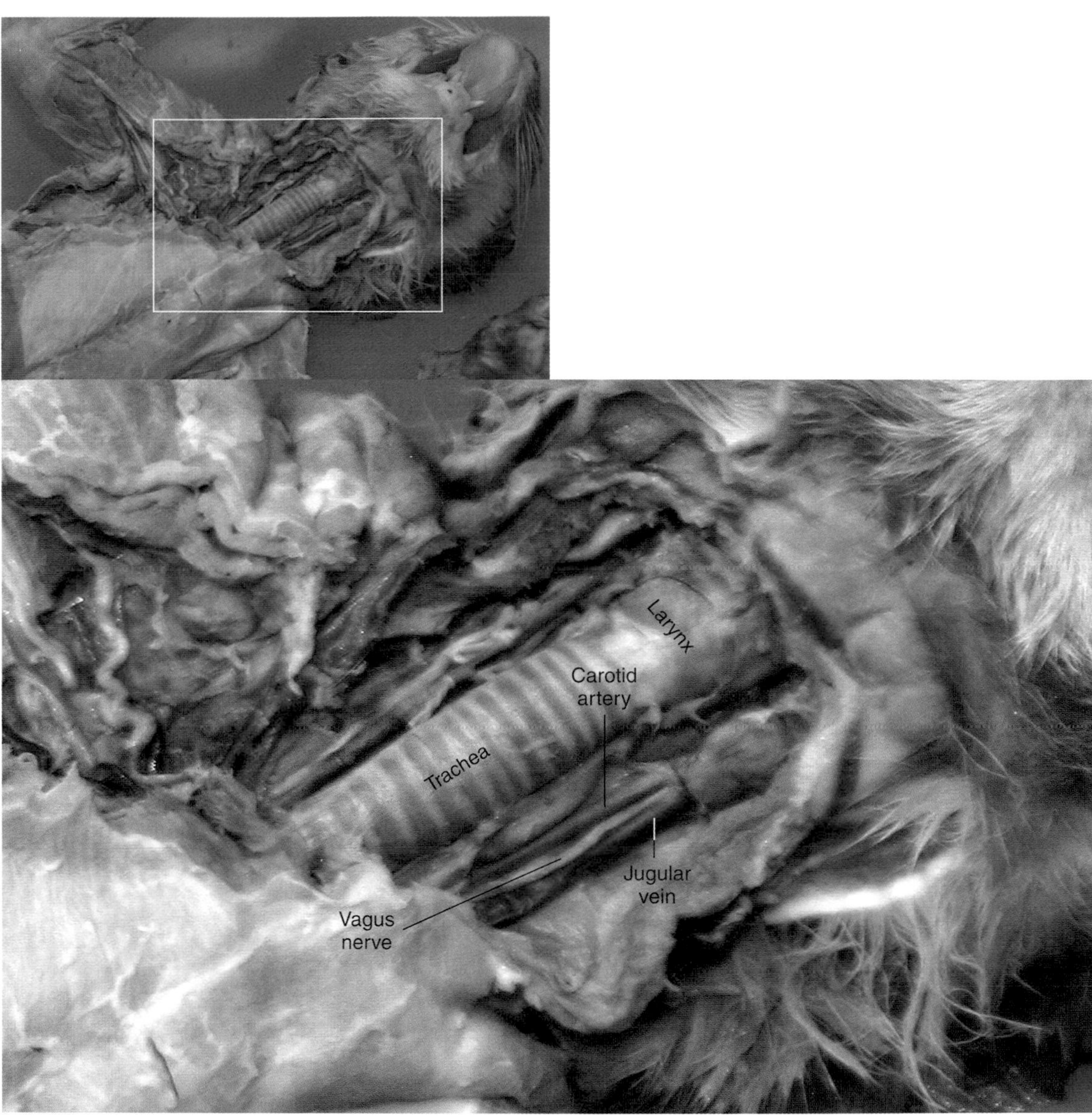

• **Fig. 8.26** Vagus nerve. Cervical area of a cat.

Brachial Plexus, Radial Nerve, Median Nerve, and Ulnar Nerve

The brachial plexus is a group of nerves in the axillary (armpit) region formed from branches of the sixth cervical to the second thoracic nerve roots. It forms many branches, but the three of most clinical significance are the radial nerve, the median nerve, and the ulnar nerve (Fig. 8.27). The **radial nerve** is the largest nerve branch from the brachial plexus. It passes between the triceps muscle and the humerus and supplies motor impulses to muscles of the elbow, carpus, and digits. It also carries sensory impulses to the brain from the dorsal and lateral forearm and dorsal area of the paw. Damage to the radial nerve results in loss of the ability to extend the paw and loss of sensation on the dorsal surface of the paw, causing it to be dragged. The median and ulnar nerves together supply motor impulses to the flexors of the forearm. The **median nerve** is the middle of the three branches and runs to the elbow and forearm regions. The ulnar nerve is the most caudal of the three brachial plexus branches. It is most easily seen near the olecranon process of the ulna at the point of the elbow. Both nerves carry sensory impulses to the brain from the foot pads.

The **ulnar nerve** also carries sensory information from the skin on the caudal forearm. Damage to either the median or the ulnar nerve does not affect the animal's gait, but if both nerves are damaged, the carpus and fetlock sink owing to loss of muscle tone. (Note: We call the human ulnar nerve our "funny bone." Because it is located very superficially near the olecranon process [point of the elbow], we can easily bump it, resulting in the usual tingly sensation.)

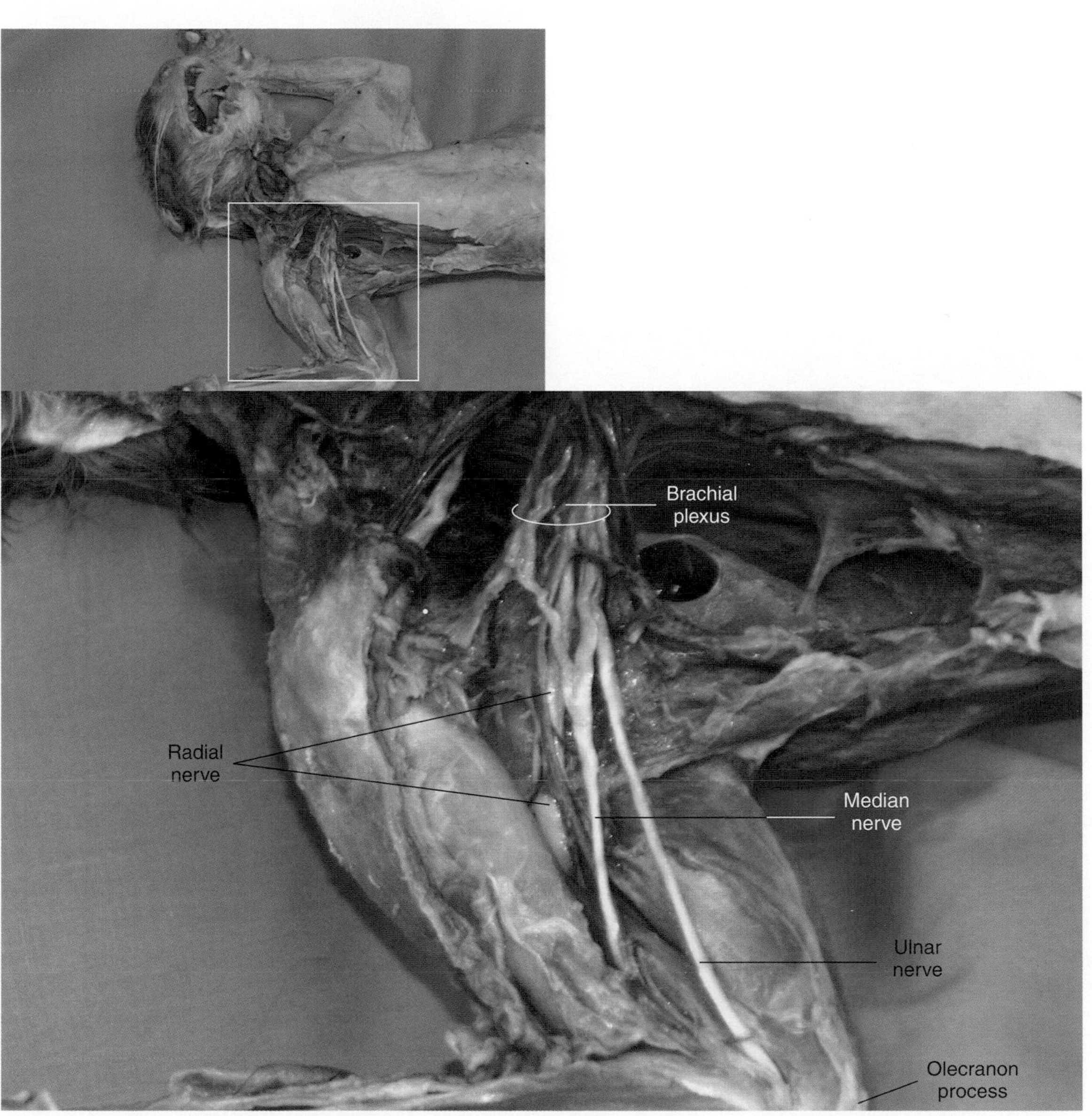

• **Fig. 8.27** Brachial plexus, radial nerve, median nerve, and ulnar nerve of a cat.

Cat Declaw Nerves

Branches of the radial, median, and ulnar nerves transmit sensations from the digits to the brain (Fig. 8.28). These nerves can be blocked with local anesthetic at the numbered sites before declaw surgery. This helps control pain in the immediate postoperative period.

Femoral Nerve

The **femoral nerve** is most easily found on the medial surface of the thigh, running with the femoral artery and vein (Fig. 8.29). It supplies motor function to the muscles of the thigh and carries sensory impulses from the skin of the hip, thigh, leg, and knee. Injury to the femoral nerve can be

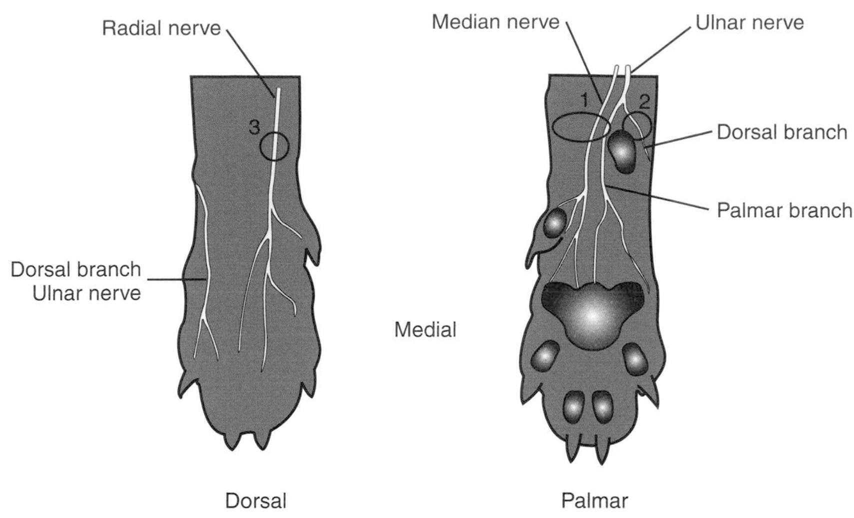

• **Fig. 8.28** Cat declaw nerves.

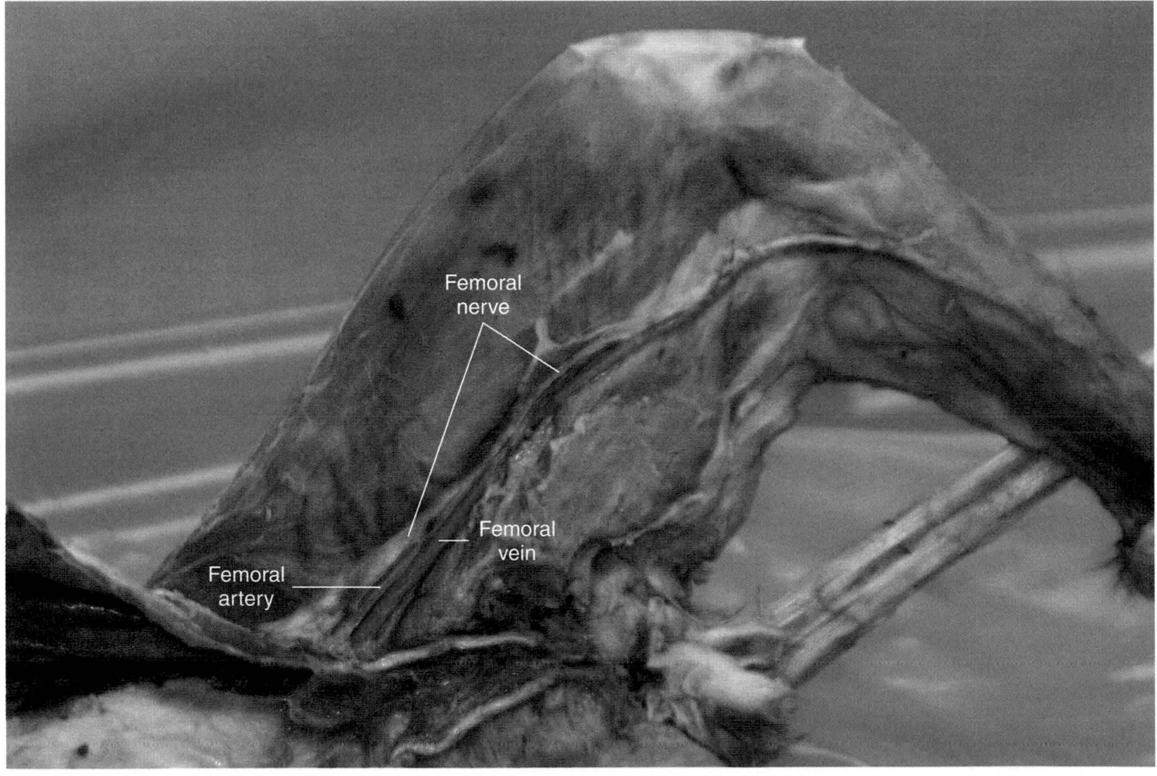

• **Fig. 8.29** Femoral nerve of the cat. Feline hind leg. Medial view.

significant in calves and foals if strong traction is applied to the hindlimbs during a difficult birth. The affected limb(s) show an inability to extend the stifle joint to support weight.

Sciatic Nerve

The **sciatic nerve** is found on the lateral thigh beneath the biceps femoris muscle (Fig. 8.30). It carries motor impulses to the flexor muscles of the stifle joint and the digits, and to the flexor muscles of the hock. The sciatic nerve can be injured by pelvic or femoral fractures, during surgery to repair femoral fractures, or by improper intramuscular injections.

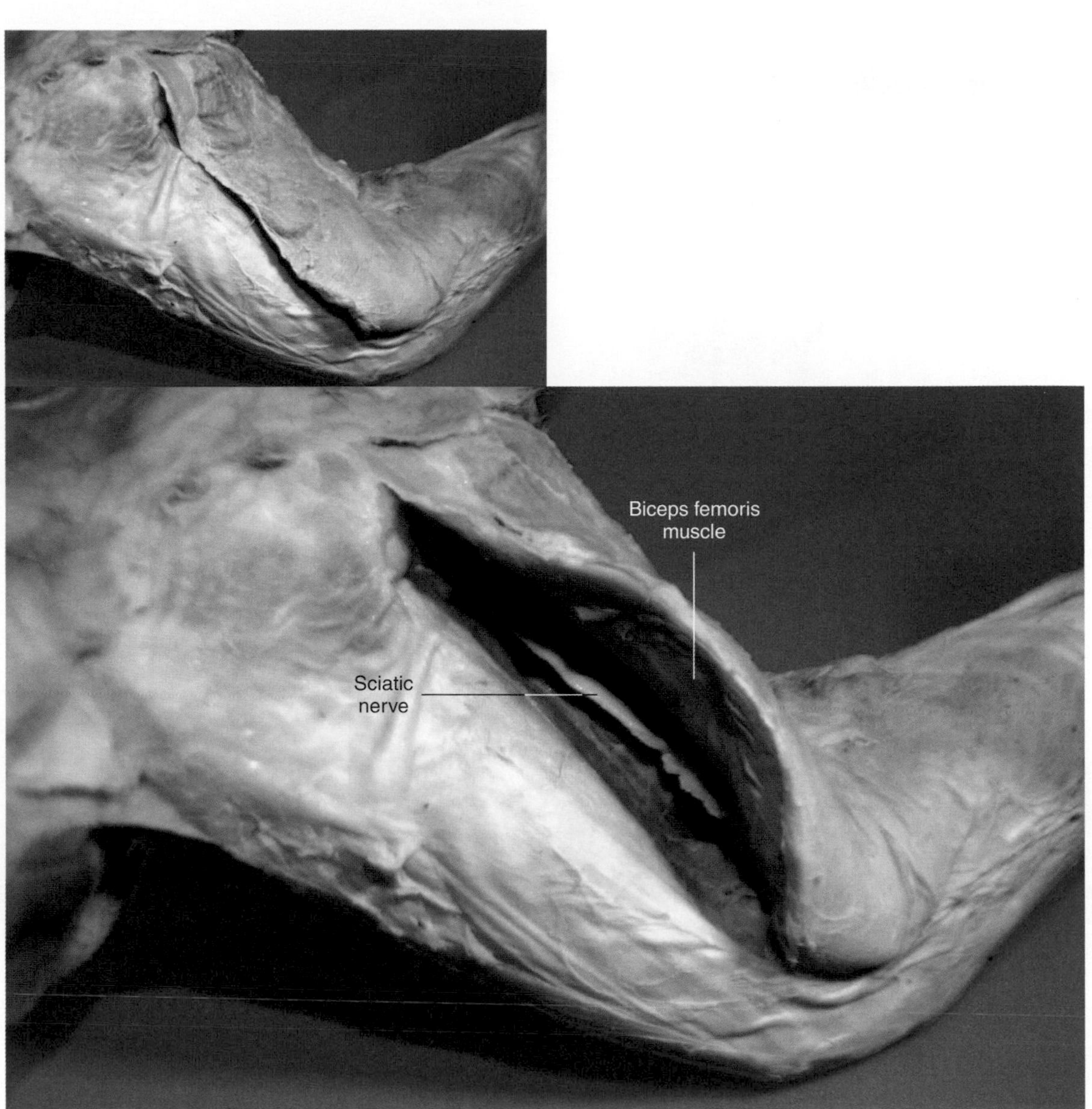

• **Fig. 8.30** Sciatic nerve of the cat. Feline hind leg. Lateral view.

EXERCISES

The Brain

Exercise 1

Label the Indicated Divisions/Structures of the Sheep Brain

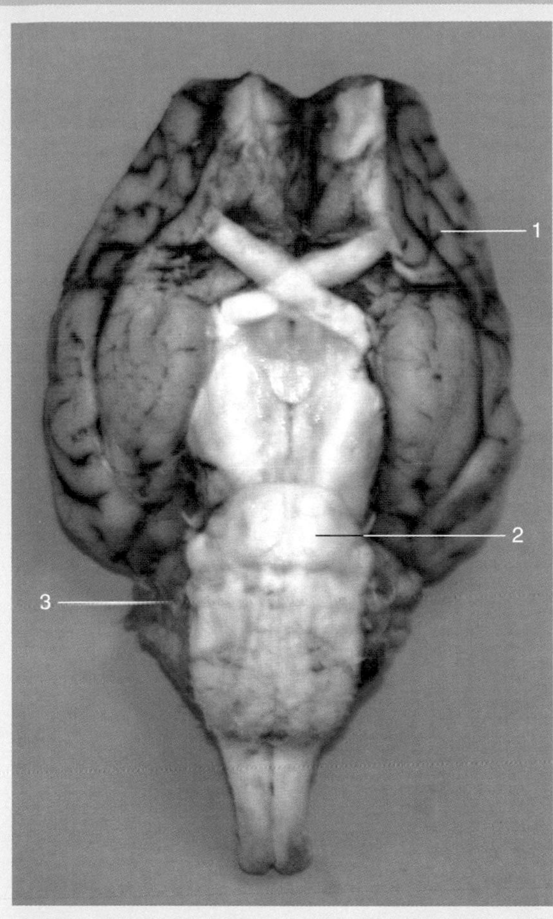

1. ______________________
2. ______________________
3. ______________________

Exercise 2

Label the Indicated Divisions/Structures of the Sheep Brain

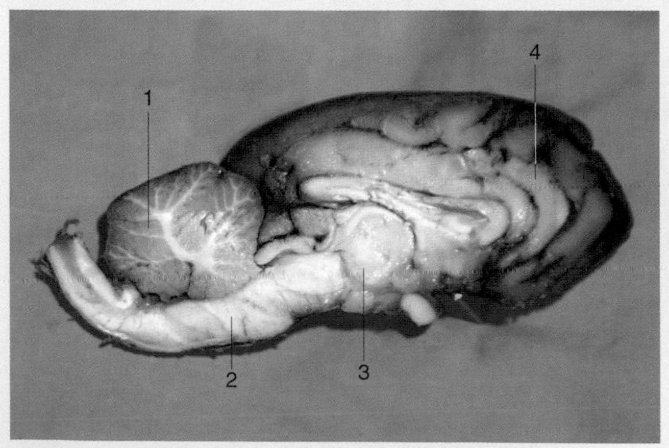

1. ______________________
2. ______________________
3. ______________________
4. ______________________

Exercise 3

Label the Indicated Structures of the Sheep Brain

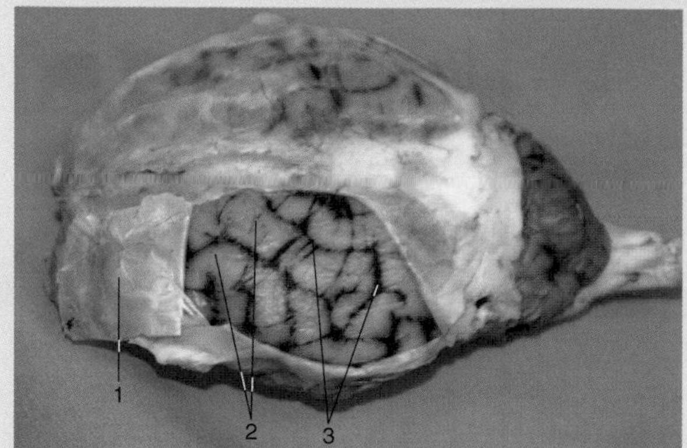

1. ______
2. ______
3. ______

Exercise 4

Label the Indicated Divisions/Structures

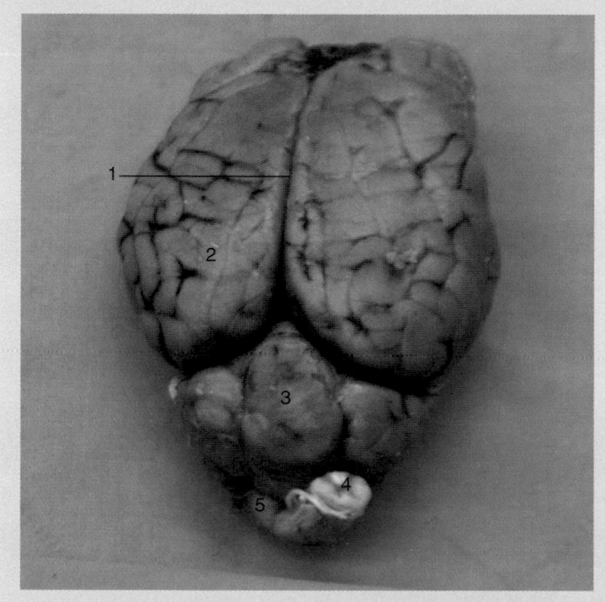

1. ______
2. ______
3. ______
4. ______
5. ______

Exercise 5

Label the Indicated Structures

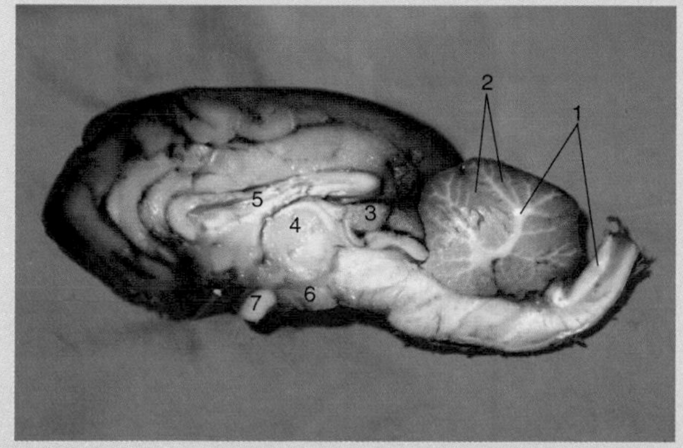

1. ______
2. ______
3. ______
4. ______
5. ______
6. ______
7. ______

Exercise 6

Label the Indicated Structures

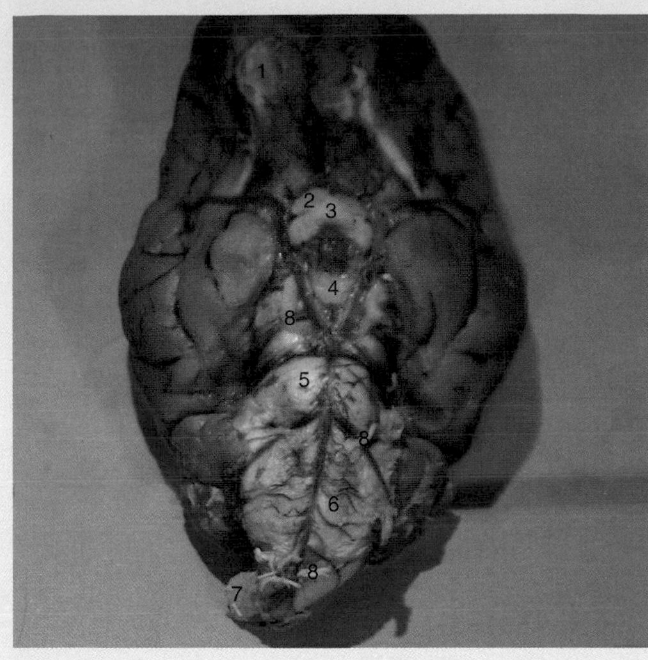

1. ______________________________
2. ______________________________
3. ______________________________
4. ______________________________
5. ______________________________
6. ______________________________
7. ______________________________
8. ______________________________

Exercise 7

Photo Quiz

What section of the brain has been removed from this dorsal view? What structures are more visible now that the section has been removed?

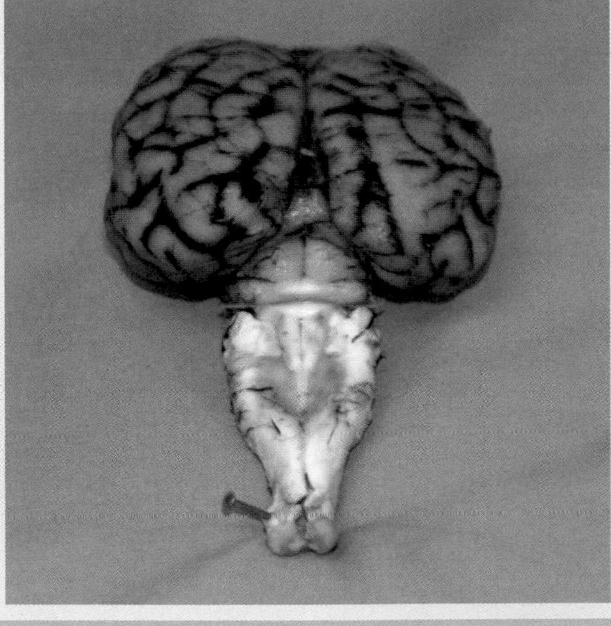

Peripheral Nerves of Clinical Importance

Exercise 8

Identify the Twelve Pairs of Cranial Nerves

Provide the missing information on the chart for the cranial nerve name and type.

Cranial Nerve Names and Functions

Cranial Nerve	Nerve Name	Type of Nerve
I	______________	______________
II	______________	______________
III	______________	______________
IV	______________	______________
V	______________	______________
VI	______________	______________
VII	______________	______________
VIII	______________	______________
IX	______________	______________
X	______________	______________
XI	______________	______________
XII	______________	______________

Exercise 9

Identify the Effect of the Sympathetic and Parasympathetic Nervous Systems

In the reception area of a veterinary clinic, two dogs begin to posture toward each other. Hackles are raised; a low growl emits from the throat of the larger dog. The smaller of the two dogs begins to snarl and show its teeth. The larger dog makes a move toward the smaller dog and, even though it is leashed, pulls the handler off the chair. The smaller dog rolls on its back, showing its belly. The incident is over within a matter of a minute. Indicate on the chart the likely effect of the incident on the sympathetic and parasympathetic nervous systems of the dogs.

	Sympathetic Effect	Parasympathetic Effect
Heart rate	__________	__________
Force of heart contraction	__________	__________
Diameter of bronchioles	__________	__________
Diameter of pupils	__________	__________
Gastrointestinal motility, secretions, and blood flow	__________	__________
Diameter of skin blood vessels	__________	__________
Diameter of muscle blood vessels	__________	__________
Diameter of blood vessels to kidney	__________	__________

Exercise 10

Identify the Nerve Indicated (Feline Groin Area)

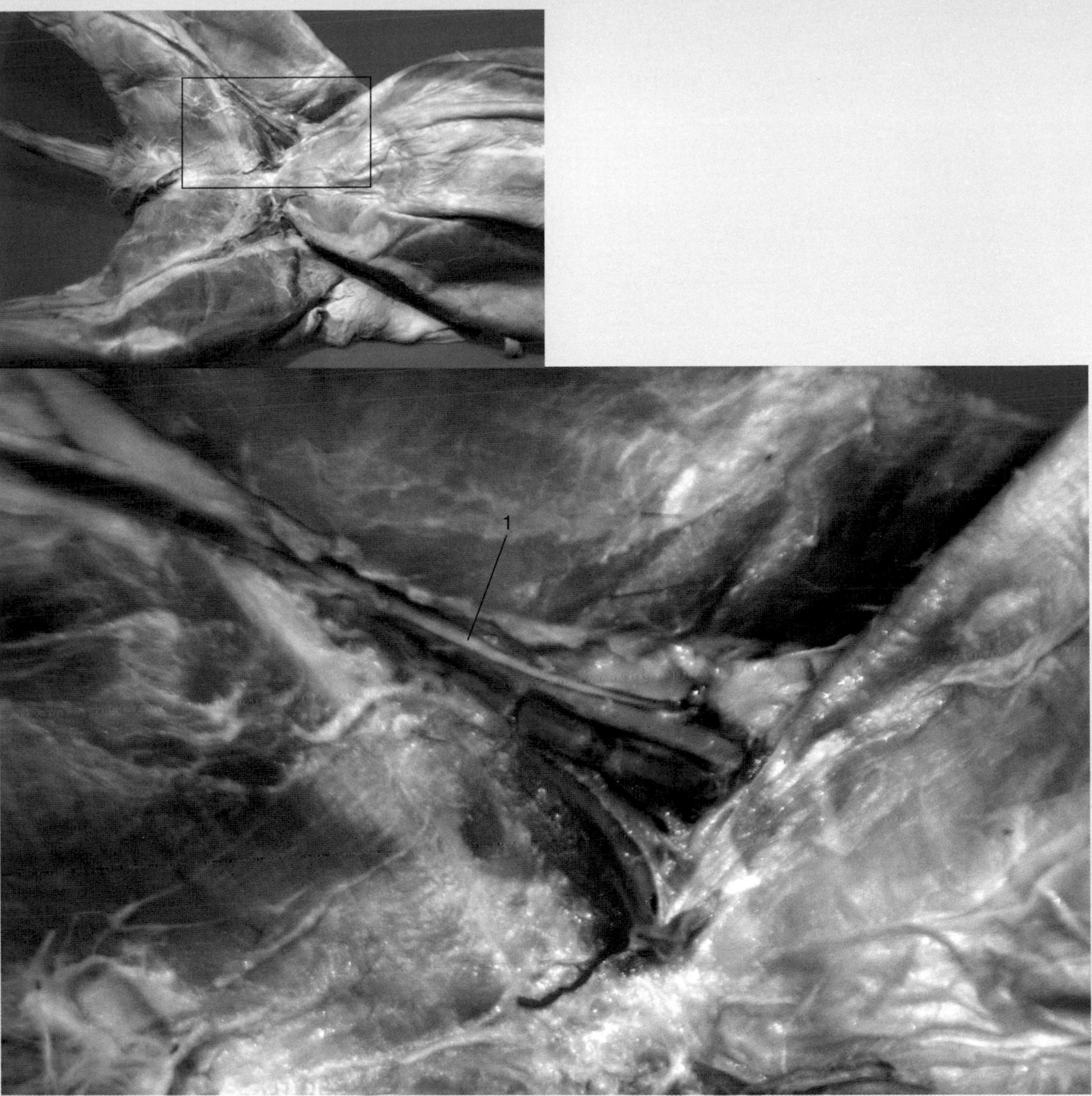

1. ______________________________

Exercise 11

Identify the Three Nerves Indicated (Medial Surface of a Cat Forelimb)

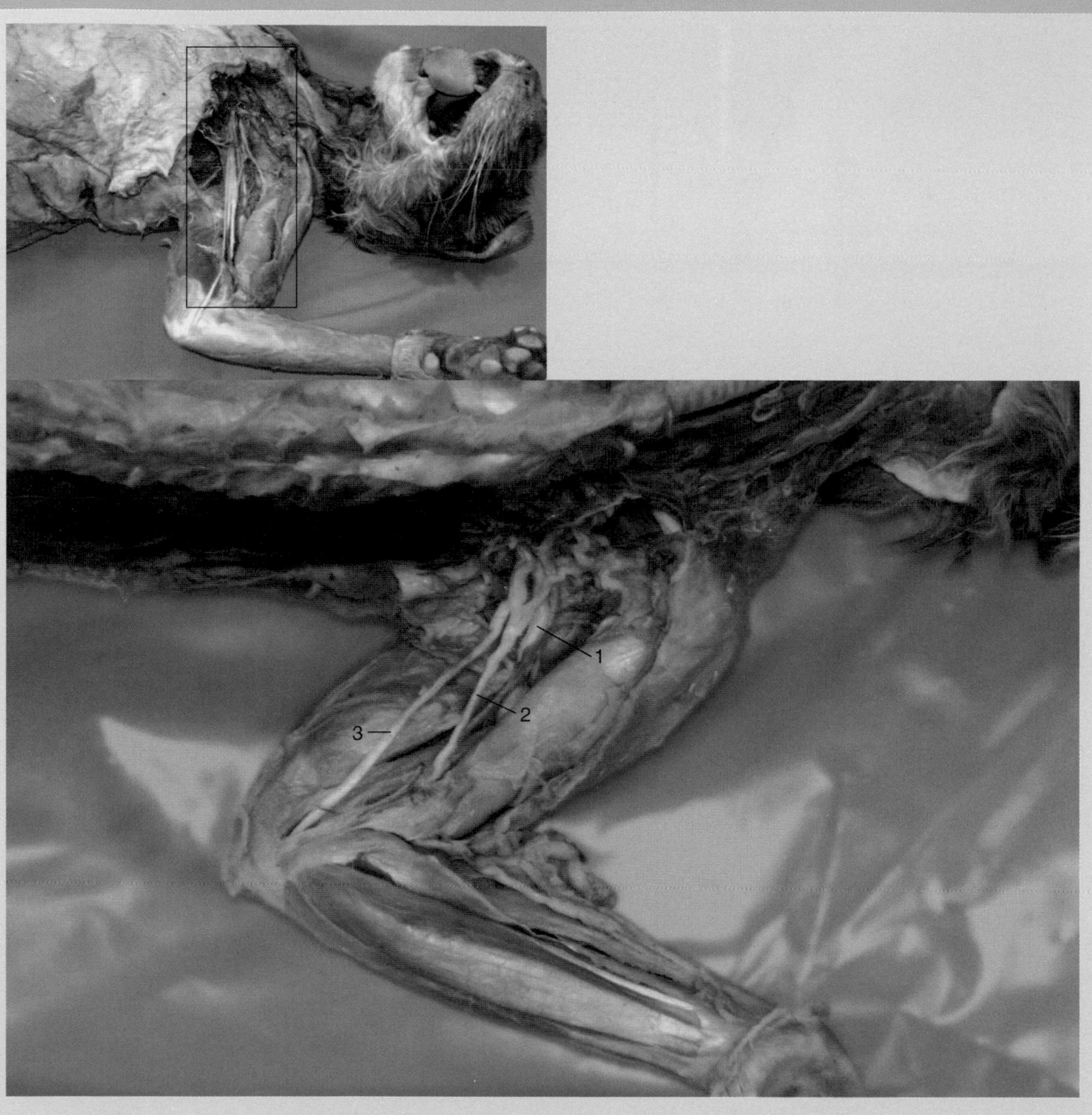

1. ______________________________

2. ______________________________

3. ______________________________

Exercise 12

Identify the Nerve Indicated (Lateral View of Cat Thigh)

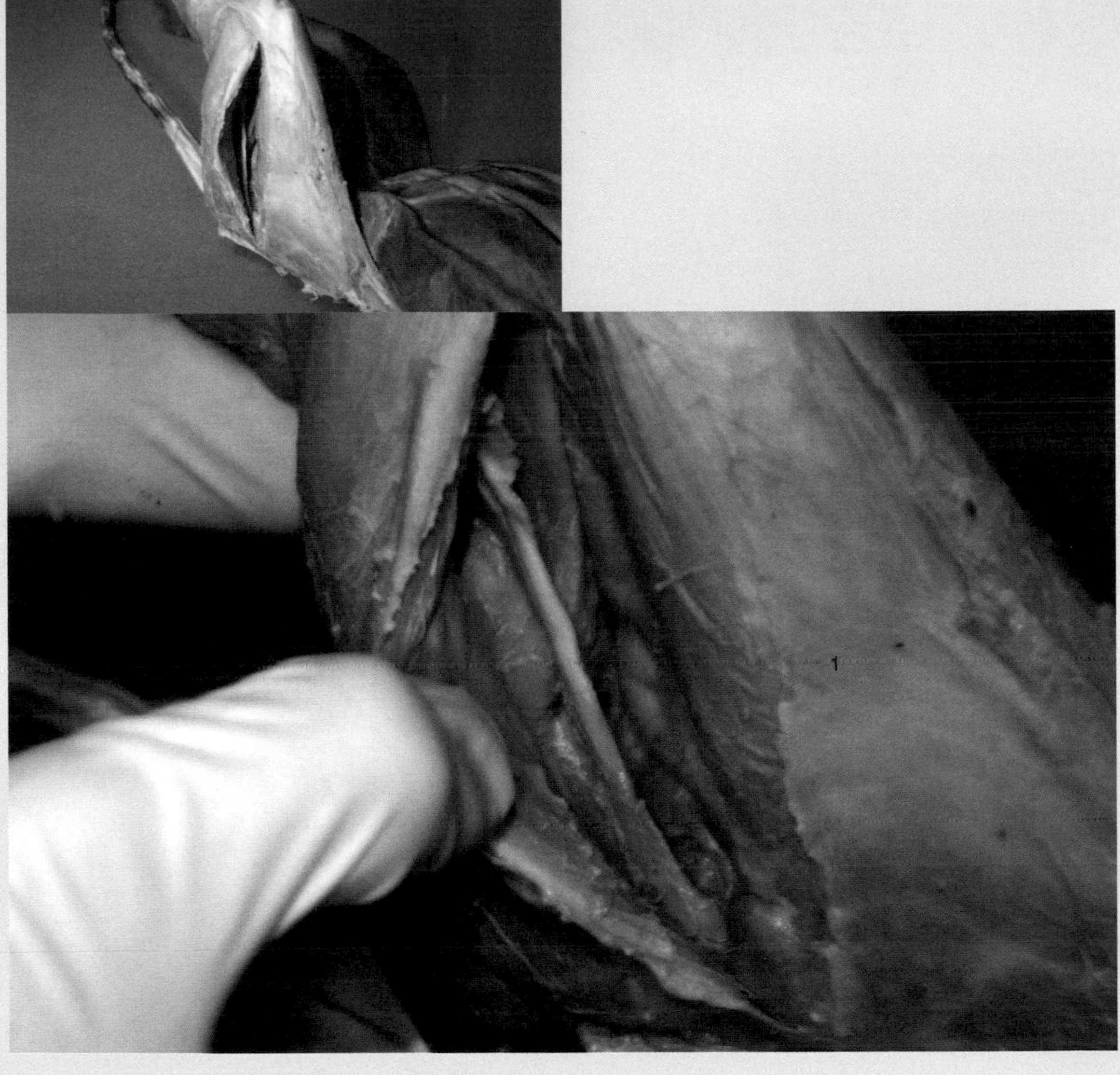

1. ______________________________

Critical and Clinical Thinking

Exercise 13

Define Clinical Terms

Write the definition for each term:

1. Arachnoid ______________________________

2. Brainstem ______________________________

Exercise 13—cont'd

Define Clinical Terms

3. Central nervous system ______________________________

4. Cerebellum ______________________________

5. Cerebrum ______________________________

6. Corpus callosum ______________________________

7. Cranial nerves ______________________________

8. Diencephalon ______________________________

9. Dorsal horn of spinal cord ______________________________

10. Dura mater ______________________________

11. Facial nerve ______________________________

12. Femoral nerve ______________________________

13. Gray matter ______________________________

14. Gyrus ______________________________

15. Hypothalamus ______________________________

16. Median nerve ______________________________

17. Meninges ______________________________

18. Mixed nerve ______________________________

19. Motor nerve ______________________________

20. Neuron ______________________________

21. Peripheral nervous system ______________________________

22. Pia mater ______________________________

23. Radial nerve ______________________________

24. Sciatic nerve ______________________________

25. Sensory nerves ______________________________

26. Spinal cord ______________________________

27. Spinal nerves ______________________________

28. Sulcus ______________________________

Continued

Exercise 13—cont'd

Define Clinical Terms

29. Thalamus ____
____
____
____

30. Ulnar nerve ____
____
____
____

31. Vagus nerve ____
____
____
____

32. Ventral horn of spinal cord ______________________________
____
____
____

33. White matter ____
____
____
____

Exercise 14

Clinical Thinking Challenge #1

1. ______________ Sensory nerve fibers carry impulses (toward, away from) the brain.
2. ______________ The ______ nerve can be found next to the carotid artery in the neck.
3. ______________ The ______ nerve is found on the medial surface of the thigh running with the femoral artery and vein.
4. ______________ The little grooves or "valleys" on the surface of the cerebrum.
5. ______________ The little folds or "hills" on the surface of the cerebrum.
6. ______________ The ______ separates the cerebrum into right and left hemispheres.
7. ______________ The ______ is a structure made up of nerve fibers that connect the two cerebral hemispheres.
8. ______________ The innermost layer of the meninges is the ______ ______.
9. ______________ The part of the brain associated with intelligence and learning ability is the ______.
10. ______________ The caudal part of the brainstem that becomes the spinal cord is the ______ ______.
11. ______________ The cortex of the cerebellum is made up of (gray, white) matter.
12. ______________ The medulla of the spinal cord is made up of (gray, white) matter.
13. ______________ The outermost layer of the meninges is the ______ ______.
14. ______________ The radial nerve is part of the (CNS, PNS).
15. ______________ The most caudal nerve of the three main nerves branching off the brachial plexus is the ______ nerve.
16. ______________ The nerve that lies just beneath (deep to) the biceps femoris muscle is the ______ nerve.
17. ______________ The ______ nerve is a cranial nerve and is the longest nerve in the body.
18. ______________ Motor nerve fibers carry impulses (toward, away from) the muscles of the body.

Exercise 15

Clinical Thinking Challenge #2

1. What are the four divisions of the brain?
____
2. Explain the difference between sensory and motor nerve fibers.
____
3. Explain the basic difference between a cranial nerve and a spinal nerve.
____

Exercise 15—cont'd

Clinical Thinking Challenge #2

4. What structures make up the PNS?

5. What structures make up the CNS?

6. What three main structures make up the diencephalon?

7. What three main structures make up the brainstem?

8. What section of the brain coordinates movements and helps an animal maintain balance and an upright posture?

9. What section of the brain controls the most primitive functions in the body? What are two of these subconscious functions?

10. What are the three layers of the meninges? How do they differ in gross appearance?

11. Which nerve must be avoided when giving an intramuscular injection in the thigh area of the hind leg? Why?

Support each of following correct statements with appropriate rationale, stating why or in what way each statement is correct.

12. The body has two communication and control systems that help keep things working properly—the nervous system and the endocrine system. Both use chemicals to carry their messages, but they do it by different means.

13. Structurally, the nervous system has two main divisions.

14. Functionally the nervous system's activities fall into three main categories.

15. Serious nervous system injuries, such as strokes and spinal cord damage, are often debilitating and have long-lasting effects.

16. Nervous tissue containing many myelinated axons is referred to as white matter.

17. Local anesthetics block the conduction of sensation from the area anesthetized.

18. It is important to understand the concepts of synaptic functioning, neurotransmitter release, and termination when treating an animal that has been poisoned.

19. The diencephalon is associated with many structures; three are of special importance to veterinary technicians.

20. Heartworm preventive drugs, such as ivermectin, are poisonous to insects and parasites but, properly dosed, do not adversely affect the dogs or cats that receive them.

9
Sense Organs[a]

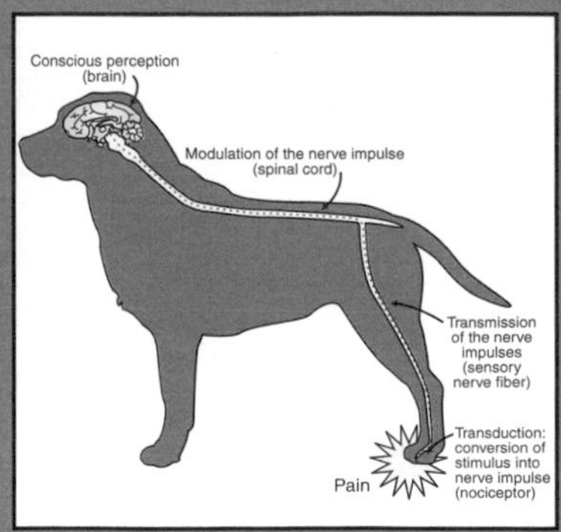

OVERVIEW AT A GLANCE

Pain 233

Taste 233

Smell 235

Hearing 235

Equilibrium 236

Vision 237

Suggested In-Class Activities 247

Exercises 250–260

Pain 250

1. *Identify Processes in Pain Perception 250*

Hearing 250–251

2. *Identify the Structures Indicated in the Canine Ear 250*
3. *Hearing Review 251*

Vision 251–255

4. *Identify Structures on the Calf Eye 251*
5. *Identify Structures of the Eye 252*
6. *Identify Structures on the Cat Eye 253*
7. *Identify Structures on the Sheep Eye 254*
8. *Identify Structures Removed from the Calf Eye 255*
9. *Identify Structures on the Rostral Half of a Transected Eyeball 255*

Critical and Clinical Thinking 256–260

10. *Matching Terms and Definitions 256*
11. *Identify Key Terms—Vision 256*
12. *Identify General and Special Senses 256*
13. *Define Clinical Terms 257*
14. *Identify Clinical Structures 260*

LEARNING OBJECTIVES

In this chapter, we will explore the basic mechanics of pain, taste, smell, hearing, and equilibrium, and the anatomy of the eye. See Chapter 10 in *Clinical Anatomy and Physiology for Veterinary Technicians* for a complete description of the sense organs.

CLINICAL SIGNIFICANCE

Understanding animals' sense organs is important for understanding their behavior. For example, it is important to know that upper respiratory infections blunt the sense of smell, which is very important to domestic animals. Because they cannot smell, affected animals often don't want to eat or drink. Another example is the exposed position of the eyes. This makes them susceptible to illnesses and injuries. Understanding their intricate structures can help us prevent and treat eye disorders. We are better able to handle and care for animals if we are familiar with the capabilities and limitations of their senses.

INTRODUCTION

Sense organs keep the central nervous system informed about what is going on inside and outside the body. They are made up of receptors that transform stimuli into sensory nerve impulses and accessory cells and structures that aid them. Some sense organs, such as those for smell and taste, are relatively simple. Others, such as hearing, balance, and sight, have complex structures that transmit the stimuli to the receptor cells.

TERMS TO BE IDENTIFIED

You will be able to Identify/define the following structures and terms when you have completed this chapter:

Pain
- Modulation
- Nociception
- Perception
- Transduction
- Transmission

Taste
- Gustatory cells
- Papilla (plural = papillae)
  - Conical
  - Filiform
  - Foliate
  - Fungiform
  - Vallate
- Taste buds

[a]The authors and publisher wish to acknowledge Joann Colville and Amy Ellwein for previous contributions to this chapter.

TERMS TO BE IDENTIFIED—cont'd

Smell
- Flehman response
- Olfactory cells
- Olfactory epithelium
- Pheromones
- Vermonasal organ

Hearing
- External ear
  - Pinna
  - External auditory canal
  - Tympanic membrane
- Middle ear
  - Eustachian tube
  - Ossicles
  - Incus
  - Malleus
  - Stapes
- Inner ear
  - Cochlea
- Equilibrium
  - Otoliths
  - Semicircular canals
  - Vestibule

The eye
- Anterior chamber
- Aqueous compartment
- Aqueous humor
- Bulbar conjunctiva
- Choroid
- Ciliary body
- Cones
- Conjunctival sac
- Cornea
- Extraocular muscles
- Eyelids
- Iris
- Lacrimal punctum (plural = puncta)
- Lateral canthus
- Lens
- Limbus
- Medial canthus
- Nasolacrimal duct
- Optic disc
- Optic nerve
- Palpebral conjunctiva
- Photoreceptors
- Posterior chamber
- Pupil
- Retina
- Rods
- Sclera
- Suspensory ligaments
- Tapetum (tapetum lucidum)
- Tarsal glands (meibomian glands)
- Tears
- Third eyelid (nictitating membrane)
- Uvea
- Vitreous compartment
- Vitreous humor (vitreous body)

MEDICAL WORD PARTS

Gustat/o = taste
Noci = pain
Ocul/o = eye
Olfact/o = smell
Ophthalm/o = eye

Pain

- **Nociception** is the process of experiencing pain.
- Pain is meant to be protective—to prevent further injury. Chronic and/or severe pain can have detrimental effects on an animal's health over and above the discomfort of the pain itself.
- Signs of pain are often suppressed by domestic animals to avoid looking weak.
- Pain perception occurs as a four-part process.
- The four parts of pain are:
  - **Transduction**—conversion of the painful stimulus to a nerve impulse.
  - **Transmission** of the impulse up to the spinal cord along nerve fibers.
  - **Modulation**—amplification or suppression of sensory nerve impulses in the spinal cord.
  - **Perception** of the painful impulses by the brain—this is when pain is consciously felt by the animal.

Taste

- The gustatory sense detects chemical substances dissolved in saliva.
- Receptors (**gustatory cells**) that detect these substances are organized into taste buds.
- **Taste buds** are found lining the mouth and pharynx but are mainly concentrated on certain papillae of the tongue.
- **Papillae** are small, elevated structures of the tongue.
- The papillae on which taste buds are commonly found include fungiform, vallate, and foliate (Figs. 9.1 and 9.2).
- **Filiform papillae**, the ones that make a cat's tongue so rough, do not have taste buds.

FUN FACTS

Foliate papillae detect salty tastes. **Vallate papillae** detect sour tastes. **Fungiform papillae** detect sweet, salty, and sour tastes.

FUN FACTS

Bitter tastes are particularly important to animals because many poisonous substances tend to be bitter, and the perception of bitter taste can allow animals to detect and avoid toxins in food.

FUN FACTS

Cats lack receptors on their taste buds that are sensitive to sweet tastes. Omnivores that chew their food have kept taste receptors sensitive to sweetness because detecting carbohydrates is essential to survival.

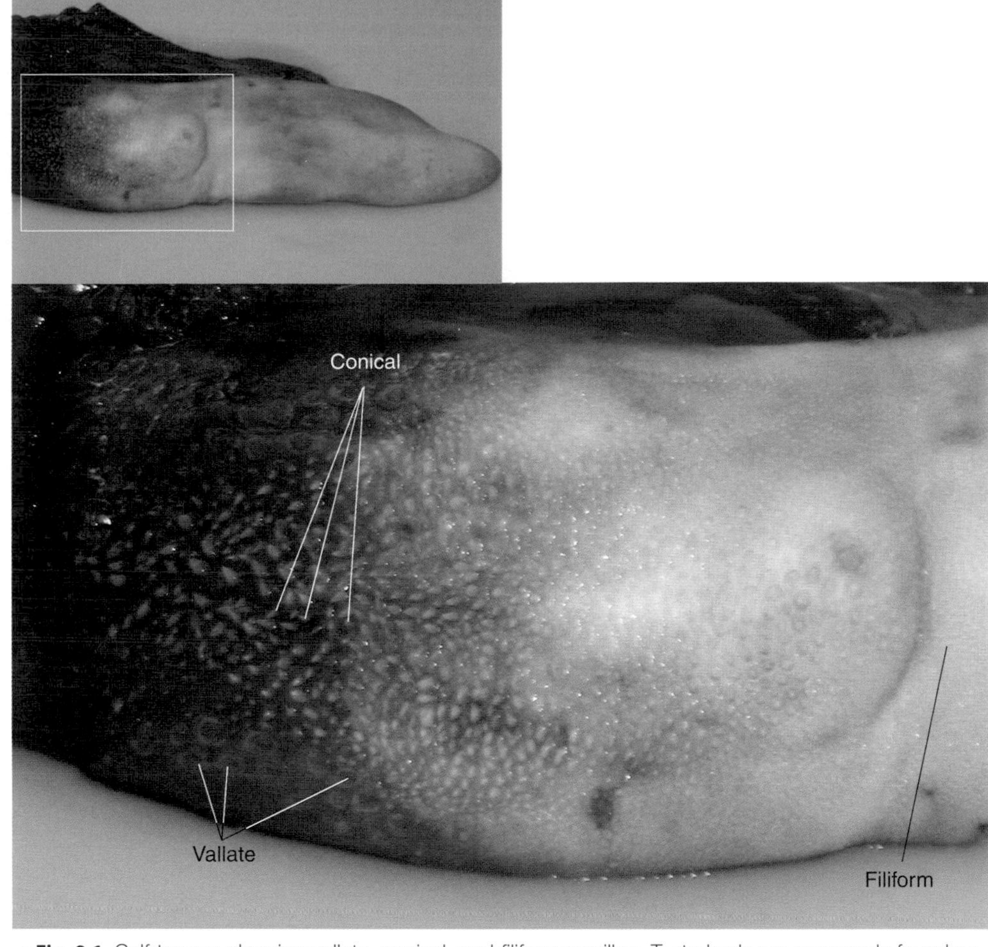

• **Fig. 9.1** Calf tongue showing vallate, conical, and filiform papillae. Taste buds are commonly found on vallate papillae.

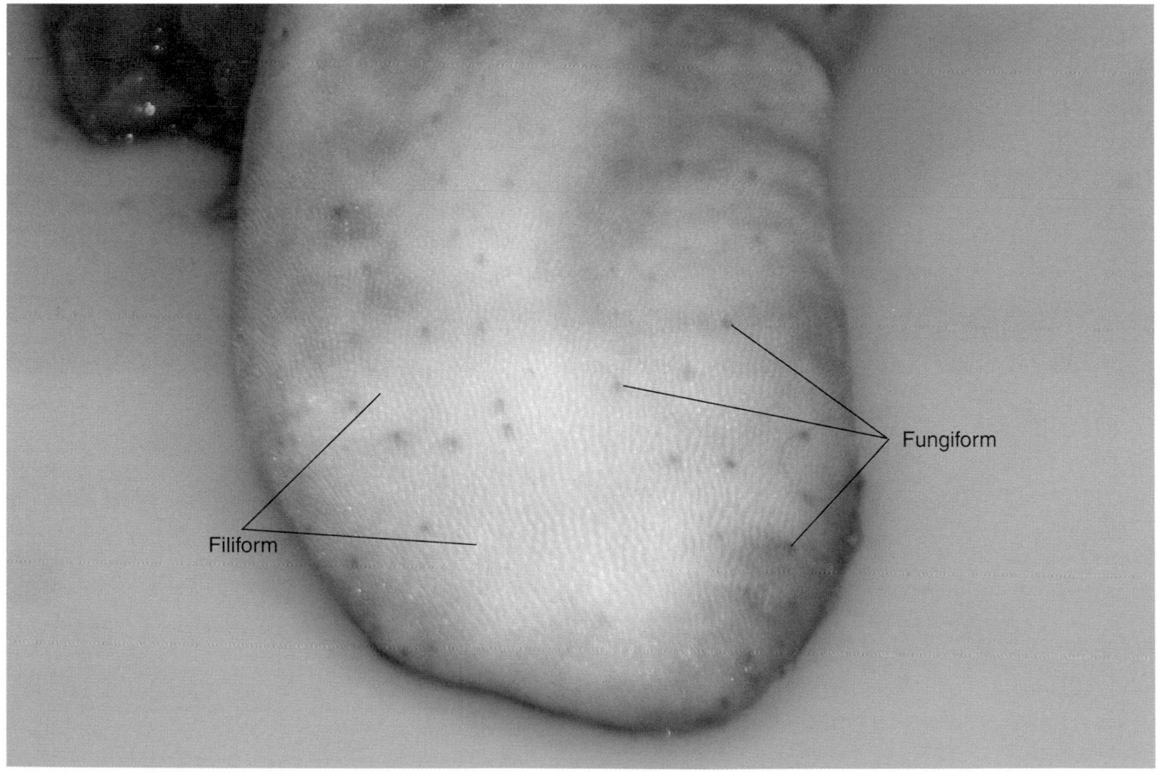

• **Fig. 9.2** Calf tongue showing fungiform and filiform papillae. Taste buds are commonly found on fungiform papillae.

Smell

- The olfactory sense detects chemical substances dissolved in the nasal mucus layer.
- Receptors (**olfactory cells**) that detect these substances are located in two patches of **olfactory epithelium** in the upper part of the nasal passages.
- The vomeronasal organ allows many species to detect the presence of pheromones through the Flehman response.

Hearing

External Ear

- The **pinna** is the earflap—the part of the ear that can be seen from the outside (Fig. 9.3). It funnels sound wave vibrations into the **external auditory canal** (external ear canal).
- In many animals, such as horses and cats, the pinna is very mobile and can be turned in the direction of sounds (Fig. 9.4). The position of the pinna can also be an indicator of the mood of the animal.
- The external auditory canal is a soft membrane-lined tube that conducts sound wave vibrations to the **tympanic membrane** (eardrum).
- The external auditory canal in domestic animals is not a straight tube. It has a lateral (outer) vertical portion and a medial (inner) horizontal portion that form an L-shaped path to the tympanic membrane.
- Sound waves striking the tympanic membrane cause it to vibrate.

Middle Ear

- The middle ear is an air-filled cavity within the temporal bone between the tympanic membrane and cochlea.
- Vibrations of the tympanic membrane are transmitted to the cochlea by three small bones, collectively called the **ossicles** (Fig. 9.5).
  - The **malleus** attaches to the tympanic membrane and forms a joint with the incus (Fig. 9.6).

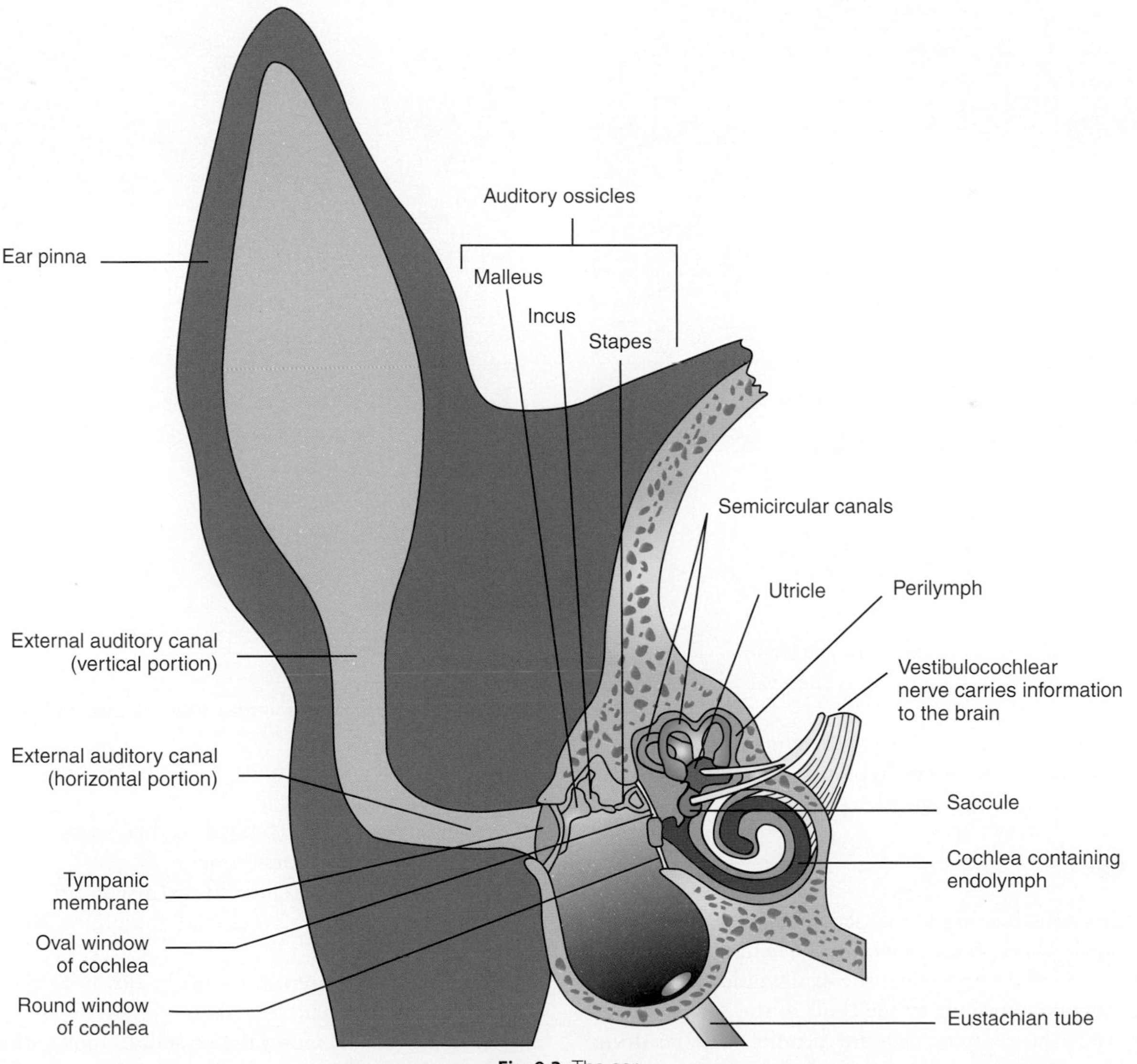

• **Fig. 9.3** The ear.

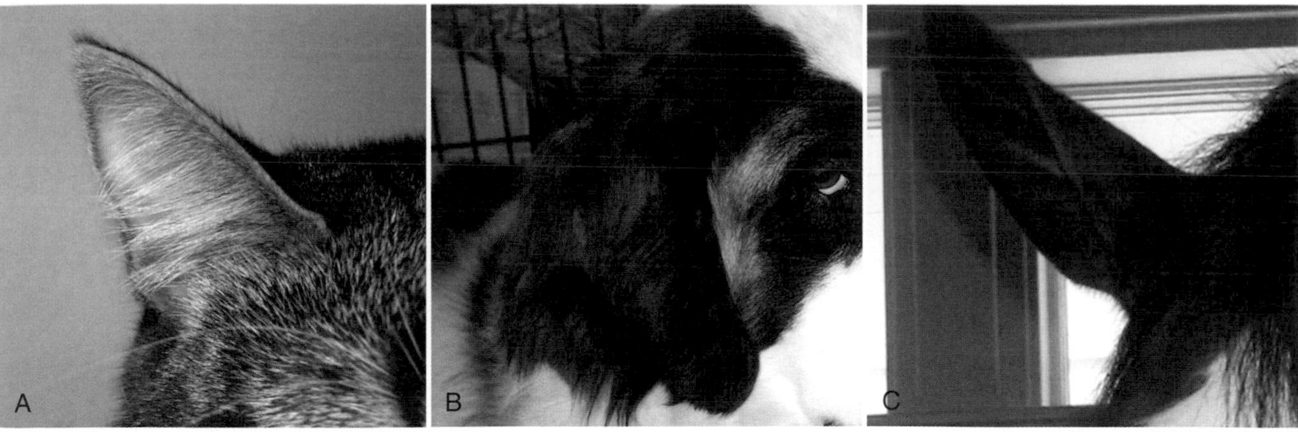

• **Fig. 9.4** The pinnas of a cat, dog, and horse. The pinnas of a cat (A), a dog (B), and a horse (C).

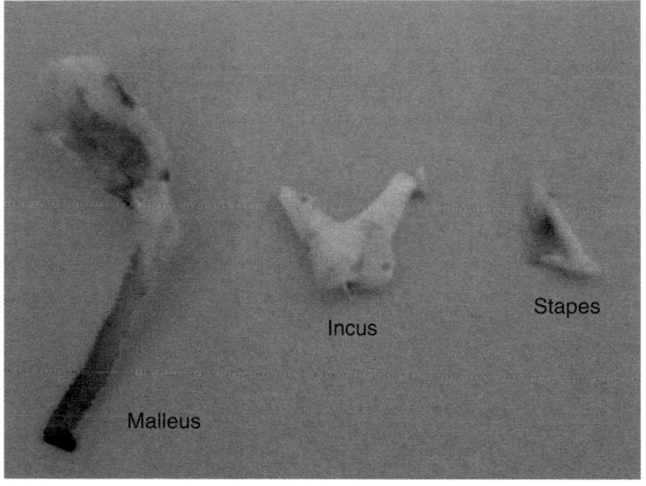

• **Fig. 9.5** The ossicles of a cat.

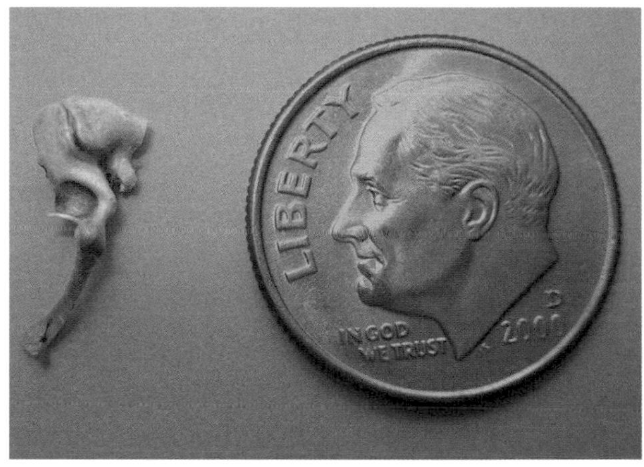

• **Fig. 9.6** Malleus of a 250-lb calf.

  - The **incus** forms a joint with the stapes.
  - The **stapes** is in contact with the oval window of the cochlea.
- Air pressure on the two sides of the tympanic membrane is equalized by the **eustachian tube** that connects the middle ear cavity with the pharynx.

Inner Ear

- Receptors for hearing are contained in the fluid-filled, snail shell-shaped **cochlea** within the temporal bone.
- The stapes vibrating against the oval window of the cochlea causes vibrations of the fluid in the cochlea. This stimulates the receptor cells for hearing. The resulting nerve impulses are interpreted by the brain as sounds.

Equilibrium

Vestibule

- The **vestibule** senses linear motion and the position of the head.
- It is located in the inner ear between the cochlea and semicircular canals.
- It consists of two fluid-filled, saclike spaces (utricle and saccule) in the temporal bone.
- A patch of sensory epithelium (macula) in each sac is covered by gelatinous material containing tiny crystals called **otoliths**.
- Gravity pulls the otoliths straight down on the sensory cells unless the head moves.
- Head movement causes the crystals to move, stimulating the sensory cells.

Semicircular Canals

- The **semicircular canals** sense rotary motion of the head.
- They are located in the inner ear medial to the vestibule.
- They consist of three fluid-filled, semicircular-shaped canals, each oriented at right angles to the other two, like the sides of a cube, coming together at each corner.
- Movement of the head in the plane of a semicircular canal causes the fluid to lag behind.
- Sensory epithelium detects movement of the fluid relative to the sensory cells.

Vision

(See Fig. 9.7.)

The Outer Fibrous Layer of the Eye

- The outer fibrous layer of the eye gives strength and shape to the eye—it is composed of the **sclera** and the **cornea** (Figs. 9.8 and 9.9).
- The cornea is the transparent "window" on the rostral surface that admits light to the interior of the eye.

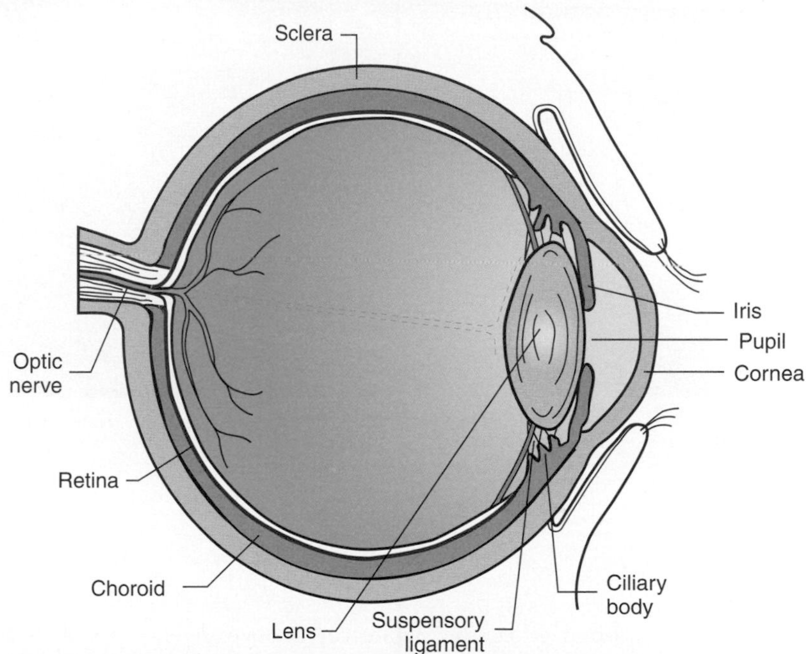

• **Fig. 9.7** Cross section of the eye.

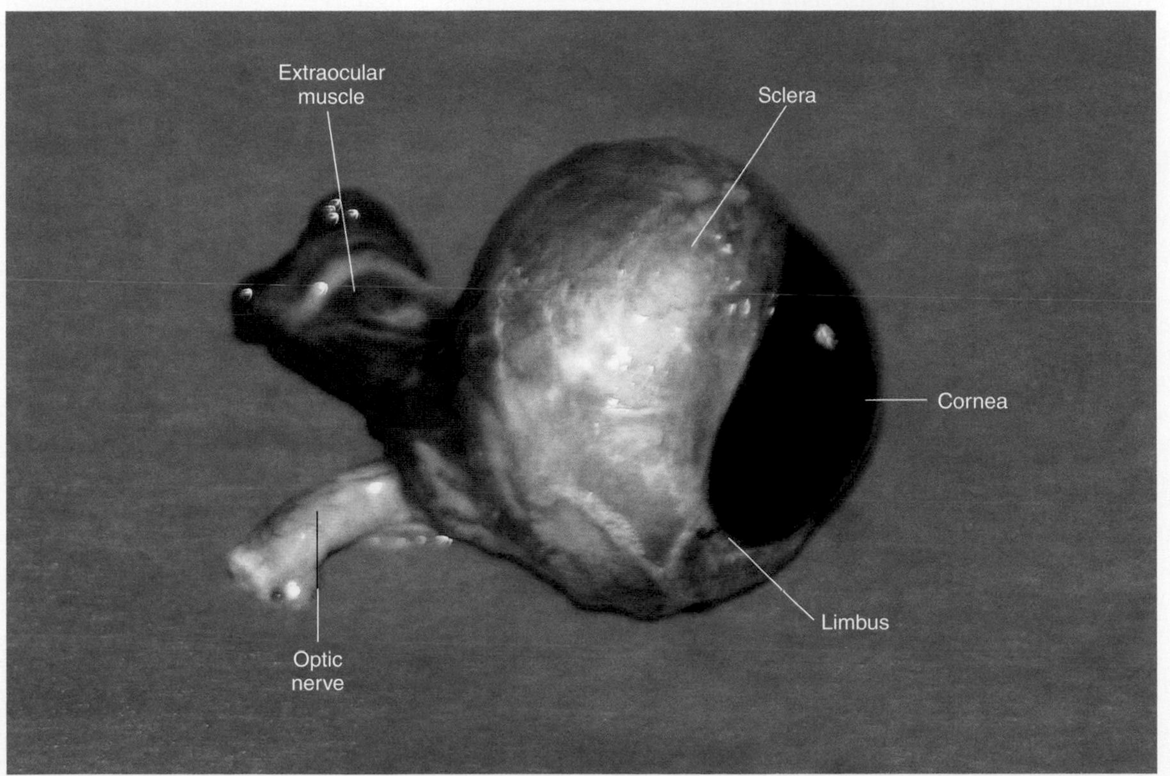

• **Fig. 9.8** The outer fibrous layer of the eye.

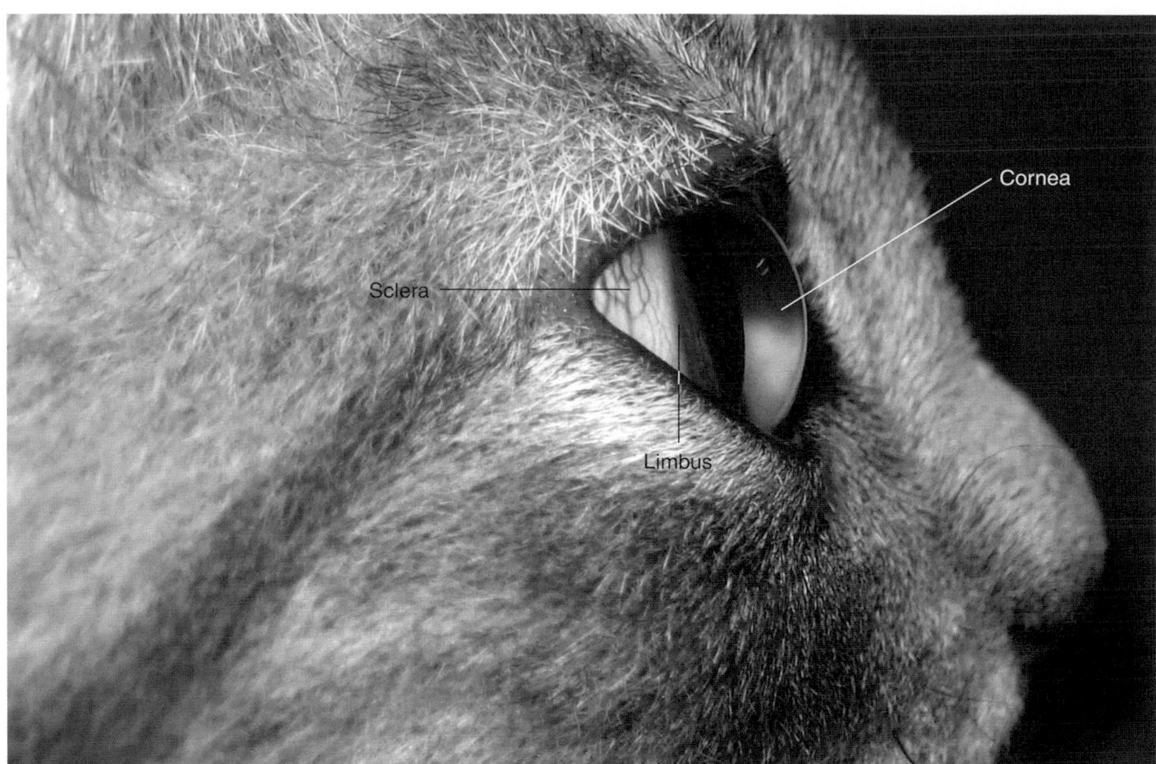

• **Fig. 9.9** Outer fibrous layer of a cat's eye. Note the rounded shape of the cornea.

- The sclera is often called the "white" of the eye. It is white in color and very tough.
- The sclera is sometimes not visible when looking directly at the eye, depending on what animal species you are observing.
- The **limbus** is the area where the sclera and cornea meet.

The Middle Vascular Layer

The middle vascular area (also called the uvea) is made up of the iris, the ciliary body, and the choroid.

Iris

- The **iris** is the colored portion of the eye.
- It is a pigmented, muscular diaphragm that controls the amount of light admitted to the eye.
- Most domestic mammals have brown eyes, but some species have a variety of colors. The iris colors of cats include yellows, greens, and blues (Fig. 9.10).
- The **pupil** is the opening or hole in the center of the iris through which light passes.
- The iris is located in the rostral (front) part of the eye behind the cornea.

Ciliary Body

- The **ciliary body** is located just behind the iris but still in the rostral part of the eye (Fig. 9.11).
- It is a ring-shaped structure that controls the shape of the lens by the pull of tiny muscles that tense and relax the suspensory ligaments attached to the periphery of the lens.

Lens

- The **lens** is made up of multiple concentric layers of tiny transparent connective tissue fibers (Fig. 9.12). If you cut an onion in half through the "equator," you will get an idea of how the layers of the lens are laid out. In a preserved lens, you can peel each layer of the lens much as you would the onion. A fresh lens is too soft to manipulate this way.
- The dark material surrounding the lens is made up of thousands of microscopic **suspensory ligaments** that attach the lens to the muscles of the ciliary body to control its shape.

Choroid

- The choroid contains dark pigment and blood vessels that supply the retina.
- The tapetum (also called the tapetum lucidum) is a highly reflective area of the choroid in many common animal species (Fig. 9.13). Its pigment has a "mother-of-pearl" look in shades of greens and blues.
- The tapetum acts as a light amplifier to aid vision in dim light.

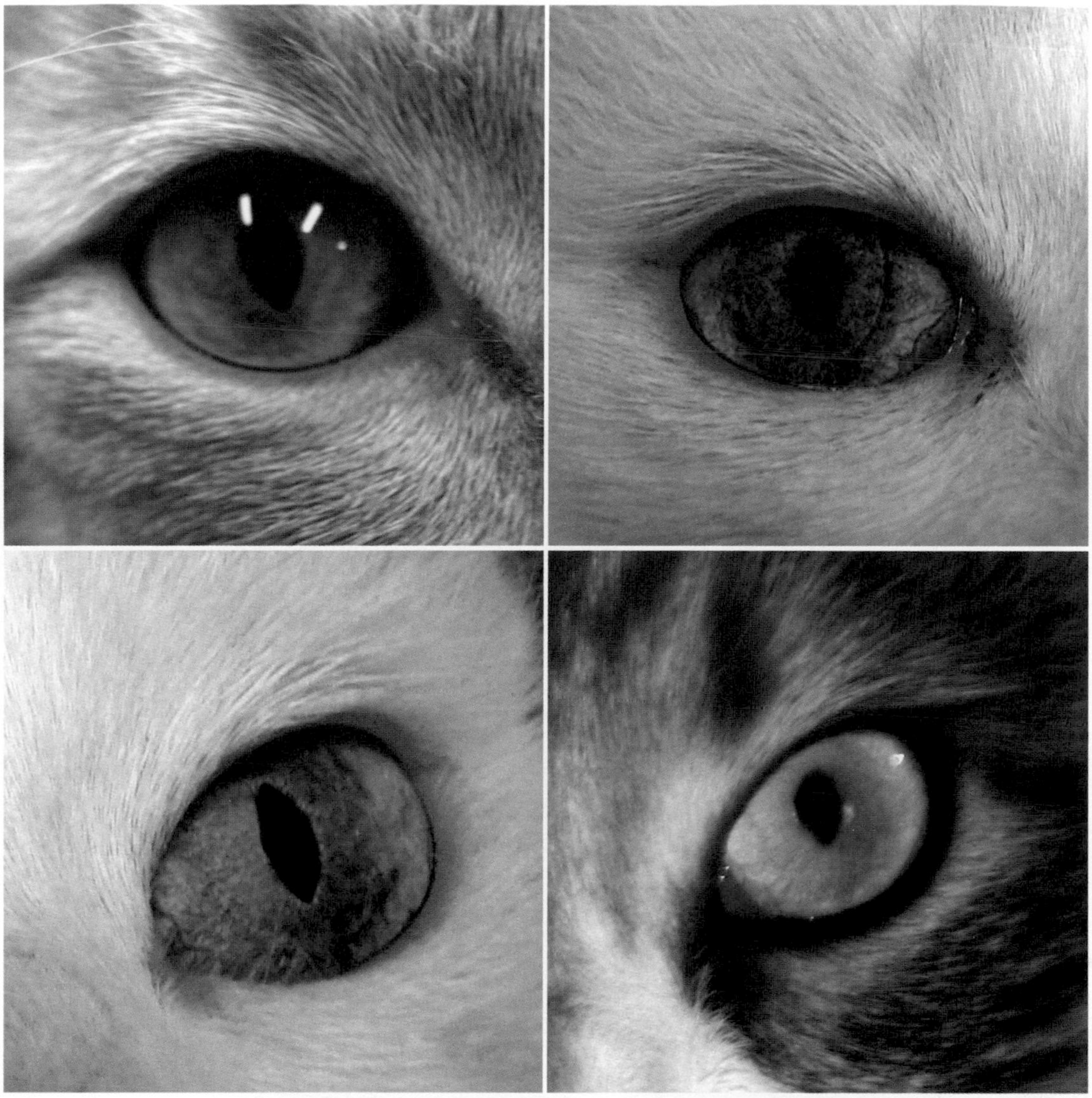

• **Fig. 9.10** Variations in the color of cat irises.

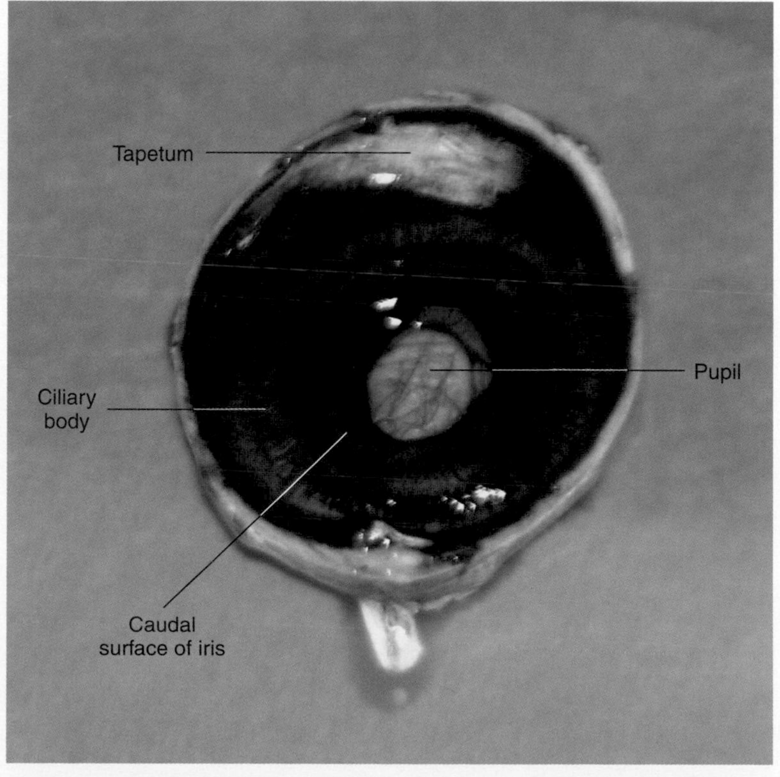

• **Fig. 9.11** Ciliary body. Rostral part of calf eye viewed from the back. The lens has been removed.

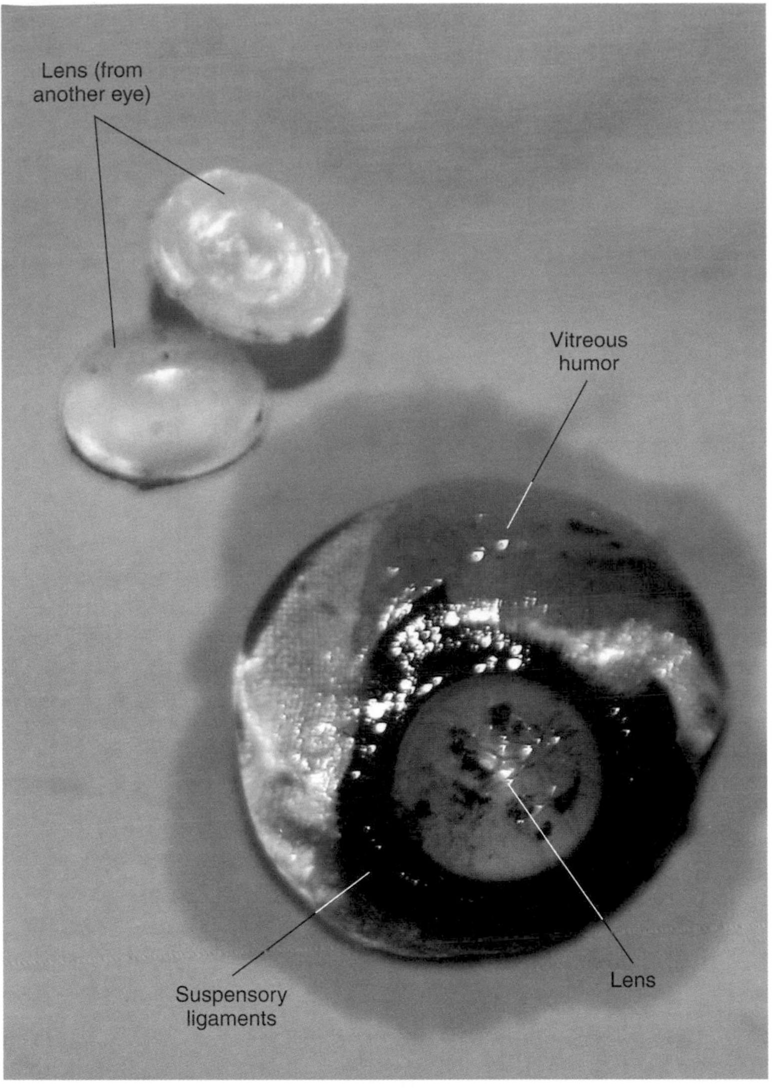

• **Fig. 9.12** The lens, vitreous humor, and suspensory ligaments of a preserved sheep eye.

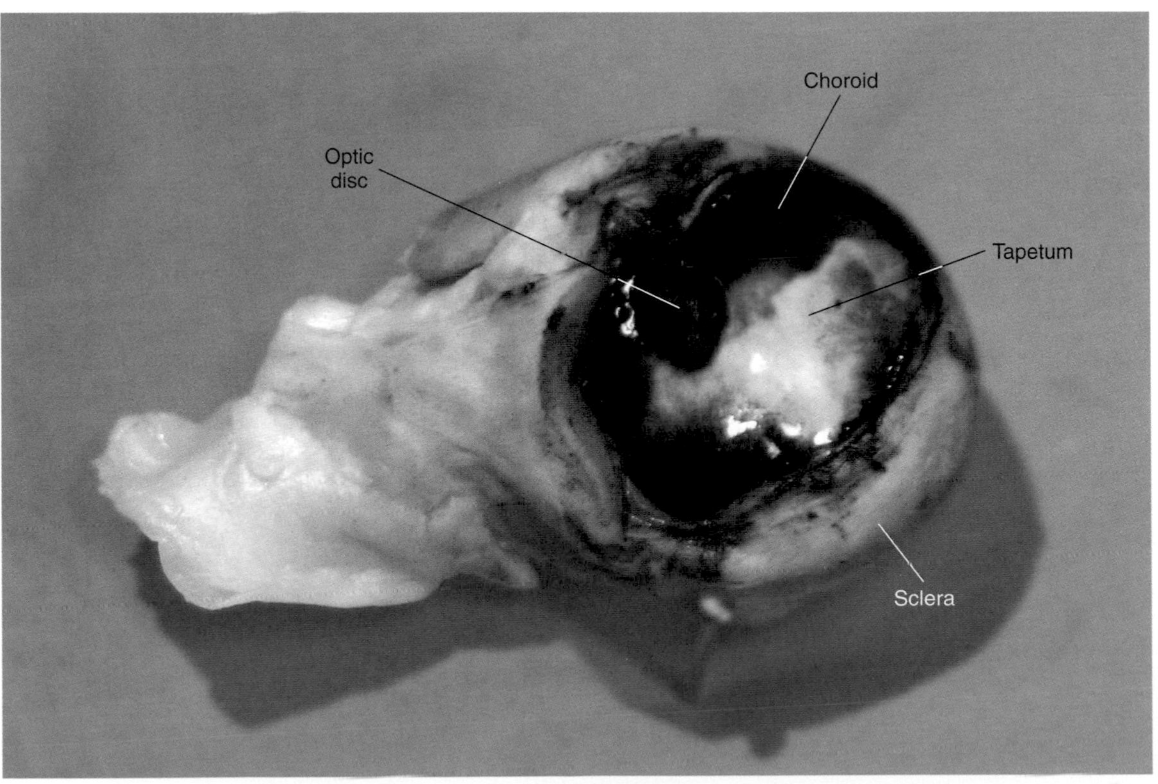

• **Fig. 9.13** The choroid layer containing the tapetum and the optic disc. The eye has been cut open and the retina and vitreous humor removed.

- When you see an animal's eyes at night reflect back a green color, you are seeing the light reflecting off the tapetum (Fig. 9.14). (The "deer in the headlights" look.)
- Humans and pigs do not have a tapetum.

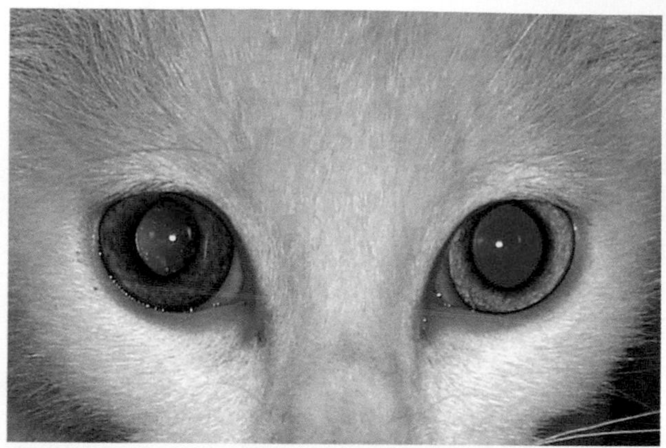

• **Fig. 9.14** Tapetum and irises. This cat has one pigmented and one non-pigmented iris.
Right eye:
- Gold colored iris
- Green colored tapetum reflecting light

Left eye:
- Pale blue colored iris
- Red color caused by light reflecting off blood vessels in the choroid layer in the back of the eye because there is no tapetum. Because humans do not have tapeta, we are frequently cursed with red eyes on flash photographs, particularly in dim light when the pupils are large

FUN FACTS

An animal with a blue-colored iris generally does not have a tapetum. The eye will reflect red (from choroidal blood vessels) like a human eye.

The Inner Nervous Layer (Retina)

- The **retina** is the working layer of the eye. It is like the film in a camera.
- It converts light rays that have been focused on it into nerve impulses that travel to the brain and are interpreted as visual images.
- The microscopic **photoreceptors,** rods and cones, are found in the retina.
- **Rods** are sensitive to dim light but cannot sense details or colors. They give the animal dim light vision in shades of gray.
- **Cones** are sensitive to color and detail, but don't work well in dim light.
- Both rods and cones send messages to the brain via the optic nerve.
- The retina lies against the choroid, lining the back of the eye (Fig. 9.15).

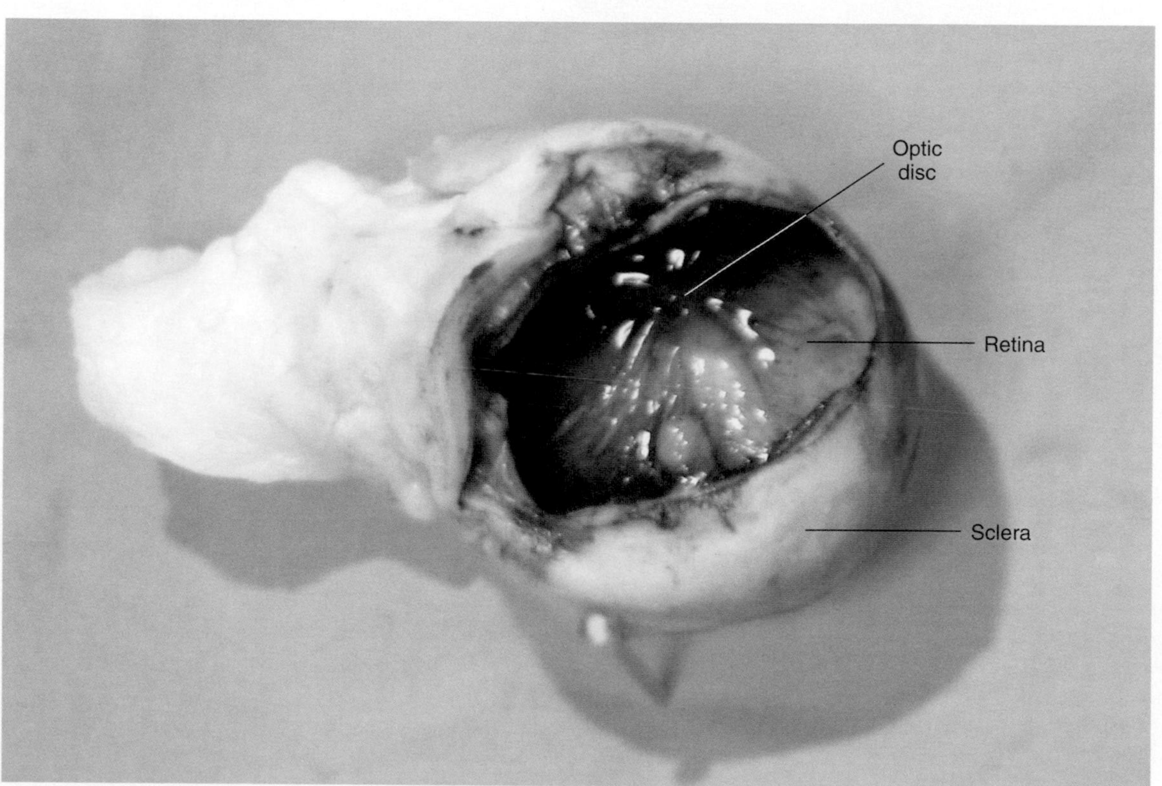

• **Fig. 9.15** Retina of a preserved sheep eye. The cornea, iris, and lens have been removed for visualization of the retina. The retina looks like a wet piece of ivory-colored tissue paper stuck flat to the back of the eye.

FUN FACTS

We often see beautiful, colored photographs of galaxies, nebulae, and star clusters taken through powerful telescopes. They are produced by taking very long exposures because their light is so dim. If we look at them directly through a telescope, they just look gray and white. Their light is too dim to activate the cones in our retinas. The colors are there, but our eyes are not sensitive enough to see them.

Optic Disc

- Nerve fibers from the retina converge to form the optic nerve at the **optic disc** (Figs. 9.16 and 9.17). There are no rods or cones in the optic disc, so this is a blind spot in the eye where no images are formed.
- When viewed in a live animal with an ophthalmoscope, the optic disc looks like a large white circle in the back of the eye. Large retinal blood vessels converge at this spot.
- The optic nerve leaves the eye just caudal to the optic disc.

Optic Nerve

The **optic nerve** (Fig. 9.18) carries the visual impulses from the eye to the optic chiasm (Fig. 9.19).

Optic Chiasm

- The optic chiasm is where half the nerve fibers carrying visual impulses from the right eye cross to go to the left side of the brain and vice versa (see Fig. 9.19).
- This ensures that visual impulses from each eye reach both sides of the brain.
- Only half the nerve fibers cross over, the other half stay on the same side as the eye of origin.

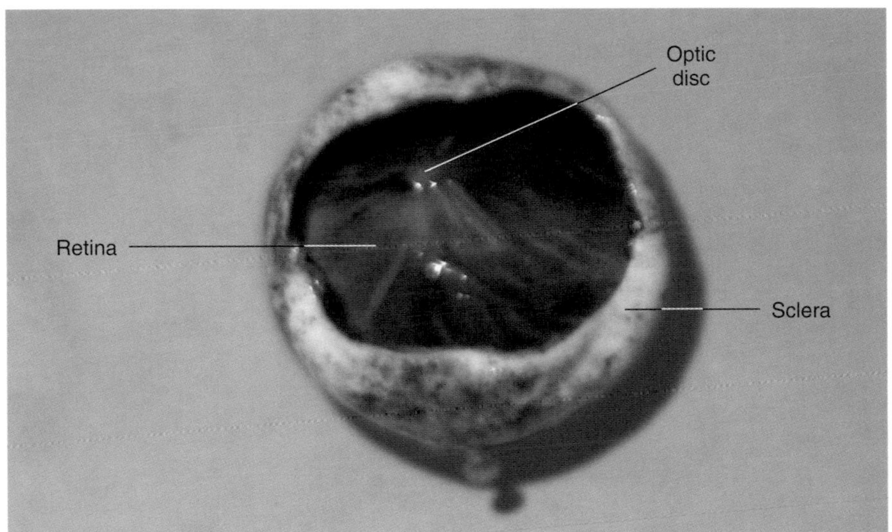

• **Fig. 9.16** Optic disc of a preserved sheep eye. If observed closely, the retina seems to bunch up in one spot. This area looks like where a button is attached to the upholstery of a sofa. The material bunches up at the attachment point. The retina bunches up slightly in a similar manner at the optic disc.

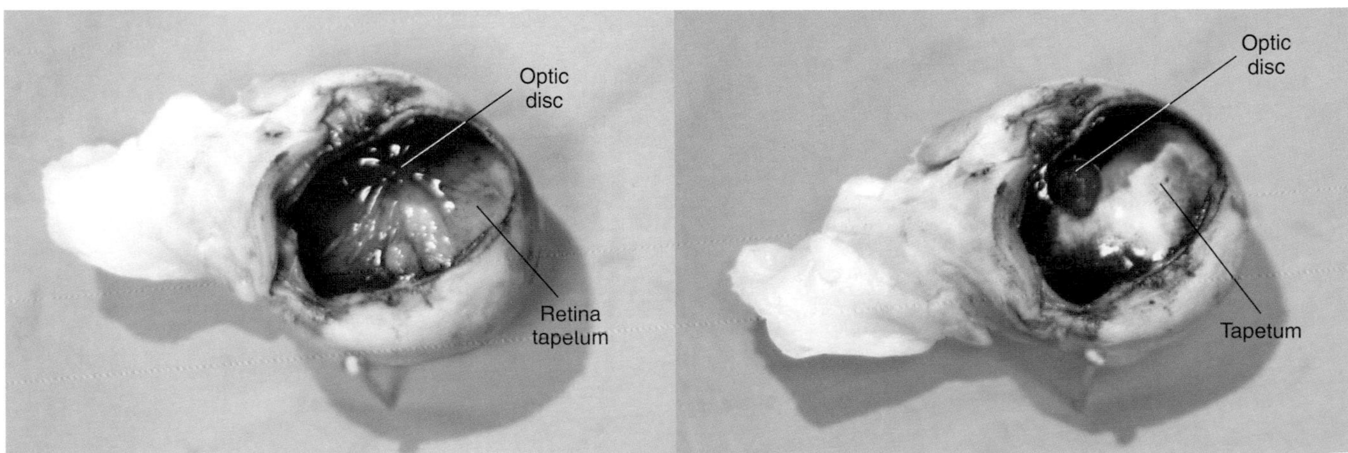

• **Fig. 9.17** Retina and tapetum of the sheep eye. In the first image, the retina is intact and lying on the choroid. In the second image, the retina has been pulled away from the choroid to expose the underlying tapetum.

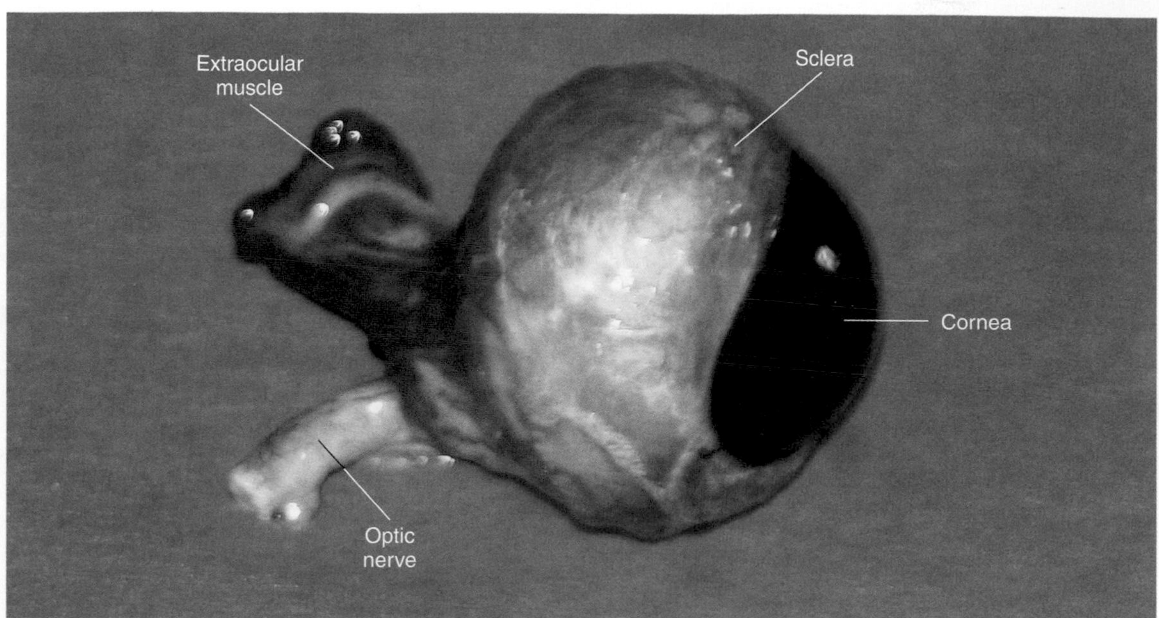

• **Fig. 9.18** Optic nerve of a calf eye.

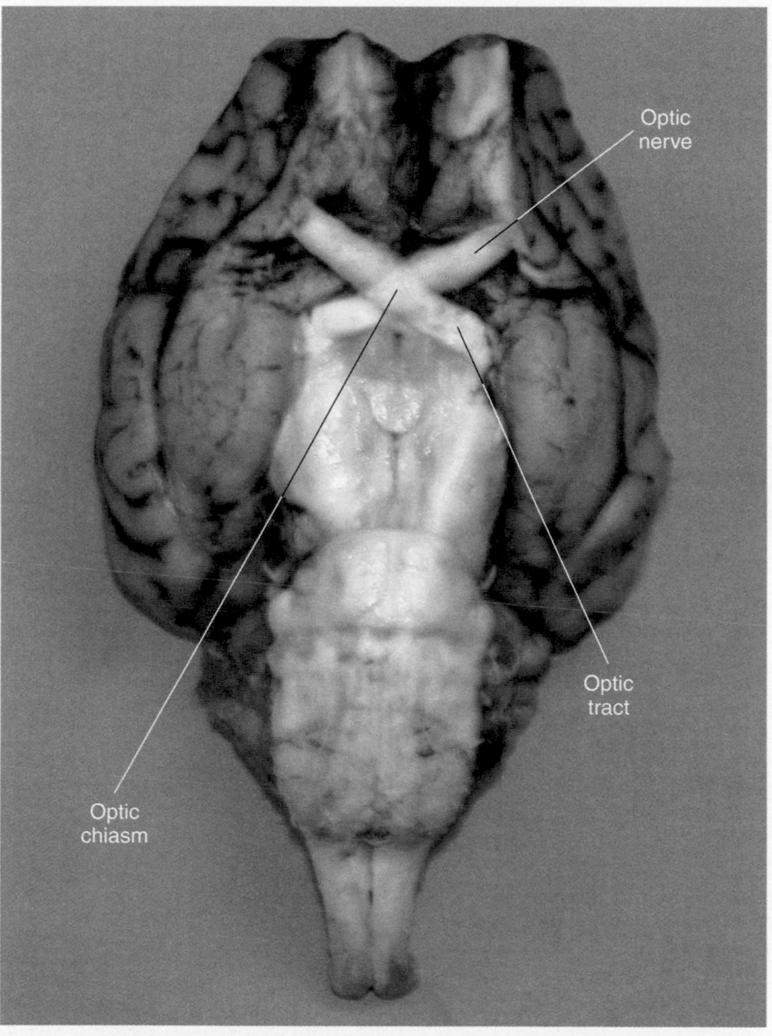

• **Fig. 9.19** Optic chiasm on the ventral surface of a sheep brain.

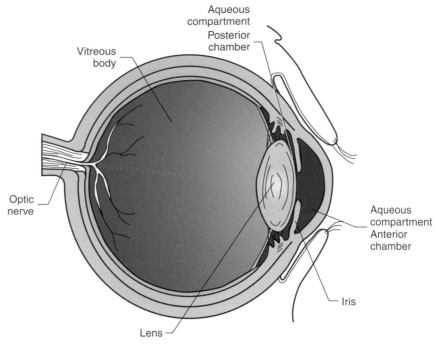

• **Fig. 9.20** Major compartments of the eye.

- This means that if an animal suffered a right-sided brain injury that affected the vision pathways, it would lose only half the vision from its right eye and half from its left eye. It would still have partial vision in both eyes.

Compartments of the Eye

The eye has two major fluid-filled compartments (Figs. 9.20 and 9.21).

- The **aqueous compartment,** located rostral to (in front of) the lens, is filled with watery **aqueous humor.** This compartment is divided into two chambers:
  - The **anterior chamber** is between the iris and the cornea.
  - The **posterior chamber** is between the iris and the lens.
- The **vitreous compartment,** located caudal to (behind) the lens, is filled with gelatinous **vitreous humor** (the vitreous body).

Eyelids and Conjunctiva

- The medial junction of the **eyelids** is called the **medial canthus,** and the lateral junction is the **lateral canthus**.
- The conjunctiva is a thin, transparent membrane that lines the eyelids and covers the "front" part of the eyeball (Figs. 9.22 and 9.23).
- The conjunctiva is a mucous membrane.
- The eyelids are lined with palpebral conjunctiva. ("Palpebral" refers to eyelid.)
- The **bulbar conjunctiva** covers the "front" part of the eyeball.
- The **conjunctival sac** is the space between the palpebral and bulbar layers of conjunctiva.

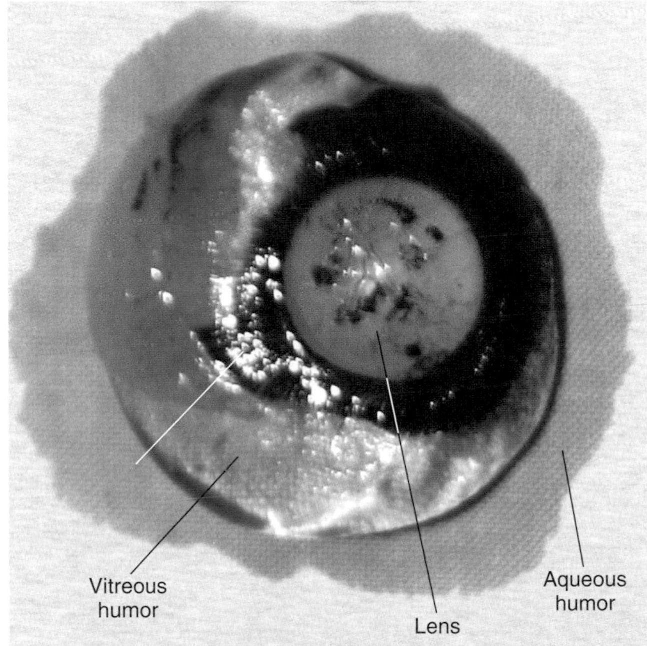

• **Fig. 9.21** Vitreous humor and aqueous humor of a preserved sheep eye. The vitreous humor that fills the vitreous compartment is a gelatinous mass. The liquid aqueous humor from the aqueous chamber has soaked into the background fabric and is seen as a wet area around the vitreous humor. If you want to view aqueous humor, you have to aspirate it from the anterior chamber before the integrity of the eyeball is broken.

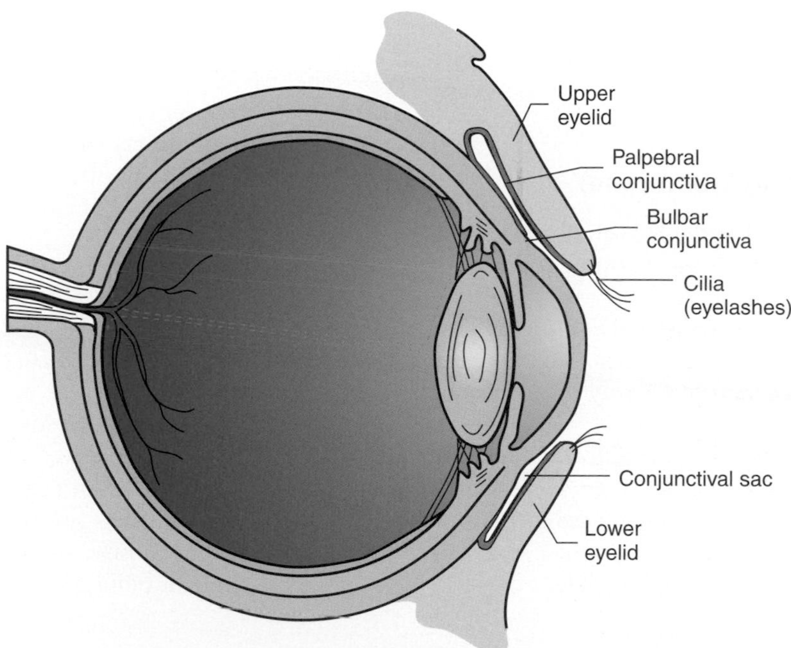

• **Fig. 9.22** The eyelids and the conjunctiva.

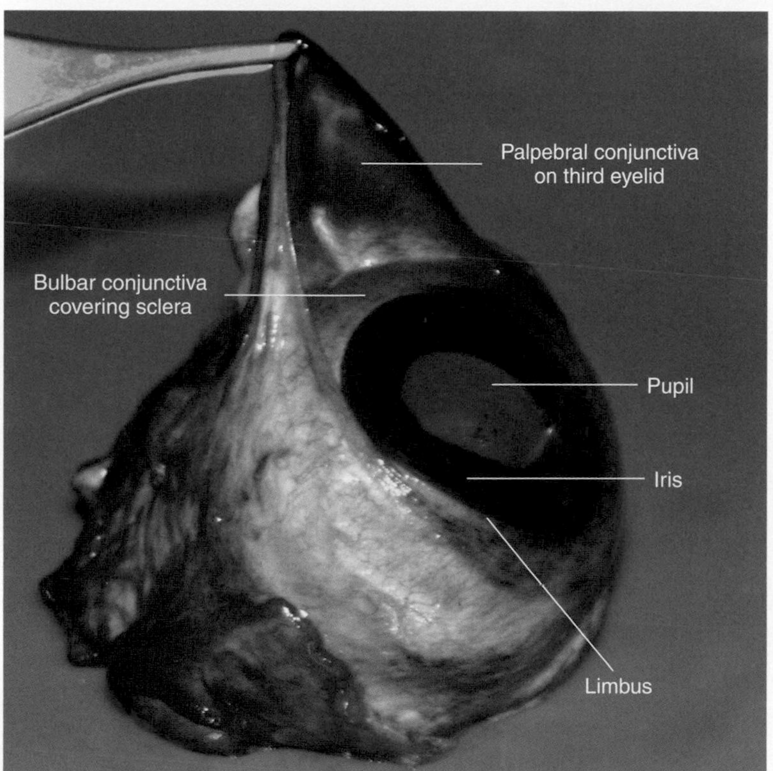

• **Fig. 9.23** Palpebral and bulbar conjunctiva of a calf eye. The palpebral and bulbar conjunctiva are one continuous membrane that folds on itself at the fold of the eyelid.

- Tiny **tarsal glands** (also known as the meibomian glands) along each eyelid margin secrete a waxy substance that helps keep tears from overflowing.

Third Eyelid (Nictitating Membrane)

- The **third eyelid** is located at the medial canthus of the eye behind the two eyelids (see Fig. 9.24).
- It contains a T-shaped plate of cartilage.
- It is covered on both sides by **palpebral conjunctiva**.
- The third eyelid is not always seen when looking at the eyes, but under certain conditions it may cover most of the visible eye.
- Its movement is passive and not controlled by muscular action. It will frequently be visible when an animal is anesthetized or if there is an irritation on the cornea.
- On its inner surface (the surface next to the eyeball), it has tear-producing glands and lymph nodules.

External Eye-Related Landmarks

- The medial canthus and lateral canthus are where the upper and lower eyelids meet (Figs. 9.24–9.27).
- The **lacrimal puncta** are openings into the **nasolacrimal system.** This system of tubes carries **tears** into the nasal passages where they can be eliminated by swallowing. (Most animals don't know how to blow their noses.)

Extraocular Muscles

- The **extraocular muscles** attach to the sclera of the eye inside the bony orbit.
- They hold the eyeball steady and produce delicate and accurate eye movements.
- Most animals have seven extraocular muscles:
  - Four rectus muscles—medial, lateral, dorsal, and ventral
  - Two oblique muscles—dorsal and ventral
  - One retractor bulbi muscle

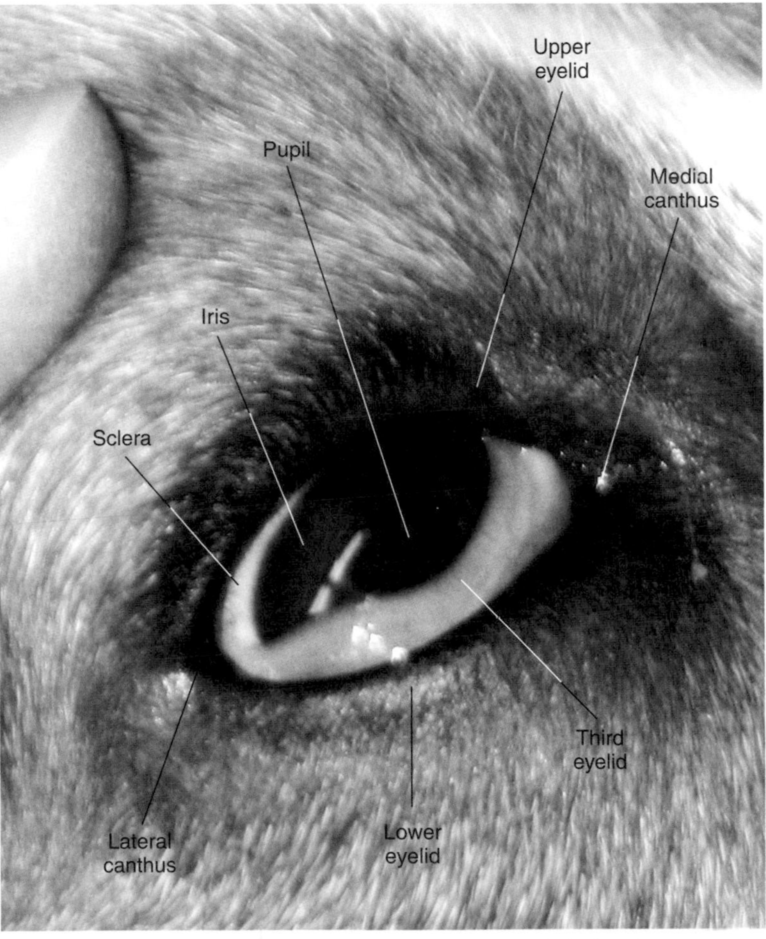

• **Fig. 9.24** The third eyelid (nictitating membrane) of a Beagle.

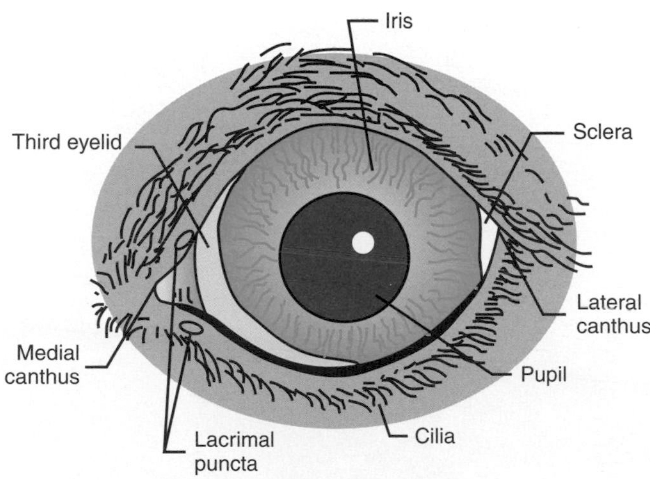

• **Fig. 9.25** External view of a dog's left eye.

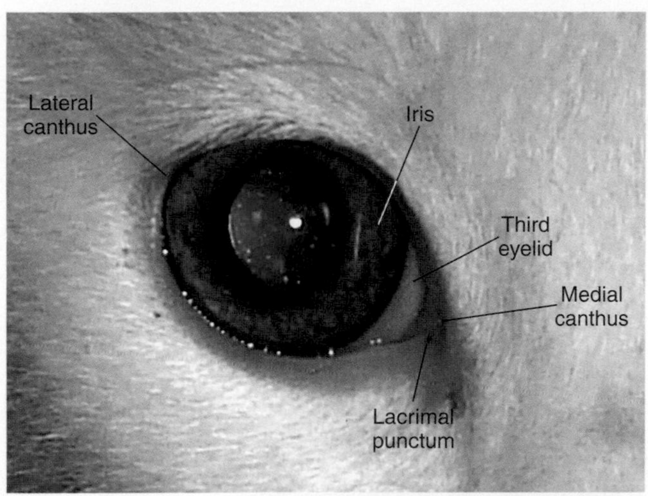

• **Fig. 9.26** Ventral lacrimal punctum of a cat.

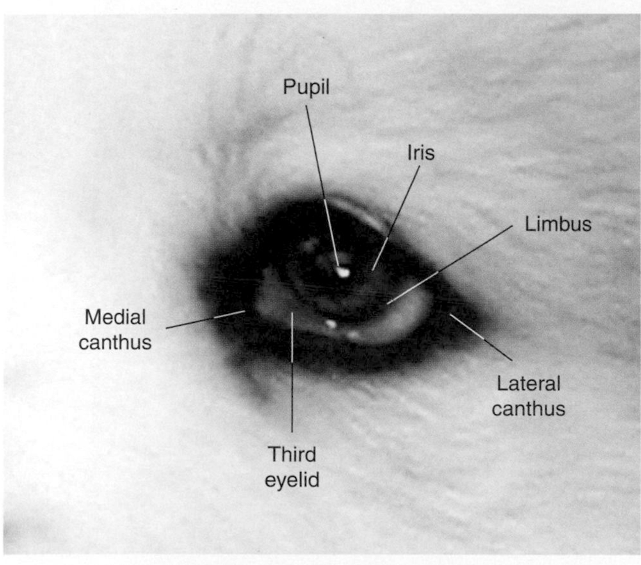

• **Fig. 9.27** External view of dog's left eye.

Suggested In-Class Activities

Dissection of a Sheep's Eye

Materials Needed

Sheep eye, scalpel handle with blade, and rat-tooth or thumb forceps.

This is an easy way to dissect your sheep eye without compromising all the structures.

1. Find these structures on the outside of your sheep eye before you make any cuts:
   Cornea
   Extraocular muscles
   Optic nerve
   Limbus
   Sclera
2. Make a circular incision in the cornea $\frac{1}{8}$ inch *inside* the line of the limbus.* Do not completely cut off the cornea. Stop with your incision when you are $\frac{1}{4}$ inch away from where you began. You will now have a "hinge" that will keep the cornea attached to the rest of the eye. (It will have a "toilet lid" type of look to it. You can open the "lid," the cornea, and look inside at the iris and pupil; Fig. 9.28).

   **Be careful when you first cut through the cornea; the aqueous humor may squirt out.*
3. Make another circular incision, this time in the sclera $\frac{1}{4}$ inch *outside* the limbus. Again, stop with your incision when you are $\frac{1}{4}$ inch away from where you began. You will now have another "hinge" that will keep the cornea and limbus attached to the rest of the eye. (Now you have a "toilet lid and seat" type of look to the eye. You can open the "seat" and look inside at the lens and the back of the eye; Fig. 9.29).

   **The lens will be resting in the vitreous humor. Using rat-tooth forceps, gently grasp the lens and remove it from the eye. The lens will come out with the entire blob of vitreous humor.*

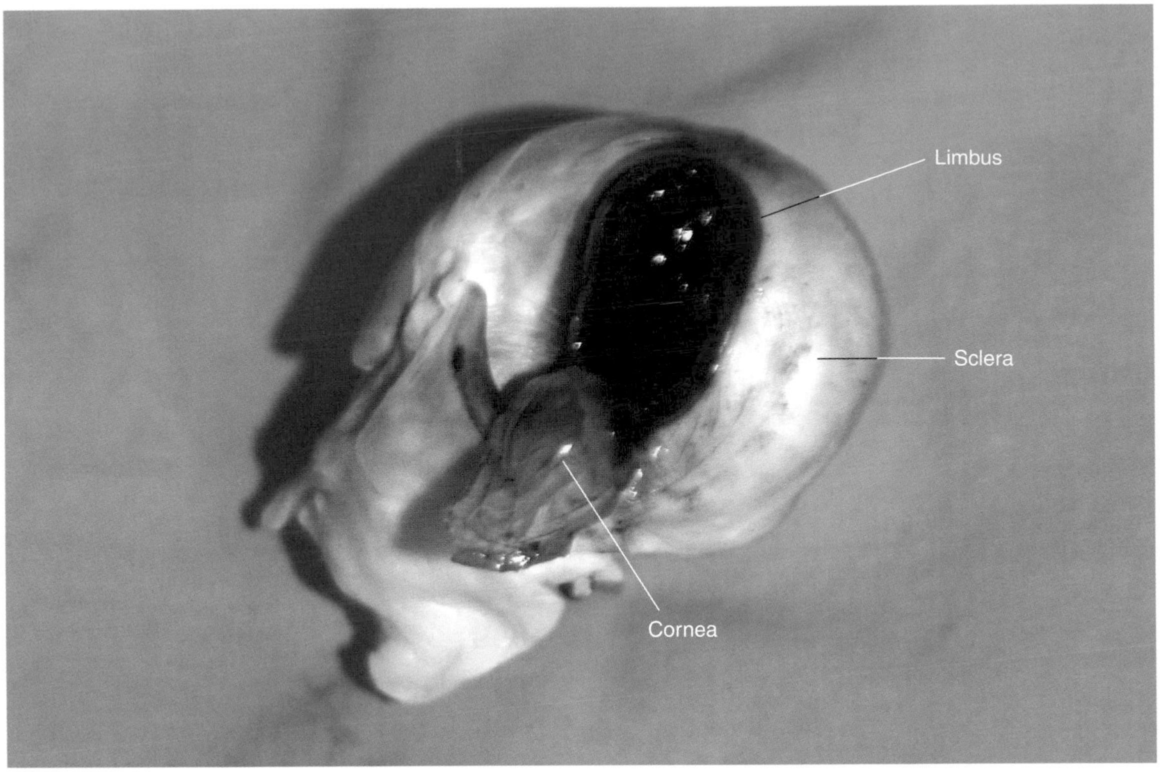

• **Fig. 9.28** The first incision to fold back the cornea.

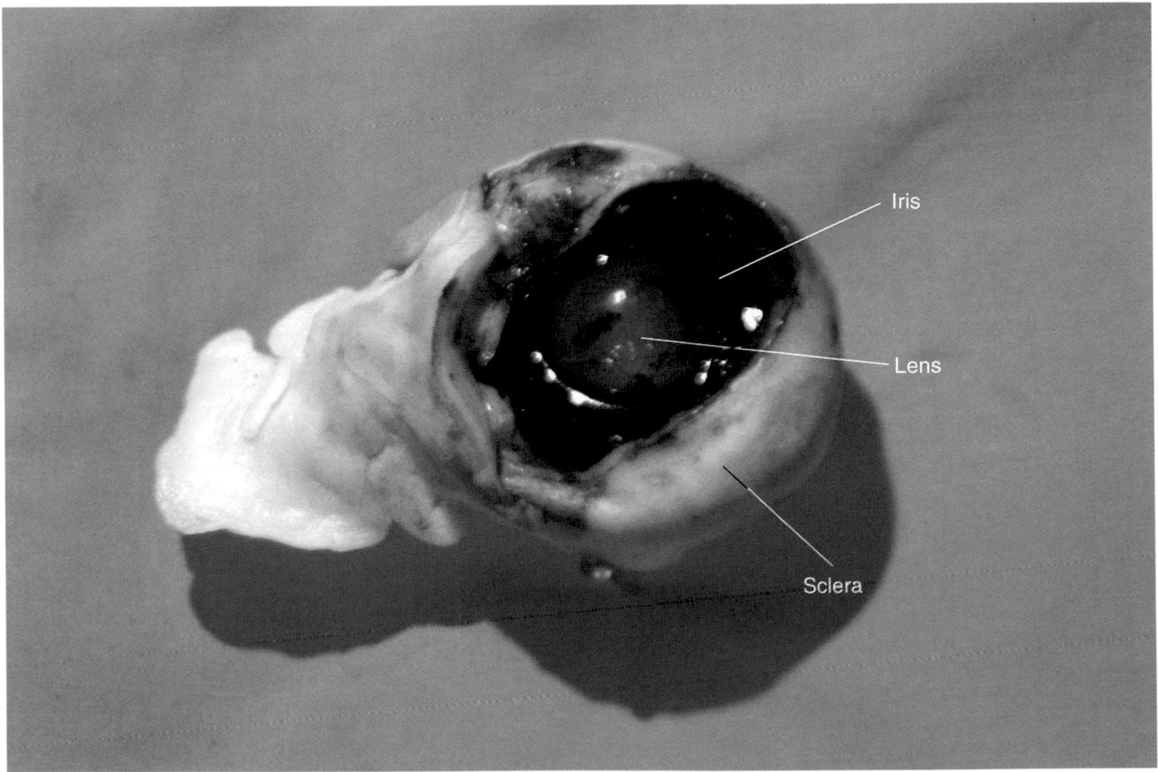

• **Fig. 9.29** The second incision to view the lens and back of the eye.

**With the lens and vitreous humor removed, you will be able to see the retina and tapetum clearly.*

Identify the following structures:

Iris
Pupil
Ciliary body
Suspensory ligaments
Choroid
Tapetum
Retina
Optic disc
Lens
Vitreous humor
Aqueous humor

4. When you have finished identifying all the structures, place the lens and vitreous humor back in the eye and close the flaps. Now the eye will stay moist, so you can come back and study the structures at a later time.

Gaze into Another's Eyes

Materials Needed

Ophthalmoscope, a human partner/restrainer, and a live animal.

In this activity, you will be identifying structures and looking into both human and animal eyes. We will begin with the human eye because you can usually tell a human not to move and he/she won't. Have your partner look straight ahead while you observe their eyes from the side. You will notice how the cornea bulges away from the sclera. This is much easier to notice in a human because you can see more of the sclera.

Next, go to a darkened room, shine the ophthalmoscope into your partner's eye, and watch how the pupil reacts. The pupil will enlarge in the dark and constrict when light shines on it.

The third, and most exciting part of this exercise is looking into the back of your partner's eye. Using the ophthalmoscope, get very close to your partner and gaze through the scope into the back of the eye. What you will see is red blood vessels running along the choroid. Follow a vessel to the optic disc. The optic disc is a large white spot. If "Oh wow!" or some similar expression does not escape from your lips, you are not seeing what you should be seeing.

Now for the challenge... Do the same three examinations on a live animal. The hard part is getting it to hold still while you are that close to its face, but it is worth it when you see the tapetum and the optic disc.

Clinical Significance

By understanding the structures of the eye and being able to examine the eye, you will be able to notice abnormalities that need to be brought to the veterinarian's attention.

Take a Trip Into the Depths of the Ear Canal

Materials Needed

Live dogs and an otoscope

We will do this one with dogs because most people don't appreciate folks touring their ear canals.

Gently grasp the ear and pull up and out on the base of the pinna. This will straighten the external auditory canal so you will be able to see the tympanic membrane. Choose the correct cone size for the otoscope. As you travel down the external canal, always watch where you are going with the cone tip. Do not just cram the otoscope into the ear and then look to see where it landed. Use the otoscope as "headlights" to guide your way down the canal to the tympanic membrane (eardrum). The eardrum looks like a thin, transparent, cream-colored piece of cellophane stretched across the canal. Do not touch the eardrum with the otoscope. It is very sensitive. If you look really closely through the tympanic membrane, you will be able to see the malleus on the other side.

Clinical Significance

Veterinary technicians must be familiar with the anatomy of the external ear down to the eardrum. Not only do they perform ear swabs looking for parasites and yeast, but they must be able to clean and treat ears without causing damage or harm.

Witness the Amazing Nasolacrimal Ducts

Materials Needed

Live cats, proparacaine ophthalmic solution, and ophthalmic fluorescein stain. Cats with pink noses work best for this exercise.

Place two drops of proparacaine ophthalmic solution on the surface of the cat's eye. Wait 2 to 3 minutes for the numbing to take effect. Place a drop or two of proparacaine solution on a sterile fluorescein strip, then gently touch the strip and the liquid on it to the cornea of the eye. Observe the nostrils. Around one nostril, an orange color will start to show as the proparacaine and dye travel down the nasolacrimal duct.

Clinical Significance

It is important to understand how the nasolacrimal ducts function so anything abnormal, such as a plugged duct, can be brought to the veterinarian's attention.

EXERCISES

Pain

Exercise 1

Identify Processes in Pain Perception

Identify each step in pain perception by filling in the chart with the missing information.

Name of Pain Process	Process (Action)
Transduction	______________________
______________	Transmits the nerve impulse up the sensory nerve fibers to the spinal cord.
______________	Amplification or suppression of the nerve impulse in the spinal cord.
Perception	______________________

Hearing

Exercise 2

Identify the Structures Indicated in the Canine Ear

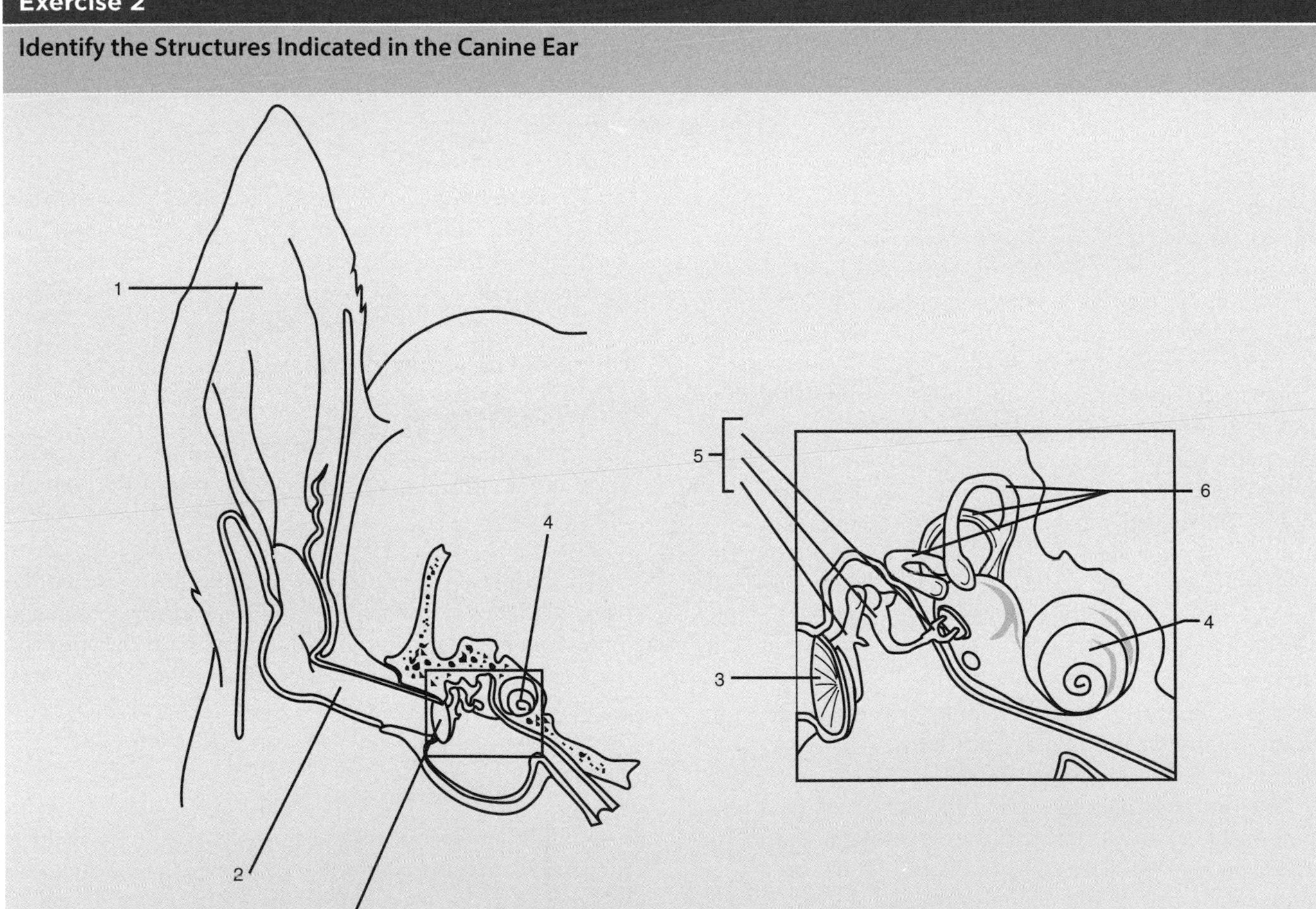

1. ______________________
2. ______________________
3. ______________________
4. ______________________
5. ______________________
6. ______________________

Exercise 3

Hearing Review

1. In what structure are the sensory receptors for hearing located? ______
2. What is the external flap of the ear called? ______
3. The ______ connects the middle ear with the pharynx.
4. What is the tiny membrane of connective tissue at the end of the external ear canal that vibrates in response to sound waves?
______
______
5. In what area of the ear are ear mites most commonly found? ______

Vision

Exercise 4

Identify Structures on the Calf Eye

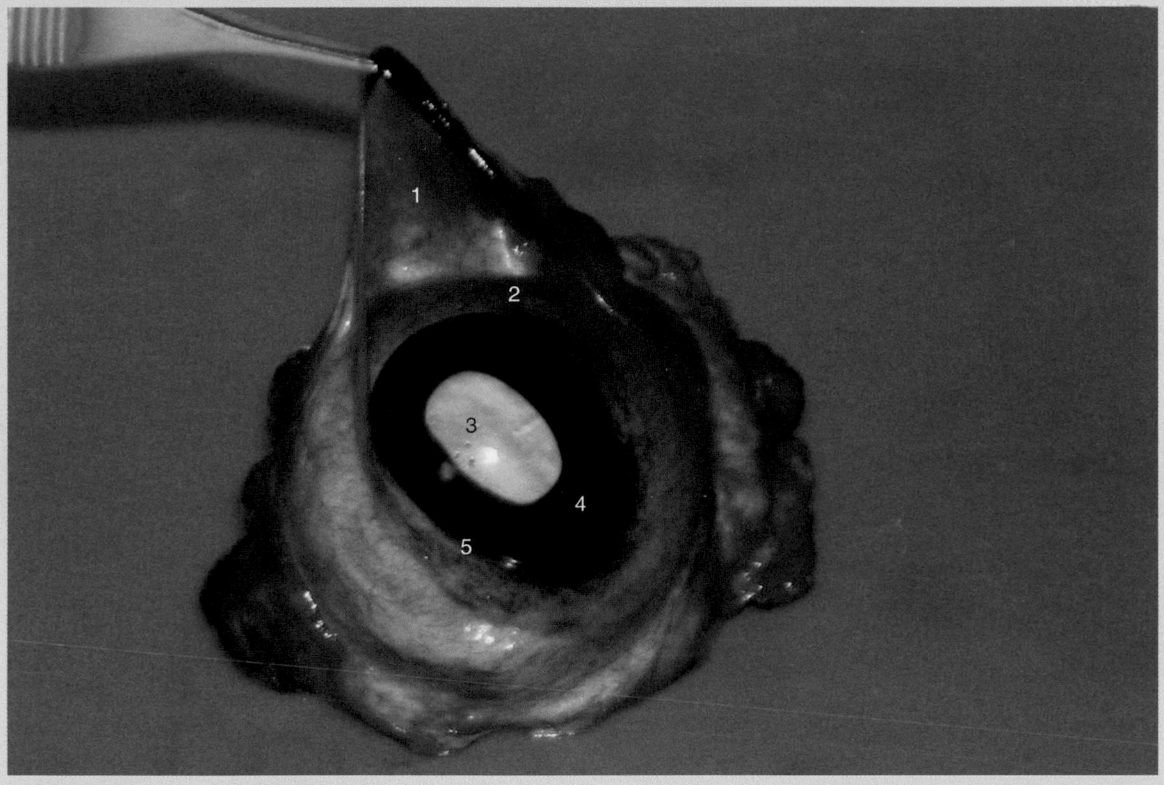

1. ______
2. ______
3. ______
4. ______
5. ______

Exercise 5

Identify Structures of the Eye

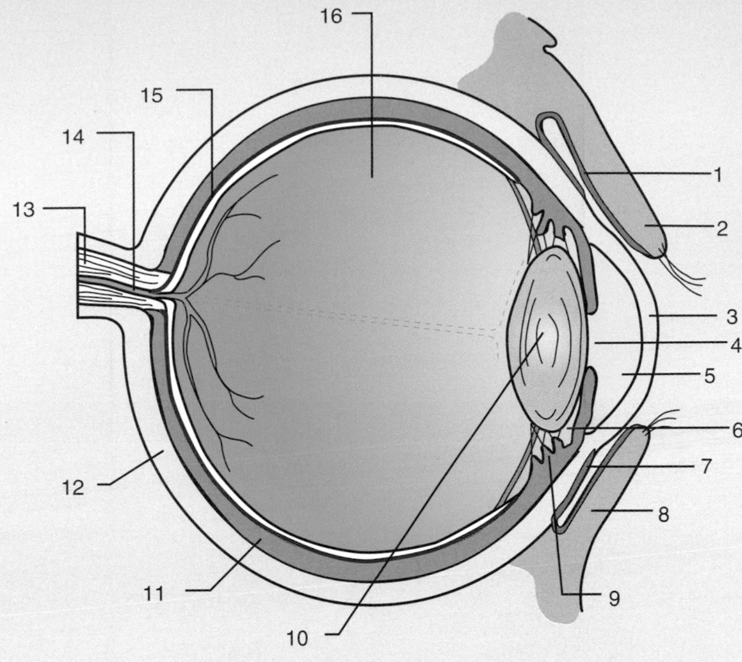

1. ______________________
2. ______________________
3. ______________________
4. ______________________
5. ______________________
6. ______________________
7. ______________________
8. ______________________
9. ______________________
10. ______________________
11. ______________________
12. ______________________
13. ______________________
14. ______________________
15. ______________________
16. ______________________

Exercise 6

Identify Structures on the Cat Eye

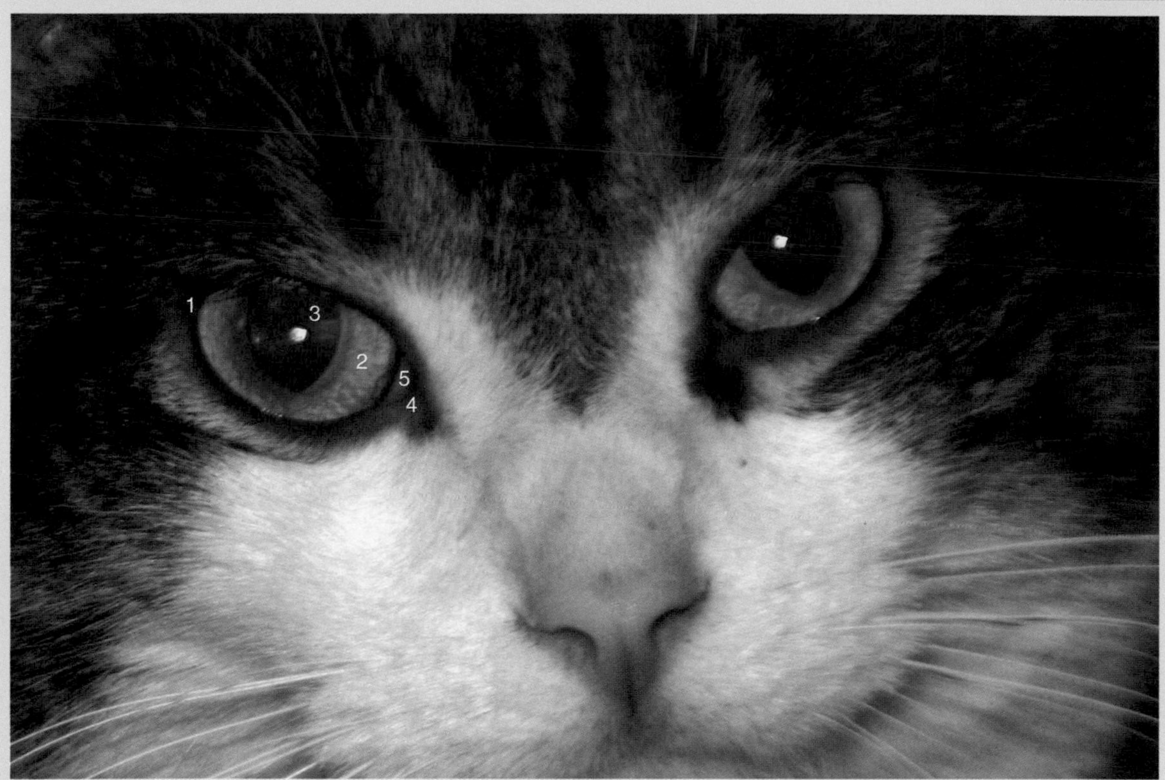

1. ______________________
2. ______________________
3. ______________________
4. ______________________
5. ______________________

Exercise 7

Identify Structures on the Sheep Eye

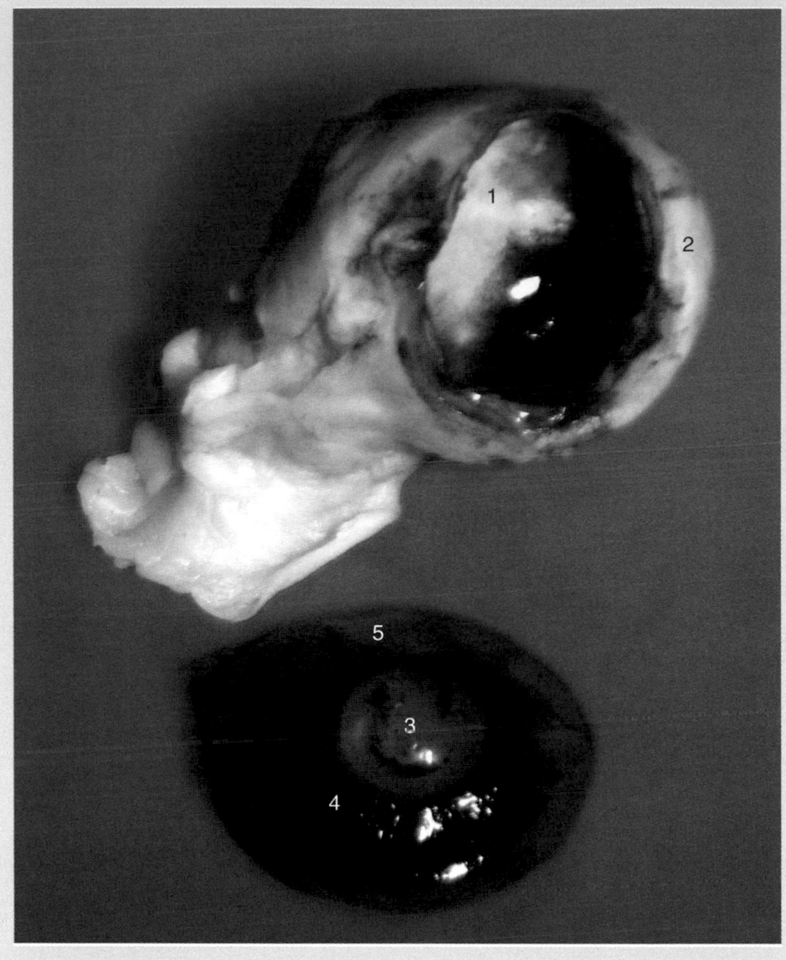

1. ______________________
2. ______________________
3. ______________________
4. ______________________
5. ______________________

Exercise 8

Identify Structures Removed from the Calf Eye

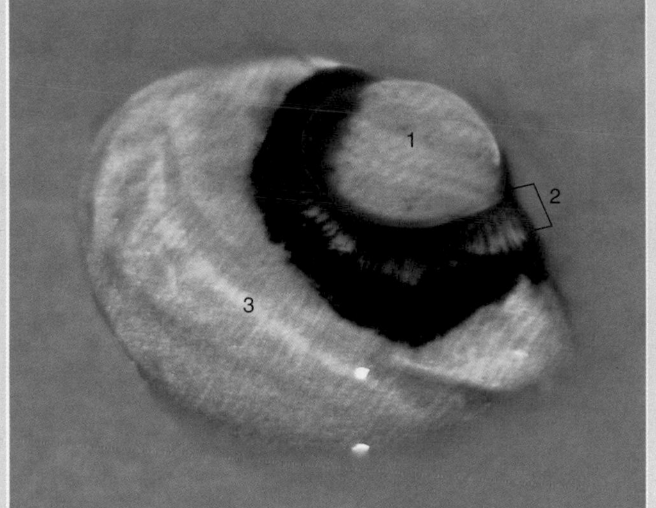

1. ______
2. ______
3. ______

Exercise 9

Identify Structures on the Rostral Half of a Transected Eyeball

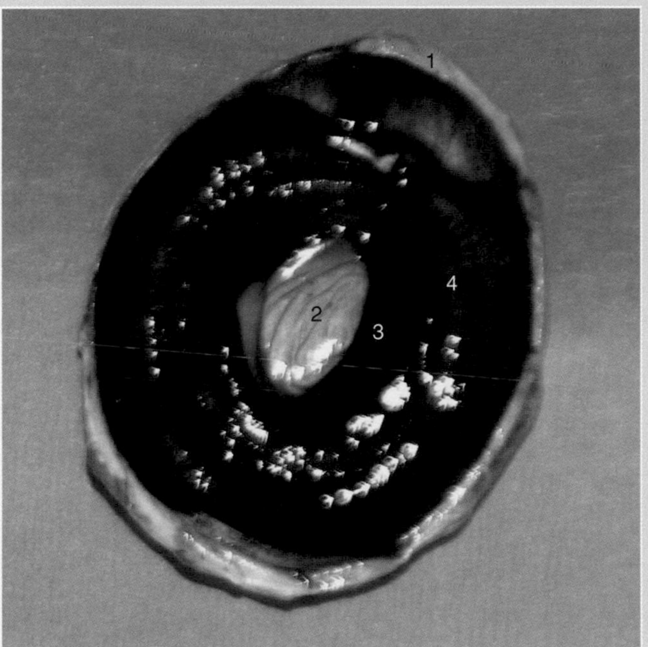

1. ______
2. ______
3. ______
4. ______

Critical and Clinical Thinking

Exercise 10

Matching Terms and Definitions

_____________ Space behind the iris but in front of the lens.

_____________ Clear watery fluid that fills the anterior and posterior chambers.

_____________ Area behind the ciliary body and lens.

_____________ Space in front of the iris.

_____________ Clear soft gelatin-like fluid that fills part of the eyeball behind the lens and ciliary body.

_____________ Area in front of the ciliary body and lens.

a. Aqueous compartment
b. Anterior chamber
c. Posterior chamber
d. Vitreous compartment
e. Vitreous humor
f. Aqueous humor

Exercise 11

Identify Key Terms—Vision

1. What causes the green reflection from the eyes of an animal in photographs or at night? _____________
2. Do domestic animals have more rods or cones in their retinas? _____________
3. Are rods used for detail and color or dim light vision? _____________
4. The _____________ is the "colored part" of the eye that is visible externally.
5. What is the name for the junction between the cornea and the sclera of the eye? _____________
6. The _____________ is the tiny hole in the medial canthus of the eyelid that allows tears to drain away from the eyes.
7. What is the "blind spot" of the eye? _____________
8. The _____________ is the muscular ring of tissue that surrounds the lens and adjusts its shape.
9. What adjustable eye structure helps focus a clear image on the retina? _____________
10. What is the clear "window" that admits light to the interior of the eye? _____________
11. What structure of the eye contains the rods and cones? _____________
12. What is the third eyelid covered with? _____________

Exercise 12

Identify General and Special Senses

Identify the missing information from the chart indicating the sense, sensation, and type of stimulus.

Sense	What Is Sensed	Type of Stimulus
General Senses		
Visceral sensations	_____________	Chemical, mechanical
Touch	Touch and pressure	_____________
Temperature	Heat and cold	Thermal
_____________	Intense stimuli of any type Thermal	Mechanical, chemical, or thermal
_____________	Body position and movement	Mechanical
Special Senses		
Taste	Tastes	_____________
Smell	Odors	_____________
Hearing	Sounds	_____________
Equilibrium	_____________	_____________
Vision	Light	_____________

Exercise 13

Define Clinical Terms

Write the definition for each term

1. Anterior chamber
2. Aqueous compartment
3. Aqueous humor
4. Bulbar conjunctiva
5. Canthus
6. Choroid
7. Ciliary body
8. Cochlea
9. Cones
10. Conjunctival sac
11. Cornea
12. Eustachian tube
13. External auditory canal
14. External ear
15. Extraocular muscles
16. Flehman response
17. Gustatory sense
18. Incus
19. Internal ear
20. Iris
21. Lacrimal glands
22. Lacrimal puncta
23. Lateral canthus

Continued

Exercise 13—cont'd

Define Clinical Terms

24. Lens ______________________________

25. Limbus ______________________________

26. Malleus ______________________________

27. Medial canthus ______________________________

28. Middle ear ______________________________

29. Modulation (pain pathway) ______________________________

30. Nasolacrimal duct ______________________________

31. Nociception ______________________________

32. Olfactory sense ______________________________

33. Optic chiasm ______________________________

34. Optic disc ______________________________

35. Optic nerve ______________________________

36. Ossicles ______________________________

37. Otoliths ______________________________

38. Palpebral conjunctiva ______________________________

39. Perception (pain pathway) ______________________________

40. Pheromones ______________________________

41. Photoreceptors ______________________________

42. Pinna ______________________________

43. Posterior chamber ______________________________

44. Pupil ______________________________

45. Retina ______________________________

Exercise 13—cont'd

Define Clinical Terms

46. Rods ______________________________

47. Sclera ______________________________

48. Semicircular canals ______________________________

49. Stapes ______________________________

50. Tapetum (tapetum lucidum) ______________________________

51. Tarsal glands (meibomian glands) ______________________________

52. Taste buds ______________________________

53. Third eyelid (nictitating membrane) ______________________________

54. Transduction (pain pathway) ______________________________

55. Transmission (pain pathway) ______________________________

56. Tympanic membrane ______________________________

57. Uvea ______________________________

58. Vermonasal organ ______________________________

59. Vestibule ______________________________

60. Vitreous compartment ______________________________

61. Vitreous humor ______________________________

Exercise 14

Identify Clinical Structures

1. ______________ The opening in the center of the iris.
2. ______________ The soft, gelatinous substance that fills the vitreous compartment of the eye.
3. ______________ The transparent membrane that lines the inner portion of the eyelid.
4. ______________ The lateral corner of the eye where the upper and lower eyelids come together.
5. ______________ The inner nervous layer of the eye where the photoreceptors are located.
6. ______________ The snail shell-shaped cavity in the temporal bone of the skull that contains the hearing portion of the inner ear.
7. ______________ Another name for the middle vascular layer of the eye.
8. ______________ A portion of the middle vascular layer of the eye. It consists mainly of pigment and blood vessels and is located between the sclera and the retina.
9. ______________ The clear "window" on the front of the eye that admits light to the interior of the eye. It is part of the outer fibrous layer of the eyeball.
10. ______________ Photoreceptors in the retina of the eye that perceive color and detail.
11. ______________ The highly reflective area of the choroid in the back of the eye of most domestic animals.
12. ______________ The ossicle in the middle ear that is shaped like a stirrup.
13. ______________ The process of experiencing pain.
14. ______________ Photoreceptors in the retina of the eye that perceive dim light images in shades of gray.
15. ______________ The openings into the nasolacrimal drainage system that help carry tears away from the surface of each eye. They are located near the medial canthus on both the upper and lower eyelid margins.
16. ______________ The paper-thin connective tissue membrane that is tightly stretched across the opening of the external ear canal into the middle ear.
17. ______________ The compartment of the eye rostral to (in front of) the lens.
18. ______________ The pigmented, muscular diaphragm that controls the amount of light that enters the caudal (posterior) part of the eyeball.
19. ______________ The tube that connects the middle ear cavity with the pharynx.
20. ______________ The white portion of the eye that is part of the outer fibrous layer of the eyeball.

10 The Endocrine System[a]

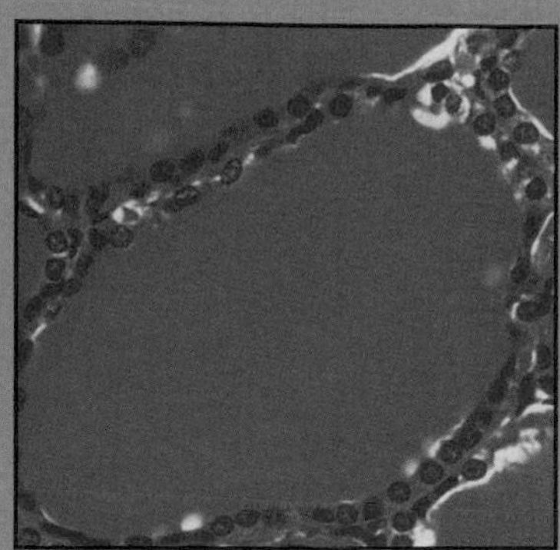

OVERVIEW AT A GLANCE

Control of Hormone Secretion 262

Hypothalamus and Pituitary Gland 262

Thyroid Gland 265

Parathyroid Gland 268

Adrenal Gland 270

Endocrine Pancreas 270

The Gonads 273

Other Endocrine Tissues 273

Exercises 273–284

Control of Hormone Secretion 273–274

1. *Explore the Exocrine and Endocrine Glands 273*
2. *Compare the Endocrine and Nervous Systems 274*

Hypothalamus and Pituitary Gland 274–275

3. *Identify and Color the Hypothalamus and Pituitary Gland Components 274*
4. *Identify the Target Organs of Eight Pituitary Hormones 274*
5. *Describe the Relationship Between the Hypothalamus and Anterior and Posterior Pituitary Glands 275*
6. *Critical Thinking: Match the Hormone With the Action 275*
7. *Clinical Thinking: Explore the Use of Oxytocin 275*

Thyroid Gland 275–277

8. *Critical Thinking: Label the Cells 275*
9. *Critical Thinking: Label the Negative Feedback Diagram 276*
10. *Clinical Thinking: Identify Thyroid Anatomy 276*
11. *Clinical Thinking: Identify Clinical Symptoms #1 276*
12. *Clinical Thinking: Identify Clinical Symptoms #2 276*
13. *Clinical Thinking: Case Study—Hyperthyroidism 277*

Parathyroid Gland 278

14. *Identify Parathyroid Anatomy 278*
15. *Critical Thinking: Identify Hormones 278*
16. *Clinical Thinking: Case Study—Follow-up (Hyperthyroidism) 278*
17. *Clinical Thinking: Case Study—Secondary Nutritional Hyperparathyroidism in the Iguana 278*

Adrenal Gland 279–280

18. *Identify the Anatomy and Structure of the Adrenal Gland 279*
19. *Identify and Describe the Effect of Hormones Released by the Adrenal Gland 279*
20. *Clinical Thinking: Identify Glucocorticosteroid Side Effects 280*
21. *Clinical Thinking: Identify Effects of Epinephrine and Norepinephrine During Fight or Flight Response 280*
22. *Clinical Thinking: Case Study—Canine Hyperadrenocorticism 280*

Endocrine Pancreas 281–282

23. *Critical Thinking: Identify Pancreatic Hormones 281*
24. *Clinical Thinking: Identify Hormones Associated With Hyperglycemia 281*
25. *Clinical Thinking: Identify Insulinoma Protocol 281*
26. *Clinical Thinking: Case Study—Feline Diabetes Mellitus 282*

Other Endocrine Tissues, 282–284

27. *Critical Thinking: Identify True and False Statements 282*
28. *Clinical Thinking: Identify and Label the Glands of the Endocrine System 283*
29. *Clinical Thinking: Identify Hormones Released by the Endocrine Glands 283*
30. *Clinical Thinking: Identify Diseases Associated With the Endocrine System 284*

LEARNING OBJECTIVES

After reading this chapter, performing the class activities, and completing the exercise questions, you will be able to:

1. Locate and identify the major endocrine glands of the cat.
2. Describe the relationships between the hypothalamus and the anterior and posterior portions of the pituitary gland.
3. Name the pituitary gland hormones, describe their functions, and identify their target organs.
4. List the hormones produced by the thyroid, parathyroid, adrenal glands, and pancreas and describe their effects on the body.
5. Describe a positive and negative feedback system.
6. List the hormones associated with the pineal gland, thymus, stomach, small intestine, kidney, and placenta.
7. Describe common endocrine diseases of animals.

[a]The authors and publisher wish to acknowledge Kathianne Komurek for previous contributions to this chapter.

CLINICAL SIGNIFICANCE

The endocrine and nervous systems are vital communication networks throughout the body which provide regulation and control of its many functions. These two systems allow all cells, tissues, and organs to communicate with one another and work together to maintain homeostasis. The endocrine system is comprised of many endocrine glands located throughout the body; these glands release their chemical messengers, or hormones, directly into the bloodstream, which carries them to various target cells. Those cells that are meant to respond to the call of a particular hormone possess specific receptors that recognize and bind that chemical messenger (Fig. 10.1). Once bound, that hormone causes the desired change within that cell, which will contribute to returning balance in the body. Hormones help to control many bodily functions, including maintaining fluid balance, directing growth and metabolism, regulating sexual reproduction, and playing a role in the "fight or flight" response.

INTRODUCTION

This chapter primarily addresses material on the endocrine system covered in Chapter 11 of *Clinical Anatomy and Physiology for Veterinary Technicians*; however, additional content from Nervous System (Chapter 9), Reproductive System (Chapter 19), and Pregnancy, Development, and Lactation (Chapter 20) is also covered in this lab manual chapter. Be sure to read Chapter 11, Endocrine System, in the textbook and be prepared to refer to the other chapters as needed before continuing.

MATERIALS NEEDED

- Preserved cat for dissection
- Preserved cat or sheep brain
- Dissection kit
- A lab coat and examination gloves
- Cat dissection guide (and good skills of observation)
- A medical dictionary

TERMS TO BE IDENTIFIED

Hypothalamus
Pituitary gland
Thyroid glands
Parathyroid glands
Adrenal glands
Pancreas

Control of Hormone Secretion

Regulation of hormone production and secretion is accomplished through three main mechanisms:

- Negative feedback systems
- Positive feedback systems
- Direct nervous system stimulation

Negative feedback pathways correct a deviation from normal and ensure that hormone production is inhibited once homeostasis is achieved, thereby preventing excessively high hormone levels. In positive feedback pathways, the desired effect of the hormone stimulates more hormone production, thus encouraging a deviation from normal. Fig. 10.2 illustrates some examples of negative and positive feedback. Nervous system stimulation is a way to provide an immediate response to an urgent stimulation, as happens with the release of catecholamines from the adrenal medulla.

Hypothalamus and Pituitary Gland

In-class Activity

Locate and identify the hypothalamus and pituitary gland in the preserved cat or sheep brain.

Anatomy

The **hypothalamus** is located in the diencephalon area of the brain, below the thalamus, and caudal to the optic chasm. The **pituitary gland** (hypophysis) is attached ventrally to the hypothalamus by a slender stalk of nervous tissue called the infundibulum (Fig. 10.3). The anterior portion of the pituitary gland (adenohypophysis) is glandular and communicates with the hypothalamus through a network of blood vessels called a portal system. The posterior pituitary gland (neurohypophysis) is derived from nervous tissue and is connected to the hypothalamus through a system of nerve fibers.

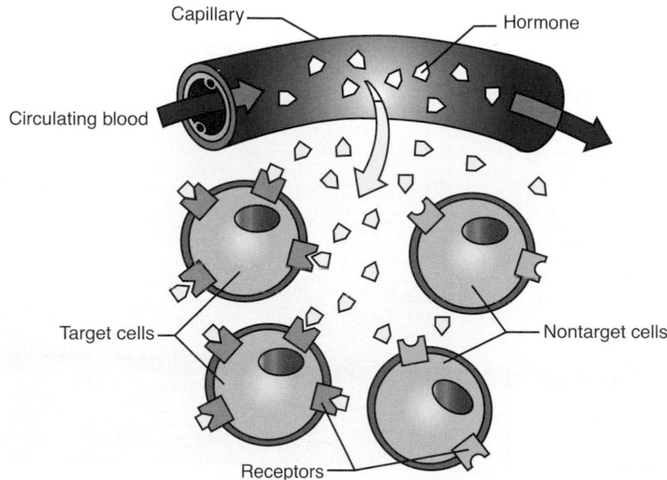

• **Fig. 10.1** Hormones and target cells. Only cells that possess the specific receptors can bind the desired hormone. (Redrawn from Thibodeau GA, Patton KT: *Anatomy and physiology*, ed. 6, St Louis, 2007, Mosby.)

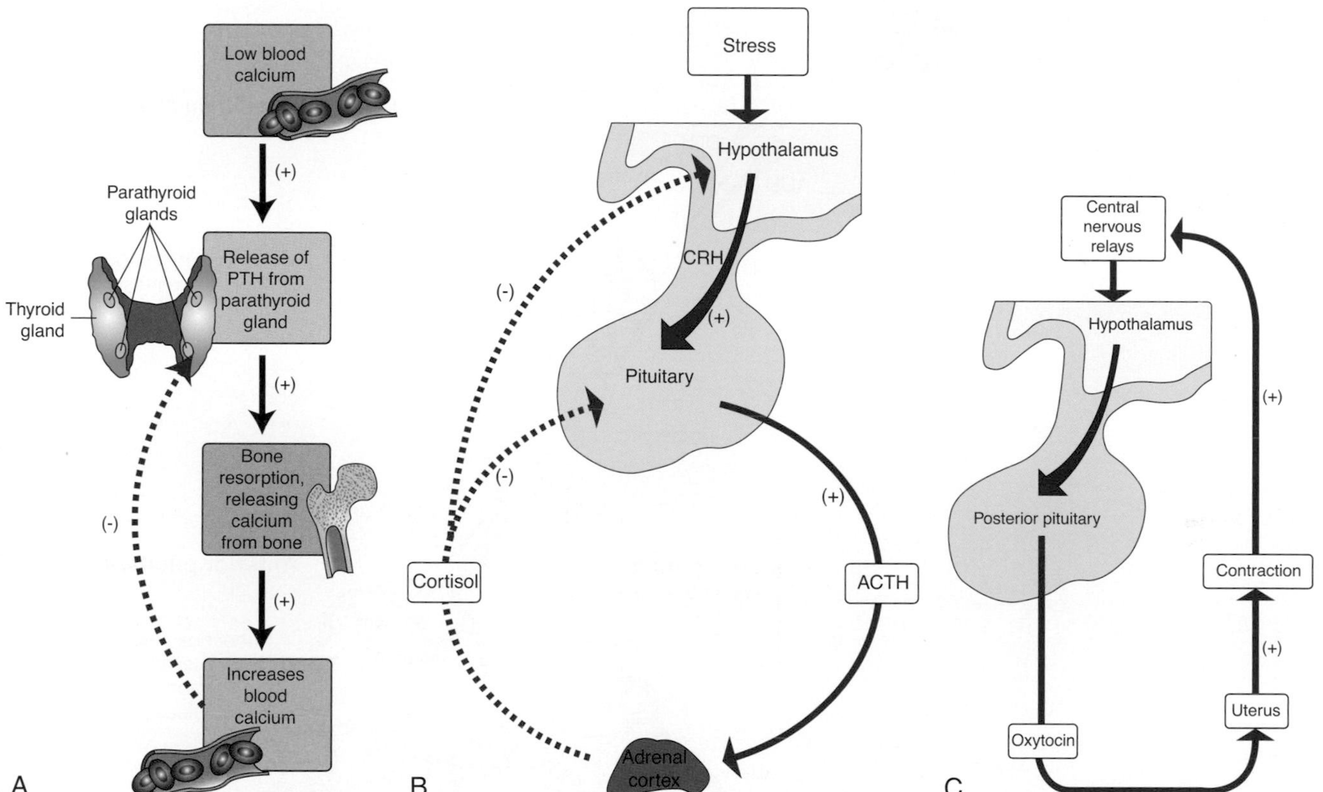

• **Fig. 10.2** (A) A simple negative feedback system. Regulation of parathyroid hormone (PTH). When blood levels of calcium drop below normal, this signals the cells of the parathyroid gland to release PTH, which promotes bone resorption, thus releasing more calcium into the bloodstream. As the calcium levels rise above the set point, the parathyroid gland cells stop producing more PTH; *(–)* inhibition, *(+)* stimulation. (B) A complex negative feedback system. Regulation of cortisol. Environmental stress signals the hypothalamus to release corticotropin-releasing hormone (CRH), which stimulates the anterior pituitary gland to secrete adrenocorticotropic hormone (ACTH). ACTH travels to the adrenal glands and causes the adrenal cortex to release cortisol. Rising cortisol levels feed back to inhibit the production of CRH and ACTH from the hypothalamus and pituitary gland; *(-)* inhibition, *(+)* stimulation. (C) A positive feedback system. Regulation of oxytocin. Uterine contractions during parturition stimulate the posterior pituitary gland to release oxytocin, which causes additional uterine contractions, leading to further oxytocin secretion.

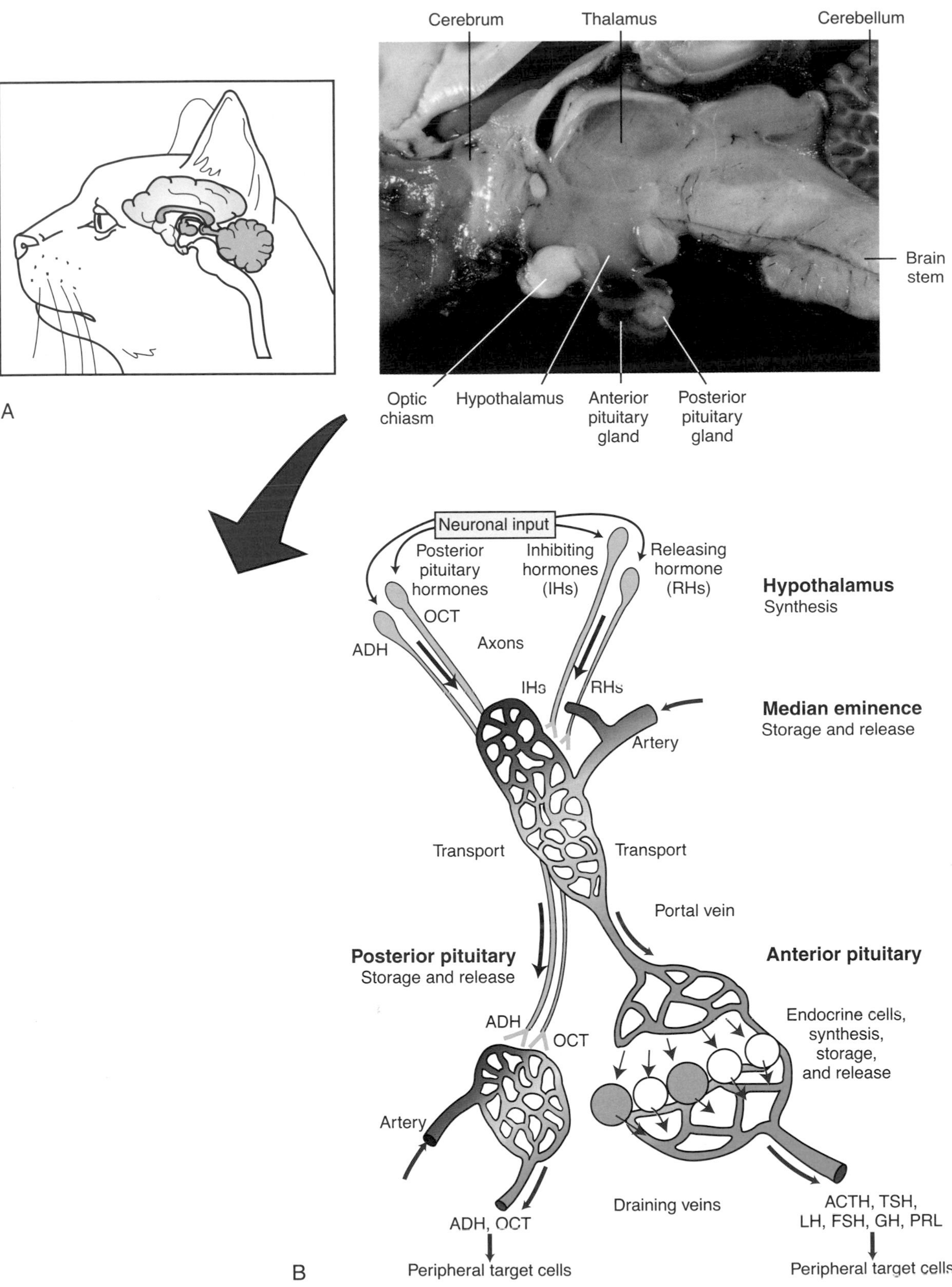

• **Fig. 10.3** Anatomic and functional relationship of the hypothalamus and pituitary gland. (A) Gross anatomy of the hypothalamus, pituitary gland, and brainstem (longitudinal section). (B) The hypothalamus produces antidiuretic hormone (ADH) and oxytocin (OCT), which travel down nerve fibers to the posterior pituitary gland, where they are stored. The hypothalamus also produces a variety of releasing and inhibiting hormones, which are released into the portal blood vessels to stimulate the production of the anterior pituitary hormones: adrenocorticotropin hormone (ACTH), thyroid-stimulating hormone (TSH), luteinizing hormone (LH), follicle-stimulating hormone (FSH), growth hormone (GH), and prolactin (PRL). (*A*, Courtesy Dr. C. Capen, College of Veterinary Medicine, The Ohio State University.)

Hormone Physiology

Hypothalamus

In response to environmental changes, the neurons of the hypothalamus produce a number of releasing and inhibiting hormones that travel through the portal system to affect the production and secretion of anterior pituitary gland hormones directly. Examples include thyrotropin-releasing hormone (TRH), which stimulates the release of thyroid-stimulating hormone (TSH), and corticotropin-releasing hormone (CRH), which promotes the release of adrenocorticotropic hormone (ACTH). The hypothalamus also produces oxytocin and antidiuretic hormone (ADH) (see Fig. 10.3).

Anterior Pituitary Gland

There are seven hormones produced by the anterior pituitary gland (see Fig. 10.3) which produce a variety of effects on the tissues and cells of the body and stimulate the growth and development of the endocrine glands in the body. These hormones are:

- Growth hormone (GH)
- Prolactin
- Thyroid-stimulating hormone (TSH)
- Adrenocorticotropic hormone (ACTH)
- Follicle-stimulating hormone (FSH)
- Luteinizing hormone (LH)
- Melanocyte-stimulating hormone (MSH)

Posterior Pituitary Gland

Acting as a storage house, the posterior pituitary gland contains the hormones oxytocin and ADH, which are produced in the hypothalamus.

Thyroid Gland

In-class Activity

Locate and identify the thyroid gland in your preserved cat. Note that, as a result of the preservation process, the appearance, and sometimes the presence, of the thyroid gland and parathyroid gland is altered, which can make them difficult to locate and identify.

Anatomy and Histology

The **thyroid gland** is a large gland located in the cranial cervical neck region under the sternothyroideus muscles (refer to the muscles of the neck in Chapter 8). It consists of two lateral lobes, one on each side of the trachea, caudal to the larynx. Blood is supplied to the thyroid from the cranial thyroid artery and drained by the caudal thyroid vein (Fig. 10.4). Also, note that the recurrent pharyngeal nerve, which runs parallel to the trachea, is in close proximity to the thyroid gland. Depending on the species, the lobes of the thyroid gland may be connected by a narrow band of connective tissue called an isthmus (Box 10.1).

The thyroid gland is primarily composed of many thyroid follicles, tiny spheres that are composed of a single layer of follicular cells that secrete a gel-like substance called colloid into the lumen of the follicle (see Fig. 10.4). These follicles are responsible for producing and releasing the thyroid hormones T_3 (triiodothyronine) and T_4 (tetraiodothyronine or thyroxine). Dispersed among the follicles are the parafollicular or C cells, which produce calcitonin (we will discuss calcitonin more in the following section).

Hormone Physiology

The thyroid gland is unique in that it stores large amounts of thyroglobulin (hormone precursor) in the colloid of the thyroid follicles. Each thyroglobulin molecule contains iodine, protein, and the preliminary forms of the thyroid hormones. When the follicular cells are stimulated by TSH from the anterior pituitary gland, the thyroglobulin molecules enter the follicular cells, where they are broken down into T_3 and T_4 and then released into the bloodstream. Regulation of thyroid hormone is accomplished through a negative feedback system involving the hypothalamus, the anterior pituitary, and the thyroid gland. Fig. 10.5 summarizes some of the effects of thyroid hormone on the body.

Clinical Applications

Review the discussion of goiter (Fig. 10.6), hypothyroidism, and hyperthyroidism in Chapter 11 of the textbook as clinically significant thyroid gland dysfunctions.

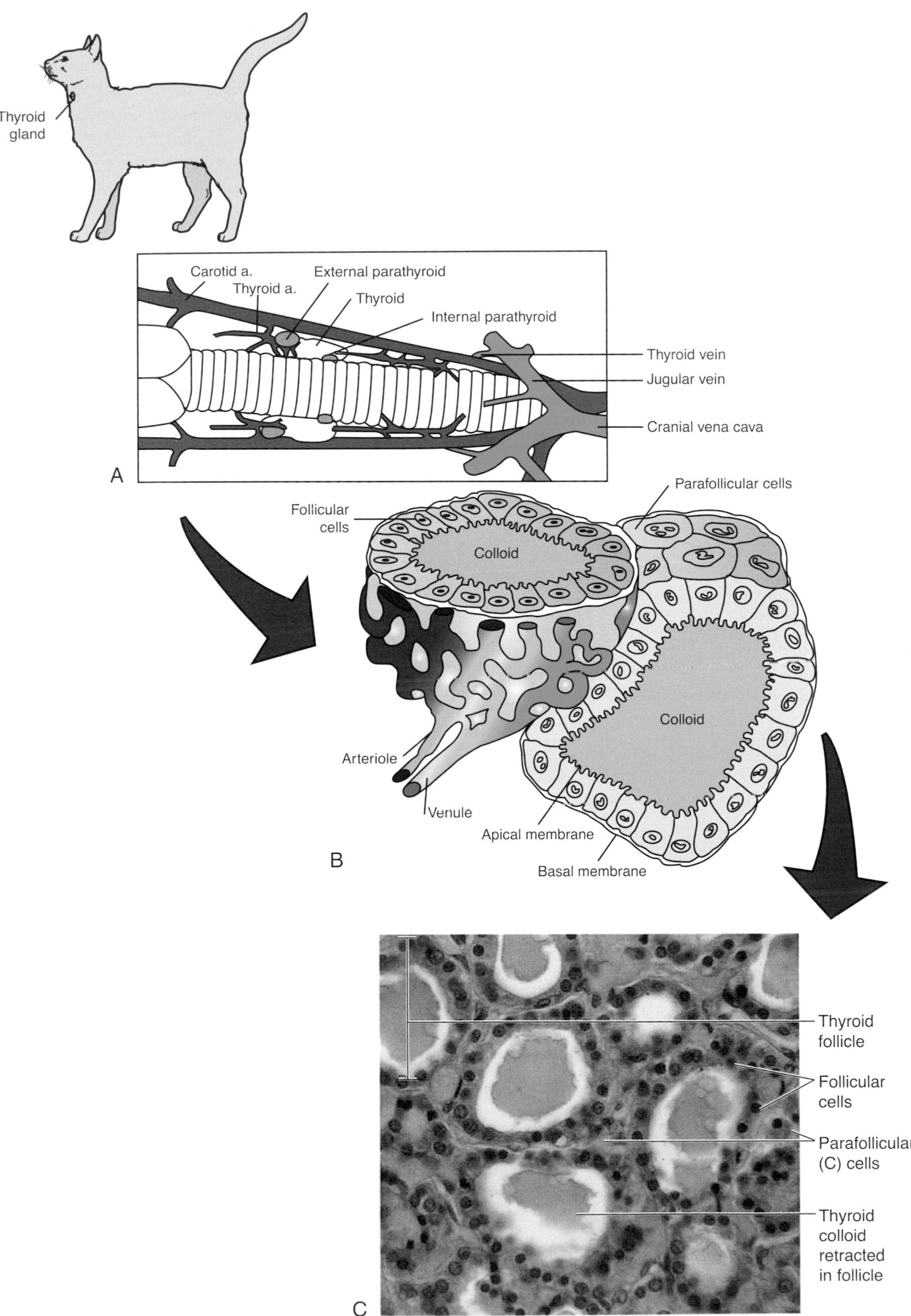

• **Fig. 10.4** Anatomy, structure, and histology of the thyroid gland. (A) The thyroid gland is located in the cranial cervical neck region. It consists of two lateral lobes, one on each side of the trachea, caudal to the larynx. Blood is supplied to the thyroid from the cranial thyroid artery and drained by the caudal thyroid vein. (B) A thyroid follicle is composed of follicular and parafollicular cells surrounding colloid, which is a gel-like substance that stores thyroid hormone precursors. (C) Histology of the thyroid gland. (*A* and *B*, From Ruckebusch Y, Phaneuf L: *Physiology of small and large animals*, ed 1, Philadelphia, 1991, Mosby. *C,* From Thibodeau GA, Patton KT: *Anatomy and physiology*, ed. 8, St Louis, 2013, Mosby.)

• BOX 10.1 Comparative Anatomy of the Thyroid and Parathyroid Glands

Whereas in most species the lobes of the thyroid are lateral to the trachea, in the pig the main lobe is in the midline on the trachea. In the cat and dog, the isthmus is thin or absent; however, in the horse, cow, and human it is very substantial. The exact number and location of the parathyroid glands vary greatly among species. The pig is unique, having only one pair of parathyroid glands. In the cat and dog, the parathyroid glands are usually attached to the capsule; in humans they are embedded within the gland. In ruminants the internal parathyroid glands are often associated with the thyroid gland, but the external glands are found cranial to the thyroid gland, sometimes embedded in the thymus. The horse has the greatest distance between the parathyroid glands, with the caudal pair located farther down the trachea at the level of the first rib.

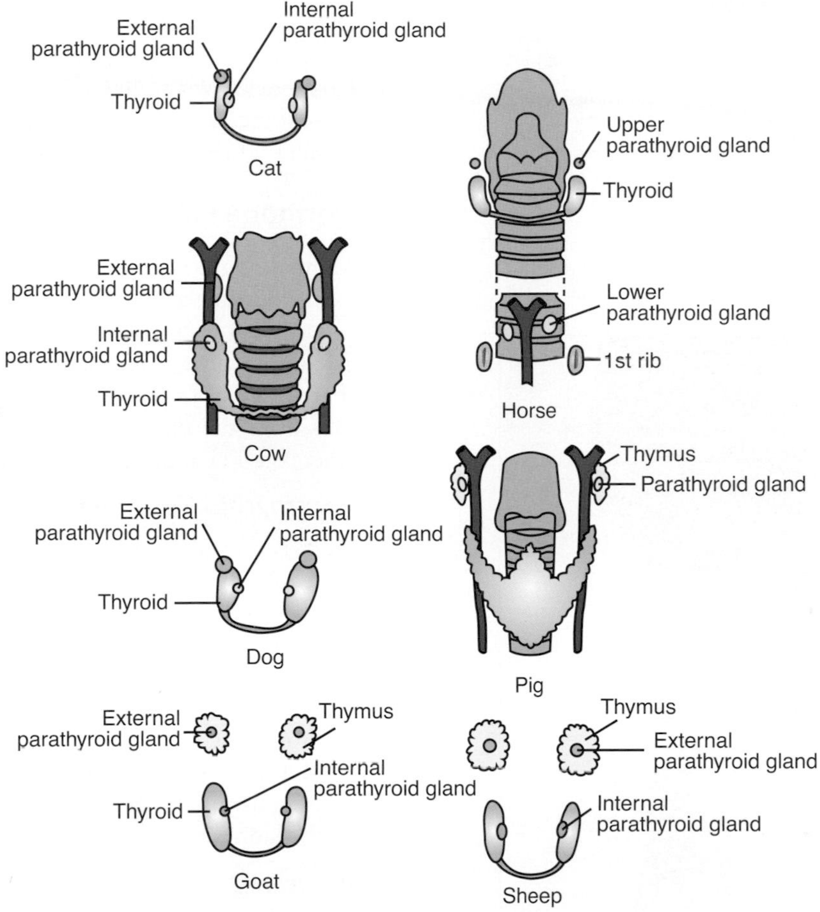

Schematic representation of the relationship between the thyroid and parathyroid glands in domestic animals. The thyroid gland is colored blue, the thymus yellow, the parathyroid gland green, and the larynx and trachea pink. (From Nelson RW, Couto CG: *Small animal internal medicine*, ed. 3, St Louis, 2003, Mosby.)

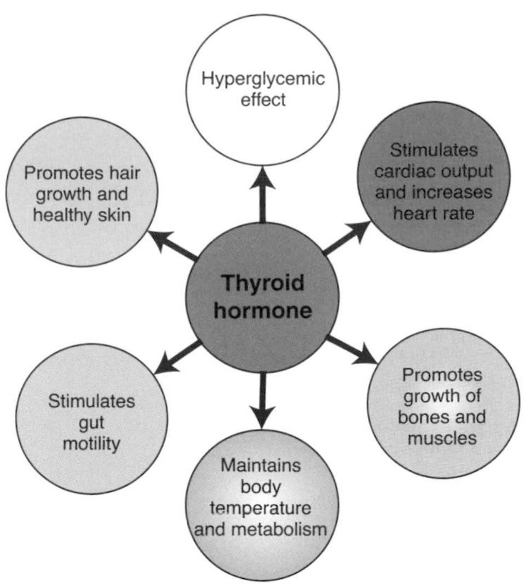

• **Fig. 10.5** The systemic effects of thyroid hormone.

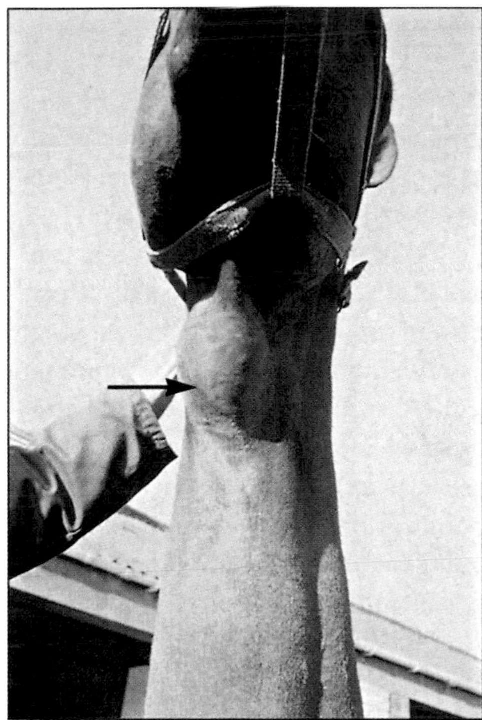

• **Fig. 10.6** Thyroid goiter in a horse. (From Knottenbelt D, Pascoe RR: *Color atlas of diseases and disorders of the horse*, ed. 2, St Louis, 1994, Mosby.)

Parathyroid Gland

In-class Activity

Locate and identify the parathyroid glands in your preserved cat.

Anatomy and Histology

The **parathyroid gland** is actually a set of two pairs of glands with a total of four separate nodules. Depending on the species, they are referred to as the external or cranial and the internal or caudal parathyroid glands. The parathyroid glands are situated in, on, or around the thyroid gland. In young animals, the external pair may be embedded in the thymus. In contrast to the thyroid gland, they are often pale (Fig. 10.7). The exact number and location of the parathyroid glands vary significantly among species (see Box 10.1).

The chief cell is the primary functional cell of the parathyroid gland and is responsible for synthesizing and secreting parathyroid hormone (PTH) (see Fig. 10.7). In humans and horses, a second cell type is found: the oxyphil cell. Oxyphil cells are larger than the chief cells and at this time have no known function. The number of oxyphilic cells present increases with age, so it is thought that these may be "retired" chief cells.

Hormone Physiology

Maintaining a normal calcium level in the body is of utmost importance because too much (hypercalcemia) or too little (hypocalcemia) can be life-threatening. Regulation of calcium involves three main hormones: calcitonin from the thyroid, PTH from the parathyroid, and calcitriol (vitamin D3) from the kidney. Calcitonin prevents hypercalcemia, whereas PTH and calcitriol prevent hypocalcemia.

Parathyroid Hormone

PTH is the primary hormone regulating calcium levels in the body. Hypocalcemia triggers the chief cells to synthesize and release PTH, which increases the amount of calcium in the bloodstream by:

- Withdrawing calcium from bone by stimulating osteoclasts to break down the bone matrix
- Promoting calcium reabsorption by the kidney
- Increasing phosphorus secretion by the kidney
- Stimulating the production and release of calcitriol from the kidneys

Vitamin D

Vitamin D is synthesized in the skin when the dermis is exposed to the sun's ultraviolet light. It is then transported to the liver, where it undergoes further metabolism before it is converted to its active form, calcitriol (vitamin D3), in the kidney. Calcitriol prevents hypocalcemia by increasing calcium absorption from food in the small intestines.

Calcitonin

Calcitonin is produced and released by the thyroid gland's parafollicular (C) cells in response to hypercalcemia. It reduces the amount of calcium in the bloodstream by stimulating the osteoblasts to deposit more bone, thereby moving the excess calcium out of the bloodstream and into the bone.

Clinical Applications

Equine Secondary Nutritional Hyperparathyroidism

Secondary nutritional hyperparathyroidism is a disease characterized by excessive parathyroid hormone levels that

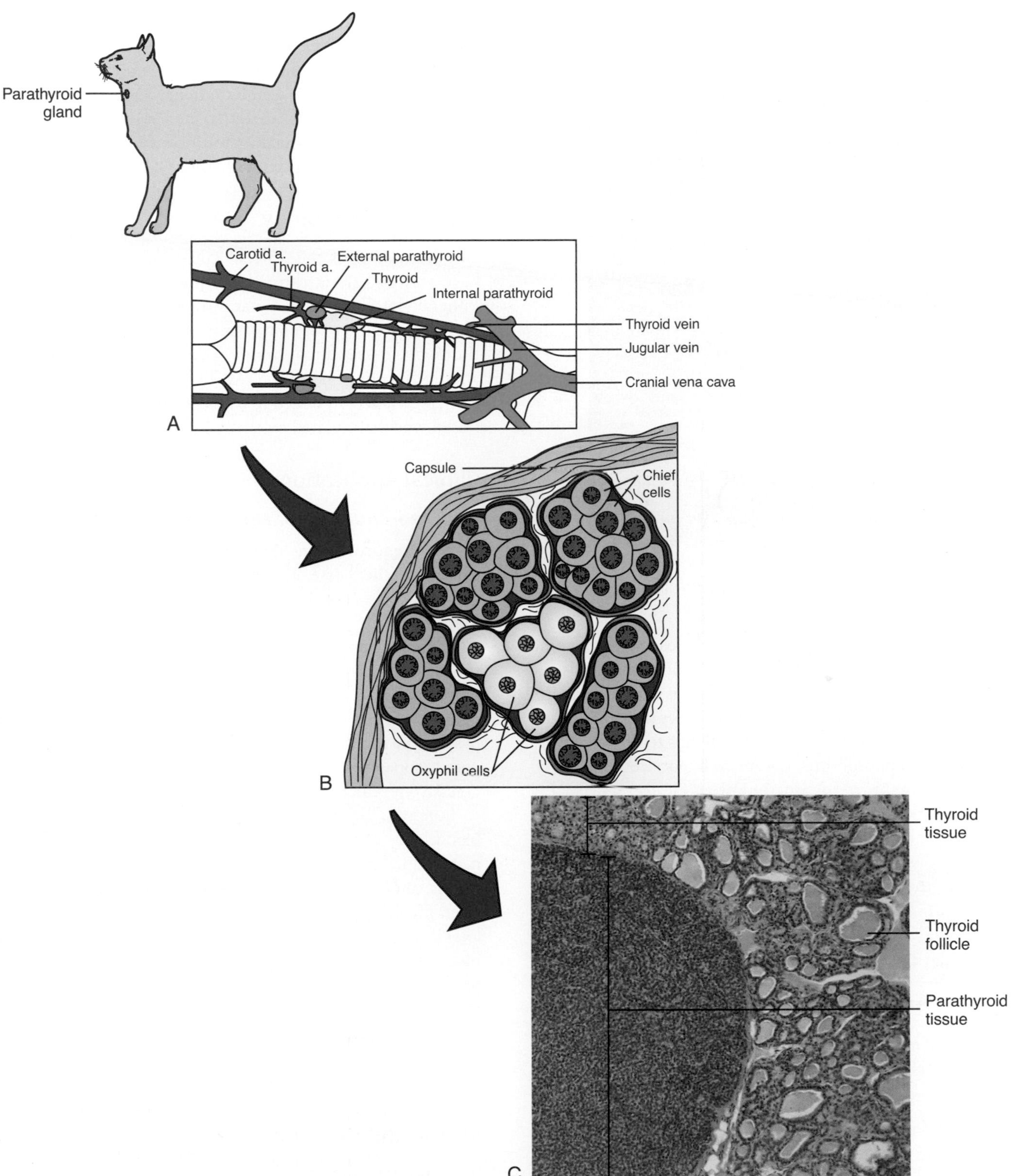

• **Fig. 10.7** Anatomy and histology of the parathyroid glands. (A) The parathyroid gland is two pairs of glands associated with the thyroid gland. (B) The main functional cell of the parathyroid gland is the chief cell, which produces parathyroid hormone. Oxyphil cells are only found in humans and horses. (C) Parathyroid tissue. This microscopic specimen shows a portion of a parathyroid gland bordered by the surrounding thyroid tissue. (*A,* From Ruckebusch Y, Phaneuf L: *Physiology of small and large animals*, ed. 1, Philadelphia, 1991, Mosby. *B,* From Goodman MH: *Basic medical endocrinology*, ed. 3, London, 2003, Academic Press. *C,* From Thibodeau GA, Patton KT: *Anatomy and physiology*, ed. 6, St Louis, 2007, Mosby.)

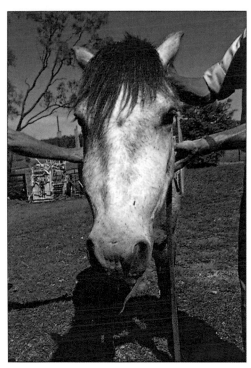

• **Fig. 10.8** A horse with hyperparathyroidism. (From Knottenbelt D, Pascoe RR: *Color atlas of diseases and disorders of the horse*, ed. 2, St Louis, 1994, Mosby.)

are caused by an underlying dietary deficiency of calcium. Before advances were made in equine nutrition, this was a very common disease seen in horses and is often referred to as Bran Disease or "Big Head." These horses are fed an excessive amount of wheat bran, which contains too little calcium and too much phosphorus, leading to hypocalcemia and triggering a constant overproduction of PTH. Too much PTH causes an increase in bone resorption and leads to massive bone loss and remodeling. Characteristic of this disease is the thickening of the flat bones of the head caused by cartilage replacing the bone, giving the appearance of a "big head" (Fig. 10.8). These horses are also at risk for bone fractures.

Adrenal Gland

In-class Activity

Locate and identify the adrenal glands in your preserved cat. Hint: First, locate the kidneys.

Anatomy and Histology

The left and right **adrenal glands** are located just cranial and slightly medial to each kidney. The left gland is situated close to the aorta, whereas the right gland is situated close to the caudal vena cava. In humans, each adrenal gland sits on top of the kidney like a cap. A thin layer of connective tissue forms the capsule that surrounds each gland. Branches of the aorta supply blood and nutrients to the adrenal glands (Fig. 10.9).

The adrenal gland is actually two glands in one, each with different origins and functions. The outer layer—the adrenal cortex—is composed of glandular tissue and is further divided into three different layers: the zona glomerulus, which produces mineralocorticoids; the zona fasciculata, responsible for the synthesis of glucocorticoids; and the zona reticularis, which secretes adrenal sex hormones. The inner layer, the adrenal medulla, is derived from nervous tissue and contains specially modified neurons that release catecholamines during times of stress (see Fig. 10.9).

Hormone Physiology

The hormones of the adrenal cortex are many, and they have various effects throughout the body. Aldosterone, a mineralocorticoid, is important in regulating urine volume. Cortisol, a glucocorticoid, has a hyperglycemic effect in the body; its production and release is stimulated by the anterior pituitary hormone, ACTH. Epinephrine and norepinephrine are produced in the adrenal medulla and are released when stimulated by the sympathetic nervous system.

Clinical Applications

Hyperadrenocorticism in Domestic Animals

Hyperadrenocorticism is the most common endocrine disease of the horse, usually affecting older animals and almost always caused by an ACTH-secreting anterior pituitary gland tumor. One of the hallmark clinical signs is a curly, dense, long coat (hirsutism) which is not shed in the summer (Fig. 10.10). Other symptoms include weight loss, polyuria, polydipsia, poor wound healing, excessive sweating, and recurrent laminitis (see Chapter 6, Integumentary System, in the textbook for more on laminitis). Treatment with a dopamine-like drug called Pergolide helps to control excessive production of cortisol from the adrenal cortex.

In ferrets, hyperadrenocorticism is responsible for elevated blood levels of the adrenal sex hormones. Typically affecting neutered ferrets of both sexes over the age of 3 years, this disease is caused by a primary problem of the adrenal cortex, often involving a tumor. Bilaterally symmetric alopecia (hair loss) is the main symptom (Fig. 10.11) and is often accompanied with a potbellied appearance and weight loss. The excess production of adrenal estrogen leads to swelling of the vulva in the female, whereas in the male adrenal androgen causes prostate enlargement, leading to difficulty urinating. Although medical treatment is available, the current treatment of choice is to remove the affected adrenal gland (adrenalectomy).

Endocrine Pancreas

In-class Activity

Locate and identify the pancreas in your preserved cat.

Anatomy and Histology

The **pancreas** is a flat, elongated organ with two lobes that is situated between the descending duodenum and the stomach (Fig. 10.12). Please refer to Chapter 11 of the textbook, where the anatomy of the pancreas is described.

• **Fig. 10.9** Anatomy, structure, and histology of the adrenal gland. (A) The adrenal glands are located just cranial and slightly medial to each kidney. (B) The adrenal gland is surrounded by a thin layer of connective tissue, which forms the capsule. The two layers of the adrenal gland are the adrenal cortex and the adrenal medulla. (C) Major regions of the adrenal gland are shown in a light micrograph of a stained specimen. (*C,* From Kierzenbaum AK: *Histology and cell biology: an introduction to pathology*, St Louis, 2002, Mosby.)

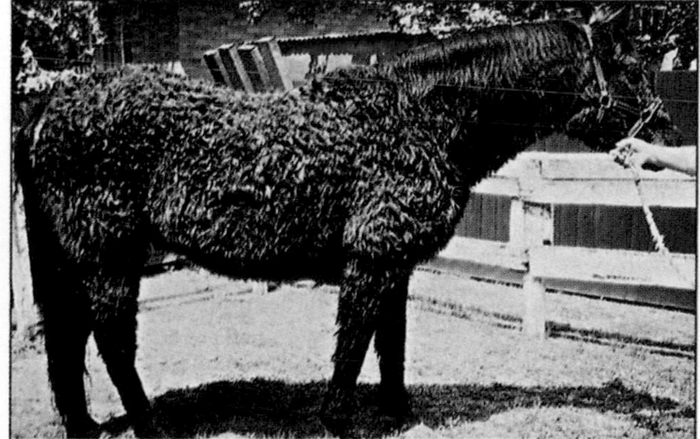

• **Fig. 10.10** Hirsutism in a horse with hyperadrenocorticism. (From Knottenbelt D, Pascoe RR: *Color atlas of diseases and disorders of the horse*, ed. 2, St Louis, 1994, Mosby.)

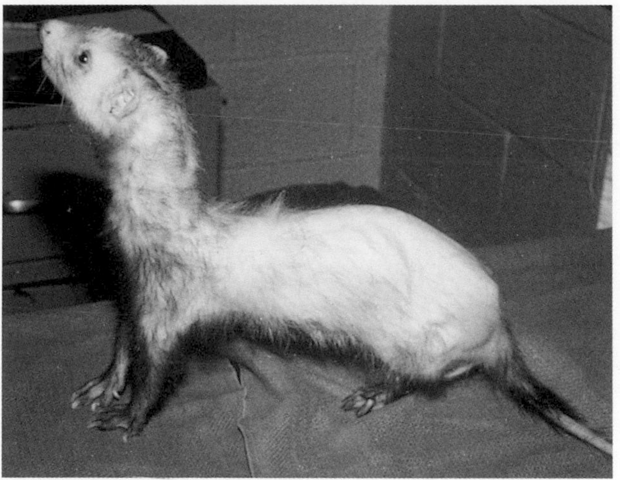

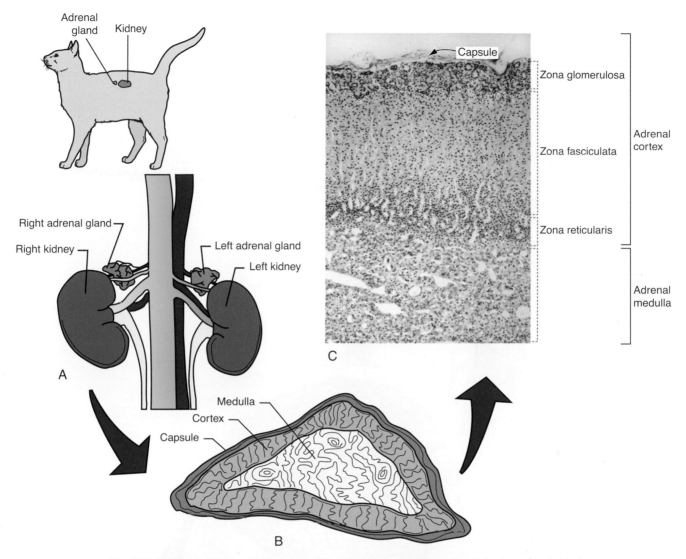

• **Fig. 10.11** Ferret with alopecia due to hyperadrenocorticism. (From Quesenberry KE, Carpenter JW: *Ferrets, rabbits, and rodents: clinical medicine and surgery*, ed. 2, St Louis, 2004, Saunders.)

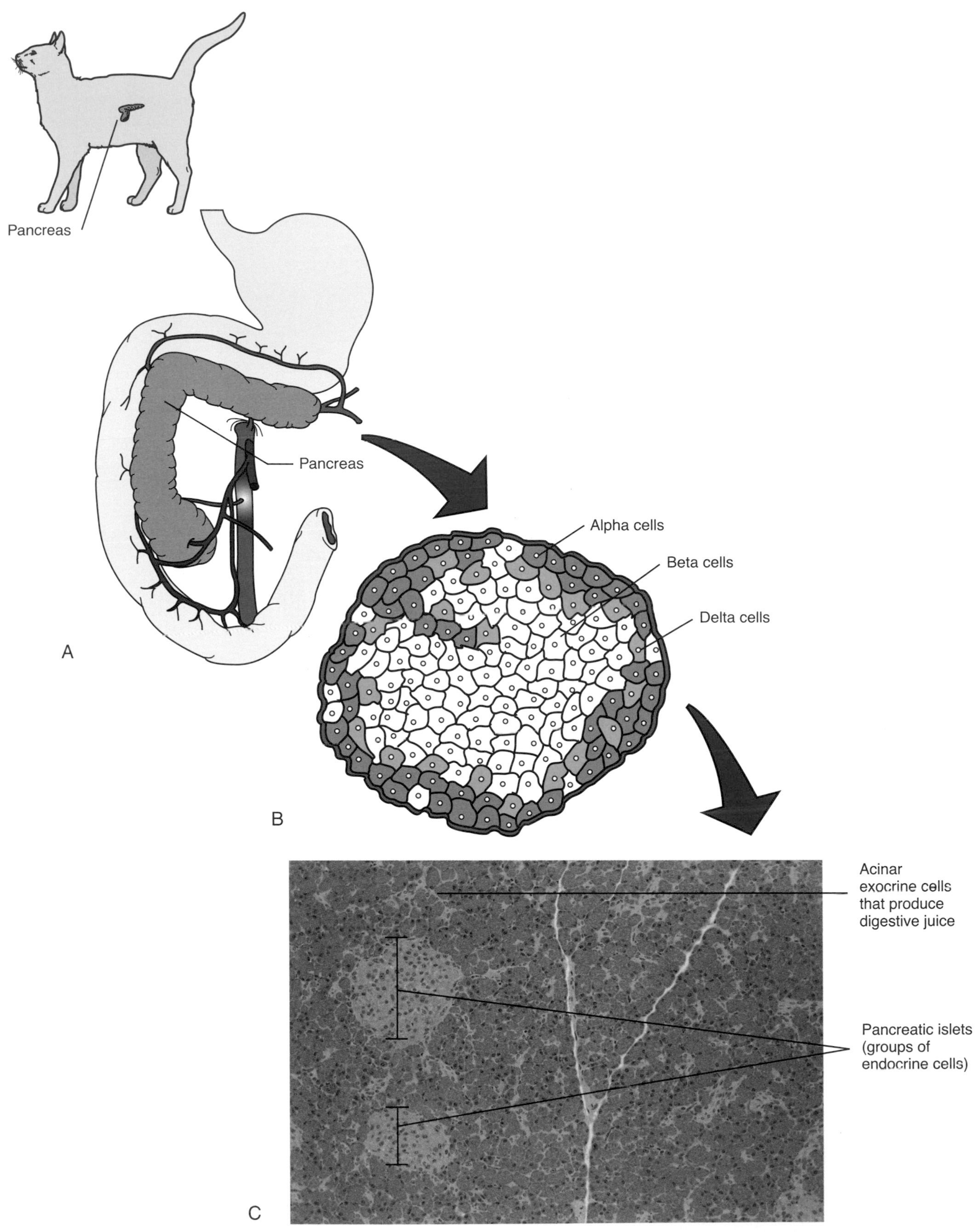

• **Fig. 10.12** Anatomy and histology of the pancreas. (A) The pancreas is located between the stomach and the descending duodenum. (B) Islets of Langerhans. The islets are composed of alpha cells, which release glucagon; beta cells, which secrete insulin; and delta cells, which produce somatostatin. (C) Two pancreatic islets, or hormone-producing areas, are evident among the pancreatic cells that produce the pancreatic digestive juice. (*C*, From Thibodeau GA, Patton KT: *Anatomy and physiology*, ed. 6, St Louis, 2007, Mosby.)

TABLE 10.1 Summary of Other Endocrine Glands, Tissues, and Organs

Organ	Hormone	Action
Kidney	Erythropoietin	Stimulates red blood cell production in the bone marrow
Stomach	Gastrin	Stimulates the gastric glands to secrete acid and digestive enzymes; increases gastric motility
Small intestine	Secretin	Stimulates the pancreas to release sodium bicarbonate; slows gastric motility
Small intestine	Cholecystokinin (CCK)	Stimulates the pancreas to release its digestive enzymes; slows gastric motility
Placenta	Chorionic gonadotropin	Stimulates the ovaries to release progesterone to maintain the uterine lining and hence, pregnancy
Thymus	Thymosin	Stimulates T-cell development
Thymus	Thymopoietin	Stimulates T-cell development
Pineal body	Melatonin	Influences moods, wake–sleep cycles, and seasonal estrus
Many body tissues	Prostaglandins (tissue hormones)	Inflammatory response, luteolysis

The functional units of the endocrine pancreas are the pancreatic islets (islets of Langerhans), which are clumps of cells scattered among the acini or exocrine pancreatic cells. Each islet is composed of three different cell types: the alpha cells, which form the periphery; beta cells, which compose the center; and delta cells, which are spread through the islet (see Fig. 10.12).

Hormone Physiology

Hypoglycemia triggers the alpha cells to release glucagon, which stimulates the liver to release glucose. The beta cells release insulin when the blood glucose levels are too high, causing glucose to be absorbed into body cells. Delta cells secrete somatostatin, which inhibits insulin and glucagon secretion in the pancreas, and also inhibits the release of growth hormone from the anterior pituitary gland.

Clinical Applications

Diseases of the endocrine pancreas result from problems with the insulin-secreting beta cells. A deficiency of insulin causes diabetes mellitus and is discussed in the textbook. An excess of insulin is produced by a tumor of the beta cells and causes profound and life-threatening hypoglycemia. This type of tumor is called an insulinoma and is commonly seen in the ferret and occasionally found in the dog. Symptoms often include staring blankly into space, drooling, nausea, seizures, and coma. Treatment consists of removing the tumor.

The Gonads

The gonads are the reproductive glands—the testes in the male and the ovaries in the female—and are discussed in Chapter 19 of the textbook. The testes produce the male sex hormone testosterone, whereas the female sex hormones estrogen and progesterone are produced by the ovaries.

Other Endocrine Tissues

Table 10.1 summarizes some of the other organs in the body that have endocrine functions.

EXERCISES

Control of Hormone Secretion

Exercise 1

Explore the Exocrine and Endocrine Glands

Define the exocrine gland and endocrine gland. Be sure to give an example of each in your definitions.

Exocrine gland ______________________________

____

Endocrine gland ______________________________

____

Exercise 2

Compare the Endocrine and Nervous Systems

Complete the table below comparing the endocrine and nervous systems.

Characteristic	Endocrine System	Nervous System
General function	______________ ______________	______________ ______________
Reaction to stimuli	______________	______________
Duration of effect	______________	______________
Chemical messenger	______________	______________
Messenger-producing cells	______________ ______________	______________

Hypothalamus and Pituitary Gland

Exercise 3

Identify and Color the Hypothalamus and Pituitary Gland Components

Color the pituitary gland yellow, the hypothalamus blue, the optic chiasm red, the cerebellum green, and the brainstem orange.

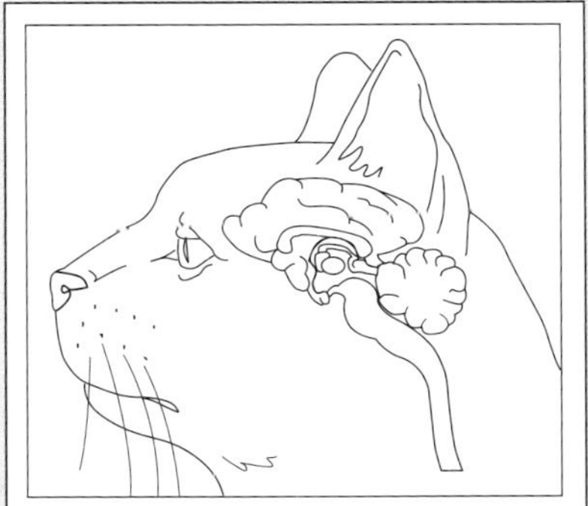

Exercise 4

Identify the Target Organs of Eight Pituitary Hormones

On the lines provided, enter the name of the target organ(s) affected by the pituitary hormone indicated.

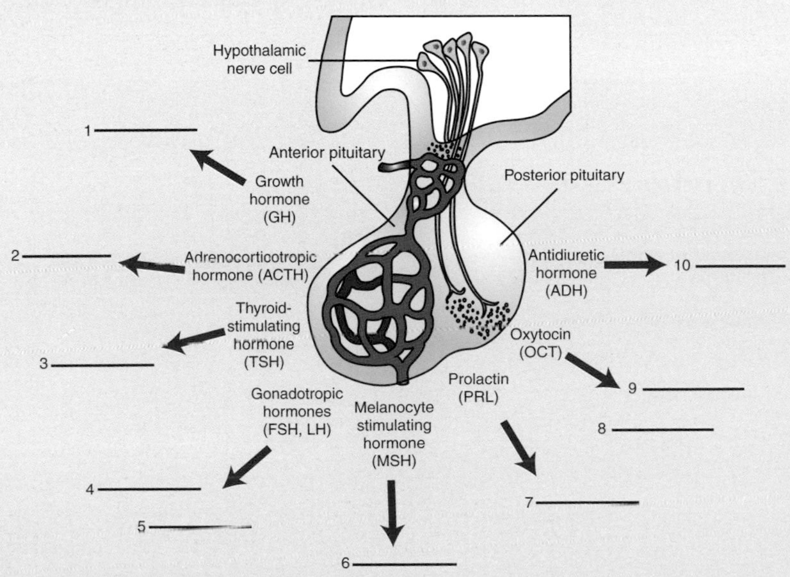

Exercise 5

Describe the Relationship Between the Hypothalamus and Anterior and Posterior Pituitary Glands

How do the hypothalamus and anterior pituitary glands communicate with one another? How does the hypothalamus communicate with the posterior pituitary and vice versa?

____

____

____

____

Exercise 6

Critical Thinking: Match the Hormone With the Action

Match each statement with the correct hormone. (Answers may be used more than once.)

________ Stimulates uterine contractions during parturition
________ Stimulates growth of bone and muscle
________ Stimulates lactation
________ Stimulates oogenesis and the production of estrogen
________ Promotes water reabsorption in the kidney
________ Called interstitial cell-stimulating hormone (ICSH) in the male
________ High levels of thyroid hormone inhibit the release of this hormone
________ High levels of adrenal hormones inhibit the release of this hormone
________ Excess of this hormone causes acromegaly
________ These two hormones are produced in the hypothalamus
________ These two hormones are called gonadotropins

a. FSH
b. TSH
c. GH
d. ACTH
e. Prolactin
f. LH
g. Oxytocin
h. ADH

Exercise 7

Clinical Thinking: Explore the Use of Oxytocin

Hormones are often used as drugs in veterinary medicine. Oxytocin is one such hormone. In what situation would giving the drug oxytocin be helpful to an animal? Be sure to explain why.

____

____

____

Thyroid Gland

Exercise 8

Critical Thinking: Label the Cells

Match the number on the figure below with the following structures:

________ Colloid
________ Thyroid follicle
________ Follicular cells
________ Parafollicular cells

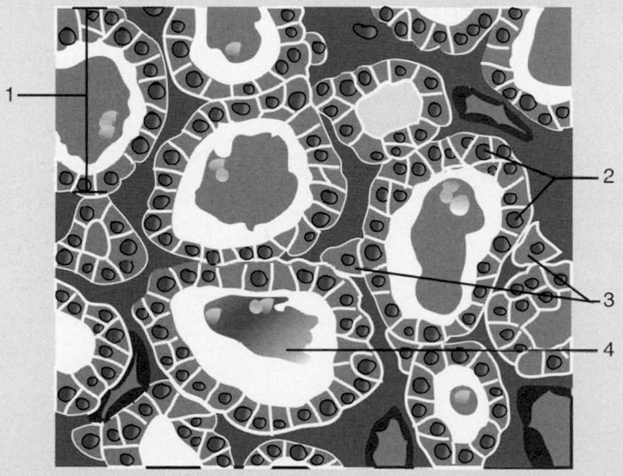

Exercise 9

Critical Thinking: Label the Negative Feedback Diagram

Label the following negative feedback diagram with the correct hormones released from each gland. On the feedback lines, indicate inhibition with a minus (–) sign and stimulation with a plus (+) sign.

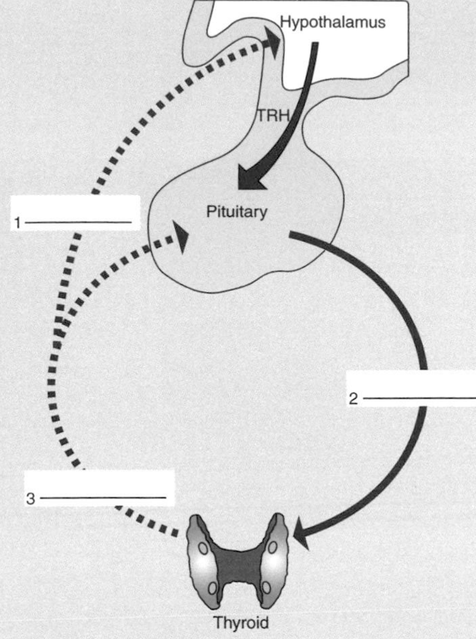

Exercise 10

Clinical Thinking: Identify Thyroid Anatomy

List three species that have a prominent thyroid isthmus.

1. ______________________________
2. ______________________________
3. ______________________________

Exercise 11

Clinical Thinking: Identify Clinical Symptoms #1

Circle the correct answers and complete the following: Deficient thyroid hormone secretion causes increased/decreased heart rate, increased/decreased appetite, and increased/decreased weight. This disease is called ________ thyroidism.

Exercise 12

Clinical Thinking: Identify Clinical Symptoms #2

Fig. 10.6 shows a horse with a goiter. Fill in the blanks with words from the Word Key below to explain how a dietary imbalance may cause a goiter.

When fed a diet ________ in the mineral ________, the thyroid gland is unable to produce proper amounts of ________ and ________. Low levels of thyroid hormone signal the ________ ________ gland to secrete more ________ hormone. Excessive levels of TSH cause hyperplasia of the thyroid gland. This ________ of the thyroid gland is called a goiter.

Word Key

Anterior	Iodine
Deficient	T_3
Pituitary	Thyroid-stimulating
Enlargement	T_4

Exercise 13

Clinical Thinking: Case Study—Hyperthyroidism

Fig. 10.13 shows a picture of Queenie taken at her appointment last week. A thorough examination was performed, and blood and urine samples were obtained for testing. Queenie's lab work showed a very elevated thyroxine level, and the doctor diagnosed her with hyperthyroidism. After considering the options, her owners decided to pursue surgical treatment, and Queenie has been admitted to the hospital today for her thyroidectomy surgery.

In reviewing Queenie's medical record, which symptoms would you expect to find in her history and physical examination? (Circle all that apply.) You will need a medical dictionary for this exercise.

Weight gain	Increased appetite	Constipation
Tachycardia	Weight loss	Increased thirst
Vomiting	Lethargy	Cold intolerance
Easily overheating	Bradycardia	Hypotension
Hypertension	Hemorrhage in fundus	Palpably enlarged thyroid gland
Decreased appetite	Diarrhea	

Fig. 10.14 is a picture of Queenie at surgery. Circle each lobe of the thyroid gland. Does one lobe look larger than the other? If so, put an "X" through the larger lobe.

Six months after her surgery, Queenie is back for a recheck examination (Fig. 10.15). Her thyroxine levels are normal, and she is feeling much better.

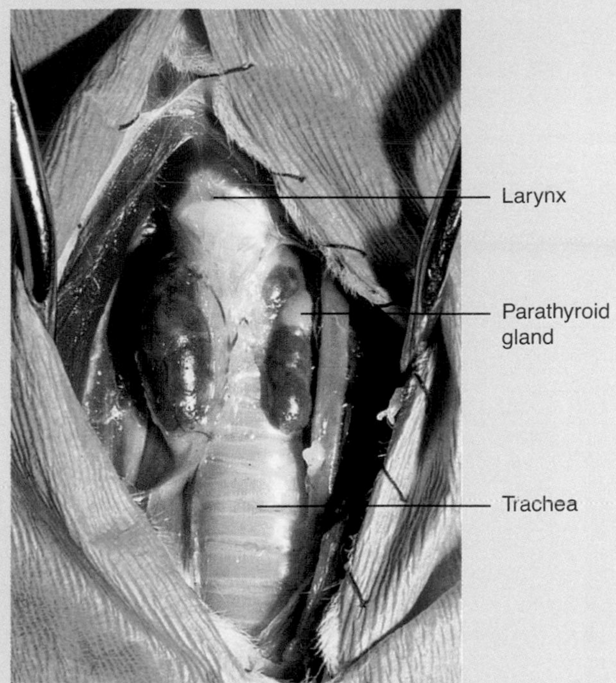

• **Fig. 10.14** "Queenie" at surgery. (From Feldman EC, Nelson RW: *Canine and feline endocrinology and reproduction*, ed. 3, St Louis, 2004, Saunders.)

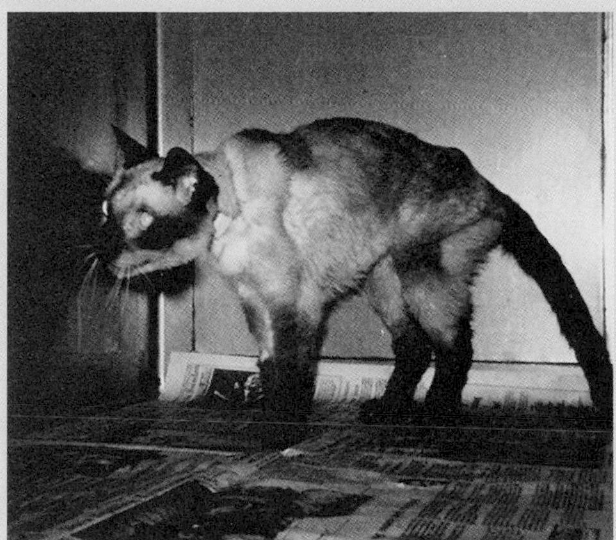

• **Fig. 10.13** "Queenie." (From Feldman EC, Nelson RW: *Canine and feline endocrinology and reproduction*, ed. 3, St Louis, 2004, Saunders.)

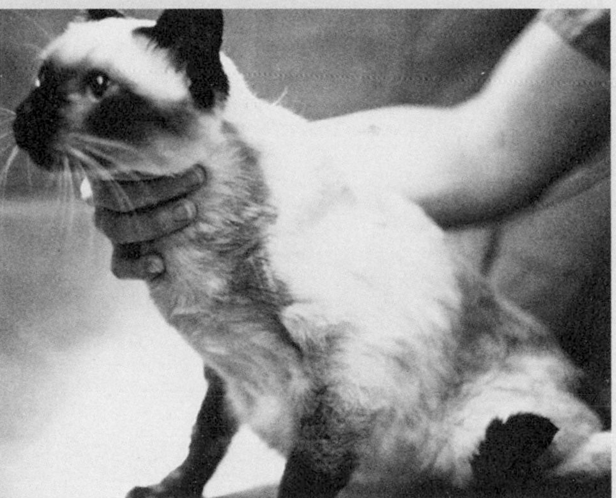

• **Fig. 10.15** "Queenie" after treatment for hyperthyroidism. (From Feldman EC, Nelson RW: *Canine and feline endocrinology and reproduction*, ed. 3, St Louis, 2004, Saunders.)

Parathyroid Gland

Exercise 14

Identify Parathyroid Anatomy

How many pairs of parathyroid glands does the pig have? ____________________

Exercise 15

Critical Thinking: Identify Hormones

Match each statement with the correct hormone. (Answers may be used more than once.)

________	Prevents hypocalcemia	a. PTH
________	Lowers calcium levels in the bloodstream	b. Calcitriol
________	Primary target organ is the small intestines	c. Calcitonin
________	Produced in the kidneys	
________	Produced by the parafollicular cells	
________	Produced by the chief cells	
________	Promotes bone resorption	
________	Promotes bone deposition	
________	Promotes the kidneys to reabsorb calcium	

Exercise 16

Clinical Thinking: Case Study—Follow-up (Hyperthyroidism)

Queenie is back in the hospital again. It has been 18 months since her thyroidectomy for hyperthyroidism. The owner is concerned because her symptoms have returned. Sure enough, blood tests confirm that her hyperthyroidism has returned. Yesterday, the surgeon removed her remaining thyroid lobe, which was enlarged. Today, as you perform your morning treatments, you notice that Queenie is weak and is having muscle tremors. The veterinarian is concerned that the parathyroid glands were removed along with the thyroid gland. You draw a blood sample from Queenie at the doctor's request. If Queenie's parathyroid glands have been removed, would you expect the blood calcium levels to be high or low? Explain why.

____

____

____

____

____

____

Exercise 17

Clinical Thinking: Case Study—Secondary Nutritional Hyperparathyroidism in the Iguana

The iguana is particularly susceptible to metabolic bone disease (MBD), a form of secondary nutritional hyperparathyroidism, because of its stringent vegetarian dietary needs and requirement for direct ultraviolet (UV) light to produce vitamin D.

Mrs. Morely and her son Mike have brought in Iggy Pop for an examination. Iggy was a birthday present given to Mike 6 months ago. They are concerned because Iggy Pop's face "looks funny." Fig. 10.16A is a picture of Iggy Pop; Fig. 10.16B a healthy iguana, is provided for comparison. In speaking with the owners, you discover that Iggy Pop has been fed an inappropriate diet. You notice that Iggy has a deformed lower jaw, and when you gently push on the lower jaw the bone is rubbery and soft. Suspecting MBD, the doctor reminds you to handle the iguana carefully as he is at risk for bone fractures. What dietary deficiency is likely causing Iggy Pop's problem?

____

____

Explain why Iggy has a deformed and soft jaw. ____________________

____

____

Exercise 17—cont'd

Clinical Thinking: Case Study—Secondary Nutritional Hyperparathyroidism in the Iguana

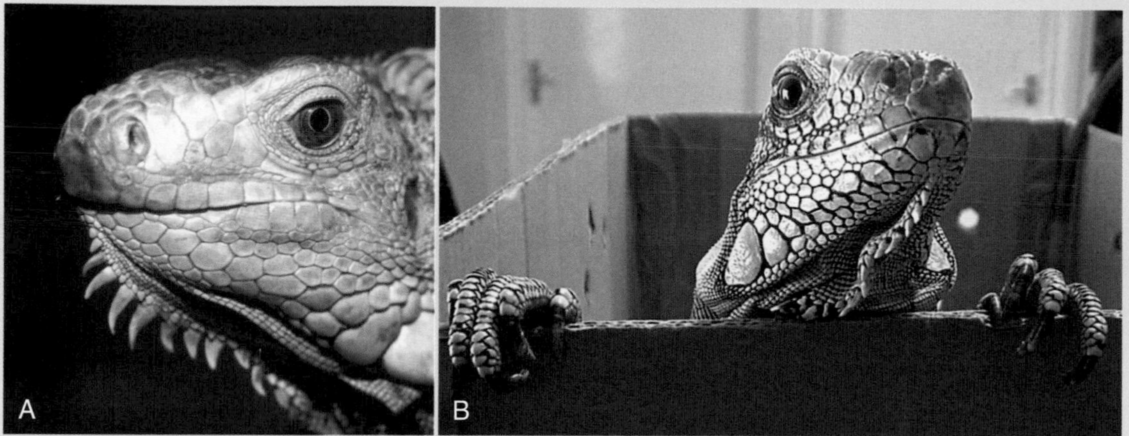

• **Fig. 10.16** (A) "Iggy Pop," a sick juvenile green iguana. (B) A healthy juvenile green iguana. (From Mader DR: *Reptile medicine and surgery*, ed. 2, St Louis, 2006, Saunders.)

Adrenal Gland

Exercise 18

Identify the Anatomy and Structure of the Adrenal Gland

Color the capsule red, the adrenal cortex blue, and the adrenal medulla yellow.

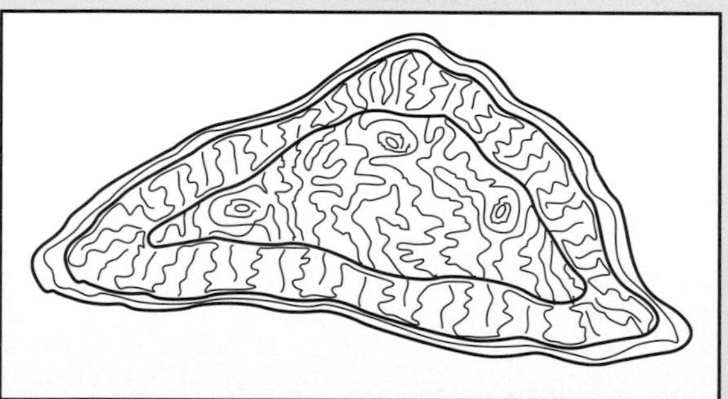

Exercise 19

Identify and Describe the Effect of Hormones Released by the Adrenal Gland

Complete the table below, which summarizes the hormones released by the adrenal gland and their effects.

Source	Group	Hormone	Target organ	Effect
________________ Zona glomerulosa	________________	Aldosterone	Kidney	Promotes ________________ reabsorption and ________________ elimination
Cortex zona ________________	________________	________________ Cortisone Corticosterone	Whole body	________________ glycemic effect; protein and lipid ________________
Cortex zona reticularis	Sex hormones	________________ Estrogen	Sex organs	Minimal effect
________________	Catecholamines	________________ Norepinephrine	Whole body	"________________" response

Exercise 20

Clinical Thinking: Identify Glucocorticosteroid Side Effects

List four potential side effects of glucocorticosteroid drugs.

1. ______________________________
2. ______________________________
3. ______________________________
4. ______________________________

Exercise 21

Clinical Thinking: Identify Effects of Epinephrine and Norepinephrine During Fight or Flight Response

List four effects of epinephrine and norepinephrine on the body as part of the "fight or flight" response.

1. ______________________________
2. ______________________________
3. ______________________________
4. ______________________________

Exercise 22

Clinical Thinking: Case Study—Canine Hyperadrenocorticism

It is Wednesday morning, and the staff is gathered in the meeting room for morning rounds. Today's case is that of Mack Small, an 18-month-old mixed-breed dog who was diagnosed last week with hyperadrenocorticism. Mr. Small had brought Mack to the clinic because Mack was losing his hair and his belly looked swollen (Fig. 10.17).

Define hyperadrenocorticism: ______________________________

____

____

In addition to a poor hair coat, what other symptoms do you expect Mack to have? Circle all that apply:

Weight gain	Coughing	Decreased appetite	Polyuria
Weight loss	Delayed wound healing	Increased thirst	Hypoglycemia
Hyperglycemia	Increased appetite	Anuria	Flaky skin

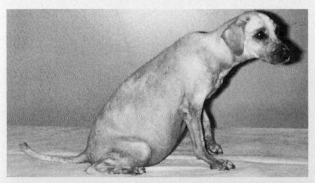

• **Fig. 10.17** "Mack." (From Feldman EC, Nelson RW: *Canine and feline endocrinology and reproduction*, ed. 3, St Louis, 2004, Saunders.)

The doctor informs you that about 80% of cases of canine hyperadrenocorticism are caused by a tumor of the anterior pituitary gland; the remaining 20% are caused by a tumor of the adrenal cortex. She also reminds you that hyperadrenocorticism (Cushing's syndrome) can be caused by the prolonged use of glucocorticosteroid drugs, but this was not the case with Mack, who has never taken any medication.

How can a tumor of the pituitary gland cause hyperadrenocorticism? ______________________________

____

____

In addition to routine lab work and abdominal x-rays, the doctor also performed a dexamethasone suppression test. This test involves measuring the cortisol level in the blood, administering an injection of dexamethasone (a glucocorticosteroid drug), and then measuring the blood cortisol level again in 8 h.

Review Fig. 10.2B. In a normal dog, would giving an injection of dexamethasone (which acts like cortisol in the body) cause a decrease or an increase in the amount of cortisol released from the adrenal cortex? ______________________________

____

____

In a dog with Cushing's syndrome caused by a pituitary gland tumor, the negative feedback system is disrupted, and suppression of cortisol production is not seen at the 8-h mark following the injection of dexamethasone. Mack's cortisol levels were above normal, confirming the diagnosis of hyperadrenocorticism. Now that Mack's condition has been diagnosed, he will be started on a medication called Lysodren, which acts on the adrenal glands to decrease its production of glucocorticoids. Fig. 10.18 shows Mack 5 months later at his recheck.

Exercise 22—cont'd

Clinical Thinking: Case Study—Canine Hyperadrenocorticism

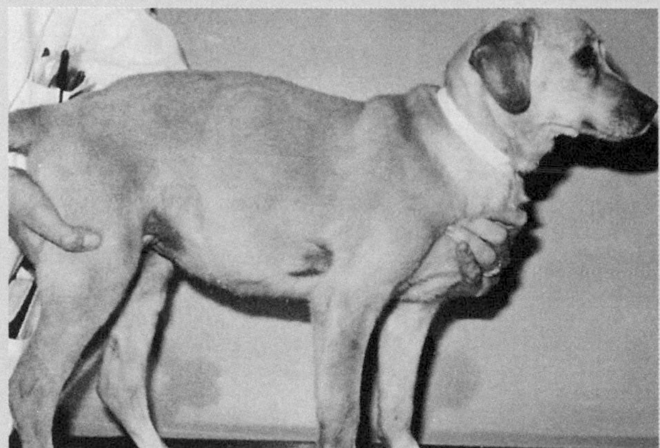

• **Fig. 10.18** "Mack" after treatment for Cushing's syndrome (From Feldman EC, Nelson RW: *Canine and feline endocrinology and reproduction*, ed. 3, St Louis, 2004, Saunders.)

Endocrine Pancreas

Exercise 23

Critical Thinking: Identify Pancreatic Hormones

Match each statement with the correct hormone. (Answers may be used more than once.)

_______ Prevents hyperglycemia by increasing glucose uptake into cells
_______ Secreted by the delta cells of the pancreatic islets
_______ Promotes gluconeogenesis
_______ Secreted by the alpha cells of the pancreatic islets
_______ Inhibits the release of insulin and glucagon
_______ Secreted by the beta cells of the pancreatic islets
_______ Causes glycogen stored in the liver to be converted into glucose

a. Insulin
b. Glucagon
c. Somatostatin

Exercise 24

Clinical Thinking: Identify Hormones Associated With Hyperglycemia

List three hormones that have a hyperglycemic effect in the body.

1. _______________
2. _______________
3. _______________

Exercise 25

Clinical Thinking: Identify Insulinoma Protocol

In an emergency situation, would feeding a ferret with an insulinoma sugary food such as corn syrup help or hurt the ferret? Why?

____
____
____
____

Exercise 26

Clinical Thinking: Case Study—Feline Diabetes Mellitus

Mr. Greene has brought his cat, Boots, to the clinic today (Fig. 10.19A). He is worried because Boots has lost weight. You place Boots on the scale, and sure enough he has lost 5 lbs since his examination 6 months ago. Upon obtaining a history from Mr. Greene, you discover that Boots is eating more, drinking more, and urinating more than usual. You obtain blood and urine samples for routine testing. The next day, the veterinarian informs you that Boots has diabetes mellitus and reviews the lab work with you.

What glucose abnormalities in the blood and in the urine were found in the test results that indicated Boots has diabetes mellitus?

1. ____

____

2. ____

____

The doctor asks you to schedule an appointment with Mr. Greene to explain the disease and show him how to administer the prescribed insulin injections that Boots will need twice a day for the rest of his life.

Why will insulin given as an injectable drug help treat diabetes mellitus?

3. ____

____

____

____

____

After 2 weeks of receiving insulin injections, Boots returns to have his blood glucose levels checked throughout the day to see how he is responding to the insulin. The normal blood glucose range in the cat is 70 to 150 mg/dL. After receiving his morning insulin, Boots' blood glucose results are:

9 a.m.: 600 mg/dL

12 p.m.: 550 mg/dL

3 p.m.: 536 mg/dL

6 p.m.: 540 mg/dL

4. Based on these results, is Boots getting too much or too little insulin?__________________

The doctor adjusts Boots' insulin dose appropriately. Two weeks later, Boots is back again to have his levels checked. After receiving his morning insulin, Boots' blood glucose results are:

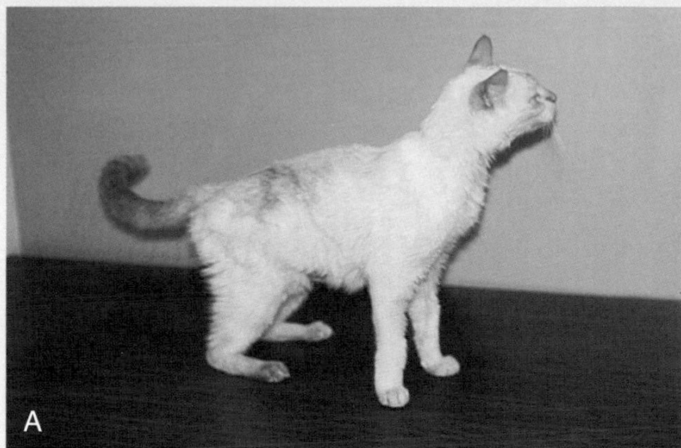

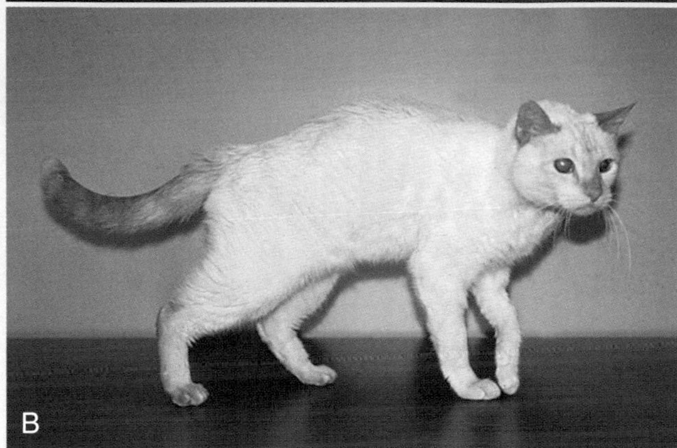

• Fig. 10.19 (A) "Boots" at initial exam. (B) "Boots" following treatment for diabetes mellitus.

9 a.m.: 120 mg/dL

12 p.m.: 101 mg/dL

3 p.m.: 60 mg/dL

6 p.m.: 42 mg/dL

5. Based on these results, is Boots getting too much or too little insulin?__________________

After a few more visits, the proper dose of insulin is achieved, and Boots' blood glucose levels are normalizing. Fig. 10.19B shows Boots after 6 months of treatment.

Other Endocrine Tissues

Exercise 27

Critical Thinking: Identify True and False Statements

________ A deficiency in erythropoietin caused by kidney failure leads to anemia.

________ Secretin helps to maintain the acidic environment of the stomach.

________ In the female, once fertilization has occurred, the ovaries release large amounts of chorionic gonadotropin to help maintain the pregnancy.

________ Melatonin helps to maintain the body's cyclic activities.

________ CCK and gastrin slow gastric motility.

Exercise 28

Clinical Thinking: Identify and Label the Glands of the Endocrine System

Identify and label the glands of the endocrine system.

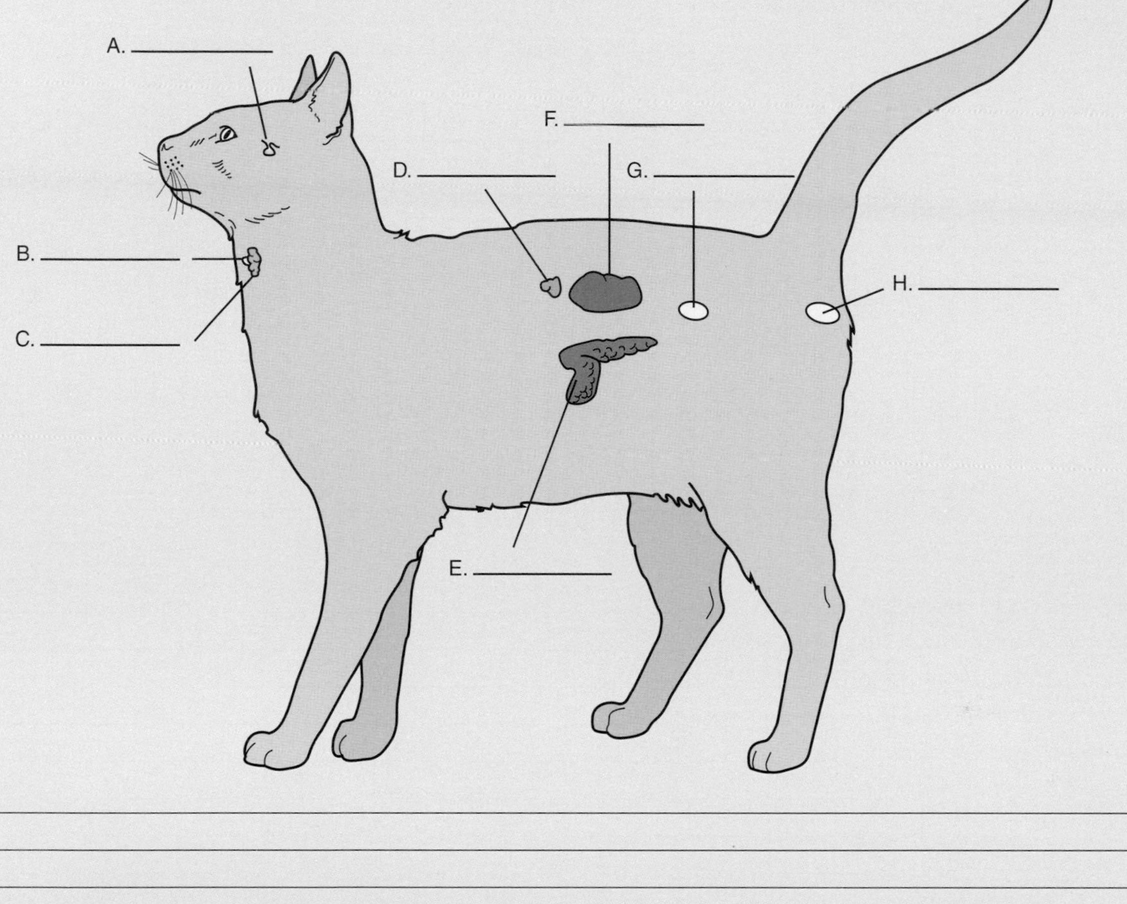

A. ______________________________

B. ______________________________

C. ______________________________

D. ______________________________

E. ______________________________

F. ______________________________

G. ______________________________

H. ______________________________

Exercise 29

Clinical Thinking: Identify Hormones Released by the Endocrine Glands

Using your answers A–H from Exercise 28, place the correct letter of the endocrine gland that releases the hormones listed below:

________ ACTH	________ Aldosterone	________ ADH
________ Calcitonin	________ Calcitriol	________ Cortisol
________ Epinephrine	________ Erythropoietin	________ Estrogen
________ FSH	________ Glucagon	________ GH
________ Insulin	________ LH	________ MSH
________ Norepinephrine	________ Oxytocin	________ PTH
________ Progesterone	________ Prolactin	________ Testosterone
________ T_3	________ T_4	________ TSH

Exercise 30

Clinical Thinking: Identify Diseases Associated With the Endocrine System

Find the answers in the word search.

Word Search for Exercise 30

```
R Y L B R W H Y O A T V B J R D R A G L P A N J S
A Y R I Y X Y S M Y Q K R X W P N D Q Y H M T E Y
V E W T J R K B H A M O N I L U S N I Q X P P O B
T D N K A R Y B J U B V W J L N F M I D S C Y C G
F I K H X A E M O R D N Y S S G N I H S U C X N O
F E X J E G V C M X I U N R U C R C G K I Q D K D
H Y P E R P A R A T H Y R O I D I S M T J S O T K
U A D H H E H P U H B H Q O A T L R Q O E U G W Q
C G D N A M F K W G H C D F M F M H M L W D U F D
Q C C D Q R C R Y P E W M F B Q Y G D P W I E M A
I L W O I X L E C R I C K Y O P K W U N I P E S G
R X F R H S E U F I G W A D E I P F C T P I N I W
W U D U B F O M F J H B O R Y S P N Q V P S H D I
V I C W E J V N F U Q S T T R Q J U D K Q N C I Q
P V A E A I B J S Y R H C O G D I F B N R I P O Q
J G K R O R H V L D Y I J U J G F N P R Y S I R W
U I L N S C F A M R I P J K I G K T Y R K E E Y E
L W M S Y W G I O R H S A P R M B F U T I T W H S
R O C R M E W I S B O X E M F U F M U W A E I T O
M P A U M L D Y R M W G A A O Y P T R M O B I O E
A U X O I I S U T T M Y F I S U L S K C Q A T P Q
R U R A S T N J M O B M A G N E U I T N H I G Y Y
Q C F M E X B R T N W J O V U Q M F U E U D J H H
A E S Y Y X T A C Y V U K T A M P C R U O Y R Q X
D K S U T I L L E M S E T E B A I D V H D X J L V
```

Key

A deficiency of insulin (two words) ____________________

An excess of adrenal cortex hormones (two words) ____________________

A deficiency of thyroid hormone ____________________

A deficiency of adrenal cortex hormones (two words) ____________________

A tumor that produces too much insulin ____________________

An excess of thyroid hormone ____________________

An excess of PTH ____________________

A deficiency of ADH (two words) ____________________

A deficiency of growth hormone ____________________

An excess of growth hormone ____________________

11 Blood, Lymph, and Lymph Nodes

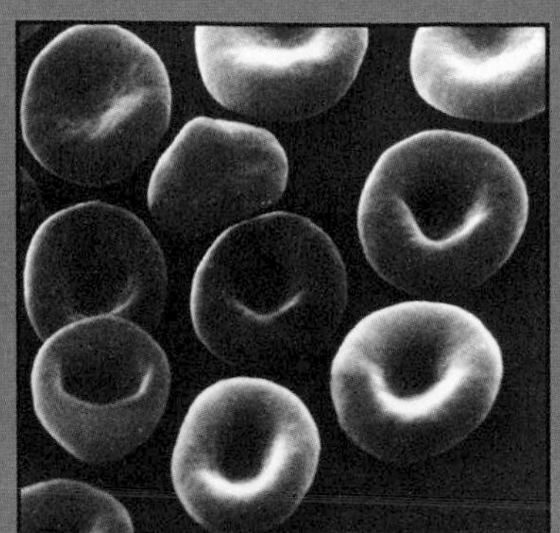

OVERVIEW AT A GLANCE

The CBC: A Veterinary Technician's Responsibilities 286

The Blood Smear 287

Hematology Stains 287

Transfusions 288

Immunoassays 291

Exercises 293–298

The CBC: A Veterinary Technician's Responsibilities 293–294

1. *Clinical Thinking I: Blood Draw Checklist 293*
2. *Clinical Thinking II: Lab Procedures for Processing Blood 294*

The Blood Smear 294–295

3. *Content Assessment of a Spun Microhematocrit Tube 294*
4. *Content Assessment of a Stained Blood Smear 295*

Hematology Stains 295–296

5. *Clinical Thinking III: Identify the Blood Component and Testing Elements 295*
6. *Identify Function, Shape, Staining, and Site of Action of White Blood Cells 296*

Transfusions: Blood Types or Groups 296–297

7. *Clinical Thinking IV: Transfusions and Blood Types 296*

Transfusions: Crossmatch Testing 297

8. *Clinical Thinking Versus Crossmatch Testing 297*

Immunoassays 297

9. *Clinical Thinking Challenge 297*

LEARNING OBJECTIVES

When you have completed this chapter, you will understand the importance of accurate blood analyses and the techniques involved, the importance of blood typing for transfusions, the need for crossmatching to detect the presence of antigen and antibodies in blood, and the use of immunoassays to detect the presence of disease antigens or antibodies against the antigens of an infected animal.

CLINICAL SIGNIFICANCE

Blood is a good indicator of what is going on in an animal. If an animal's liver is damaged, enzymes that are normally found inside liver cells will spill into the blood, raising the blood level of the enzyme. If the pancreas is not producing enough of the hormone insulin to metabolize glucose, the blood glucose levels will rise, and diabetes mellitus can develop. When the kidney is not adequately getting rid of waste material such as urea (normally excreted in the urine), increased urea levels will show up in the blood. An animal suffering from acute inflammation will have increased numbers of neutrophils in its blood as the neutrophils use the blood to travel to the site of inflammation. An animal that has slowly lost a lot of blood internally or externally may suffer from anemia, and the red blood cell numbers and morphology could indicate whether the red bone marrow is keeping up with red blood cell production to cover the loss.

For these reasons and many more, a blood sample mirrors the state of health of an animal. So, if you are asked to draw a blood sample and analyze it for its various components, or you are asked to transport a blood sample to a laboratory for analysis, you are responsible for the overall quality of the sample.

In an animal, blood is a living fluid. Once blood leaves an animal, the animal begins to change because it slowly begins to die. It had living components (the blood cells) when they left the animal and, without the constant supply of essential nutrients found in systemic blood, the cells begin to die in the tube. Also, some of the substances in the plasma will begin to break down. It is important to handle in vitro blood (blood removed from the body) in a manner that will keep it as close as possible to the in vivo blood (blood left in the animal).

- If you want a serum sample, make sure the blood goes into a plain tube and not one containing an anticoagulant. When using a vacuum tube system, this would most often be a red-top tube.
- If you want a plasma sample, make sure the blood is immediately placed into a tube with an anticoagulant. When using a vacuum tube system, this would most often be a purple/lavender-top tube (ethylenediaminetetraacetic acid, EDTA) or a green-top tube (heparin). Blood starts to clot as soon as it leaves the body when it is not mixed with an anticoagulant.
- If possible, blood smears to be used for the analysis of the blood cells need to be made immediately following the blood draw, before the blood goes into an anticoagulant. Smears cannot be made from blood that has been allowed to clot because the blood cells are trapped in the clot.

CLINICAL SIGNIFICANCE—cont'd

- Separate the cells from the plasma as soon as possible. Cells are living objects and obtain their nutrients, especially glucose, from plasma. If cells are allowed to sit in the plasma for too long, they may utilize some of the nutrients, for example, glucose, resulting in a lower glucose level in the in vitro plasma than in the in vivo plasma.
- Analyze the blood as soon as possible. Refrigerate or freeze the plasma or serum if you cannot do it right away. Refrigerate whole blood, but do not freeze it. Freezing and thawing will rupture the blood cells.

INTRODUCTION

Without blood, there would be no life. As a veterinary technician, you will be drawing, handling, and analyzing blood on a daily basis. It is important that you complete all these tasks correctly. In this chapter, you will learn what makes blood so important and how your actions when dealing with a patient's blood can directly affect the patient's health.

Blood is the transport system of the body. It carries cells, nutrients, hormones, enzymes, chemicals, drugs, proteins, and waste materials to and from all areas of the body. And yet, to look at it, all you see is a red, opaque liquid. That's because everything blood carries, except the cells, is dissolved in the liquid portion of blood, plasma.

MATERIALS NEEDED

Animal blood
Slides
Latex gloves
Laboratory goggles
Microscope
Diff-Quick (or another rapid dipping stain)
Manual Wright's stain (or the equivalent)
Spun microhematocrit tube

TERMS TO BE IDENTIFIED

Before you can work with blood, you must understand a few key terms and principles relating to blood.

- **Whole blood** is blood as it is flowing through the animal's body and blood as it leaves the animal's body before it is put in an anticoagulant. It contains plasma and cellular components.
- **Plasma** is the liquid portion of whole blood after the blood cells have been removed. If a whole blood sample is allowed to sit with an anticoagulant added, it will not clot (Fig. 11.1). The cells will settle to the bottom of the sample tube and a clear, colorless to light yellow fluid will remain. This is plasma. When the sample is gently mixed, the cells will go back into suspension.
- **Serum** is not found in a natural state in an animal's circulatory system. It is the liquid portion of whole blood if no anticoagulant is added to a blood sample. The blood sample is allowed to clot after it has been removed from the animal's body. The clot is made up of the cells of whole blood; the remaining fluid is serum. The clot that has formed holds the cells together in the clot. If the sample is gently mixed, the cells will not go back into suspension because they are trapped in the clot.
- The difference between plasma and serum is the presence or absence of **clotting factors**. Clotting factors are proteins and other chemicals normally dissolved in the plasma portion of whole blood. Once activated, the clotting factors work together to clot blood. In the animal, this is important when a blood vessel is damaged and blood leaks out of the vessel. Clotting factors create a plug (scab on the external surface) that stops blood from leaving the blood vessel. Without clotting factors, no plug would form, and blood would continually seep out of the vessel.

  When a blood sample has clotted in a syringe or test tube, the clotting factors are removed from the plasma. They can't be replaced because there is no source of fresh blood. The fluid that remains after the clotting process is completed is serum.
- The **cellular component** of whole blood is made up of erythrocytes (RBCs, red blood cells), leukocytes (WBCs, white blood cells), and thrombocytes (platelets).

The CBC: A Veterinary Technician's Responsibilities

"The buck stops here!" That saying is especially true when discussing the role the veterinary technician plays in producing results from the tests that make up the complete blood count (CBC). Below is a list of responsibilities with some questions you need to ask yourself and some pitfalls you may encounter:

- Obtaining the blood sample. If you are the person responsible for drawing the blood sample, consider the following:
  - Do you have the correct animal? Check. Then double check.
  - Do you have all the supplies you need to draw the blood sample before you start the procedure?
  - Which vein are you going to use? How much blood do you need? How much serum/plasma can you harvest from the blood sample?

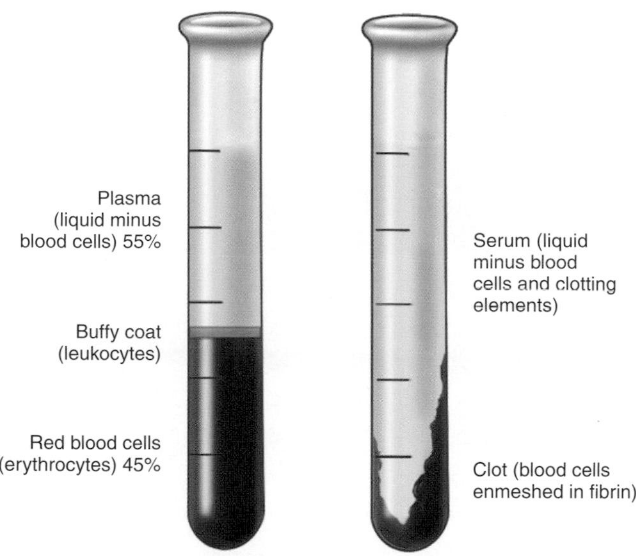

• **FIG. 11.1** Difference between blood plasma and blood serum. (From Patton K, Thibodeau G: *Anatomy & physiology*, ed. 8, St Louis, 2013, Mosby.)

- Do you have someone to restrain the animal? Do not ask or rely on clients to do this. Use trained personnel.
- If you are using a needle and syringe to draw the sample, have an EDTA tube (purple-top Vacutainer tube) available to put the blood in as soon as it is drawn. Gently mix the blood with the anticoagulant. Label the tube with at least the patient's name and the date.
- Make sure the blood sample gets to the laboratory as quickly as possible. Any delay can affect the final analytical results.

- The blood sample. After you have the blood sample in the lab:
  - Make sure it is in EDTA if you are using the sample for a CBC.
  - Make at least five blood smears right away. Blood that has been in EDTA for a long time may have cellular morphology and staining issues. Label everything, including the smears.
  - If you can't stain the smears right away, fix them in a methanol fixative. You do not have to stain all five smears at one time. Stain two smears and save the other three (make sure they are fixed) in case you need to reevaluate the smear.
  - Complete the analyses of the blood sample and smears. This can be done manually or by an automated hematology analyzer. Do not forget to include units of measure for the tests.
  - Check your results for obvious errors. If something does not look right, try to figure out why or repeat the test.
  - Report your results to the veterinarian. He or she is going to trust you and depend on you to provide accurate results. The results are used to help diagnose an illness, plan a course of treatment, or provide a prognosis for the outcome of the illness.

The Blood Smear

Automated hematology instruments in some veterinary practices are used to evaluate the blood sample. If used and maintained properly, these instruments can save time and provide accurate results. Some of these instruments will report up to 22 parameters and a five-part differential count of the white blood cells. But these instruments do not have eyes to see the morphology of the cells. They may give you numbers, but you have no idea whether the cells that were counted are normal or abnormal cells. For that, you have to look at a stained blood smear. It is a good idea to remain competent in manually evaluating a blood sample even if you are using an automated hematology instrument. Eventually the instrument will be out of commission for some reason, and you will have to perform manual tests. When this happens, you can get a lot of information from a spun hematocrit tube (packed cell volume, PCV) and evaluation of a stained blood smear.

- The hematocrit tube will show a relative red blood cell count by the height of the packed red blood cells. The width of the buffy coat on top of the packed red blood cells will indicate a relative white blood cell count. The color and height of the plasma layer will show the presence of jaundice, lipemia, and dehydration. Although you don't have actual values, you can see relative abnormalities.
- From the stained blood smear, you can estimate the total white blood cell count, do a differential white blood cell count, evaluate the morphology of the red blood cells and white blood cells, evaluate platelet numbers and morphology, and look for blood parasites or other foreign organisms.

A good blood smear will have distinct regions (Fig. 11.2A): the body, the counting area, and the feathered edge (see Fig. 11.2B and D). The counting area is where the cells are spaced so that you can evaluate the morphology of the red and white blood cells and count the white blood cells. In this area, the red blood cells are close together, but not clumped or overlapping, and the white blood cells are evenly spaced. In the body of the smear, the red blood cells are too cramped so their morphology can't be analyzed, and the white blood cells are compressed by the cramped red blood cells. In the feathered edge, all the cells are spaced too far apart, and the white blood cells and the red blood cells tend to form clumps.

Hematology Stains

Most blood smears are stained with a Romanowsky-type hematology stain. Dr. Romanowsky discovered his original stain in 1891. He was looking for a way to stain malarial parasites in blood, and when he developed the stain, he noticed it also stained white blood cells very clearly. So, the Romanowsky stain became the standard hematology stain until 1902, when Drs. Wright and Giemsa separately made improvements to the stain. This resulted in two Romanowsky-type stains, Wright's stain and Giemsa stain.

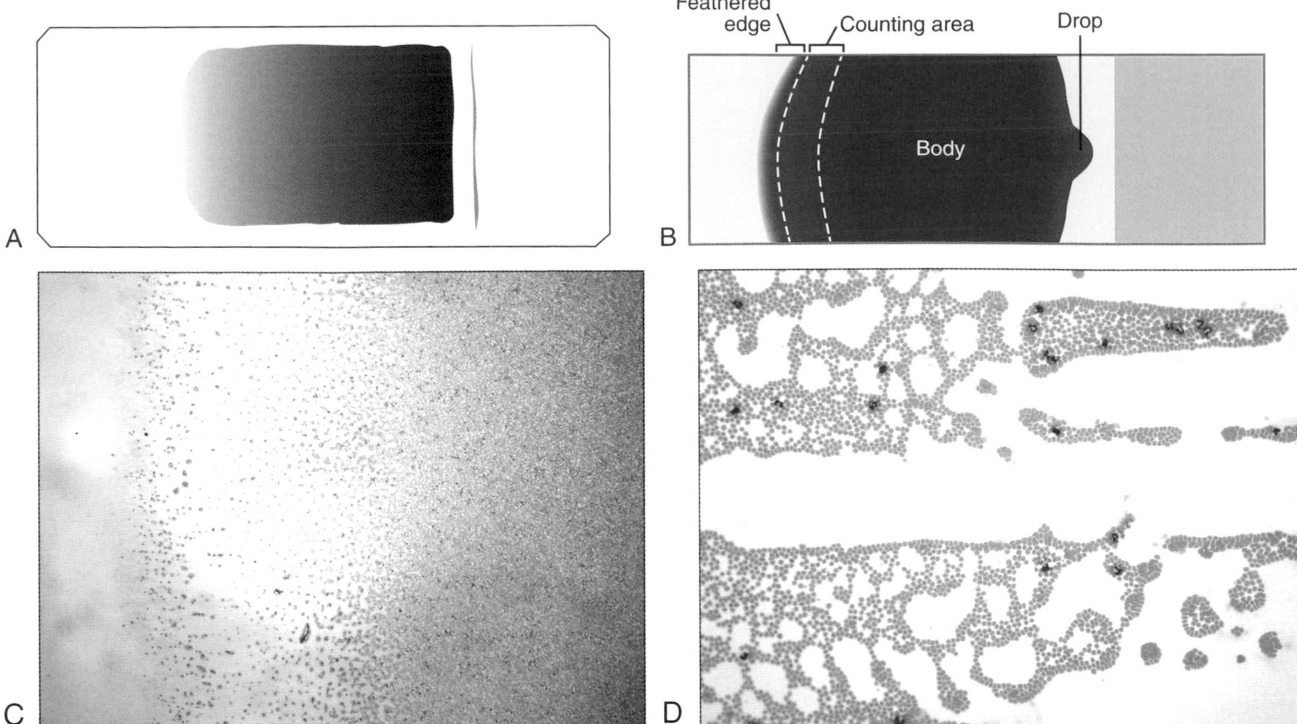

• **FIG. 11.2** (A) Well-made peripheral blood film. (B) Regions of a blood smear. (C) Feathered edge (left side of smear) of a blood smear (10×). (D) Feathered edge of a blood smear (40×). (**A,** From Rodak BF: *Hematology: clinical principles and applications*, ed. 4, Philadelphia, 2012, Saunders. **B,** From Bassert J, Thomas J: *McCurnin's clinical textbook for veterinary technicians*, ed. 8, Philadelphia, 2014, Saunders. **C** and **D,** From Valenciano A, et al: *Atlas of canine and feline peripheral blood smears*, St Louis, 2014, Mosby.)

There are other Romanowsky-type stains, but Wright's and Giemsa are the two most commonly used.

The Romanowsky stain is based on the basic stain, methylene blue. With the addition of an acidic stain, usually eosin, a polychromatophilic stain is produced. The basic or alkaline (cationic) stain, methylene blue, stains basophilic structures that contain RNA and DNA blue (i.e., the nucleus and some cytoplasmic inclusions and structures such as basophil granules; Fig. 11.3). The acidic (anionic) stain, eosin, stains proteins with amino groups red–orange (i.e., hemoglobin and some cytoplasmic structures, especially eosinophil granules; Fig. 11.4). Do you see the connection between the name of the cell and the stain that stains its granules?

If a structure is stained by both the basic and acidic stains, a light purple/pink color develops. This is a neutrophilic reaction. The granules of a neutrophil stain with a neutrophilic reaction (Fig. 11.5). Do you see that same connection?

There are commercially available reagents and kits for manual techniques using Wright's stain, Giemsa stain, and Wright–Giemsa stain. The staining process takes about 15 minutes plus drying time, so there is a delay in being able to evaluate the smear. Some clinics use automated slide stainers for consistent staining quality.

Commercially available staining systems are available that provide more rapid staining (less than a minute, plus drying time) than the standard Romanowsky-type stains. These systems involve dipping a blood smear in a fixative, followed by dips in an acidic stain, a basic stain, and a buffer. Although the staining quality for fine detail is not as good as with the standard Romanowsky-type stains, these systems allow you to look at a smear in a shorter amount of time.

Transfusions

A transfusion is defined as an infusion of donated blood, blood products, or other fluids. Most animals will go through their entire lives without receiving a transfusion. However, there are instances when transfusions are necessary and can save an animal's life. Whole blood transfusions are generally used in emergency situations when blood is needed immediately. For example, a dog may be hit by a car and have its spleen ruptured. This results in massive *internal* abdominal bleeding. Even though most of the blood will eventually be reabsorbed (autotransfusion), the dog may have lost enough blood that it needs an immediate whole blood transfusion just to maintain adequate tissue perfusion to keep it alive. As another example, a horse may have a traumatic injury that results in massive *external* bleeding. In this situation, the blood is lost and cannot be reabsorbed, as with internal bleeding. Again, a blood trans-

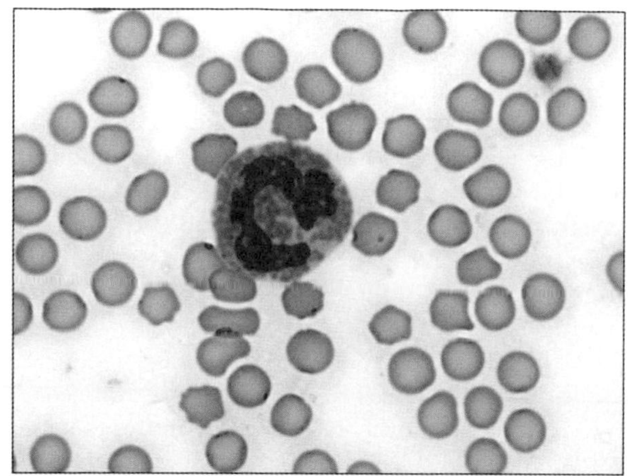
A

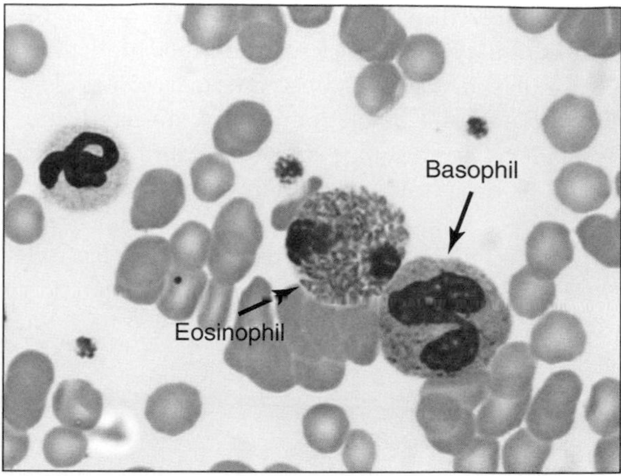

B

• **FIG. 11.3** (A) A basophil with blue staining granules (1000×). (B) Compare the staining characteristics of the granules of an eosinophil and a basophil. (From Valenciano A, et al: *Atlas of canine and feline peripheral blood smears*, St Louis, 2014, Mosby.)

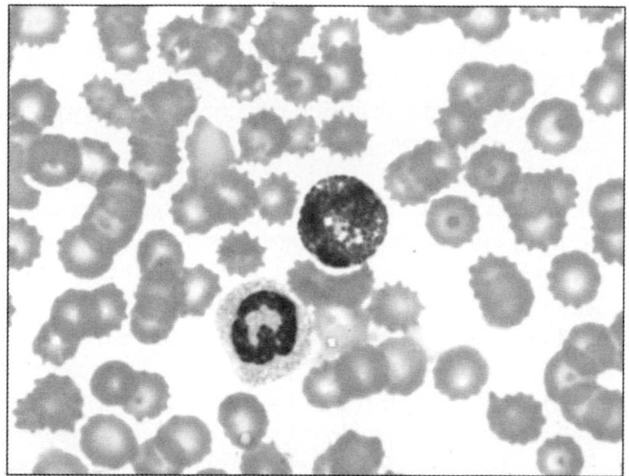

• **FIG. 11.4** Eosinophil with red–orange staining granules (1000×). (From Valenciano A, et al: *Atlas of canine and feline peripheral blood smears*, St Louis, 2014, Mosby.)

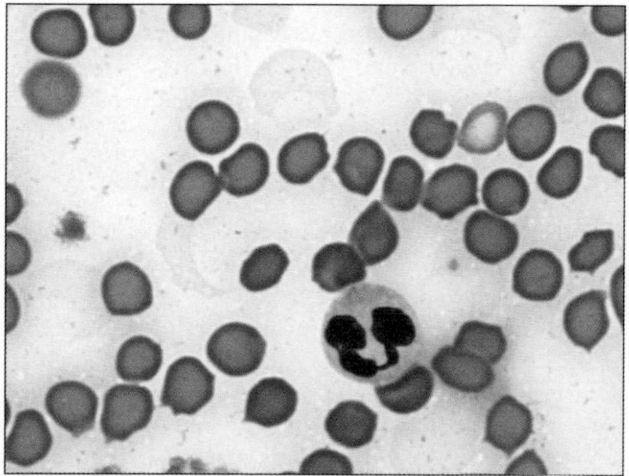

• **FIG. 11.5** Neutrophil with light purple/pink staining granules (1000×). (From Valenciano A, et al: *Atlas of canine and feline peripheral blood smears*, St Louis, 2014, Mosby.)

fusion may be necessary to maintain tissue perfusion and save the horse's life.

There are also predictable situations when transfusions can be planned. For example, an animal being treated for chronic kidney failure may need regular blood transfusions. The kidneys are the source of the hormone erythropoietin that tells the bone marrow to make red blood cells. If there is no hormonal stimulation, the bone marrow will not make red blood cells and the animal becomes anemic. Animals receiving chemotherapy may also need transfusions if the drugs used to treat the cancer adversely affect the bone marrow.

Nowadays, planned transfusions may involve transfusion of blood components rather than whole blood. This reduces the chance of a transfusion reaction and replaces only the component the patient needs. For example, packed red blood cells can be transfused into patients with nonlife-threatening anemia or bone marrow disorders. Fresh whole blood is centrifuged to separate the red blood cells and plasma. The red blood cells are harvested to produce a concentrated (hematocrit ~80%) solution that is transfused into the patient.

Plasma alone can be transfused into animals with diseases that affect clotting. Plasma contains the clotting factors that will help control hemorrhage during and after an injury or surgical procedure.

Platelet-rich plasma can be transfused into patients with uncontrolled bleeding or decreased platelet numbers or function. Platelets are found in the buffy coat of a centrifuged whole blood sample. After centrifugation, the plasma and buffy coat are harvested and transfused. This solution contains the clotting factors in plasma as well as platelets, both of which are necessary to control hemorrhage.

Whatever solution or blood component is going to be transfused, a donor animal will most likely be necessary. As of this writing (2017), there are only six commercial blood banks for domestic animals in the United States. There is a time factor involved in receiving blood from one of these blood banks so in an emergency situation they probably will not be of much help. A very busy veterinary practice may keep whole blood and blood components on hand in case of an emergency. But there are strict protocols for collecting and storing blood and blood products for transfusion that must be followed. Many veterinary facilities do not have the capability to do this. A typical veterinary practice has to rely on donor animals to provide the blood or blood components needed. However, not just any animal can be a donor animal.

Blood Types or Groups

Do you know your blood type? Do you know your cat's blood type? Or your horse's? Or your dog's? Just like humans, animals have blood types that are unique to their species. Blood types (also known as blood groups) are inherited species-specific antigens found on red blood cell surfaces. When transfusing blood, you want to make sure the blood you are giving (donor blood) is compatible with the recipient's blood. For example, an animal has antigen X on its red blood cells. Antigen X is recognized by its body as "self" and it does not produce antibodies against antigen X. If your donor animal also has antigen X on its red blood cells, and you transfuse donor blood into the recipient, the recipient's body will recognize the donated blood as "self," also. Nothing happens to the donated red blood cells and the transfusion is successful.

If your donor animal has Y antigens on its red blood cells and not X antigens, and you transfuse donor blood into the recipient with X antigens, the recipient's body will detect the "foreign" Y antigens and produce antibodies against those red blood cells that have Y antigens on their cell membranes. Because it takes time to produce the antibodies against antigen Y, the donor blood from the first transfusion is not affected. However, the recipient animal has been sensitized to antigen Y, and, if it receives another transfusion of blood with antigen Y on the red blood cells more than 4 weeks after the first transfusion, there will be a memory immune response against antigen Y and antibodies will appear almost immediately, resulting in hemolysis of the red blood cells in the transfused blood.

Dogs have anywhere from 7 to 13 blood types depending on how they are classified. The most common antigens are called DEA (dog erythrocyte antigen) 1.1, 1.2, 1.3, 3, 4, 5, 6, 7, and 8. The DEA 1.X antigens are the most antigenic and cause the most severe transfusion reactions. Dogs that are DEA 4 positive and DEA 1.1, 1.2, 1.3, 3, 5, and 7 negative are universal donors. Their blood can be safely transfused to any dog no matter its blood type.

Cats have three blood types. The antigens are called A, B, and AB. Type A cats make up about 97% of the feline population in the United States. Type B cats are usually purebred exotic breeds (Persian, Birman, Himalayan, Abyssinian, Somali, Devon rex, British shorthair, Cornish rex, Scottish fold) and make up about 2% of the cat population in the United States. Type AB cats are rare and make up only 1% of the cat population in the United States. Cats do not have to be sensitized to noncompatible blood to develop a transfusion reaction. They have naturally preformed antibodies. Type B cats have very strong reactions against type A blood. Type A cats have a milder reaction against type B blood. Type AB blood is the most antigenic.

Horses have eight blood types, designated by letters. The antigens are A, C, D, K, P, Q, U, and T. Antigens A, C, and Q are the most antigenic; therefore horses that are negative for antigens A, C, and Q make the best donor horses.

Cattle have 11 major blood groups. The antigens are A, B, C, F, J, L, M, R, S, T, and Z. Some of the antigens have subgroups. The A and F antigens are the most antigenic. Sheep have seven blood groups. The antigens are A, B, C, D, M, R, and X. Goats have five blood groups that are similar to sheep blood groups. The antigens are A, B, C, M, and J.

There are numerous reasons for knowing the blood type of an animal:

- To prevent blood transfusion reactions. Animals with the same blood type can safely be transfused.
- To identify potential blood donors. In emergency situations, you may not have time to blood type the patient. Knowing animals that may be universal donors is helpful in these situations.
- To prevent neonatal isoerythrolysis (NI). This is a condition in foals and kittens that results in destruction of their red blood cells after receiving colostrum rich in antibodies against their red blood cells from their mothers. A mare could have produced these antibodies as a result of a previous transfusion or transplacental exposure to a different blood type during a previous pregnancy. In cats, NI can be a problem if a type B queen is bred to a type A tom and type A kittens are born. The queen's colostrum will be naturally high in antibodies against type A red blood cell antigens. When the kittens receive the colostrum, they also receive the antibodies that will destroy their red blood cells. In the case of either a foal or kittens, they are born apparently healthy but develop clinical signs after nursing. If left untreated, the newborns will die. In cats, this is known as the "fading kitten syndrome."
- To determine parentage. For example, two type A cats could not produce a type B cat. Cattle breeders also use blood typing to determine parentage.

There are commercially available kits for blood typing dog (DEA 1.1) and cat (types A, B, and AB) blood (Rapid Vet-H Feline and Canine Blood Typing) (Fig. 11.6). Many veterinary practices now offer blood typing as part of a new puppy or kitten examination. This becomes part of the animal's permanent record so, if it ever needs a transfusion, its blood type is already known.

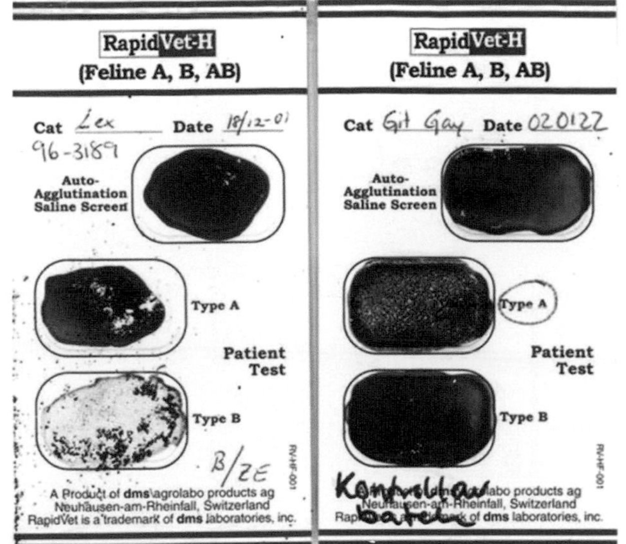

• **FIG. 11.6** Blood typing is very important before blood transfusion, especially in cats. (From Willard MD, Tvedten H: *Small animal clinical diagnosis by laboratory methods*, ed. 5, Philadelphia, 2012, Saunders.)

Crossmatch Testing

If a transfusion is necessary and the blood types of both the donor and the recipient are known, the transfusion can proceed without further testing. If, however, the blood type of the recipient and/or donor is not known, a crossmatch test must be performed before the transfusion can begin. A crossmatch test is used to detect incompatibility between donor and recipient blood.

To perform a crossmatch test, EDTA blood samples are obtained from both the donor and the recipient. Both samples are centrifuged to separate the cells from the plasma. The plasma is removed from each sample and placed in a separate clean, dry test tube. The samples must be labeled so the recipient's plasma and cells and the donor's plasma and cells are clearly identified. The packed red blood cells are removed from the bottom of each collection tube and placed in separate, clearly labeled, clean, dry test tubes. The red blood cells in each tube are washed five times in sterile, normal saline. After the final wash, the saline is decanted and a weak (2% to 4%) suspension of red blood cells is made with additional saline. You now have four clearly labeled tubes: donor plasma, washed donor red blood cells in a 2% to 4% suspension, recipient plasma, and washed recipient red blood cells in a 2% to 4% suspension.

A major crossmatch test involves putting a specified amount of the donor's washed red blood cell suspension in the recipient's plasma and incubated at room temperature for 30 minutes. If the cells stay in suspension without clumping, the donor's blood and recipient's blood are compatible and the transfusion can begin. If the red blood cells hemolyze macroscopically (you'll see red plasma) or clump together (hemagglutination) microscopically, the blood is not compatible, and the donor should not be used for the transfusion. A minor crossmatch test involves putting the recipient's red blood cells in the donor's plasma.

In emergency situations, the repeated cell washings and 30-minute incubation period may not be practical, so a slide crossmatch can be performed. In a major slide crossmatch, two drops of recipient plasma are mixed with one drop of blood from the potential donor on a clean glass slide. The slide is rotated at room temperature for 1 minute to look for signs of agglutination or clumping. If agglutination occurs, the blood is incompatible. The major drawback to this method is that potentially fatal hemolytic reactions will be missed.

The minor slide crossmatch test is performed in the same way but using two drops of potential donor plasma and one drop of recipient blood.

Using incompatible blood for transfusion can result in fatal acute hemolysis in the recipient. The signs may appear as soon as the transfusion begins and include fever, decreased blood pressure, altered heart rate, difficulty breathing, loss of bowel control, loss of bladder control, renal failure, shock, and death.

Immunoassays

Just as the crossmatch test is based on the presence of antigen and antibodies in blood samples, there are many other tests that rely on the presence of disease antigens or antibodies against the antigens that have infected an animal. If an animal gets sick and the veterinarian suspects a specific disease, for example, a cat that has been infected with the feline immunodeficiency virus (FIV), the cat's blood can be tested for the presence of antibodies against FIV. This is the basis of immunoassay testing.

- An immunoassay test is based on the formation of an antigen–antibody complex when antibodies and antigens are combined.
- In most clinical situations, immunoassays are performed using commercially available immunoassay kits.
- Commercial immunoassay kits are available for detection of either specific antibodies (antibody tests) or specific antigens (antigen tests) in a patient's blood.
- The most sensitive and specific immunoassays are primary binding tests. These are tests that detect a specific antigen or antibody directly. An example of a primary binding test is an enzyme-linked immunosorbent assay (ELISA). When performing an ELISA, wells are coated with either a specific antibody or antigen. The patient's serum is added to the well. If there is an antigen–antibody complex formed, it will stay in the well when the wells are rinsed. The amount of complex formed is measured by adding an enzyme complex that will combine with the antigen–antibody complex in the well. When the

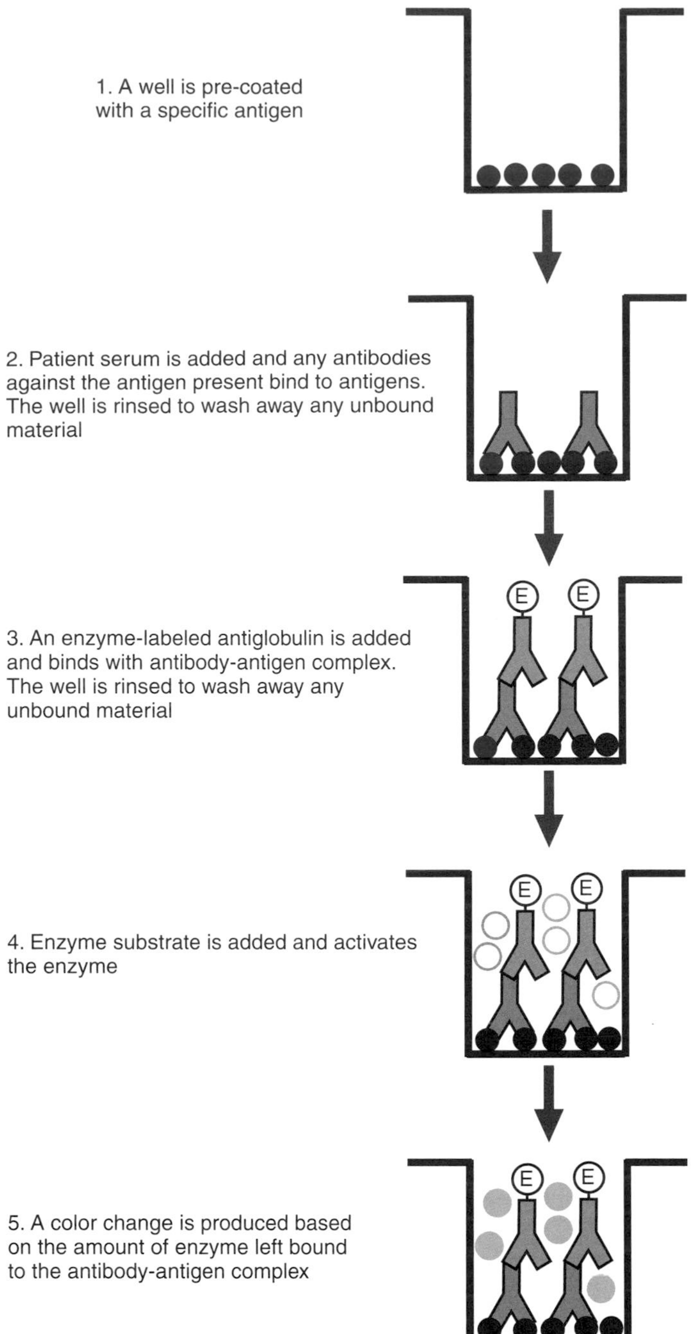

1. A well is pre-coated with a specific antigen
2. Patient serum is added and any antibodies against the antigen present bind to antigens. The well is rinsed to wash away any unbound material
3. An enzyme-labeled antiglobulin is added and binds with antibody-antigen complex. The well is rinsed to wash away any unbound material
4. Enzyme substrate is added and activates the enzyme
5. A color change is produced based on the amount of enzyme left bound to the antibody-antigen complex
E

• **FIG. 11.7** The indirect ELISA technique. Antigen is bound to the wells in a styrene plate. (From Tizard, I: *Veterinary immunology*, ed. 9, Philadelphia, 2013, Saunders.)

enzyme substrate is added to the well, a color will develop. The degree of color development is proportional to the amount of antigen–antibody complex in the well (Fig. 11.7).

- The principle of the ELISA is also used in in-practice immunoassay test kits that detect a specific antigen or antibody (e.g., ImmunoComb or SNAP tests). In these kits, the antigen or antibody is fixed to a membrane, the patient's serum, plasma, or whole blood is added, and a rapid reaction occurs at a designated area of the strip if the test is positive (Fig. 11.8).
- Secondary binding tests are easier to perform but are less sensitive than primary binding tests. These tests measure the results of antigen–antibody complex formation. Examples include precipitation and agglutination tests (Fig. 11.9).

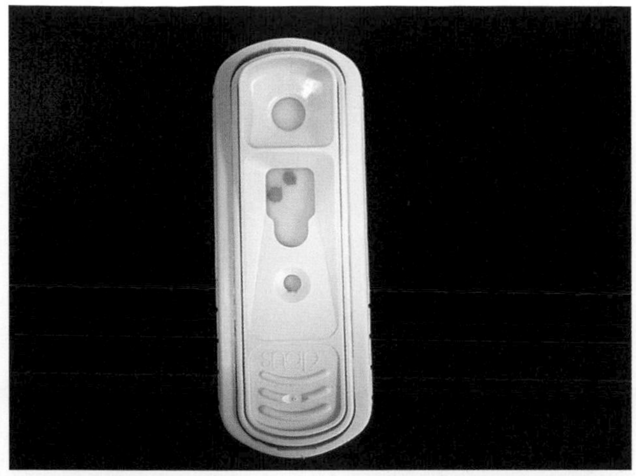

• **FIG. 11.8** A positive test result indicated on the ELISA membrane format (SNAP Test for *Ehrlichia* antibodies, IDEXX). (From Hendrix C, Sirois M: *Laboratory procedures for veterinary technicians*, ed. 5, St Louis, 2007, Mosby.)

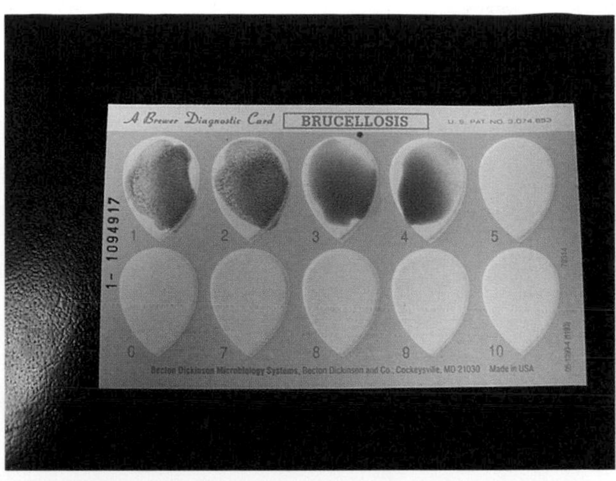

• **FIG. 11.9** Clumped latex particles representing antigen–antibody complexes. (From Hendrix C, Sirois M: *Laboratory procedures for veterinary technicians*, ed. 5, St Louis, 2007, Mosby.)

EXERCISES

The CBC: A Veterinary Technician's Responsibilities

Exercise 1

Clinical Thinking I: Blood Draw Checklist

You have been asked to create a checklist for obtaining a blood sample to establish a protocol for the practice. List the steps you would include, in the correct order, with a Y/N column for each step.

Exercise 2

Clinical Thinking II: Lab Procedures for Processing Blood

You have been asked to create a checklist for processing blood in the lab. List the steps you would include, and the correct order.

CBC:

____

Blood smear:

____

____

Staining:

____

____

Analysis:

____

____

____

____

____

Reporting:

____

The Blood Smear

Exercise 3

Content Assessment of a Spun Microhematocrit Tube

Identify the following from a spun microhematocrit tube:

- Plasma
- Serum
- Buffy coat
- Red blood cells
- Measure the packed cell volume

Determine the amount of plasma that can be harvested from a 15 mL blood sample based on the PCV ______________

Determine how much blood will have to be drawn to get 3 mL of plasma from a blood sample based on the PCV ______________

Exercise 4

Content Assessment of a Stained Blood Smear

Using prepared blood smears, stain one with Diff-Quick (or another rapid dipping stain) and another with manual Wright's stain (or the equivalent). Compare the staining results.

Identify the Following on Each of the Stained Smears:	Diff-Quik (or Another Rapid Dipping Stain)	Wright's Stain (or the Equivalent)
Red blood cells	______________	______________
White blood cells	______________	______________
Neutrophils	______________	______________
Eosinophils	______________	______________
Basophils	______________	______________
Monocytes	______________	______________
Lymphocytes	______________	______________
Platelets	______________	______________
Feathered edge of the smear	______________	______________
Counting area of the smear	______________	______________
Body of the smear	______________	______________
Estimated WBC count	______________	______________

Hematology Stains

Exercise 5

Clinical Thinking III: Identify the Blood Component and Testing Elements

Identify the blood component in each of the following "Who Am I?" statements:

1. ______________ My contents include plasma and cellular components, and I am what flows through the body and leaves the body prior to being placed in an anticoagulant.
2. ______________ I am the liquid portion of whole blood after the blood cells have been removed and am colorless to light yellow in color.
3. ______________ I am not found in a natural state in an animal's circulatory system, but I am the liquid portion of whole blood if no anticoagulant is added to a blood sample.
4. ______________ Once activated, I cooperate to form a plug to stop blood from leaving a vessel.
5. ______________ I am made up of RBCs, WBCs, and platelets.
6. ______________ When the pancreas does not produce enough of me, the blood glucose levels will rise, and diabetes mellitus can develop.
7. ______________ I can be found in great numbers in an infection.
8. ______________ I am the color topmost often found on a vacuum tube without anticoagulant, used to create a serum sample.
9. ______________ I am the color topmost often found on a vacuum tube used to make a plasma sample using heparin.
10. ______________ I am the color topmost often found on a vacuum tube used to make a plasma sample using EDTA.
11. ______________ My width on the top of the packed red cells will indicate a relative white blood cell count.
12. ______________ I was the standard hematology stain until 1902.
13. ______________ We are the two most commonly used Romanowsky-type stains.
14. ______________ In the fetus, hematopoiesis takes place in us.
15. ______________ I am the origin of all blood cells.

Continued

Exercise 5—cont'd

Clinical Thinking III: Identify the Blood Component and Testing Elements

16. ______________ I am the process by which red blood cells are created.
17. ______________ I am the production of platelets.
18. ______________ I am the process by which a pluripotential stem cell differentiates into one of three types of granulocytes.
19. ______________ Ninety percent of the destruction of senescent red blood cells occurs as a result of me.
20. ______________ I am a white blood cell.

Exercise 6

Identify Function, Shape, Staining, and Site of Action of White Blood Cells

For each of the WBCs listed, indicate the function, shape, staining, and site of action. Include all that apply.

WBC

Neutrophil ______________________

B cell ______________________

Eosinophil ______________________

T cell ______________________

Basophil ______________________

Monocyte ______________________

Function

1. Phagocytosis
2. Allergic reaction
3. Anaphylaxis
4. Antigen processing
5. Antibody production
6. Humoral immunity
7. Cytokine production
8. Cell-mediated immunity

Nuclear Shape

9. Polymorphonuclear
10. Pleomorphic
11. Mononuclear

Staining

12. Does not stain well
13. Stains red
14. Stains blue
15. Does not stain

Site of Action

16. Body tissues
17. Body tissues or blood
18. Lymphoid tissue
19. Lymphoid tissue and other body tissues

Transfusions: Blood Types or Groups

Exercise 7

Clinical Thinking IV: Transfusions and Blood Types

Identify the component in each of the following "Who Am I?" statements:

1. ______________ I am generally used in emergency situations when blood is needed immediately.
2. ______________ I only involve transfusing blood components, not whole blood.
3. ______________ When clotting is needed during or after an injury or surgical procedure, I am most often transfused.
4. ______________ When a patient has uncontrolled bleeding or decreased platelet function, I am often transfused.
5. ______________ I am the most antigenic blood type in a dog and cause the most severe transfusion reactions.
6. ______________ I am considered a universal donor blood type in a dog; I can be safely transfused into any dog no matter its blood type.
7. ______________ We are the three cat blood types.
8. ______________ My blood type makes up about 2% of the cat population.
9. ______________ We are the best horse blood type for blood donation.
10. ______________ We are the most antigenic blood types in cattle.
11. ______________ I am a condition in foals and kittens that results in destruction of the red blood cells after receiving colostrum-rich antibodies against their red blood cells from their mothers.

Transfusions: Crossmatch Testing

Exercise 8

Clinical Thinking Versus Crossmatch Testing

An injured animal has been brought to your surgery and is going to need a transfusion. You have been asked to perform a crossmatch. Detail the steps you will need to take. Indicate the type of crossmatch that will be done given the severity of the emergency situation, and the drawbacks, if any.

Immunoassays

Exercise 9

Clinical Thinking Challenge

Support each of following correct statements with appropriate rationale, stating why or in what way each statement is correct:

1. Smears cannot be made from blood that has been allowed to clot.
2. Cells must be separated from the plasma as soon as possible.
3. Whole blood can be refrigerated, but not frozen.
4. A blood sample must get to the laboratory as quickly as possible.

Continued

Exercise 9—cont'd

Clinical Thinking Challenge

5. It is a good idea to remain competent in manually evaluating a blood sample even if you use an automated hematology instrument.

6. Whatever solution or blood component is going to be transfused, a donor animal will most likely be necessary.

7. Cats do not have to be sensitized to noncompatible blood to develop a transfusion reaction.

8. There are numerous reasons for knowing the blood type of an animal.

9. One should never wipe away the blood that seeps from a venipuncture site.

10. One should always look at a stained blood smear even when using an automated analyzer.

12
The Cardiovascular System[a]

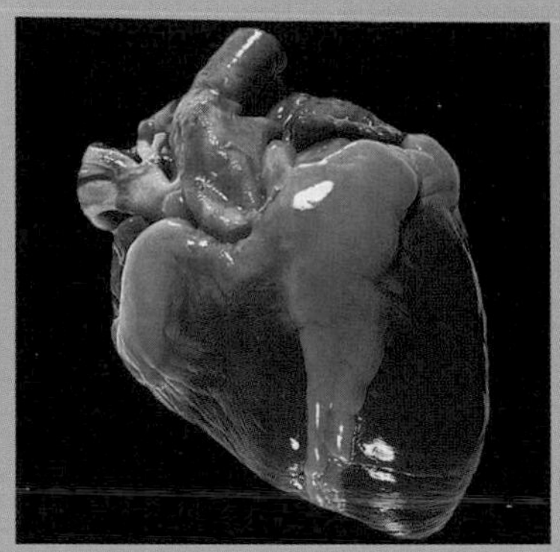

OVERVIEW AT A GLANCE

Basic Blood Flow Through the Cardiovascular System 300

Suggested In-Class Activities 315

Exercises 320–332

Basic Blood Flow Through the Cardiovascular System 320–327

1. *Identify the External Structures of the Heart 320*
2. *Identify the Structures of the Heart 321*
3. *Identify the Structures of the Heart 321*
4. *Chart the Sequence of Blood Flow 322*
5. *Trace the Flow of Blood Through the Heart 323*
6. *Identify Thoracic and Cervical Arteries and Veins 324*
7. *Identify Thoracic and Cervical Arteries and Veins 325*
8. *Identify Cardiac and Abdominal Structures 326*
9. *Identify Feline Caudal Abdominal and Proximal Hindlimb Arteries and Veins 327*
10. *Locate Veins 327*

Critical and Clinical Thinking 328–332

11. *Define Key Terms 328*
12. *Clinical Thinking Challenge 329*
13. *Identify the Cardiovascular Component 332*

LEARNING OBJECTIVES

In this chapter, we will concentrate on the heart and the major blood vessels in the body. We will also identify other blood vessels that are of clinical importance. Read Chapter 14 in *Clinical Anatomy and Physiology for Veterinary Technicians* for detailed descriptions and locations of these structures.

CLINICAL SIGNIFICANCE

As a veterinary technician, you need to understand what is normal before you can detect abnormalities. A heart with a murmur doesn't sound the same as a normal heart. You should be able to pick that up during a physical exam. You should also be able to explain to a client why her dog with congestive heart failure is coughing. And why her friend's dog with congestive heart failure due to a different cause isn't coughing but has really swollen legs.

It is also important to know which blood vessels are commonly used to collect blood samples, administer medications intravenously, or place venous or arterial catheters. When you are asked to draw a blood sample from a cat's jugular vein, you need to know where to find it. Or, when you're asked to draw an arterial sample from the carotid artery, you don't have to go running for the nearest textbook to find the location of the artery.

INTRODUCTION

The cardiovascular system is the body's internal transport system. It picks up and delivers a variety of cargo, such as nutrients, hormones, antibodies, electrolytes, waste products, and drugs, to and from all parts of the body. These various payloads are carried in the blood, which is pumped around the body by the heart.

The cardiovascular system consists of the heart and the blood vessels that carry blood from the heart to the rest of the body and then return it. The blood vessels are named according to their positions and roles in the system. Arteries carry blood outward from the heart to the extensive network of capillaries all around the body. The capillaries deliver materials to the cells and take other materials away from the cells. The veins then return the blood to the heart.

From a functional standpoint, the capillaries are the real "business end" of the cardiovascular system. It is at the capillary level that substances are actually exchanged between the blood and the cells. However, the capillaries are simply thin, porous tubes of the endothelium (simple squamous epithelium), so there is not much anatomic detail about them to learn. On the other hand, the heart has various chambers, valves, and so on that can significantly affect an animal's health and well-being if anything goes wrong with them. We will concentrate much of our examination of the cardiovascular system on the heart.

Structures of the cardiovascular system are not very obvious on external examination of an animal. Veins usually lie closer to the surface of the body than arteries do, and they have thin walls

[a] The authors and publisher wish to acknowledge Joann Colville and Amy Ellwein for previous contributions to this chapter.

INTRODUCTION—cont'd

because the blood they carry is moving along under fairly low pressure. In injected cadavers, the veins are usually filled with blue latex. Superficial veins are often used to obtain blood samples for analysis and to administer medications. Arteries usually lie deeper than veins and have thicker walls because the blood they carry is under higher pressure. The pulsations of some arteries can be palpated (felt) in specific locations where they are fairly superficial. Arteries are usually filled with red latex in injected cadavers.

TERMS TO BE IDENTIFIED

- Heart exterior
  - Aorta
  - Apex
  - Auricles—right and left
  - Base
  - Coronary vessels
  - Interventricular groove
  - Pericardial sac
  - Pulmonary artery
  - Pulmonary vein
  - Vena cava
  - Ventricles—right and left
- Heart Interior
  - Aortic valve
  - Atria—right and left
  - Chordae tendineae
  - Interatrial septum
  - Interventricular septum
  - Mitral valve
  - Myocardium
  - Pulmonary valve
  - Tricuspid valve
  - Ventricles—right and left
- Major/clinically important blood vessels
  - Aortic arch
  - Brachiocephalic trunk
  - Carotid artery
  - Caudal vena cava
  - Cephalic vein
  - Cranial vena cava
  - Femoral artery and vein
  - Iliac artery and vein
  - Jugular vein
  - Ovarian artery and vein
  - Pulmonary artery and vein
  - Renal artery and vein
  - Saphenous vein
  - Subclavian artery
  - Testicular artery and vein

MEDICAL WORD PARTS

Angi/o = blood vessel
Aort/o = aorta
Arteri/o = artery
Cardi/o = heart
Hemo/o or sanguin/o = blood
Phleb/o = vein
Ven/o = vein

Basic Blood Flow Through the Cardiovascular System

Although it appears to be one structure, the heart functions as two separate pumps, the *left* side of the heart receives oxygen-rich blood from the lungs and pumps it out through systemic arteries to capillaries in all parts of the body except the lungs. At the capillary level, oxygen moves from the blood to the cells, and carbon dioxide, produced as a waste product by the cells, moves into the blood. Systemic veins carry the now carbon dioxide-rich blood back to the *right* side of the heart, which sends it out through the pulmonary arteries to the lungs for reoxygenation. In the capillaries of the lungs, the blood dumps its carbon dioxide and takes on a new load of oxygen for delivery to the cells. The pulmonary veins carry the now oxygen-rich blood back to the *left* side of the heart to be pumped out again through the systemic arteries to the rest of the body.

This double-sided flow of blood can be visualized as "Figure 8" (Fig. 12.1).

Helpful Heart Hints: Finding Your Way on the Outside of the Heart

(Figs. 12.2 and 12.3.)

- The **base** of the heart is where all the blood vessels enter and leave. It is oriented in a generally cranial direction in the living animal, tipped dorsally and to the right.
- The **apex** of the heart is the pointed tip. It faces in a generally caudal direction in the living animal, tipped ventrally and to the left.
- The fat-filled **interventricular groove** that spirals around the heart marks the location of the **interventricular septum** (the "wall" between the left and right ventricles).
- The left **ventricle** reaches all the way to the apex of the heart. The right ventricle does not.
- The right **auricle**, located cranial to the right ventricle, is an extension of the right atrium.
- The left auricle, located cranial to the left ventricle, is an extension of the left atrium.
- The blood vessel at the cranial end of the right ventricle near the interventricular groove is the **pulmonary artery**.

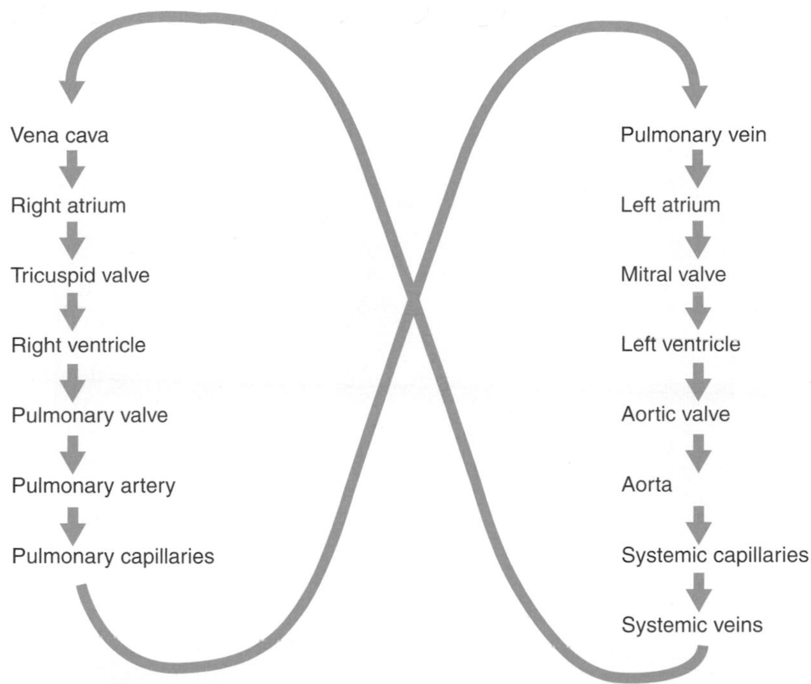

• **FIG. 12.1** The "Figure 8" of blood flow through the heart and blood vessels.

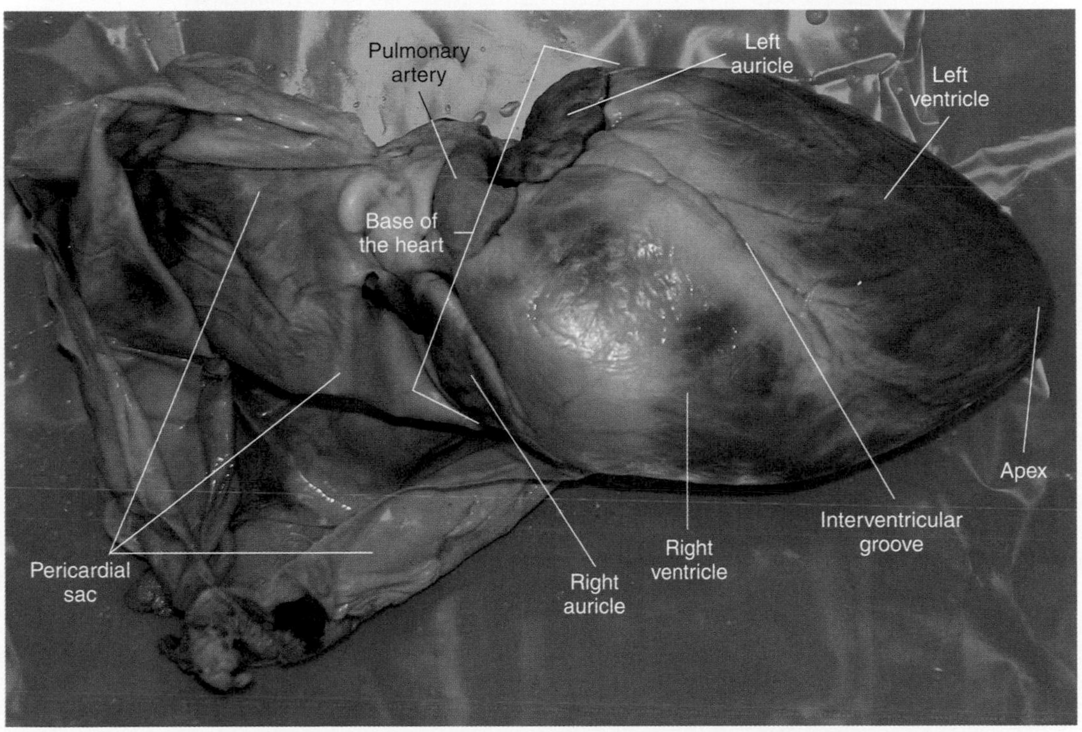

• **FIG. 12.2** Sheep heart with pericardial sac opened and reflected back.

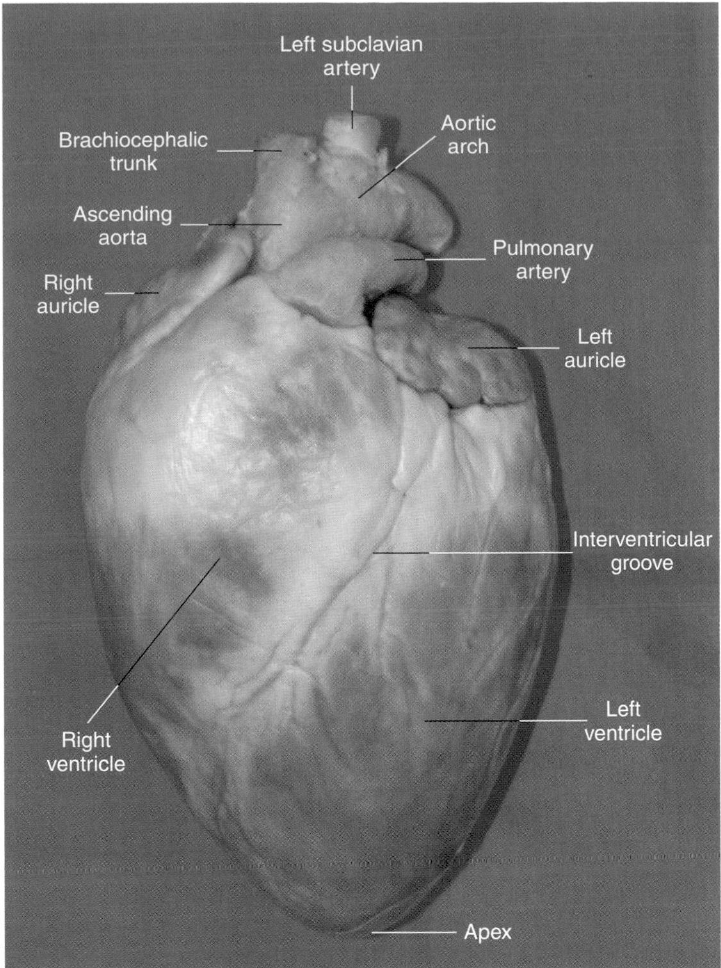

• **FIG. 12.3** Sheep heart with pericardial sac removed.

Helpful Heart Hints: Making Sense of the Inside of the Heart

(Fig. 12.4.)

- The right and left **atria** are "inside" (deep to) the right and left auricles.
- The atria are smaller, lighter in color, and have smoother walls than the **ventricles**.
- The large blood vessel that enters the right atrium is the **vena cava**.
- The large blood vessel that enters the left atrium is the **pulmonary vein**.
- The large blood vessel that leaves the right ventricle is the **pulmonary artery**.
- The large blood vessel that leaves the left ventricle is the **aorta**.
- The wall of the left ventricle is thicker than the wall of the right ventricle.
- The **tricuspid valve** (right atrioventricular valve) can be identified by its three cusps or flaps.
- The **mitral valve** (left atrioventricular valve) can be identified by its two cusps or flaps.
- The **chordae tendineae** are threadlike cords that connect the cusps of the mitral and tricuspid valves to the walls of the ventricles.
- The **aortic valve** is located where the aorta leaves the left ventricle.
- The **pulmonary valve** is located where the pulmonary artery leaves the right ventricle.

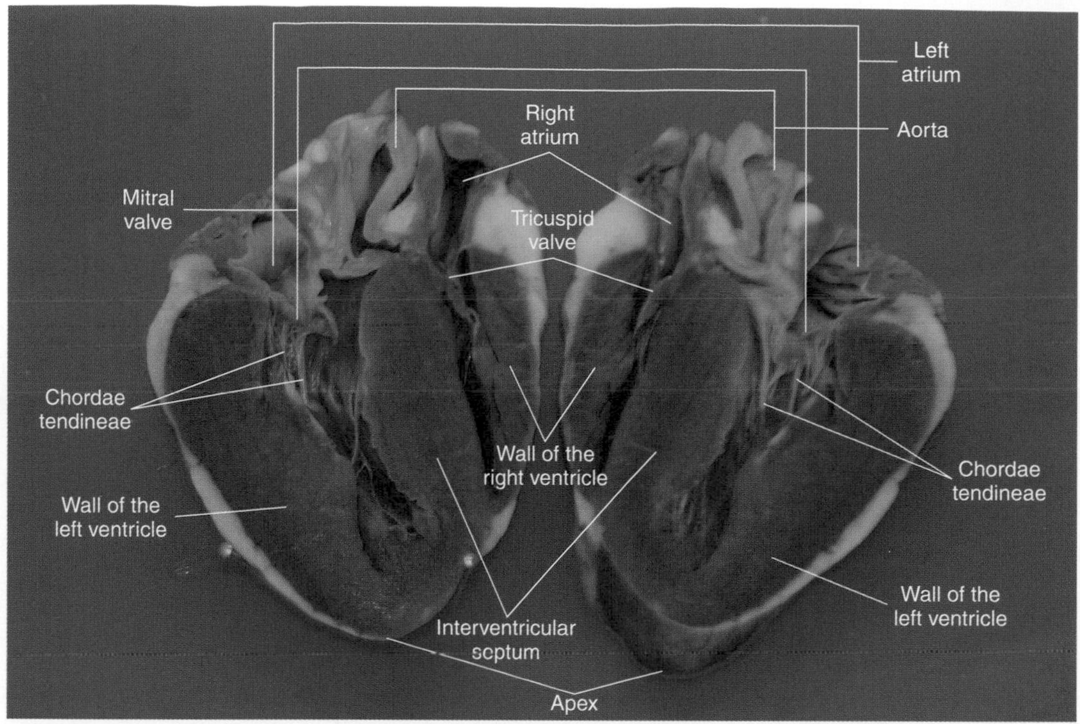

• **FIG. 12.4** Sheep heart cut in half.

Important Blood Vessels of the Neck and Thoracic Cavity

(Figs. 12.5–12.12.)

- The first two main arteries that branch off the **aortic arch are** the brachiocephalic trunk and the left subclavian artery.
  - The left **subclavian artery** supplies blood to the left front leg.
  - The right subclavian artery, which supplies blood to the right front leg, branches of the **brachiocephalic trunk**.
- The right and left **carotid arteries** branch off the brachiocephalic trunk.
- The left and right external **jugular veins** are common venipuncture sites in most domestic animals.
- The jugular veins carry blood to the cranial vena cava.
- The **cranial vena cava** returns blood to the heart from the head and front legs.
- The **caudal vena cava** returns blood to the heart from the abdomen and hind legs.

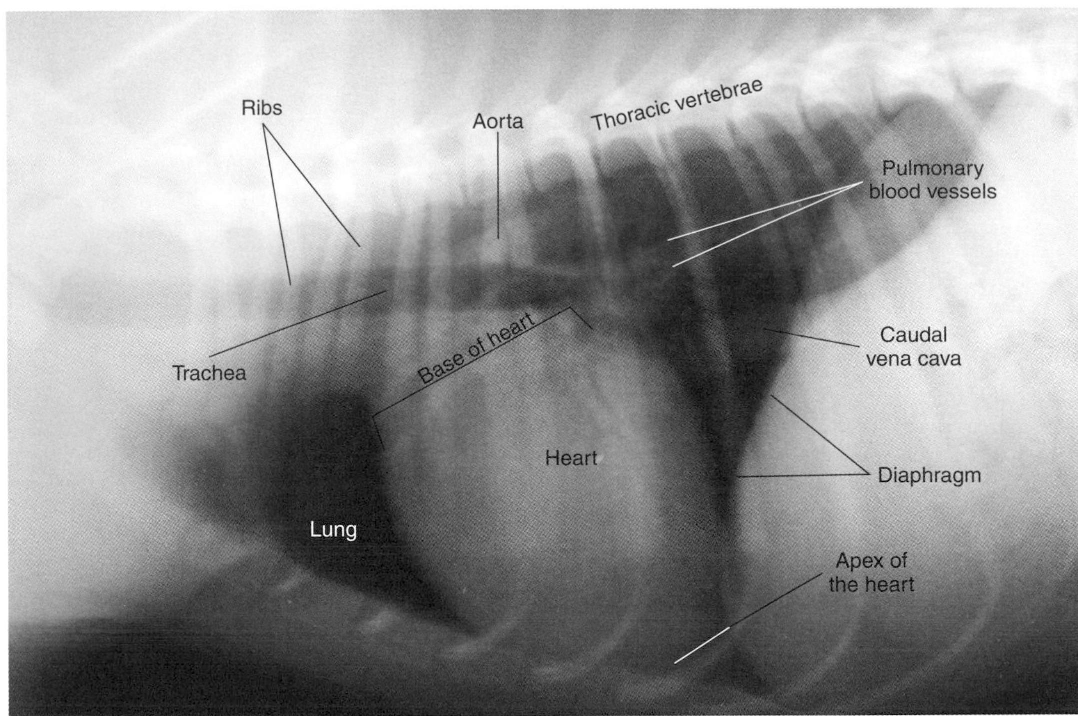

• **FIG. 12.5** Lateral radiograph of a canine thorax. Note: Structures that contain air (trachea and lungs) appear dark. Structures that contain blood (heart and large blood vessels) appear a lighter shade of gray. Bones appear white or very light gray.

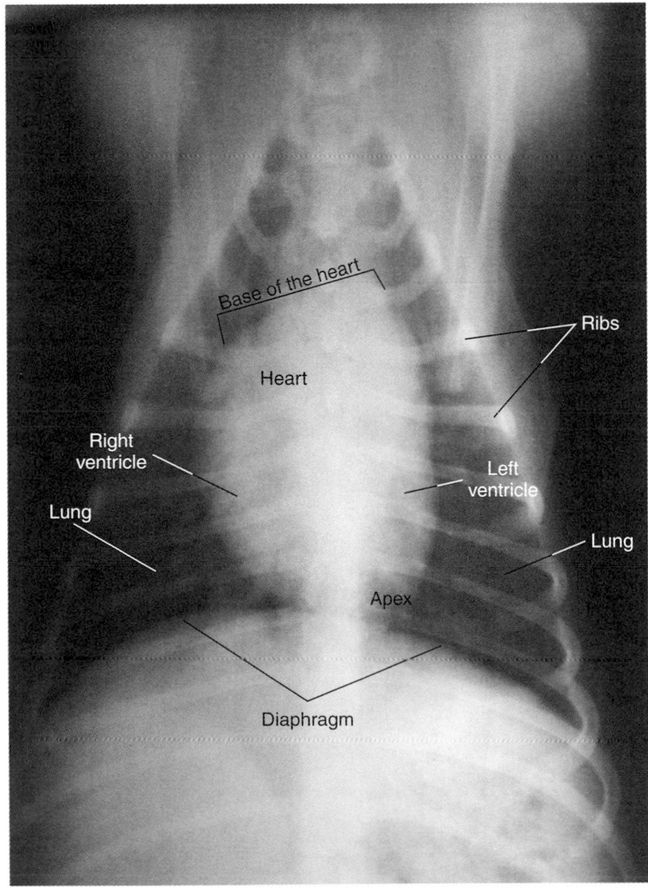

• **FIG. 12.6** Ventrodorsal (VD) radiograph of a canine thorax.

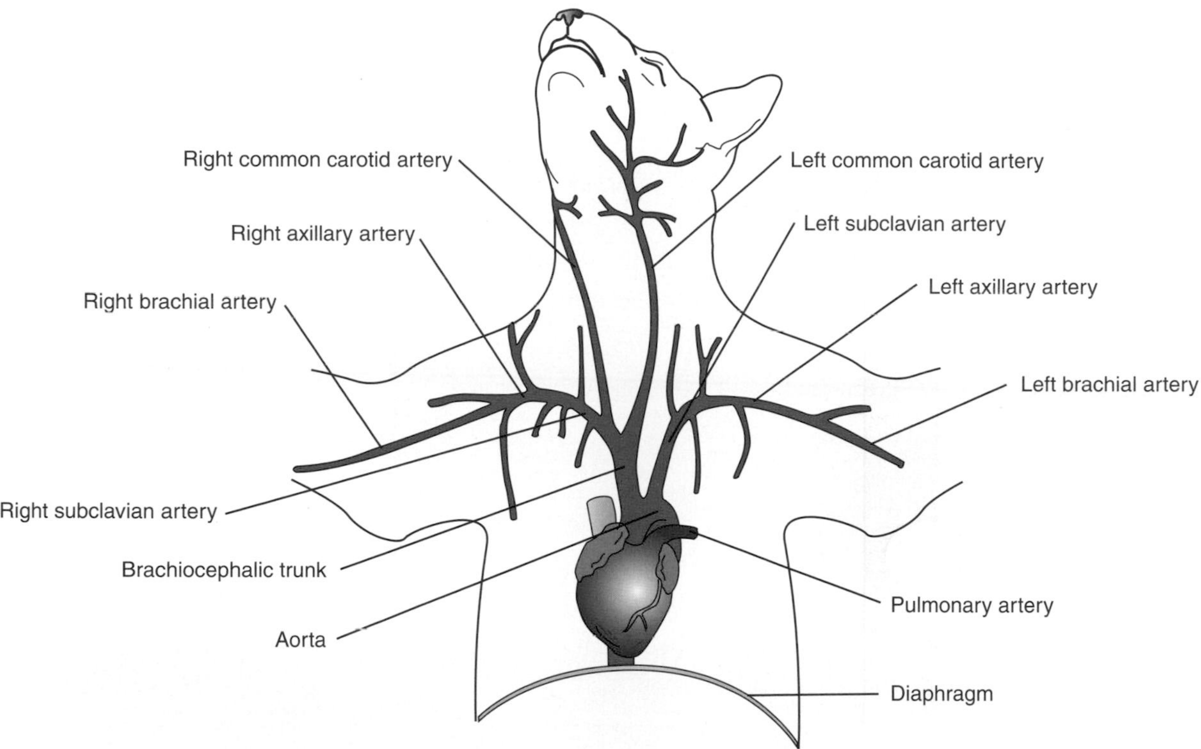

• **FIG. 12.7** Branches of the thoracic aorta in the cat.

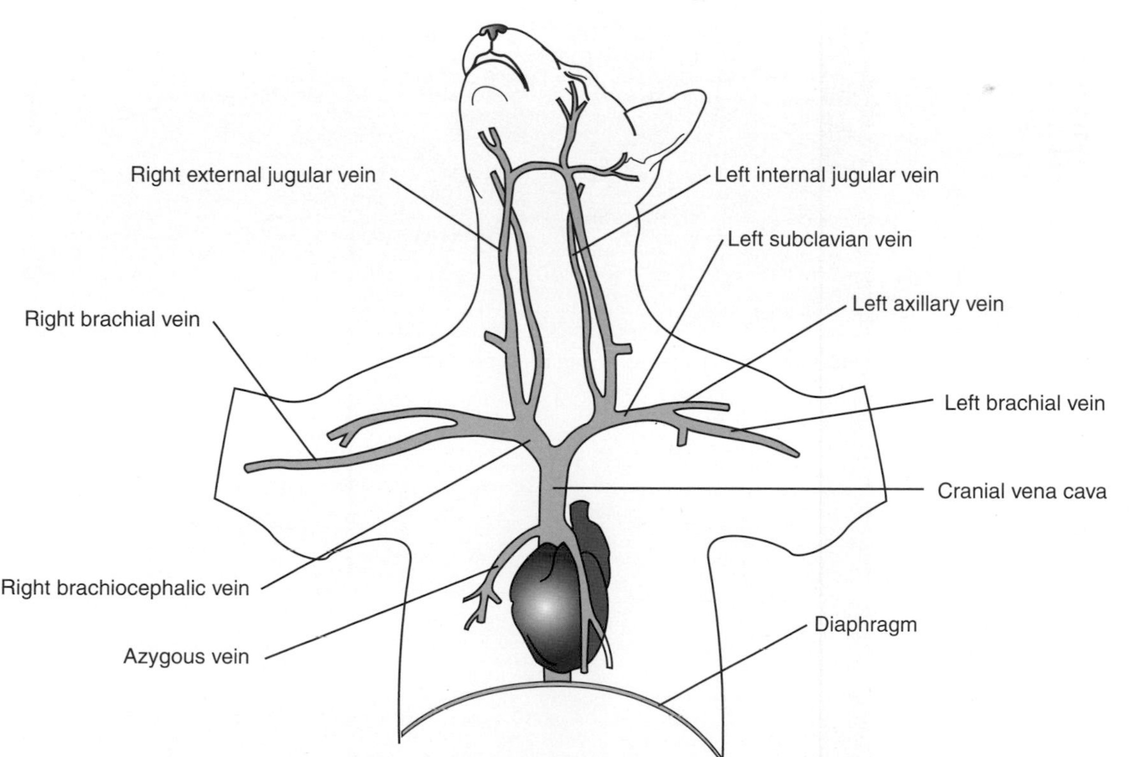

• **FIG. 12.8** Branches of the thoracic veins in the cat.

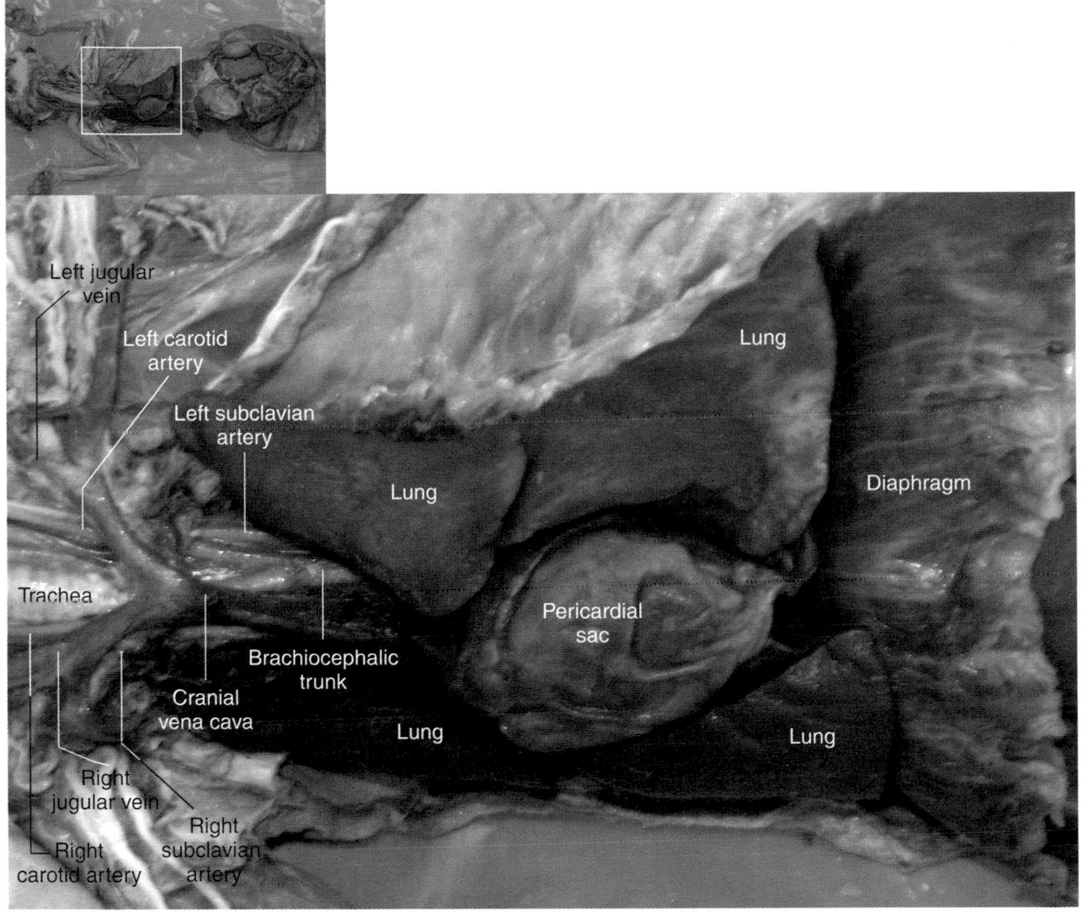

• **FIG. 12.9** Feline thorax with heart in the pericardial sac. Ventral view.

• **FIG. 12.10** Feline thorax with pericardial sac opened. This view is similar to Fig. 12.9, but the pericardial sac has been opened to expose the heart.

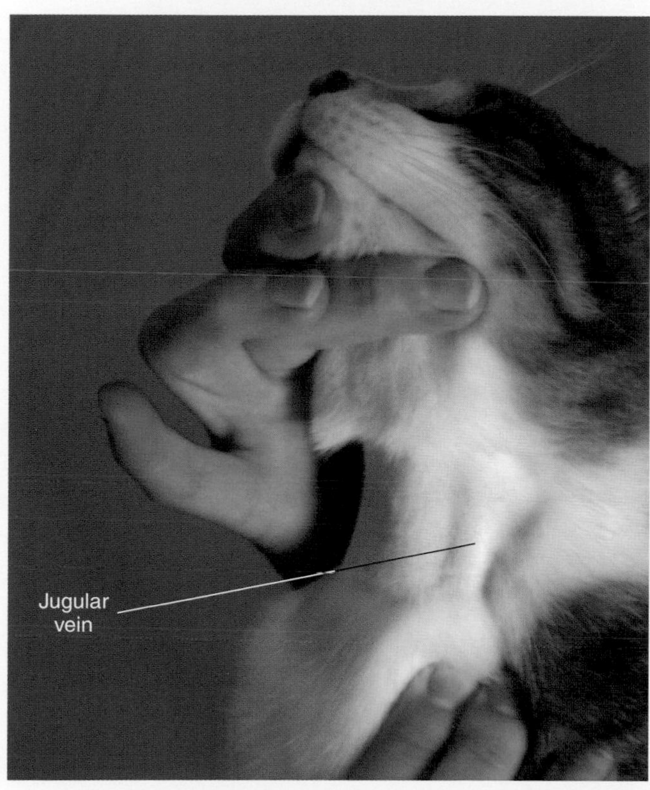

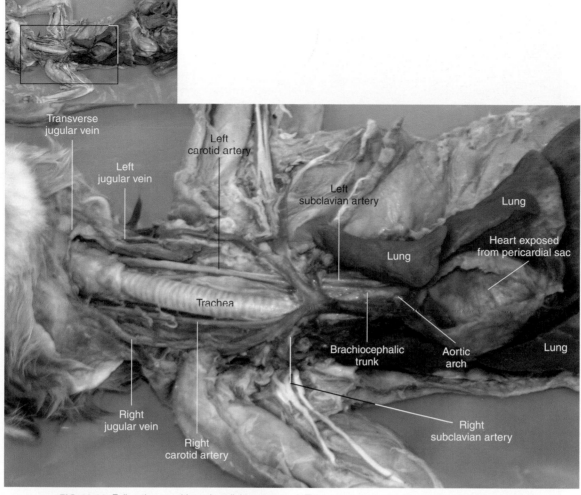

• **FIG. 12.11** Left jugular vein distended in a cat. Light digital pressure at the ventral end of the vein causes it to expand. This is often done clinically when venipuncture of the jugular vein is necessary.

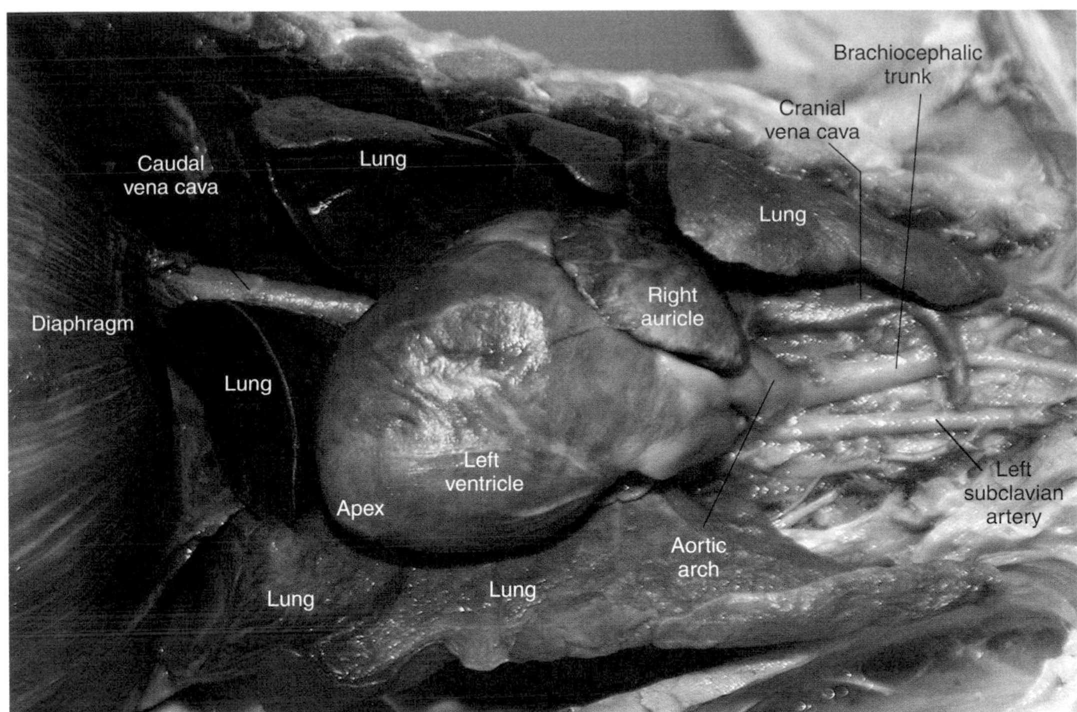

• **FIG. 12.12** Feline thorax. In this view of the thoracic cavity, the caudal vena cava is seen passing through the diaphragm.

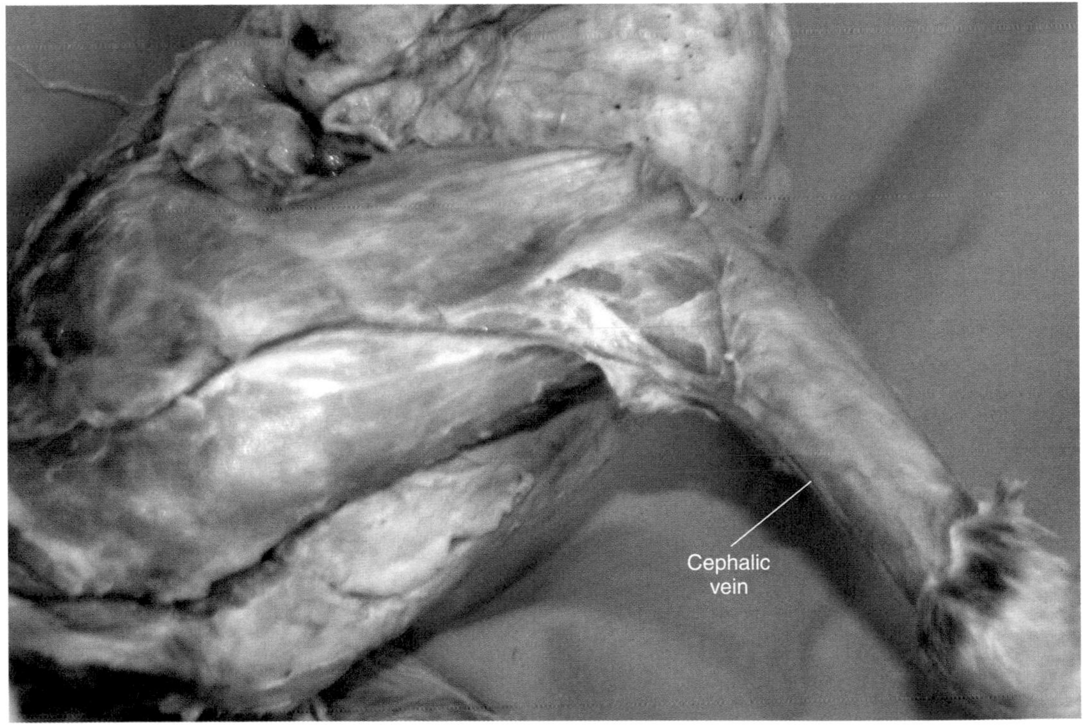

• **FIG. 12.13** Feline forelimb showing cephalic vein.

Important Blood Vessels of the Thoracic Limb

(Figs. 12.13 and 12.14.)

The **cephalic vein** is a superficial vein that runs between the elbow and the carpus on the craniomedial surface of the forearm. This is an important vein for drawing blood samples and administering intravenous substances to dogs and cats.

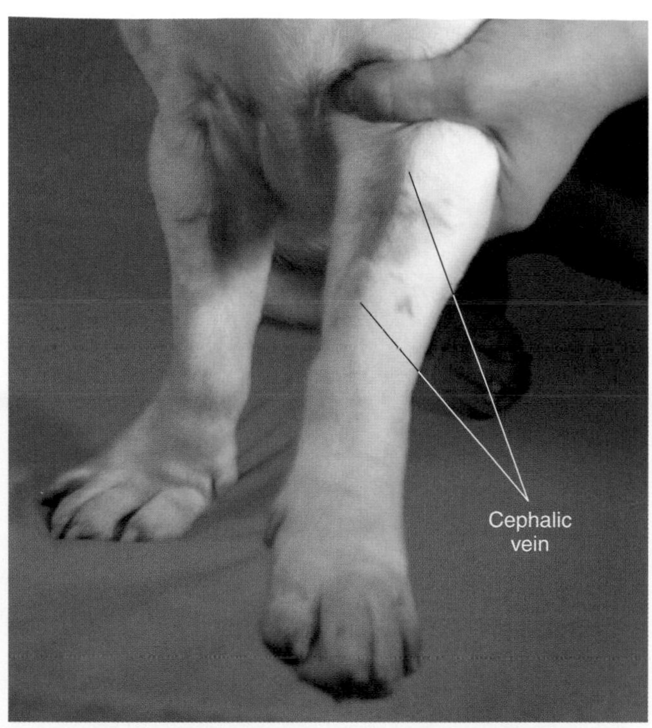

• **FIG. 12.14** Canine forelimb showing cephalic vein.

Important Blood Vessels in the Abdominal Cavity

(Figs. 12.15–12.20.)

- The aorta and caudal vena cava are located just ventral to the spinal column.
- The **renal (kidney) arteries and veins** branch directly off the aorta and caudal vena cava.
- The **ovarian arteries and veins** enlarge if the animal is in heat or pregnant and branch off the aorta and caudal vena cava.
- The **testicular arteries and veins** branch off the aorta and caudal vena cava.
- Other arteries and veins supply the digestive tract, spleen, and other abdominal organs.

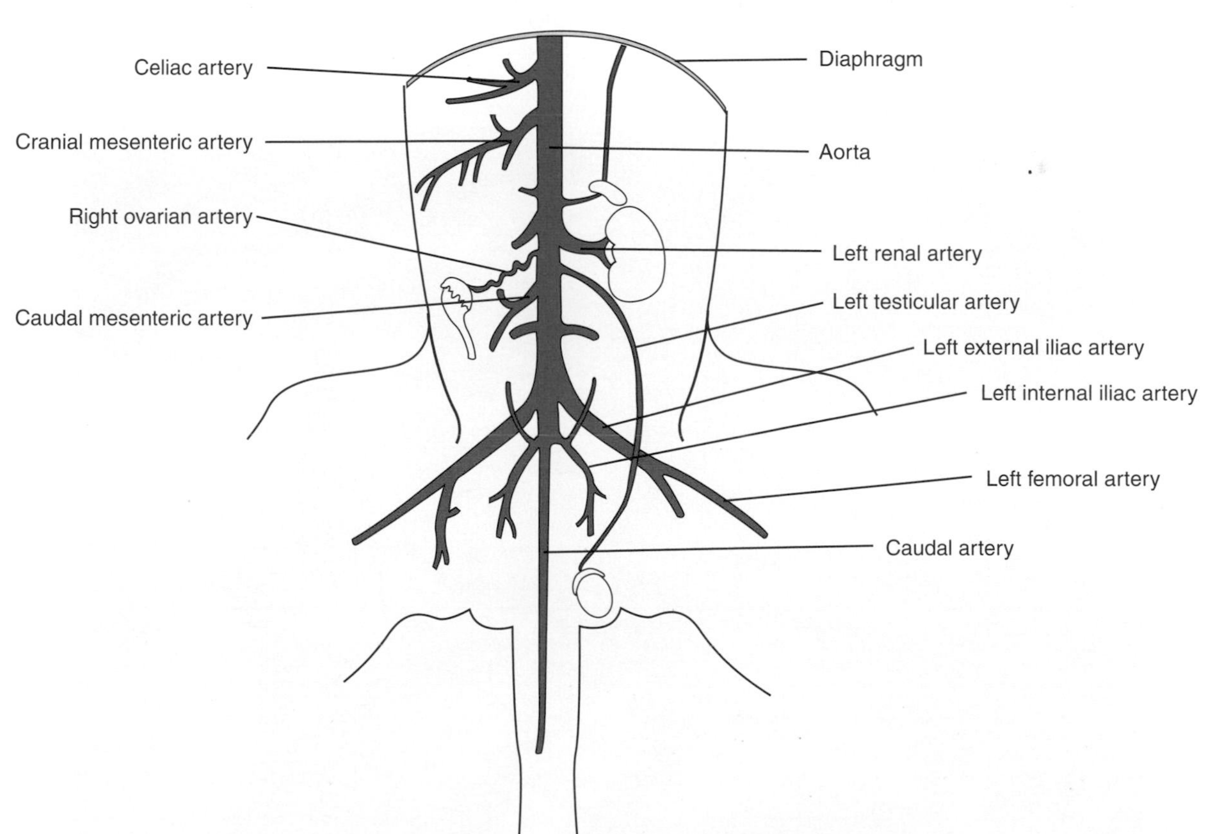

• **FIG. 12.15** Branches of the abdominal aorta in the cat.

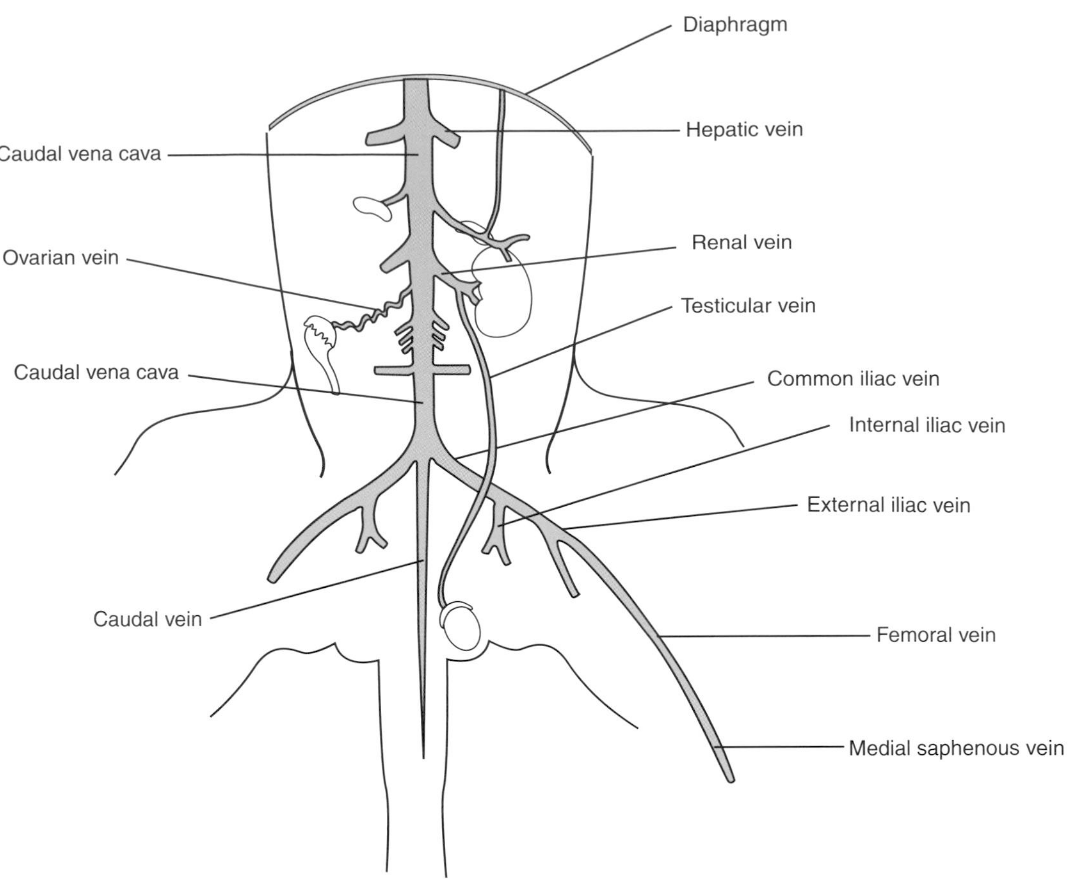

• **FIG. 12.16** Branches of the caudal vena cava in the cat.

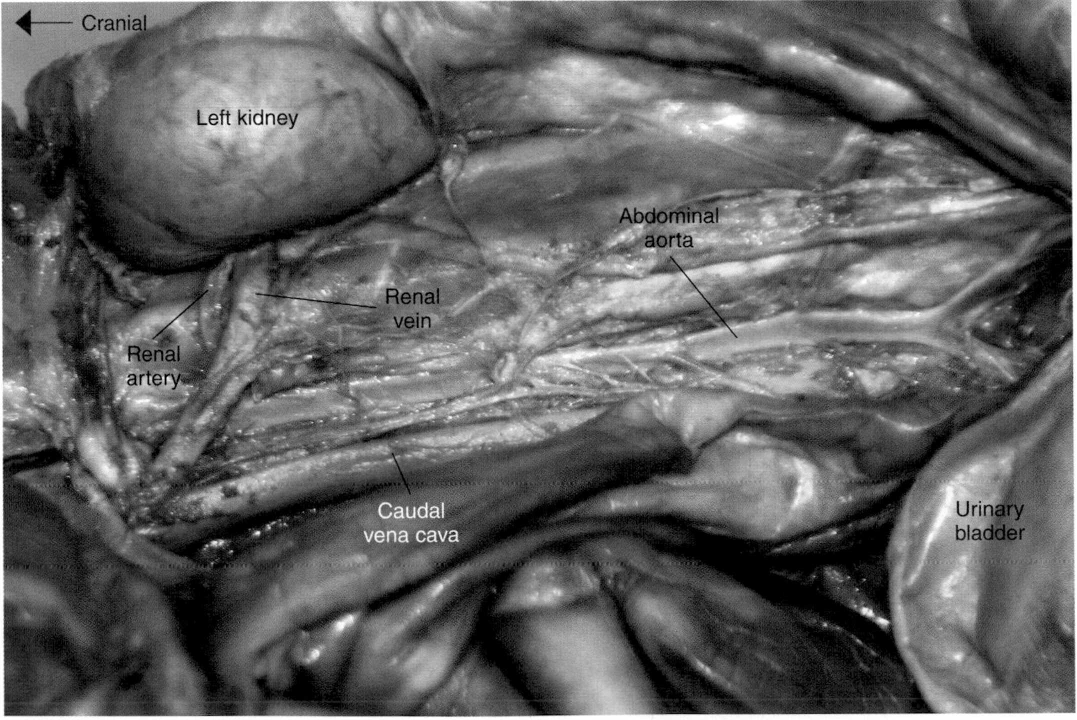

• **FIG. 12.17** Renal arteries and veins in a cat.

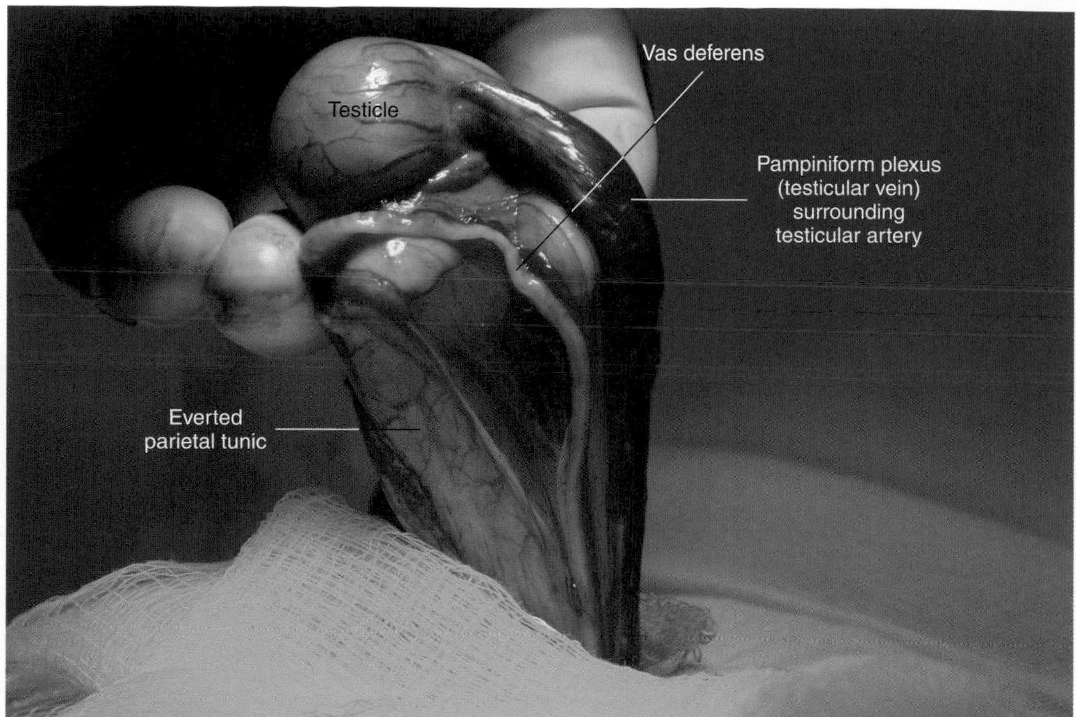

• **FIG. 12.18** Testicular blood vessels in the spermatic cord of a dog. The testicular vein forms a network called the pampiniform plexus that surrounds the testicular artery. This helps cool the blood going to the testicle and warm the blood that is returning to the body.

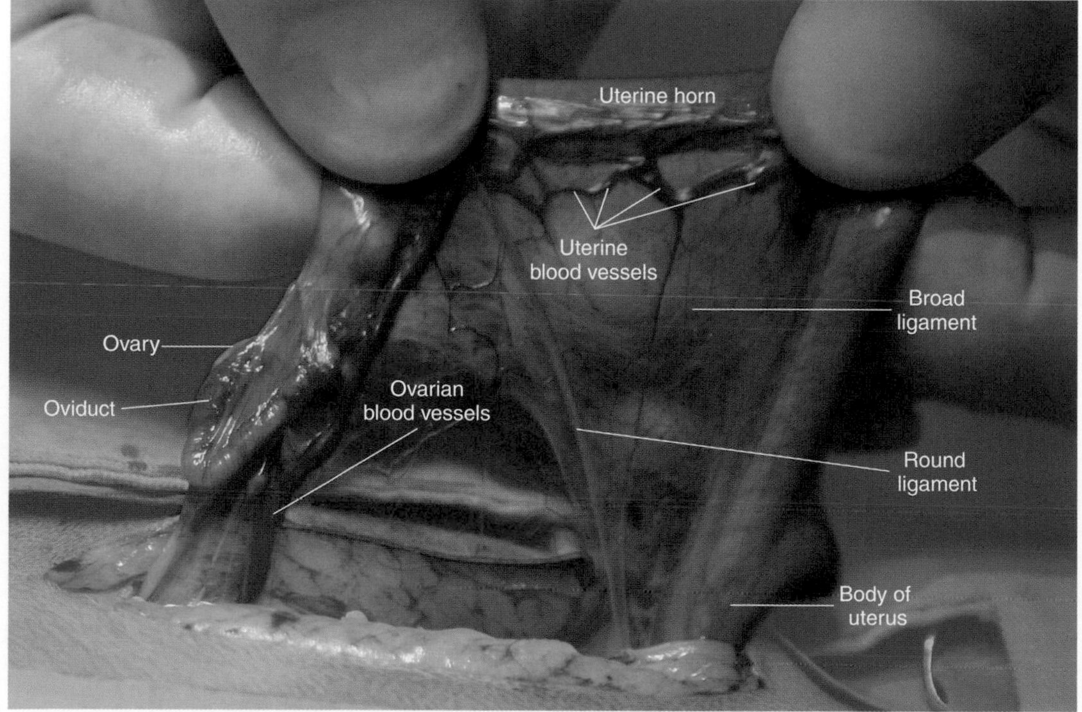

• **FIG. 12.19** Blood vessels in the reproductive tract of a nonpregnant cat.

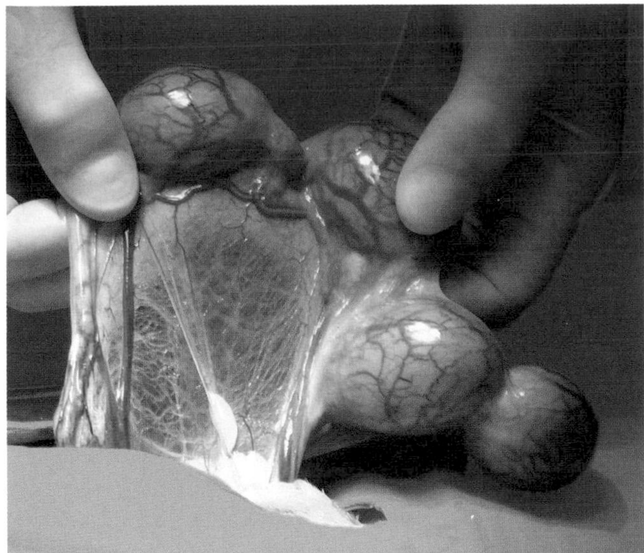

• **FIG. 12.20** Blood vessels in a cat's reproductive tract in early pregnancy (about 3 to 4 weeks). Note that the blood vessels are larger and more extensive than those in Fig. 12.19.

Important Blood Vessels of the Pelvic Limb

(Figs. 12.21–12.26.)

- The abdominal aorta bifurcates in the groin area to become the right and left iliac arteries.
- Once the **iliac artery** passes through the abdominal wall, it becomes the femoral artery, located on the medial side of each hind leg.
- The **femoral artery** is commonly used to take the pulse of an animal.
- The **femoral vein** runs superficially along the medial surface of the hindlimb between the stifle joint and the groin.
- The femoral vein is commonly used for venipuncture in the cat.
- The right and left femoral veins become the right and left **iliac veins** once the vessels have passed through the abdominal wall.
- In the abdominal cavity, the caudal vena cava is formed by the merging of the right and left iliac veins.
- The lateral **saphenous vein** is a superficial vein commonly used for venipuncture in dogs.
- The lateral saphenous vein runs along the lateral surface of the hindlimb between the hock and the stifle joint.

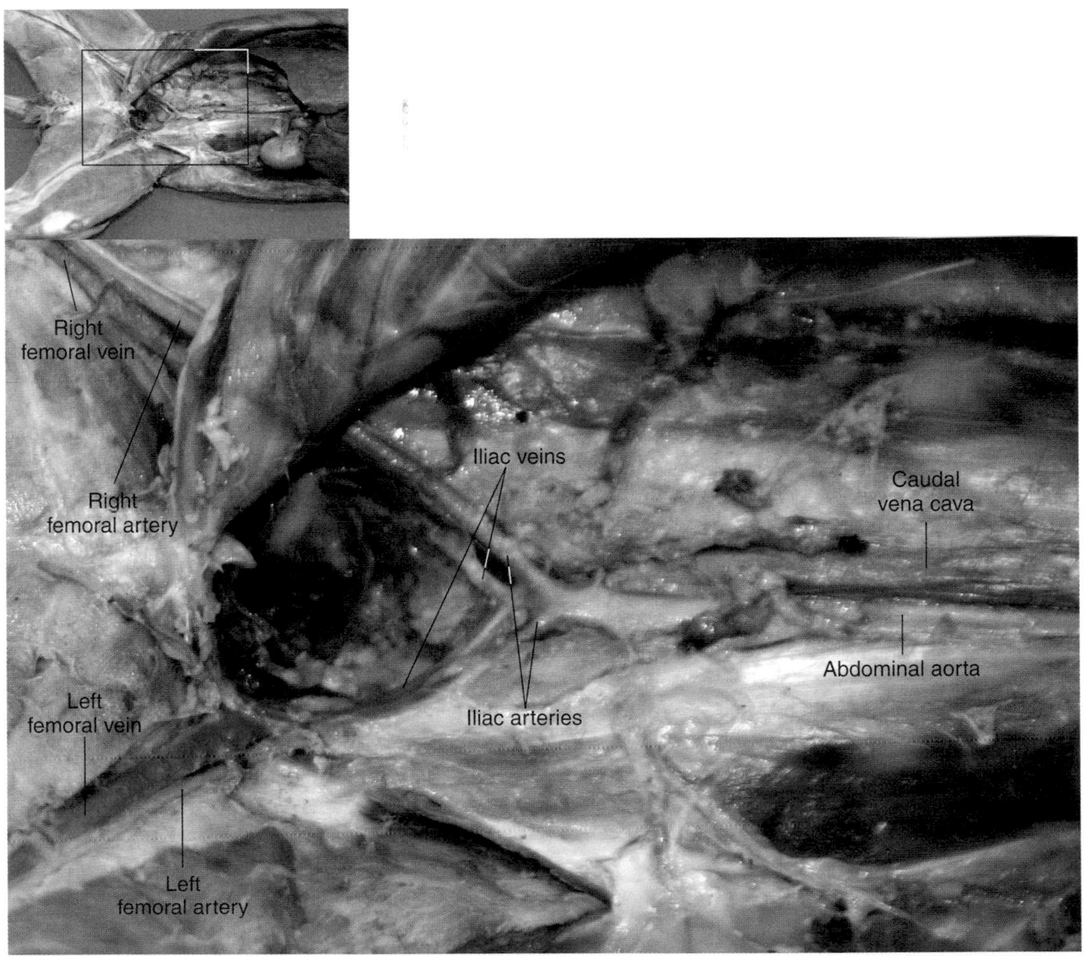

• **FIG. 12.21** Feline caudal abdomen and proximal hindlimbs. In the abdominal cavity, the caudal vena cava is formed by the merging of the right and left iliac veins. The iliac veins are formed from the femoral veins. The abdominal aorta bifurcates in the groin area to become the right and left iliac arteries. The iliac arteries become the right and left femoral arteries. The left femoral artery is not fully exposed in this view.

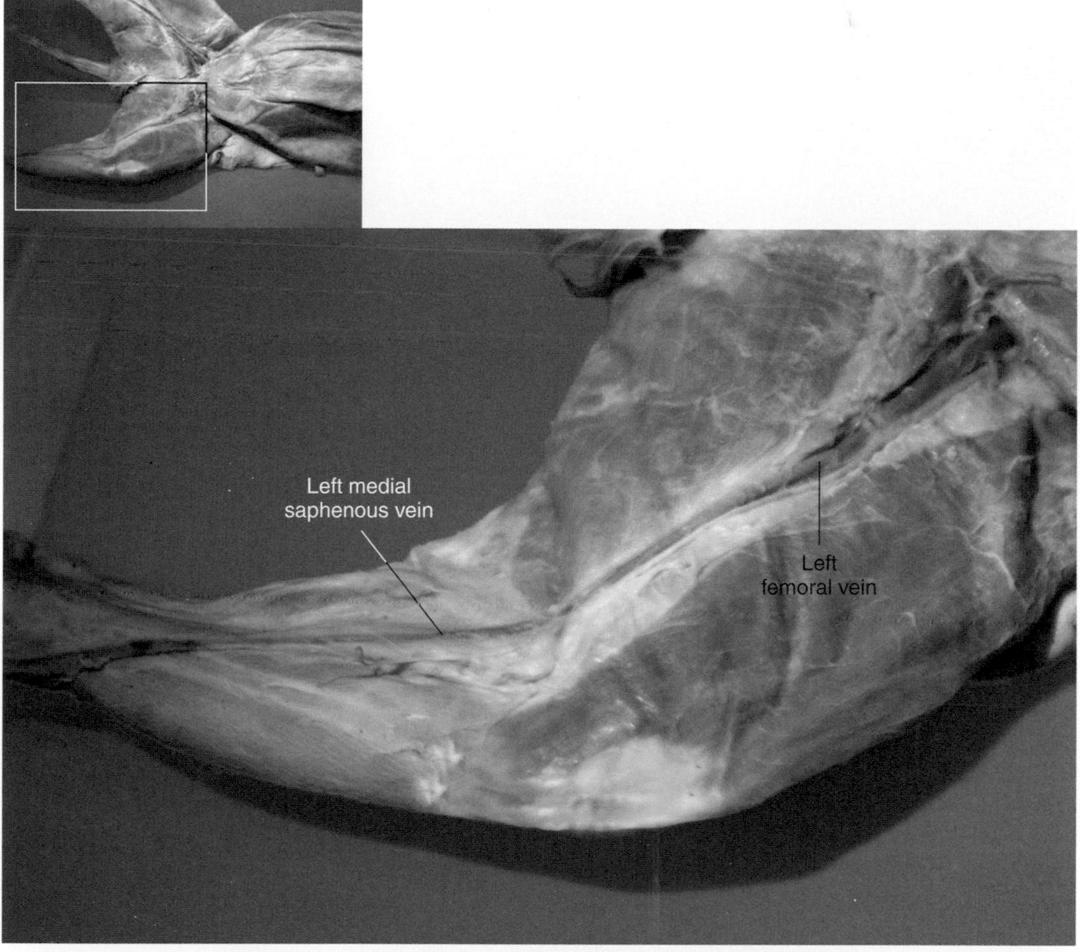

• **FIG. 12.22** Feline hindlimb. In this view, the left medial saphenous vein becomes the left femoral vein after it has passed proximal to the stifle joint.

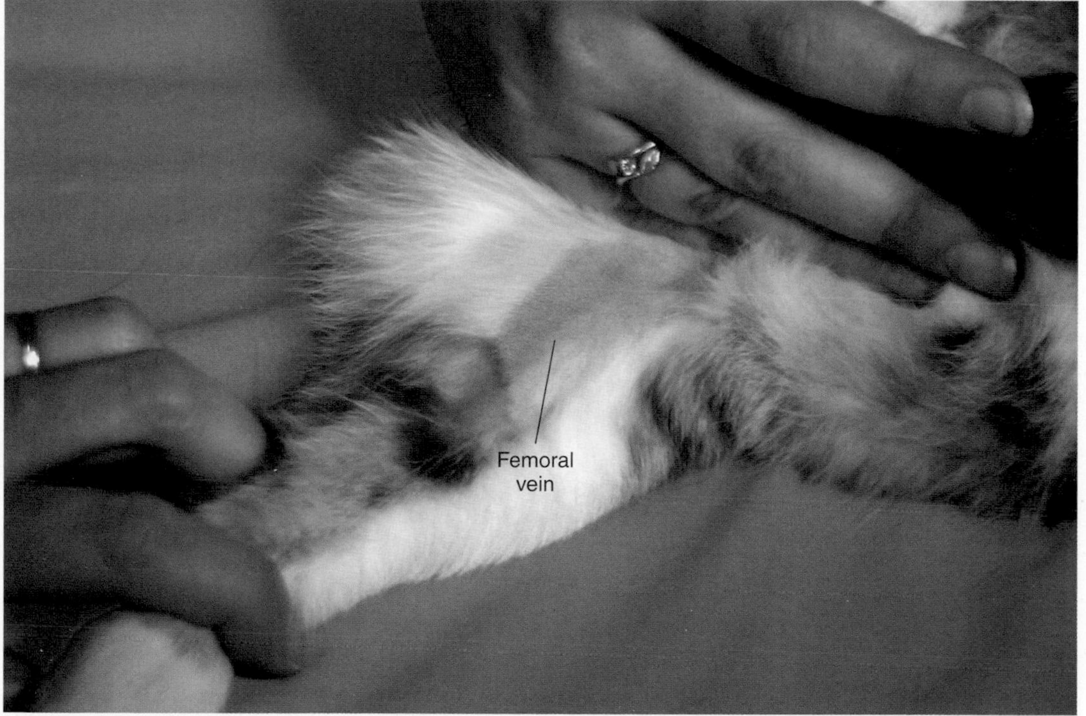

• **FIG. 12.23** Left femoral vein in a cat.

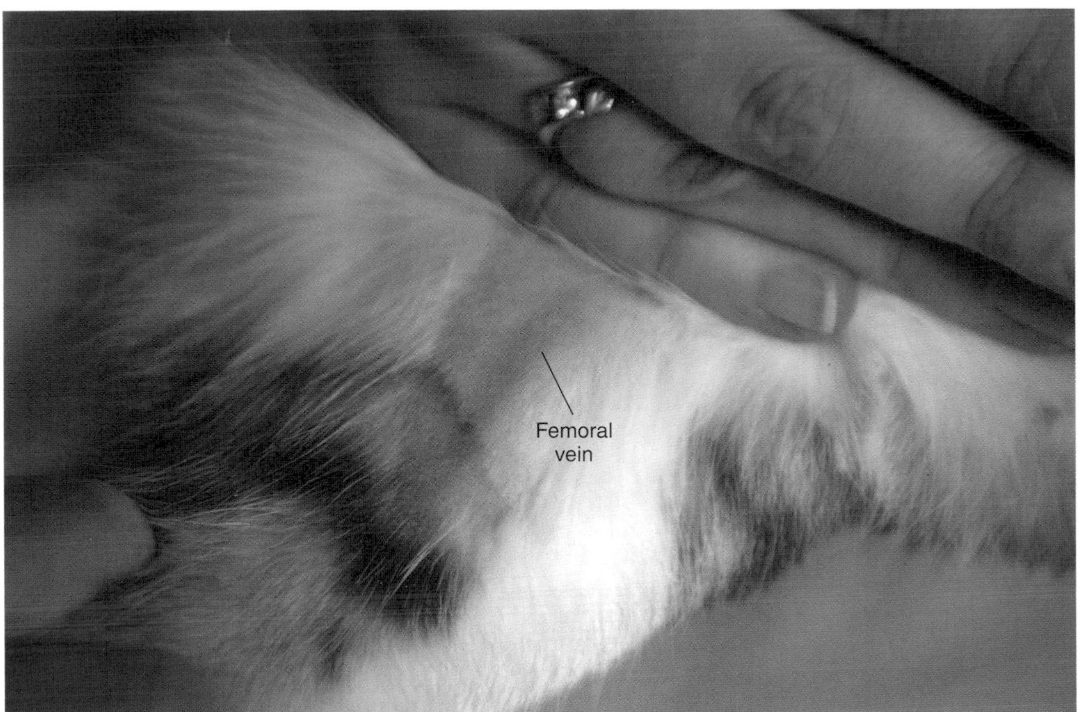

• **FIG. 12.24** Left femoral vein in a cat. Close-up view.

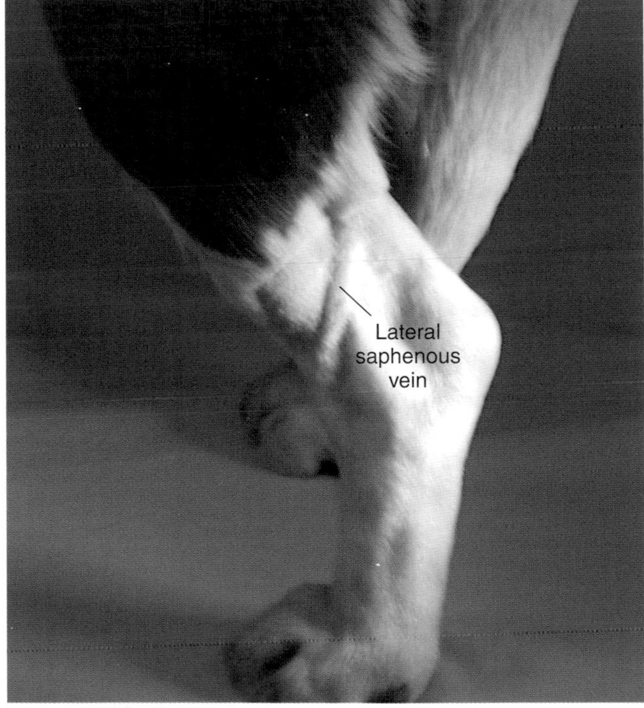

• **FIG. 12.25** Left lateral saphenous vein in a dog.

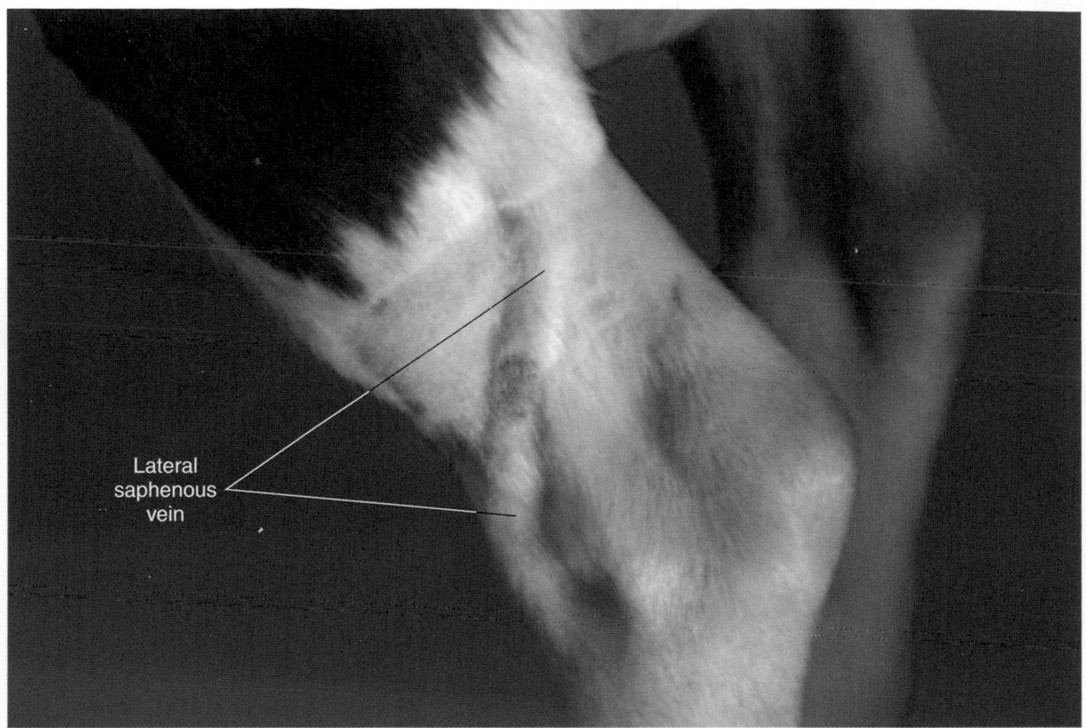

• **FIG. 12.26** Left lateral saphenous vein in a dog. Close-up view.

Suggested In-Class Activities

Materials for Suggested In-Class Activities

Trace the Flow of Blood Through the Heart

Sheep heart dissected but still in one piece, string, and forceps.

Palpate Common Venipuncture Sites

Live animals and a restrainer (partner).

Auscultate (Listen to) the Heart

Live animals and a stethoscope.

Palpate Pulse Points

Live dogs and/or cats.

Peek Inside the Living Chest

Radiographs of the thoracic cavity of various animals.

Dissection of a Sheep Heart

(Figs. 12.27 and 12.28.)

Materials Needed

Sheep heart, scalpel handle with a blade, and scalpel handle without a blade.

Procedure

There are many different ways to approach dissecting a sheep's heart. The heart can simply be cut in half to view the interior chambers and valves, or it can be dissected in a way that it remains in one piece, but all the structures can still be examined. To do this, you must first be able to identify all of the external structures before you touch a scalpel blade on them. Use the back end of a scalpel handle without a blade as a probe to locate the different vessels.

1. Find these structures on the outside of your sheep's heart:
   Apex and base
   Right and left auricles
   Right and left ventricles
   Interventricular groove
   Coronary vessels
   Vena cava
   Pulmonary vein
   Pulmonary artery
   Aorta
2. Locate the right auricle. The vena cava will be right next to it. In many preserved sheep hearts, the vena cava has been completely removed. All that may remain of this vessel is a hole into the right atrium. Remember, the vena cava brings blood from all of the body except the lungs and dumps it into the right atrium. The right atrium is directly under the right auricle.

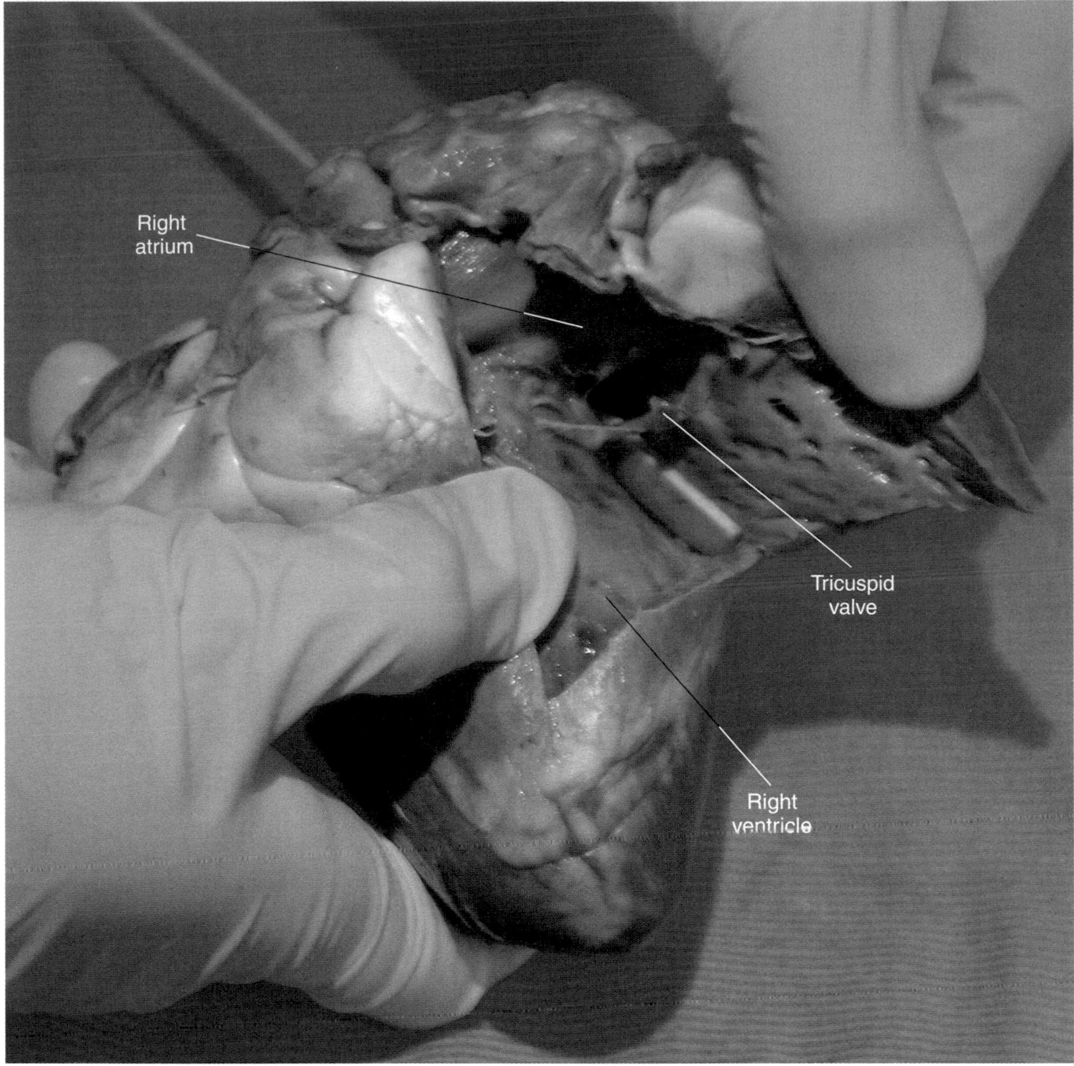

• **FIG. 12.27** Right atrium and ventricle opened.

3. Insert the probe, *not* your finger, through the vena cava into the right atrium. Position your scalpel blade over the probe to cut down from the hole left by the vena cava through the wall of the atrium down to the caudal part of the wall of the right ventricle.
   - Take care not to cut too close to the interventricular groove. Make your cut about one-third of the total width of the right ventricle from the groove. Keep the probe on the right side of the heart as a guide so you don't cut through the septum.
   - It helps to have your lab partner gently pull the incision open from both sides while you are cutting to better see the structures inside.
   - As you are making the incision, you will notice a horizontal line of fat around the base of the heart. This is where you will encounter the tricuspid valve. Try not to cut through the cusps of the valve or the chordae tendineae connected to their free edges as you continue the incision down through the wall of the right ventricle.
   - Once the incision has been made through the wall of the right ventricle, a small horizontal incision can be made off the main incision at the caudal end of the ventricle. This will allow the right ventricle to open wider to better view the internal structures.
4. Turn the heart over and repeat the process on the left side. Locate the left auricle. Next to the left auricle will be the pulmonary vein. In many preserved sheep hearts, the pulmonary veins have been completely removed. All that may remain of these vessels is a hole into the left atrium. Remember, the pulmonary vein brings blood from the lungs and dumps it into the left atrium. The left atrium is directly under the left auricle.

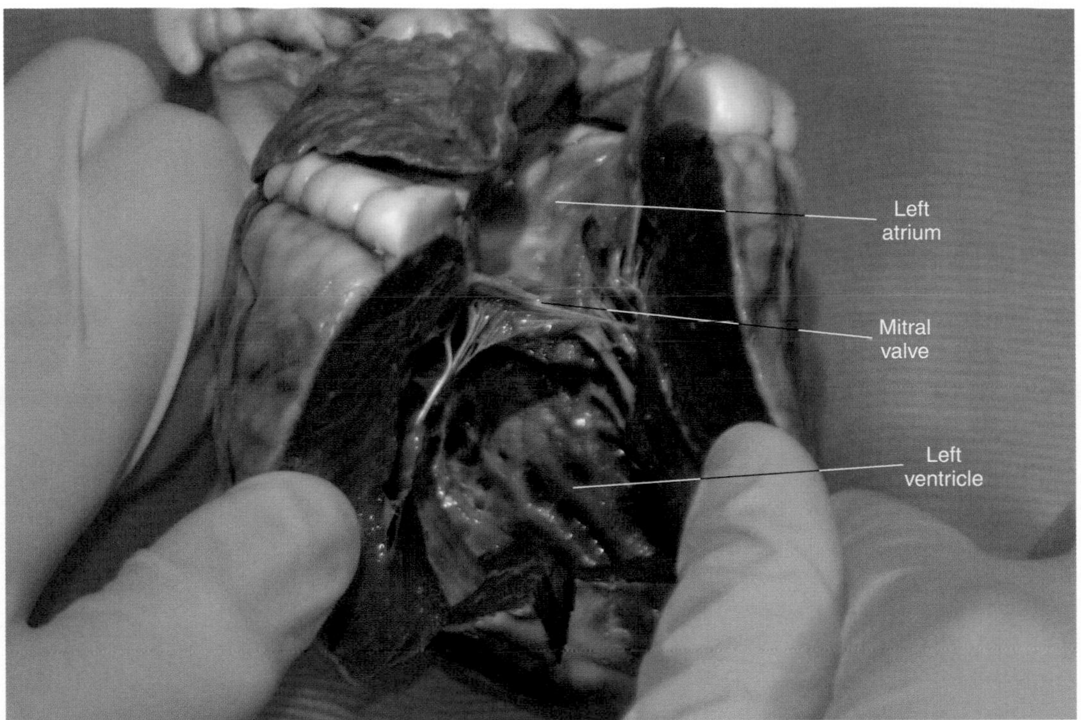

• **FIG. 12.28** Left atrium and ventricle opened.

5. Insert the probe, *not* your finger, through the pulmonary vein into the left atrium. Position your scalpel blade over the probe to cut down from the hole left by the pulmonary vein through the wall of the atrium down to the caudal end of the wall of the left ventricle.
   - Keep the probe in the left side of the heart as a guide so you don't cut through the septum. Continue your cut straight down the middle of the left ventricle. There is a ridge running down the left ventricle. That is the perfect place to make this incision.
   - It helps to have your lab partner gently pull the incision open from both sides while you are cutting to better see the structures inside.
   - As you are making the incision, you will notice a horizontal line of fat around the base of the heart. This is where you will encounter the mitral valve. Try not to cut through the cusps of the valve or the chordae tendineae connected to their free edges as you continue the incision down through the wall of the left ventricle.
   - Once the incision has been made through the left ventricle, a small horizontal incision can be made off the main incision at the caudal end of the ventricle. This will allow the left ventricle to open wider for better viewing of the internal structures.

Once your heart has been dissected in this manner, identify the following structures in your sheep heart:

Aorta
Aortic valve
Chordae tendineae
Mitral valve
Moderator band
Pulmonary artery
Pulmonary valve
Pulmonary vein
Right and left atria
Right and left ventricles
Tricuspid valve
Vena cava

Try inserting your probe into the various vessels at the base of the heart. Locate the probe on the inside of the heart. Where did it come out? Is it in a vein or an artery? Did it go into an atrium or a ventricle? Quiz, your partner.

Trace the Flow of Blood Through the Heart

Materials Needed

Sheep heart dissected but still in one piece, string, and forceps.

Procedure

To do this activity, the heart must be dissected as previously described. It must remain in one piece for this activity to be effective. Thread a piece of string through the heart in the direction that the blood flows. Begin at the vena cava and end at the aorta. Use the forceps to pull the string through the various vessels.

Clinical Significance

By understanding how blood flows through the heart, you can understand the normal cardiac cycle and how the heart sounds are produced. This also helps you learn where the different vessels, chambers, and valves are located.

Palpate Common Venipuncture Sites

Materials Needed

Live animals and a restrainer (partner).

Procedure

We usually draw blood and give intravenous injections in veins, not arteries. When drawing blood or giving an intravenous injection, the vein must be held off (occluded) between the venipuncture site (the place where the needle is going in) and the heart. This stops the venous return and makes the vein stand out.

Locate the cephalic, femoral (on a cat), and lateral saphenous (on a dog) veins on the animal. Have your partner occlude each vein and feel how it stands out. Gently squeeze the foot a few times, and the vein may stand out even more. Watch how it flattens back out once the occlusion is released.

Occlude the jugular vein. Run your index and middle fingers down the groove on either side of the trachea. Before you reach the manubrium, push in slightly to occlude the jugular vein. Feel cranial to your fingers with your other hand, and the jugular vein should be there. Try this on both the left and right sides.

Clinical Significance

Venipuncture is one of the most common procedures that veterinary technicians perform. It is critical that you are familiar with the different veins and the best way to occlude those veins to gain access to the circulatory system.

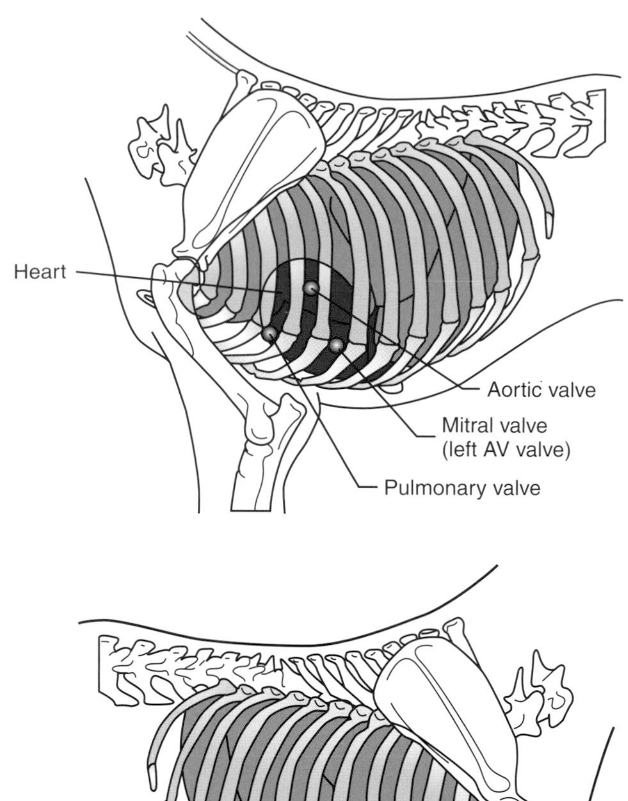

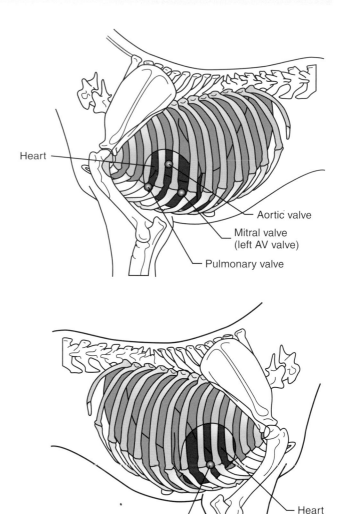

• **FIG. 12.29** Position of canine heart in the thoracic cavity.

Auscultate (Listen to) the Heart

(Fig. 12.29.)

Materials Needed

Live animals and a stethoscope.

Procedure

The four heart valves make sounds when they snap closed during each heartbeat. We can easily hear these heart sounds through a stethoscope. A normal heart produces two distinct heart sounds: a louder first sound and a softer second sound in a "LUB-dub, LUB-dub" pattern. The first heart sound (the "LUB") is produced when the mitral and tricuspid valves close as the ventricles begin to contract (the beginning of ventricular systole). The second heart sound (the "dub") is produced when the aortic and pulmonary valves close at the end of the ventricular contraction (the end of ventricular systole).

Three of the four valves can be heard best on the left side of the thorax. They are the pulmonary, the aortic, and the mitral valves. The pulmonary and aortic valves are located further cranially than the mitral valve because of the way the heart is oriented in the chest. To hear the mitral valve best, place the stethoscope near the sternum on the left side of the thorax at the level of the fourth or fifth intercostal (between ribs) space. Be sure to stay close to the sternum. The heart sound you should hear is the mitral valve closing as part of the first heart sound. Once you have heard the mitral valve, slide the stethoscope dorsally and cranially to the area of the fourth intercostal space, and you will hear the aortic valve closing as part of the second heart sound. Move the stethoscope cranially and ventrally to the level of the costochondral junction in the third intercostal space. At this level, you should hear the pulmonary valve closing as part of the second heart sound. The heart sounds heard on the left side of the thorax are produced mainly by the pulmonary, aortic, and mitral valves. A common mnemonic used to remember the order of the valves from cranial to caudal is P-A-M (Pulmonary–Aortic–Mitral).

On the right side of the thorax, the tricuspid valve can be heard best at the level of the costochondral junction in the fourth intercostal space. It makes part of the first heart sound.

Clinical Significance

By becoming familiar with normal heart sounds, you will be able to detect abnormal heart sounds when you hear them.

Palpate Pulse Points

Materials Needed

Live dogs and/or cats.

Procedure

An animal's pulse can be palpated (felt) where arteries are located superficially. A common pulse point in dogs and cats is the femoral artery. Gently place your fingertips (not your thumb—you might feel your own pulse) on the inner thigh of the animal, just at the point where the thigh meets the groin. You will feel a little groove where two muscles come together. The femoral artery lies in this groove. Count the beats for 15 seconds and multiply that number by 4 to get the animal's pulse rate per minute. Do you get the same number of beats when listening to the heart with a stethoscope? Is the pulse strong and steady, or weak and irregular?

Clinical Significance

By knowing where and how to feel for an animal's pulse, you can note changes in an animal's blood pressure. You can also count the animal's heart rate without using a stethoscope.

Peek Inside the Living Chest

Materials Needed

Radiographs of the thoracic cavity of various animals.

Procedure

View as many lateral and ventrodorsal (VD) or dorsoventral (DV) radiographs of the thoracic cavity as possible. Look at radiographs from a variety of species to identify the normal heart position, size, and shape. The caudal vena cava, aorta, and pulmonary blood vessels are often visible on lateral radiographs of the thoracic cavity as well.

Clinical Significance

Knowing the normal position and shape of the heart will enable you to evaluate the quality of the radiographs you produce.

EXERCISES

Basic Blood Flow Through the Cardiovascular System

Exercise 1

Identify the External Structures of the Heart

Heart

1. ______________________
2. ______________________
3. ______________________
4. ______________________
5. ______________________

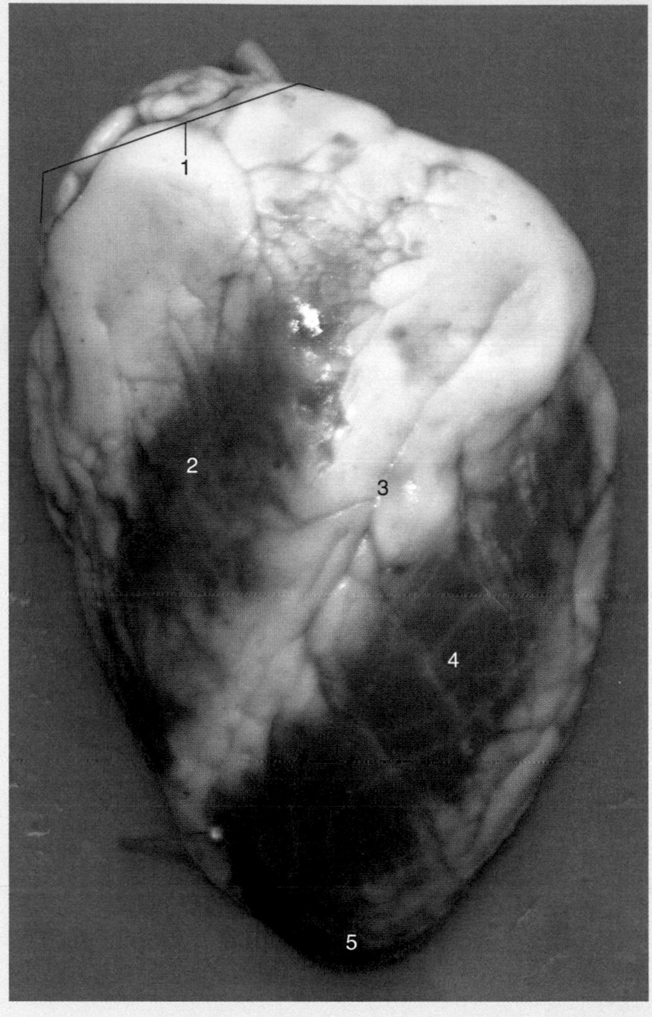

Exercise 2

Identify the Structures of the Heart

1. ______________________
2. ______________________
3. ______________________
4. ______________________
5. ______________________
6. ______________________
7. ______________________
8. ______________________
9. ______________________
10. ______________________
11. ______________________
12. ______________________

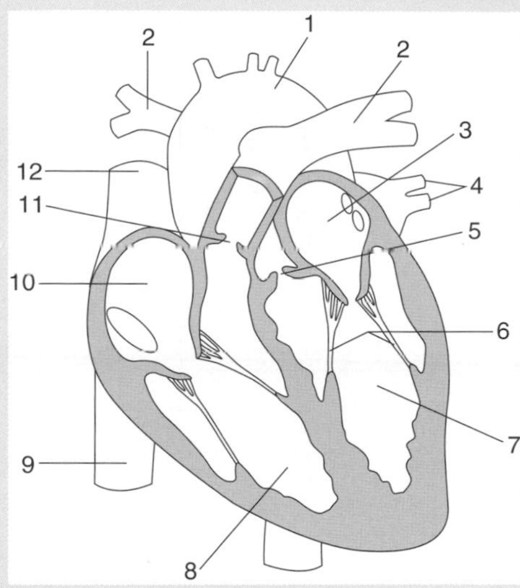

Exercise 3

Identify the Structures of the Heart

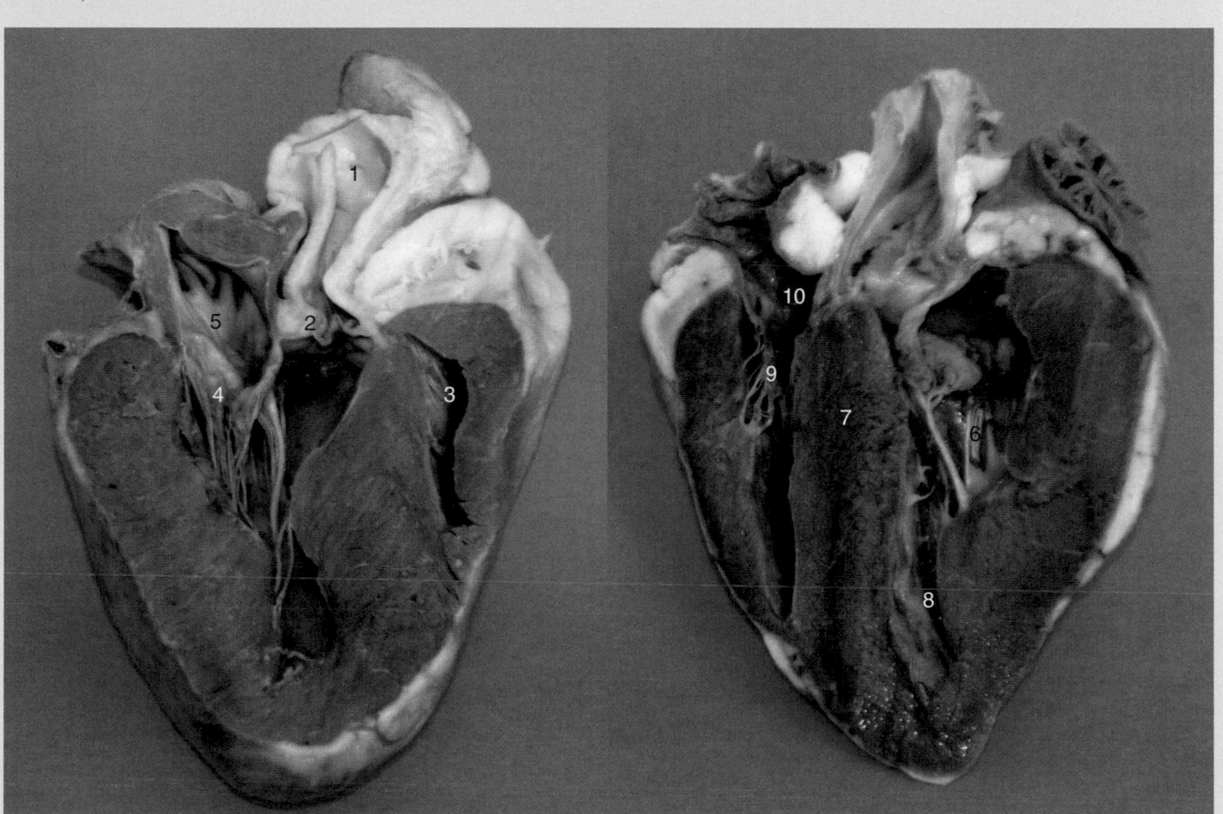

1. ______________________
2. ______________________
3. ______________________
4. ______________________
5. ______________________
6. ______________________
7. ______________________
8. ______________________
9. ______________________
10. ______________________

Exercise 4

Chart the Sequence of Blood Flow

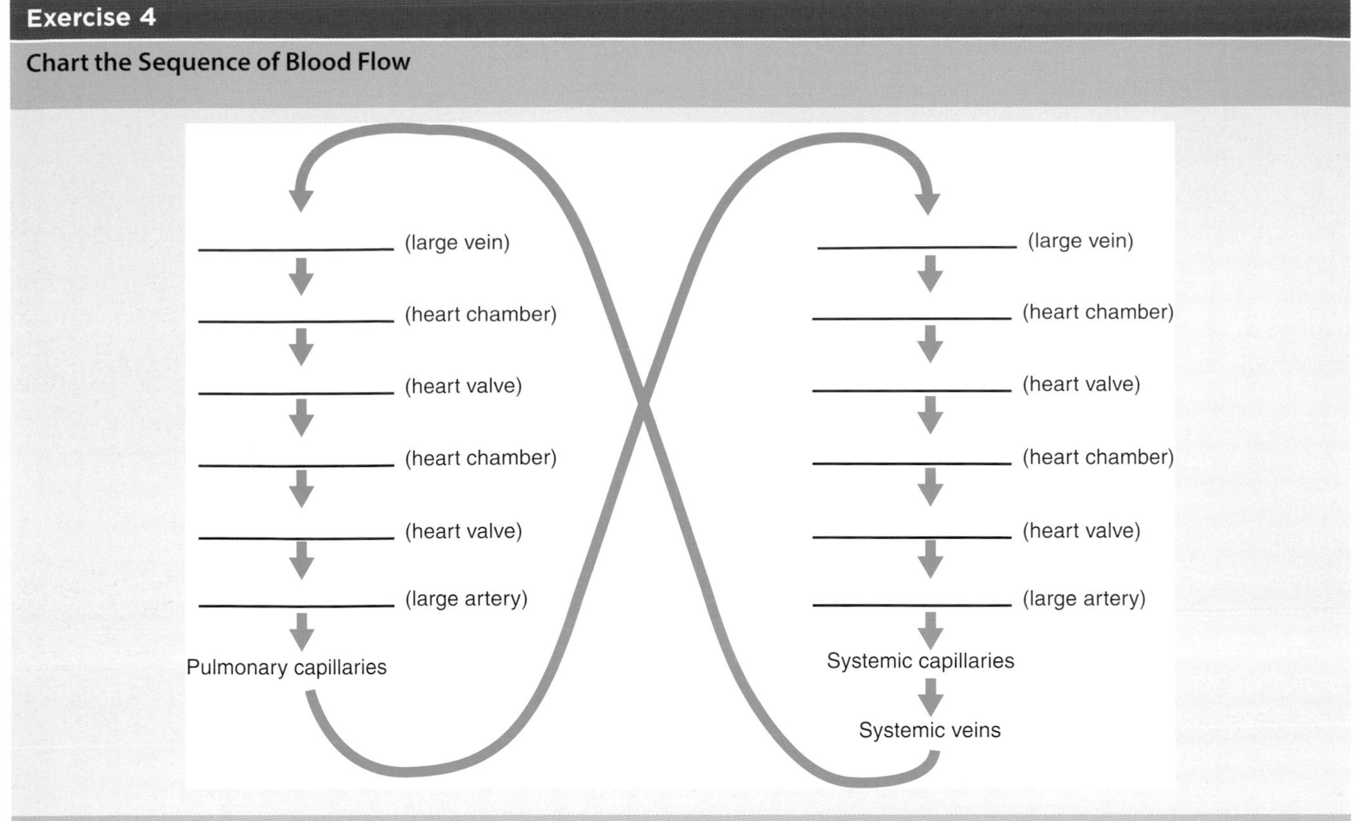

Exercise 5

Trace the Flow of Blood Through the Heart

Using a blue pen or pencil, indicate with arrows the direction of the flow of unoxygenated blood through the heart. Use a red pen or pencil to indicate with arrows the direction of the flow of the oxygenated blood. Start with unoxygenated blood arriving at the heart.

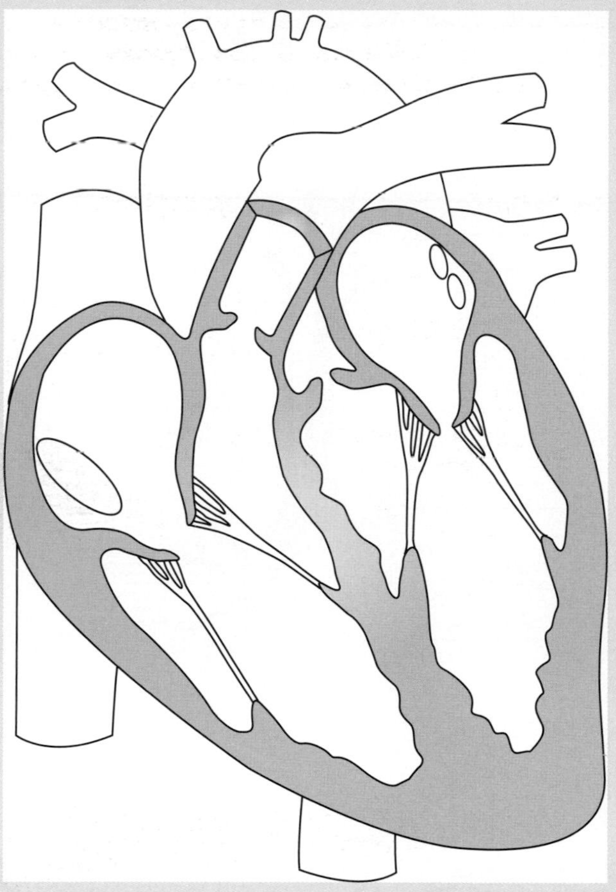

Exercise 6

Identify Thoracic and Cervical Arteries and Veins

Identify the numbered structures. Indicate right or left where applicable.

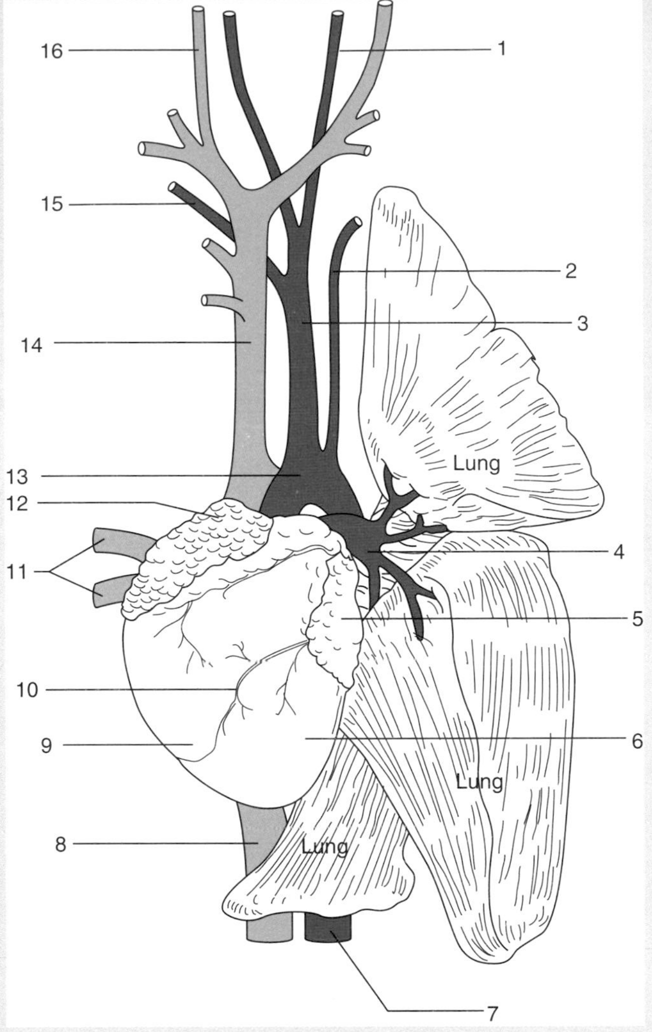

1. ____________________
2. ____________________
3. ____________________
4. ____________________
5. ____________________
6. ____________________
7. ____________________
8. ____________________
9. ____________________
10. ____________________
11. ____________________
12. ____________________
13. ____________________
14. ____________________
15. ____________________
16. ____________________

Exercise 7

Identify Thoracic and Cervical Arteries and Veins

Indicate right or left where applicable.

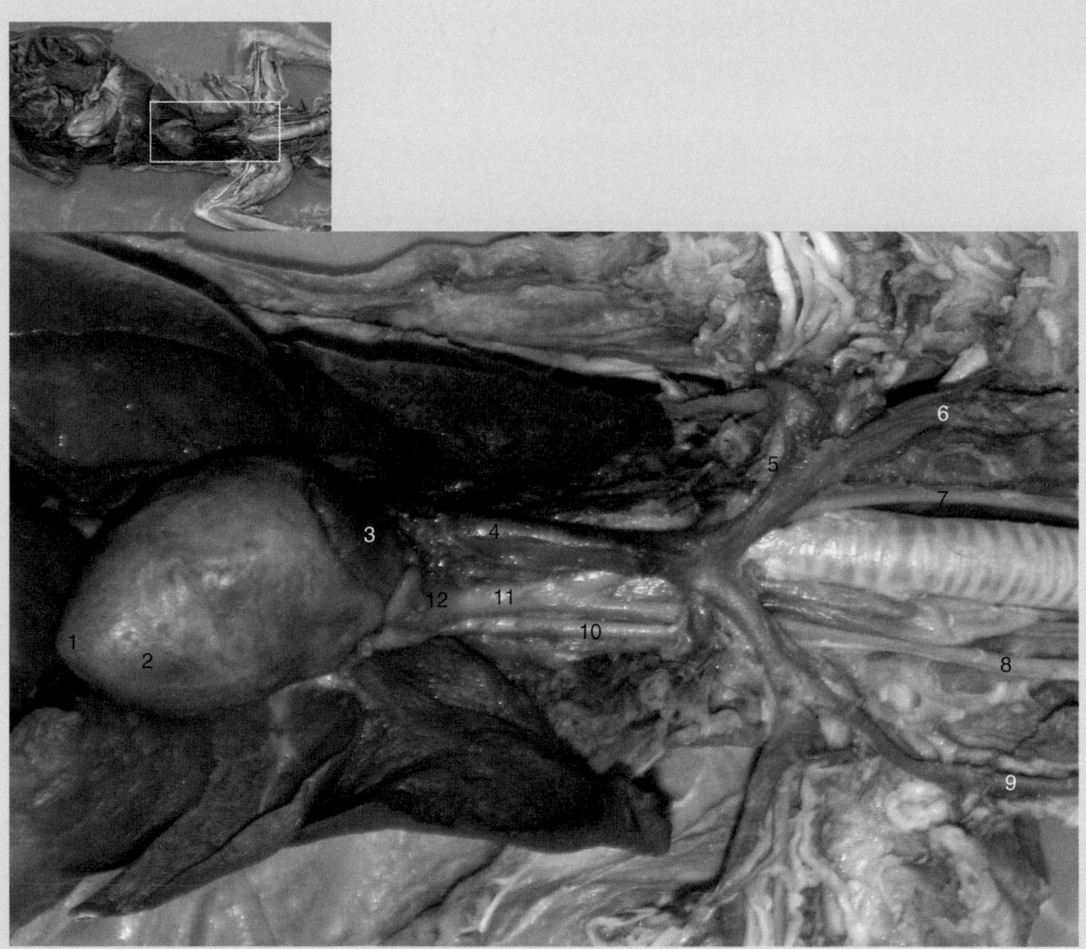

1. ______________________
2. ______________________
3. ______________________
4. ______________________
5. ______________________
6. ______________________
7. ______________________
8. ______________________
9. ______________________
10. ______________________
11. ______________________
12. ______________________

Exercise 8

Identify Cardiac and Abdominal Structures

1. ______________________
2. ______________________
3. ______________________
4. ______________________
5. ______________________
6. ______________________
7. ______________________
8. ______________________
9. ______________________

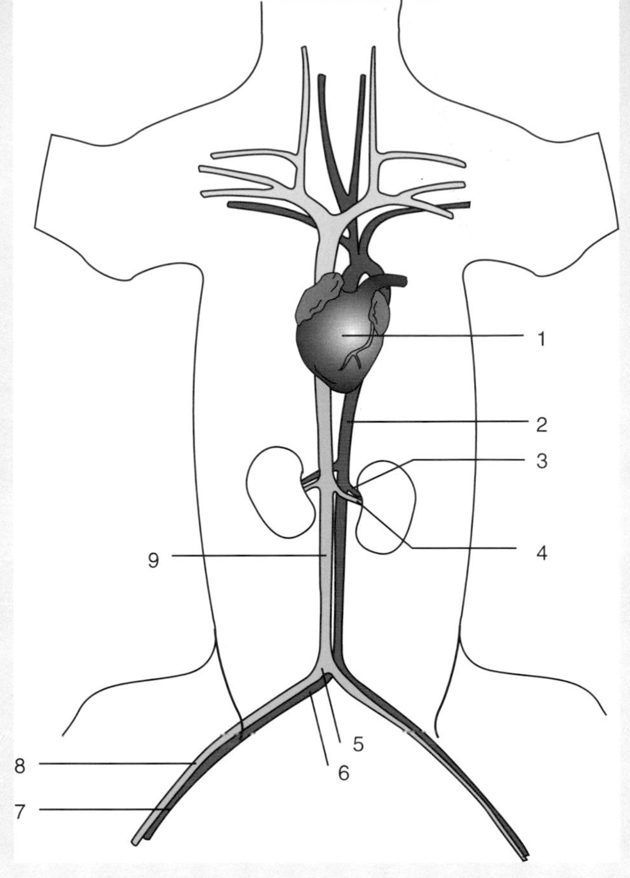

Exercise 9

Identify Feline Caudal Abdominal and Proximal Hindlimb Arteries and Veins

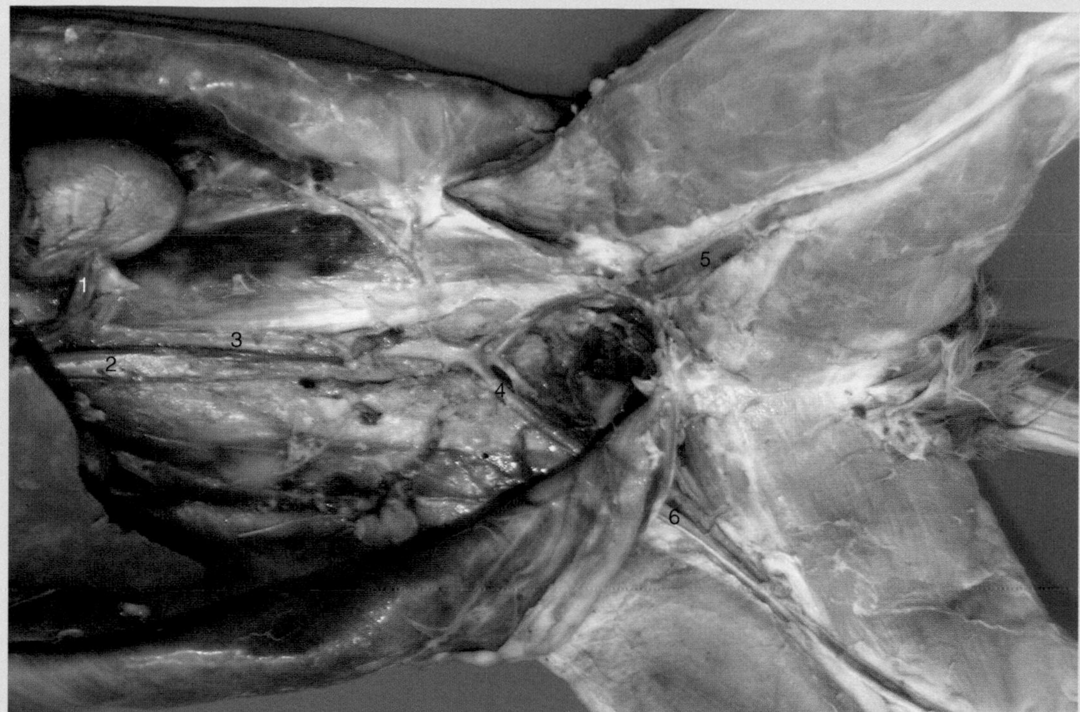

1. ______________________
2. ______________________
3. ______________________
4. ______________________
5. ______________________
6. ______________________

Exercise 10

Locate Veins

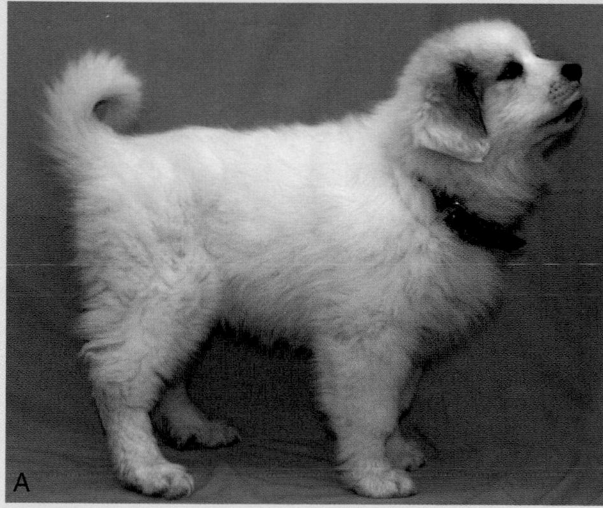

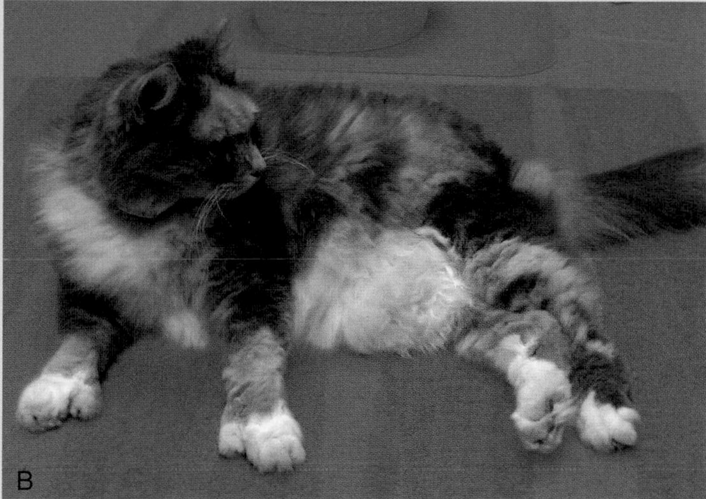

Mark numbers on the photographs for the locations of the following veins:

1. Jugular vein
2. Cephalic vein
3. Femoral vein
4. Saphenous vein

Critical and Clinical Thinking

Exercise 11

Define Key Terms

1. Aorta ______

2. Aortic arch ______

3. Aortic valve ______

4. Artery ______

5. Atrioventricular (AV) node ______

6. Atrium ______

7. Auricle ______

8. Capillary ______

9. Caudal vena cava ______

10. Chordae tendineae ______

11. Coronary circulation ______

12. Cranial vena cava ______

13. Diastole ______

14. Endocardium ______

15. Heart ______

16. Interatrial septum ______

17. Interventricular groove ______

18. Interventricular septum ______

19. Mediastinum ______

20. Mitral valve ______

21. Moderator band ______

22. Myocardium ______

Exercise 11—cont'd

Define Key Terms

23. Pericardial sac
24. Pericardium
25. Pulmonary circulation
26. Pulmonary valve
27. Pulmonary vessels
28. Renal artery and vein
29. Sinoatrial (SA) node
30. Semilunar valves
31. Systemic circulation
32. Systole
33. Tricuspid valve
34. Vein
35. Ventricle

Exercise 12

Clinical Thinking Challenge

1. What are three common venipuncture sites in cats?
2. What is the general name for the flap of connective tissue that makes up a heart valve?
3. What are the little cords of connective tissue that attach the free edges of an atrioventricular valve to the walls of a ventricle?
4. How many cusps does the mitral valve have?

Continued

Exercise 12—cont'd

Clinical Thinking Challenge

5. Does the *right* or *left* ventricle of the heart have thicker muscle? Why?

6. How many cusps does the tricuspid valve have?

7. Is the tricuspid valve located on the *right* or *left* side of the heart?

8. What valves are also known as the semilunar valves?
   ______ and ______

9. What valve is located between the right ventricle and the pulmonary artery?

10. What is the name for the wide cranial end of the heart? This is the area where the arteries and veins enter and exit.

11. What is the name for the caudal, pointed end of the heart, which contains the left ventricle?

12. Is a blood vessel carrying blood away from the heart and *afferent* or *efferent* blood vessels?

13. Is a blood vessel carrying blood toward the heart an *afferent* or *efferent* blood vessel?

14. Does the *right* or *left* side of the heart pump blood to the lungs?

15. Does the *right* or *left* side of the heart receive blood from the body (systemic circulation)?

16. What vessel carries blood from the lungs to the heart?

17. What is the valve between the left ventricle and the largest systemic artery?

18. What is the name of the largest systemic artery?

19. Is the vena cava an *afferent* or *efferent* blood vessel?

20. Is the aorta an *afferent* or *efferent* blood vessel?

21. Is the blood in the aorta *oxygen-rich* or *oxygen-poor*?

22. Is the blood in the vena cava *oxygen-rich* or *oxygen-poor*?

Exercise 12—cont'd

Clinical Thinking Challenge

23. Is the blood in the pulmonary artery *oxygen-rich* or *oxygen-poor*?

24. What artery supplies blood to the head?

25. What vessel carries blood from the heart to the lungs?

26. What is the largest vein in the body?

27. What superficial vessels (an artery and a vein) lie on the medial surface of the inner thigh?

28. What vein runs up the cranial surface of the forelimb below the elbow?

29. What vein is located just distal to the femoral vein on the hind leg?

30. What vein is most commonly used for drawing blood when a large volume is needed?

31. What vein curves up the lateral surface of the hindlimb just above the hock?

32. What blood vessels, which supply blood to the hindlimbs, does the abdominal aorta bifurcate (divide) into?

33. Is the jugular vein an *afferent* or *efferent* blood vessel?

34. Is the color of arterial blood *dark red* or *bright red?* ______
    Why? ______

35. Does venous blood *spurt* or *ooze* from a damaged vein? ______
    Why? ______

36. Does arterial blood *spurt* or *ooze* from a damaged artery? ______
    Why? ______

Exercise 13

Identify the Cardiovascular Component

Identify the cardiovascular component in each of the following "Who Am I?" statements.

1. ___________ I am the fluid in which all the elements of the cardiovascular system live.
2. ___________ We are the planes, trains, and automobiles responsible for moving oxygen from place to place.
3. ___________ We are the first responders to a vessel wall injury.
4. ___________ I have the mighty responsibility to move blood and everything it carries through an animal's body.
5. ___________ I carry blood away from the heart.
6. ___________ I carry blood toward the heart.
7. ___________ I am the side of the heart that controls the pulmonary circulation, receiving deoxygenated blood and pumping it into the lungs via the pulmonary artery where it becomes oxygenated.
8. ___________ I am the side of the heart that controls the systemic circulation and receives oxygenated blood from the lungs to pump it to the rest of the body via the aorta.
9. ___________ I am the area in the middle of the thoracic cavity where the heart sits.
10. ___________ When an animal is standing, you will find me located between the elbows.
11. ___________ I am the fibrous sac in which the heart rests.
12. ___________ I am a little loose so the heart can beat inside me, but I am not elastic enough to allow the heart to become abnormally enlarged.
13. ___________ I am the smooth, moist part of the serous pericardium.
14. ___________ I fill the pericardial space and lubricate the two membranes, preventing friction as they rub together during contractions and relaxations of the heart.
15. ___________ I am the thickest muscle layer of the wall of the heart.
16. ___________ Because of me, heart muscles do not fatigue.
17. ___________ I have two names; but by either name, I am the outermost layer of the heart wall.
18. ___________ I am composed of thin, flat simple squamous epithelium and lie on the internal surface of the myocardium.
19. ___________ I am the heart chamber that receives blood into the heart.
20. ___________ I pump blood out of the heart.
21. ___________ You could call me an ear flap or an ear. But either way, I am a blind pouch that comes off the main part of the atria.
22. ___________ I am visible on the outside of the heart, contain coronary blood vessels, and am frequently filled with fat.
23. ___________ I close at specific times to prevent backflow of blood into the chamber.
24. ___________ I open when the pressure from the amount of blood in the right atrium forces me open, allowing blood to flow into the right ventricle.
25. ___________ I am a collagen fiber cord that prevents the valve from opening backward into the atrium.
26. ___________ I am the valve that has two names; one because I resemble the headgear of a Roman Catholic bishop.
27. ___________ We have three crescent-shaped cups and control blood flow out of the ventricles and arteries.
28. ___________ I have four dense fibrous connective tissue rings and four primary functions, and I am located between the atria and the ventricles.
29. ___________ I am a channel formed by the joining of coronary veins in order to return blood to circulation.
30. ___________ As a transplanted heart, I don't have this, but I continue to function well.
31. ___________ I am an infection of the pericardium that usually progresses to heart failure and death.
32. ___________ I may occur spontaneously, but when I do, I cause excess fluid to accumulate in the pericardial sac.
33. ___________ I often accompany the answer to #32, and when I do, there is less complete cardiac filling, decreased stroke volume, and decreased cardiac output.

Exercise 13—cont'd

Identify the Cardiovascular Component

34. ____________ This activity occurs when the synchronized contraction of the heart is lost, and the heart receives electrical currents from more than one direction.
35. ____________ I am the pacemaker of the heart.
36. ____________ We are the processes by which sodium and calcium ions move through channels from the exterior to the interior of the cell, and potassium ions move through channels in the cell membrane from the interior to the exterior, and we then reverse the process to keep the heart automatically going through the cardiac cycle.
37. ____________ I am the term for contraction of the myocardium, considered the working phase of the cardiac cycle.
38. ____________ I am the term for the relaxation and repolarization of the myocardium, considered the relaxation phase of the cardiac cycle.
39. ____________ We are snapping shut when you hear a "lub" sound through a stethoscope.
40. ____________ We are snapping shut when you hear a "dub" sound through a stethoscope.
41. ____________ I am the side of the animal on which most heart sounds can be heard best.
42. ____________ I am the sound heard when cardiac valves do not close all the way.
43. ____________ I am a condition where the valves do not open all the way.
44. ____________ I am a measure of blood output from the left ventricle over a unit of time, usually 1 min.
45. ____________ The term used to answer #44 is determined by the two of us.
46. ____________ We are the smallest branches in the arterial tree.
47. ____________ I am the largest vein in an animal's body, and in yours, too.
48. ____________ Oxygenated blood flows through me from the mother to a developing fetus.
49. ____________ Blood entering the fetus via the answer to #48, oxygenated by the maternal blood, bypasses the oxygen exchange by us.
50. ____________ I am the rate of alternating stretching and recoiling of the elastic fibers in an artery as blood passes through it with each heartbeat and can be felt on superficial arteries lying against firm surfaces such as bones.
51. ____________ I am a number in a blood pressure reading, produced by the ejection of blood from the left ventricle into the systemic circulation by way of the aorta.
52. ____________ I am sometimes measured when an anesthetized animal is being monitored to check for tissue perfusion.
53. ____________ On an electrocardiogram, I am the time it takes the wave of depolarization to travel from the SA node through the aorta.
54. ____________ On an electrocardiogram, I am the time of ventricular depolarization.
55. ____________ On an electrocardiogram, I am the time of ventricular relaxation.
56. ____________ I am an especially useful method of evaluating the relative size of the heart chambers, the thickness of the myocardium, and the functioning of the valves.
57. ____________ I am the most commonly used site of venipuncture in dogs and cats and run between the elbow and the carpus on the craniomedial aspect of the forearm.
58. ____________ The two of us lie close together, and care must be taken to avoid accidental injection into one of us as we carry blood quickly to the brain—not a good idea when injecting a sedative.
59. ____________ I can be found on lactating dairy cattle along the ventral aspect of each side of the abdomen from the udder to the level of the sternum but must never be used for venipuncture. I am small, thin-walled, and prone to excessive bleeding and hematoma formation, which may lead to the development of an abscess.
60. ____________ I can be found on a rodent, along the ventral midline of the tail, and can be used for venipuncture.

13
The Respiratory System[a]

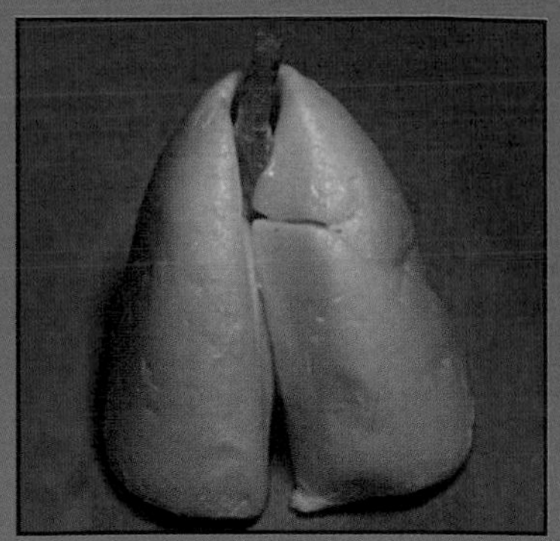

OVERVIEW AT A GLANCE

Respiratory Revelations: Structures of the Upper Respiratory Tract in the Skull 335

Respiratory Revelations: The Larynx 338

Respiratory Revelations: The Trachea 340

Respiratory Revelations: Structures of the Lower Respiratory Tract in the Thoracic Cavity 342

Suggested In-class Activities 347

Exercises 349–362

The Skull and Neck 349

1. *Label the Structures in the Skull and Neck 349*

The Larynx and Trachea 350

2. *Label the Indicated Structures 350*

Structures of the Lower Respiratory Tract in the Thoracic Cavity 351–356

3. *Label the Structures of the Respiratory Tract 351*
4. *Label the Structures in the Thorax of the Cat 352*
5. *Label the Structures in the Respiratory Tract of the Cat 353*
6. *Identify the Structures of the Lower Respiratory Tract of Cat 354*
7. *Is This the Right or Left Side of the Cat? Why? 355*
8. *Identify the Lobes of the Lung 356*

Critical and Clinical Thinking 356–362

9. *Name that Nose—Common Animals 356*
10. *Name that Nose—Exotic Animals 358*
11. *Connect the Anatomic Dots 359*
12. *Who Am I? 360*
13. *Define Clinical Terms 361*
14. *Clinical Thinking Challenge 362*

LEARNING OBJECTIVES

The objectives of this chapter are to describe and identify the organization, function, location, and appearance of clinically important structures of the upper and lower respiratory tracts.

Read Chapter 15 in *Clinical Anatomy and Physiology for Veterinary Technicians* for detailed descriptions and locations of these structures.

CLINICAL SIGNIFICANCE

An understanding of the anatomy of the respiratory system will enable you to understand how the system functions and what happens when it doesn't function properly. How would you explain respiratory tract infections to a client if you couldn't explain what structures were involved? What's involved in putting a breathing tube down a dog's throat when it's going to be anesthetized for surgery? Some clients are very curious. Why does the trachea sometimes collapse? What's the difference between a cough, a sneeze, a yawn, a sigh, and the hiccups? All these questions involve the respiratory system and you should know the answers.

INTRODUCTION

The respiratory system has many jobs, but the most fundamental one is to remove carbon dioxide (CO_2) from the blood and replace it with oxygen (O_2). To do that, it has to bring outside air into close proximity with the network of tiny capillaries in the lungs.

Our examination of the respiratory system will focus on the series of tubes that bring outside air into the lungs, and the lungs themselves. The tubes that move air to and from the lungs make up the *upper respiratory tract* and the structures within the lungs make up the *lower respiratory tract*.

[a]The authors and publisher wish to acknowledge Joann Colville and Amy Ellwein for previous contributions to this chapter.

TERMS TO BE IDENTIFIED

Upper respiratory tract
- Arytenoid cartilages
- Bifurcation of the trachea
- Epiglottis
- Larynx
- Nasal cavity and turbinates
- Nasal septum
- Nostrils (nares)
- Paranasal sinuses
- Pharynx
- Trachea
- Vocal cords

Lower respiratory tract
- Bronchi
- Diaphragm
- Hilus
- Lungs
- Thoracic cavity

MEDICAL WORDS AND WORD PARTS

Bronch/o = bronchus
Laryng/o = larynx
Nas/o = nose
Pharyng/o = pharynx
Pneumo/o = air, lung, or respiration
Pulmonary = lungs
Respir/o = respiration
Trache/o = trachea

Respiratory Revelations: Structures of the Upper Respiratory Tract in the Skull

(Figs. 13.1–13.5.)

- The **nostrils** open into the nasal cavity.
- **Paranasal sinuses** are outpouchings of the nasal passages that are contained within spaces in certain skull bones.
- The **nasal septum** separates the right and left sides of the **nasal cavity**.
- The **turbinates** increase the surface area of the nasal cavity so it can be more efficient at warming, filtering, and humidifying the air that passes through it.
- The respiratory tract (nasal passage) is dorsal to the digestive tract (mouth) in the skull. In the pharynx, the respiratory tract switches positions with the digestive tract and moves to a ventral location.

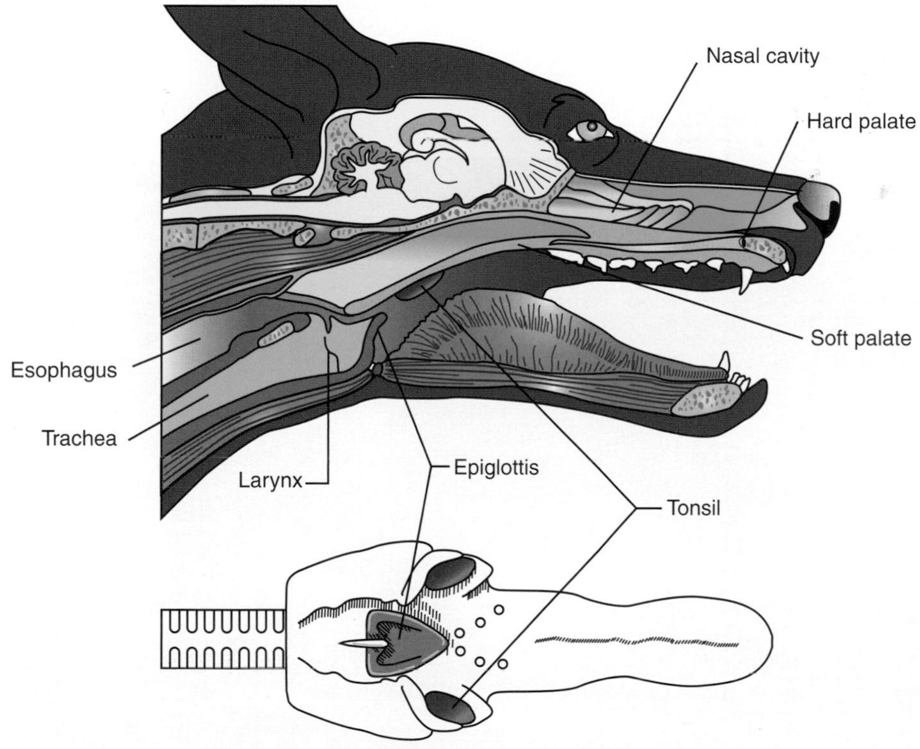

• **Fig. 13.1** The upper respiratory tract of a dog.

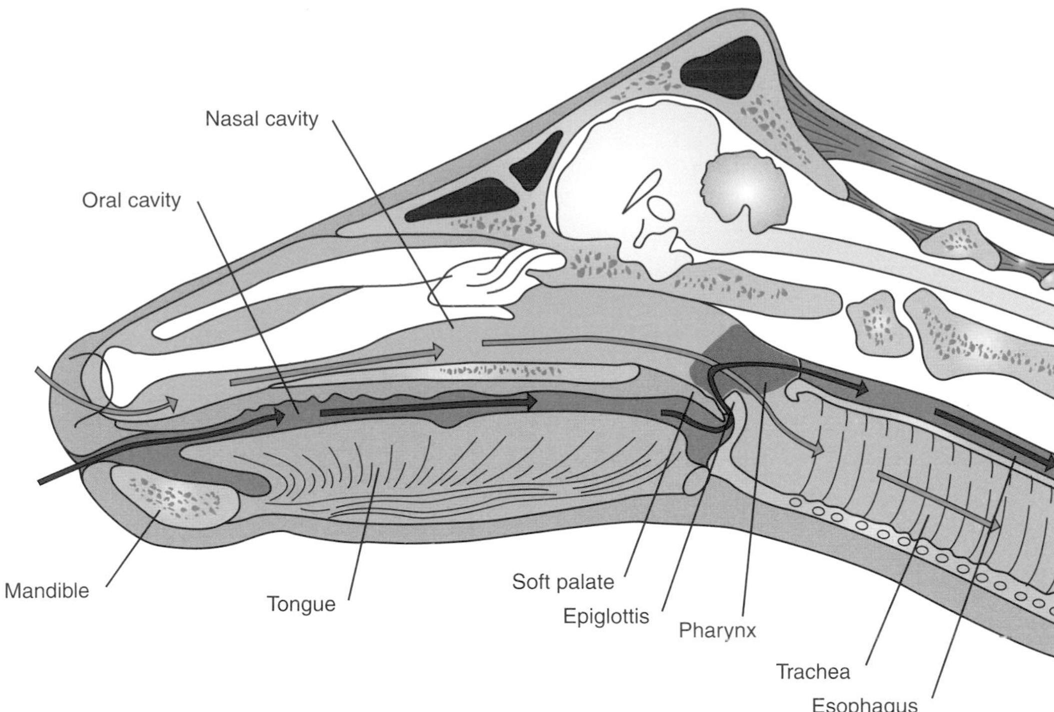

• **Fig. 13.2** The upper respiratory tract of a cow. The blue arrow follows the path of air that is breathed through the nostrils. The red arrows follow the route of food after it is taken into the mouth. Note that the two paths cross at the pharynx.

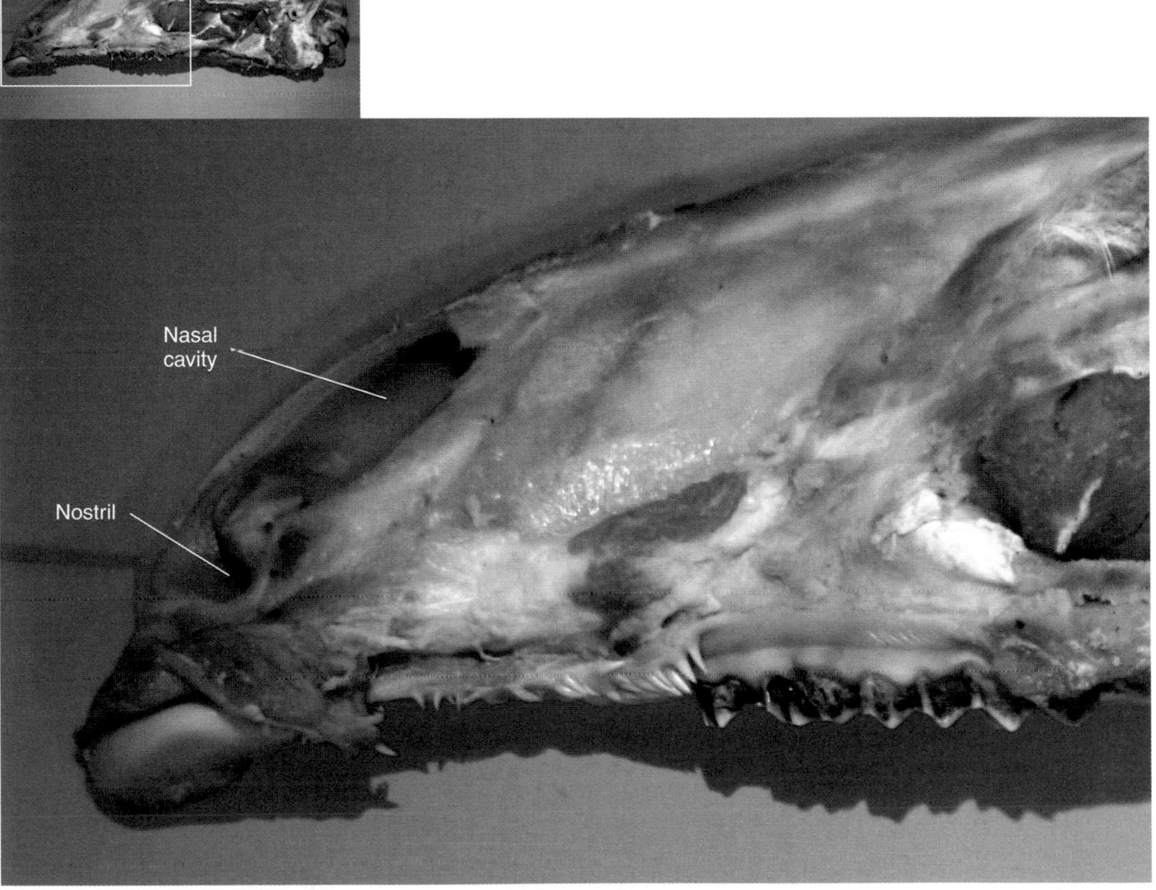

• **Fig. 13.3** Skinned ovine skull (lateral view.) The mandible has been removed. View of the nostrils and beginning of the nasal cavity in a sheep.

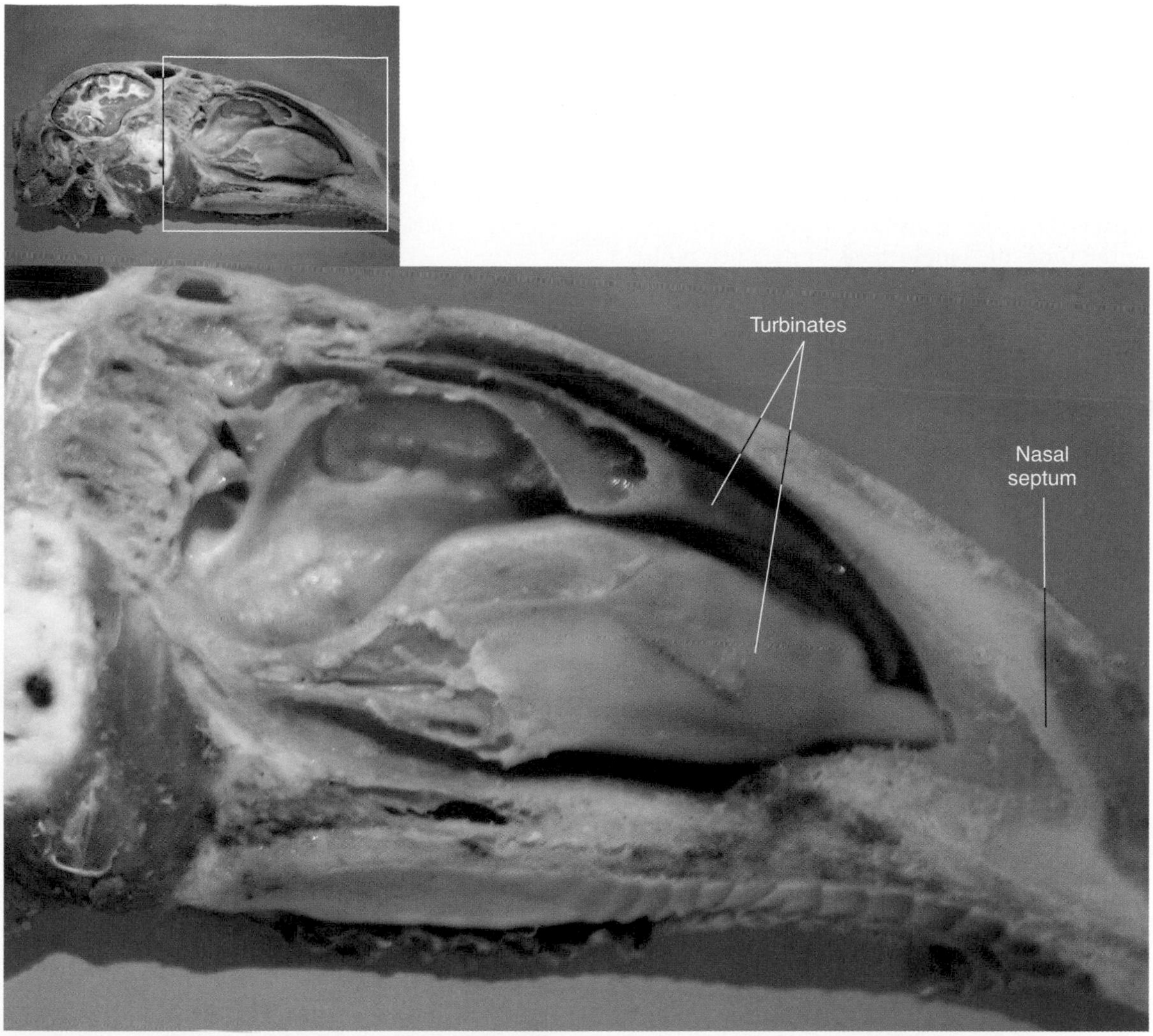

• **Fig. 13.4** Skinned ovine skull (medial view.) The mandible has been removed. View of the nasal septum and nasal turbinates in a sheep.

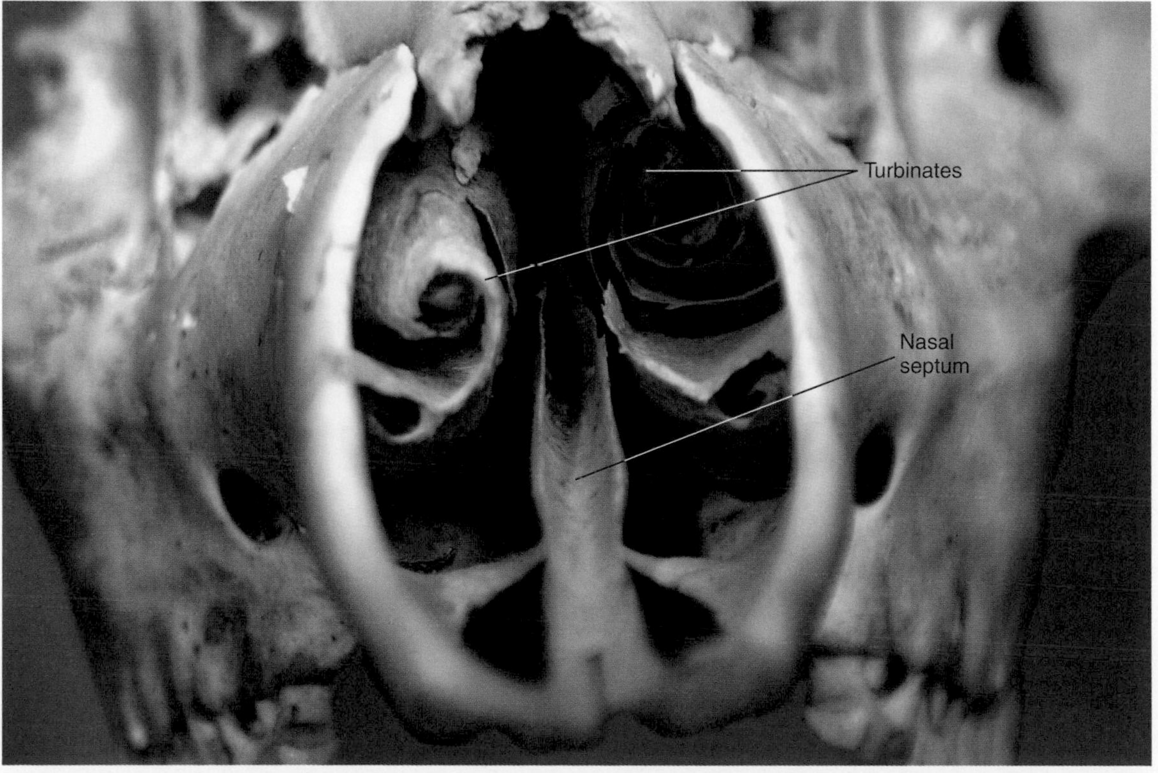

• **Fig. 13.5** Nasal turbinates and nasal septum in a deer skull (rostral view.)

Respiratory Revelations: The Larynx

(Figs. 13.6–13.10.)

- The **larynx** is located between the **pharynx** (throat) and the trachea (windpipe).
- The larynx is ventral to the esophagus.
- The glottis is the opening into the larynx.
- Most of the time, the **epiglottis** is in the open position to allow breathing. The epiglottis covers the glottis when the animal swallows, to prevent food and saliva from entering the trachea.

When placing a breathing tube (endotracheal [ET] tube) into an animal, you must press down (ventrally) on the epiglottis to expose the glottis. Otherwise, the tube will slide dorsally and enter the other opening in the back of the throat—the esophagus.

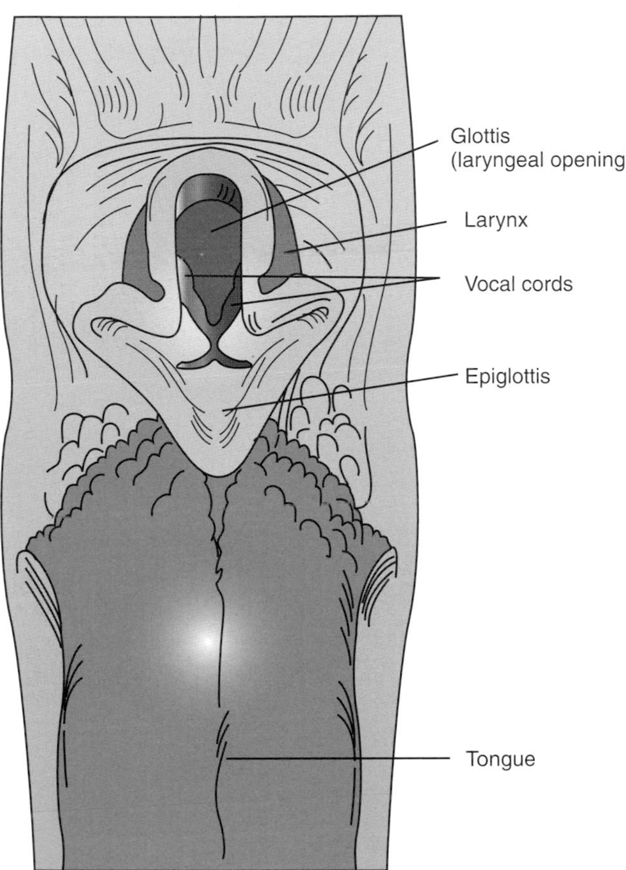

• **Fig. 13.6** Schematic drawing of the caudal pharynx and the opening to the larynx.

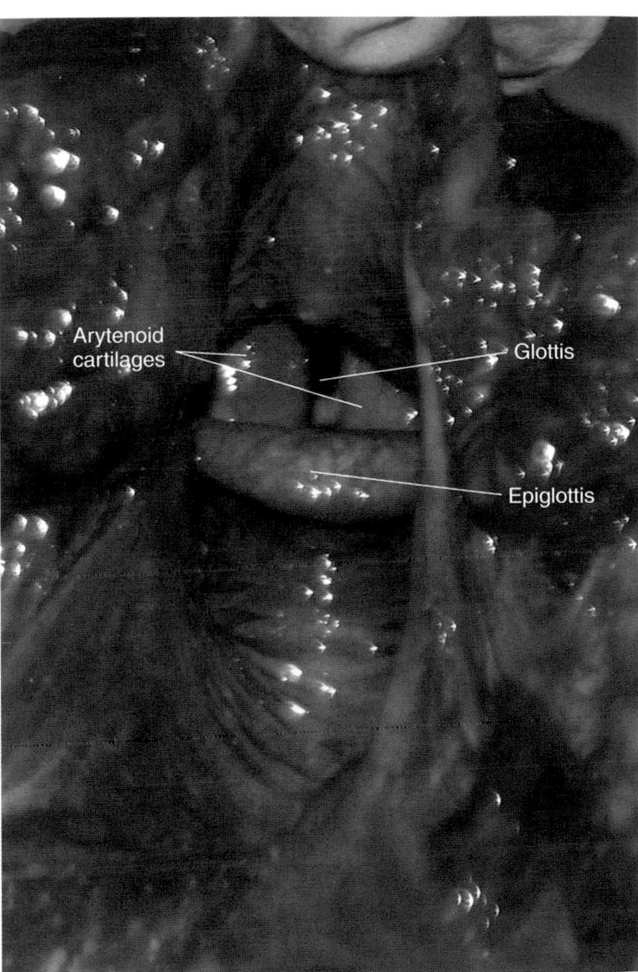

• **Fig. 13.7** Larynx of a calf. From this rostral view, the epiglottis and the arytenoid cartilages are visible.

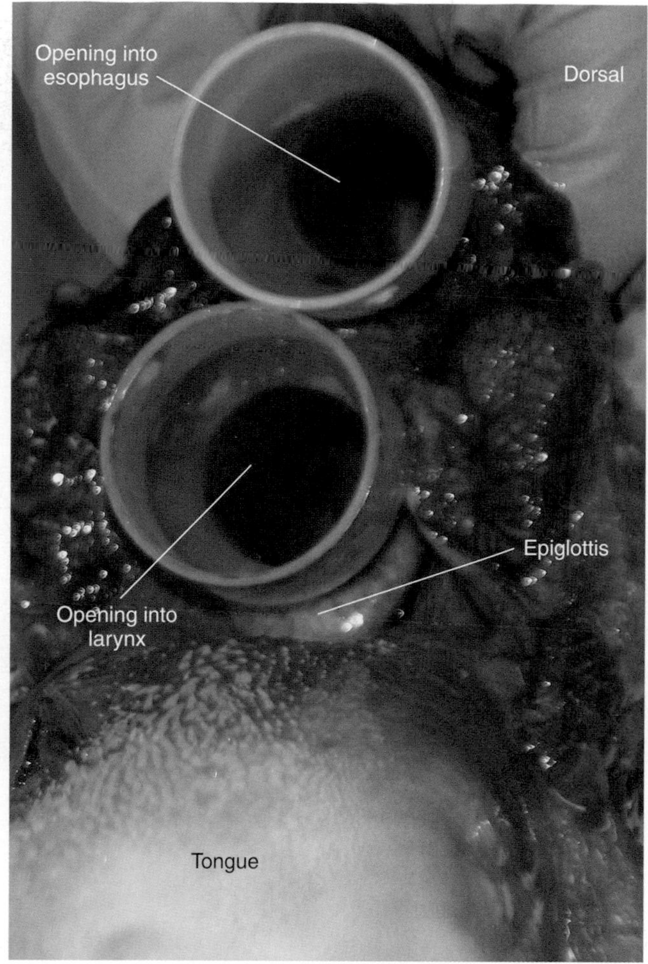

• **Fig. 13.8** Position of openings into larynx and esophagus. Syringe cases have been inserted into the openings of the larynx (ventral) and esophagus (dorsal).

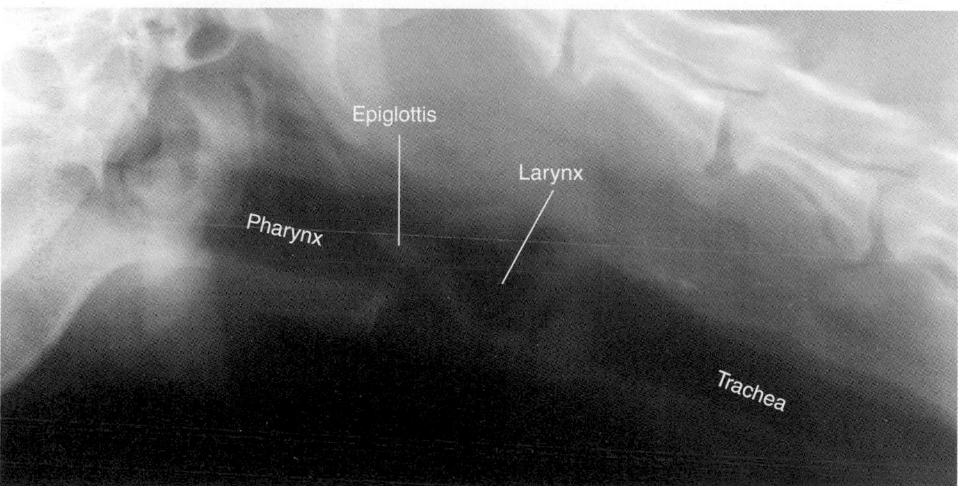

• **Fig. 13.9** Lateral radiograph of the neck of a dog. The epiglottis is visible at the entrance to the larynx and trachea.

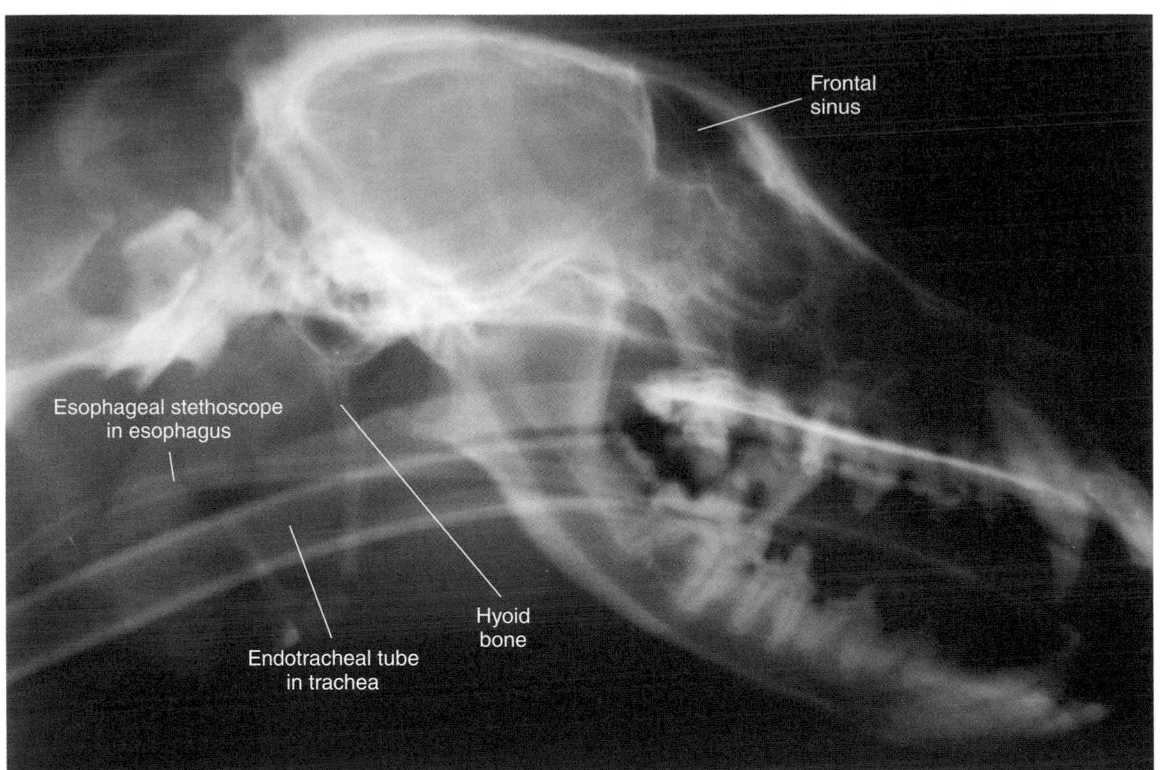

• **Fig. 13.10** Radiograph of dog with endotracheal tube and esophageal stethoscope in place. Note that the trachea is ventral to the esophagus in the neck area. The hyoid bone and frontal sinus are also visible.

Respiratory Revelations: The Trachea

(Figs. 13.11–13.13.)

- The **trachea** carries air from the larynx down through the neck region to the lungs in the thoracic cavity.
- The trachea is ventral to the esophagus in the neck.
- The hyaline cartilage rings that support the trachea appear as light-colored structures regularly spaced along the length of the trachea.

At its caudal end, the trachea **bifurcates** (divides) into two branches called primary bronchi, which enter the lungs.

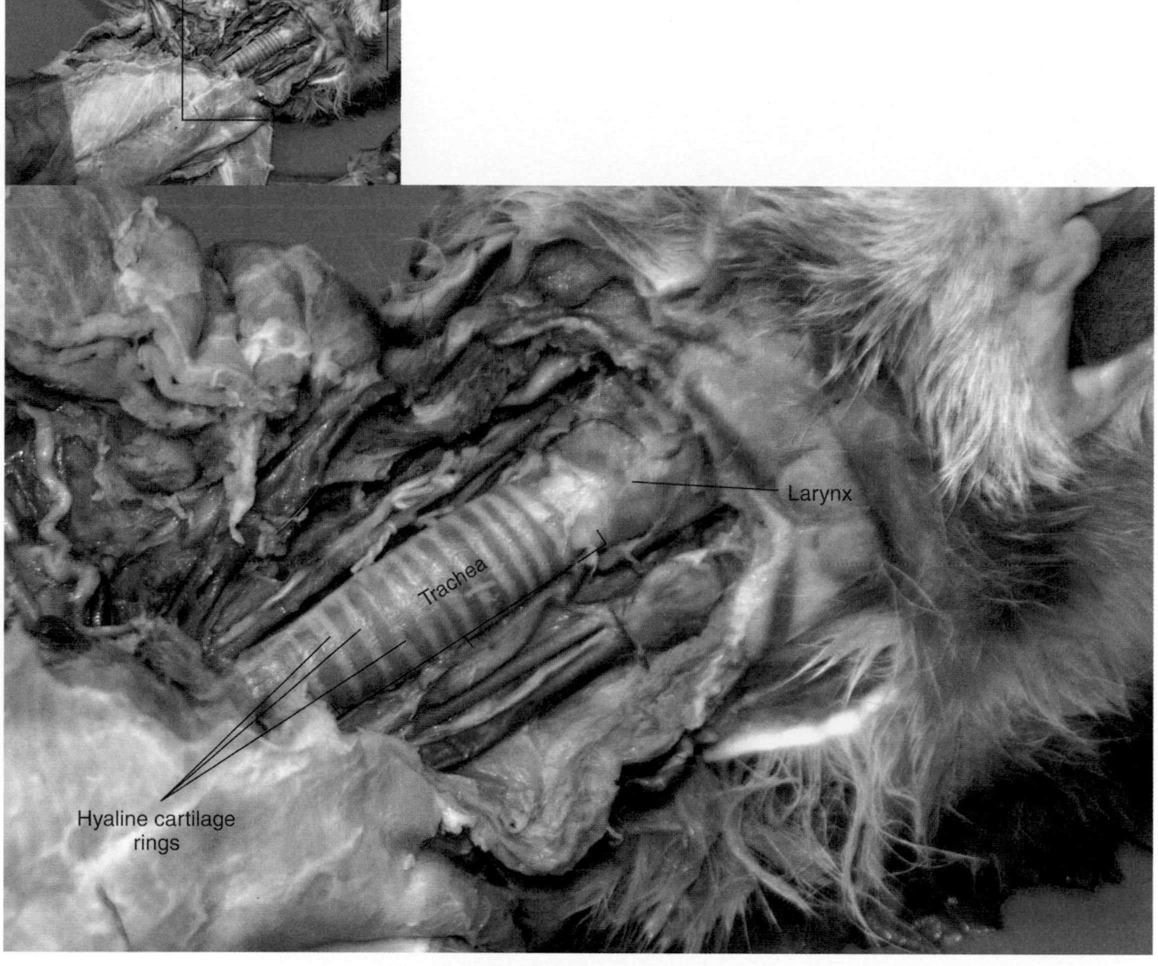

• **Fig. 13.11** The larynx and trachea of a cat.

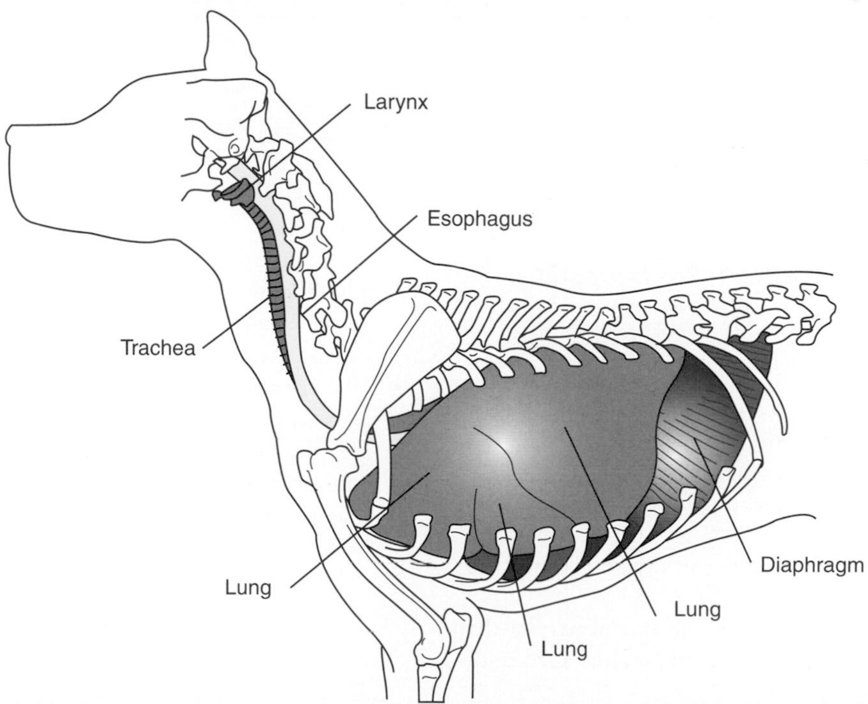

• **Fig. 13.12** Schematic drawing of the position of the respiratory system in the neck and thoracic cavity of a dog.

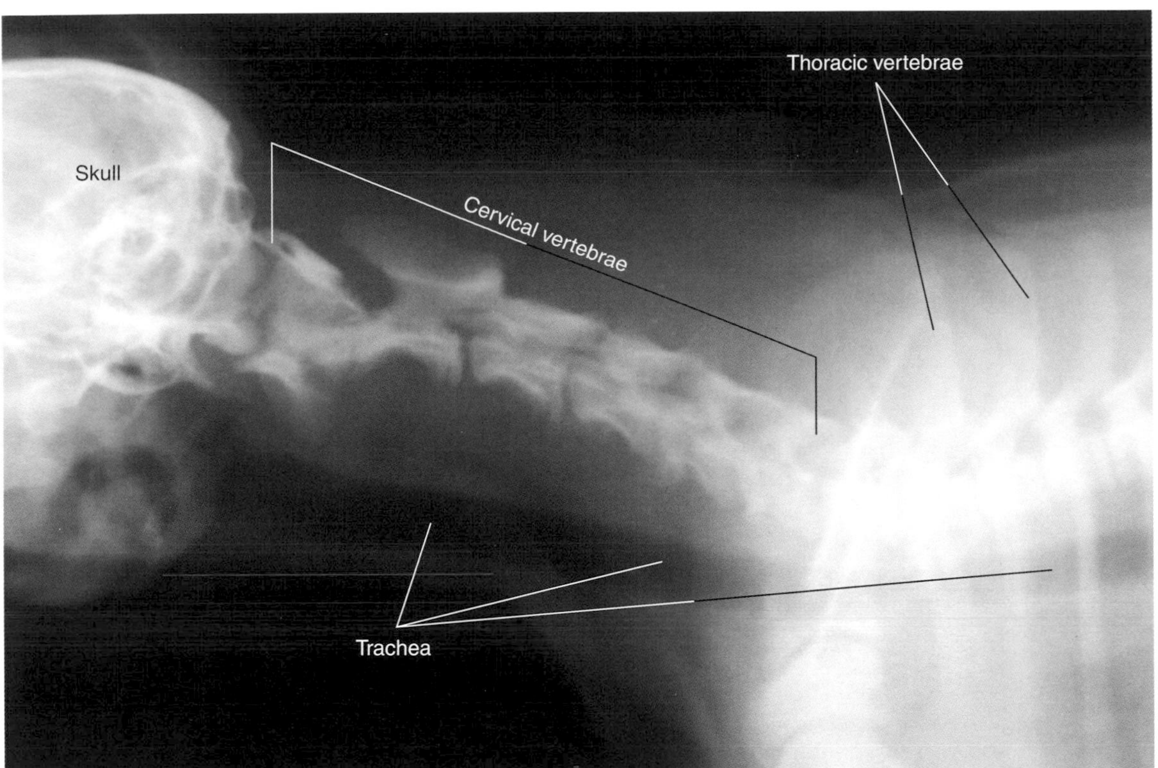

• **Fig. 13.13** Radiograph of the neck and cranial thorax of a dog showing the trachea.

TABLE 13.1 Lung Lobes

Species	Left Lung	Right Lung
Cat, cow, dog, goat, pig, sheep	Cranial lobe	Cranial lobe
	Middle lobe	Middle lobe
	Caudal lobe	Caudal lobe
		Accessory lobe
Horse	Cranial lobe	Cranial lobe
	Caudal lobe	Caudal lobe
		Accessory lobe

Respiratory Revelations: Structures of the Lower Respiratory Tract in the Thoracic Cavity

(Table 13.1 and Figs. 13.14–13.20.)

- The mediastinum is the area between the **lungs** in the thoracic cavity. It contains the heart, trachea, esophagus, blood vessels, nerves, and lymphatic structures.
- The heart fills a significant portion of the **thoracic cavity**.
- The narrow apex of each lung lies in the cranial portion of the thoracic cavity.
- The wide base of each lung is in the caudal part of the thoracic cavity, resting directly on the cranial surface of the diaphragm.
- The left lung of most animals has two lobes. The right lung of most animals has four lobes.
- The **hilum** of each lung is where air passageways, blood vessels, lymph vessels, and nerves enter and leave the lung.
- The primary bronchi divide into secondary bronchi that are sent to each **lobe** of the lungs.
- Healthy lungs have a light, spongy consistency.
- The **diaphragm** is a thin dome-shaped sheet of muscle that separates the thoracic cavity from the abdominal cavity.

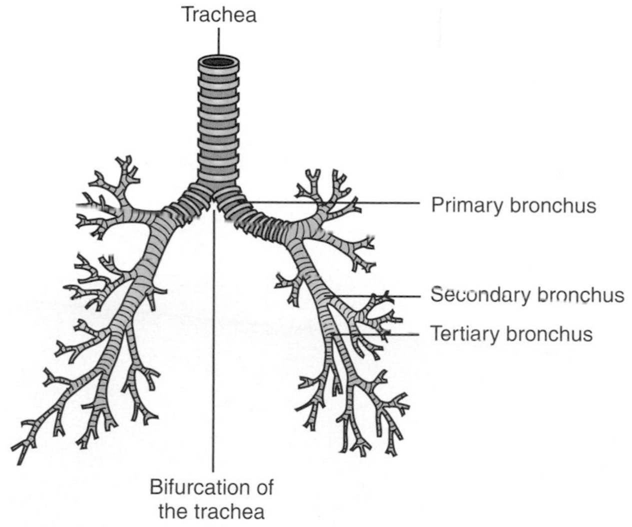

• **Fig. 13.14** The bronchial tree.

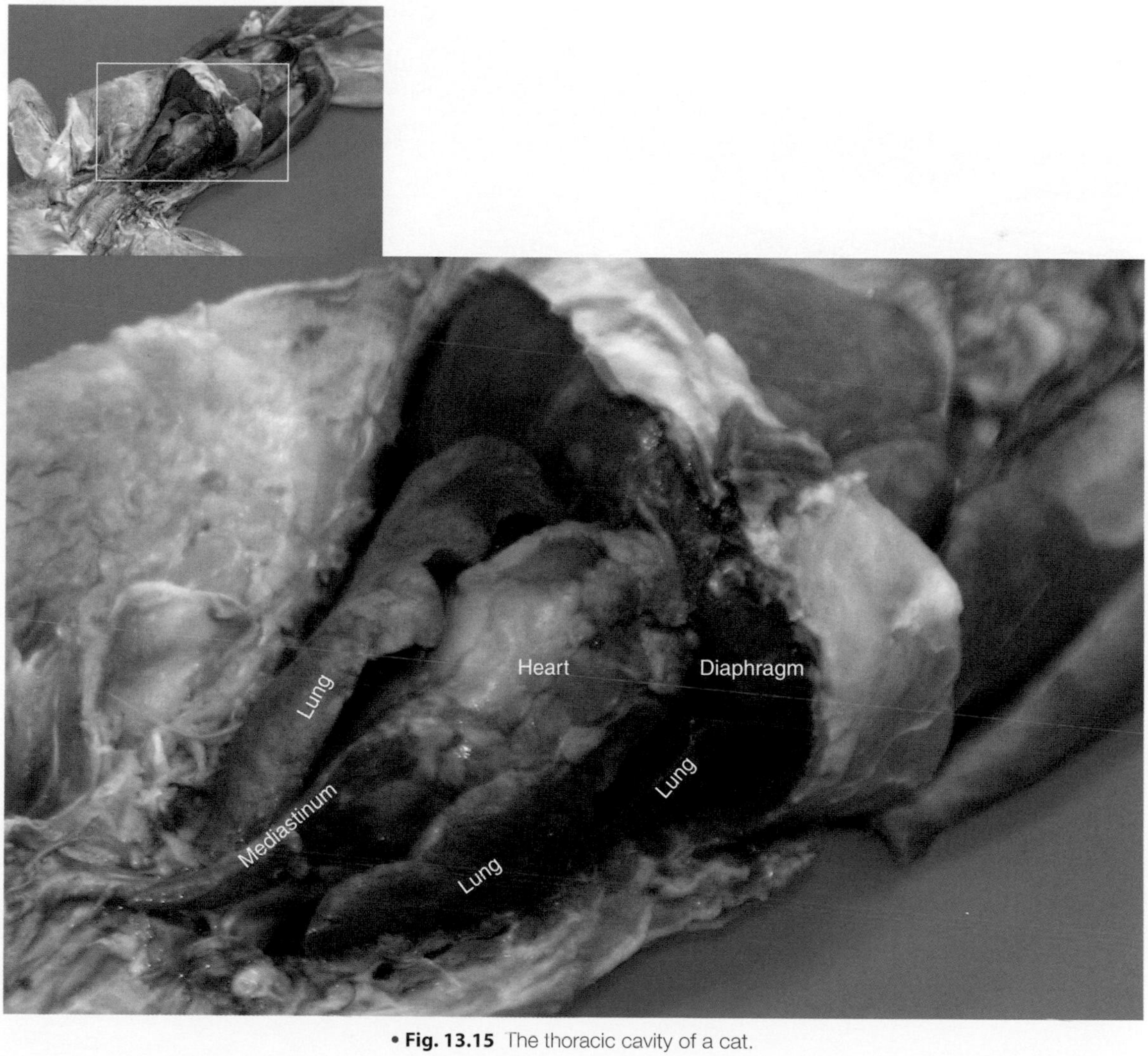

Heart
Diaphragm
Lung
Lung
Mediastinum
Lung

• **Fig. 13.15** The thoracic cavity of a cat.

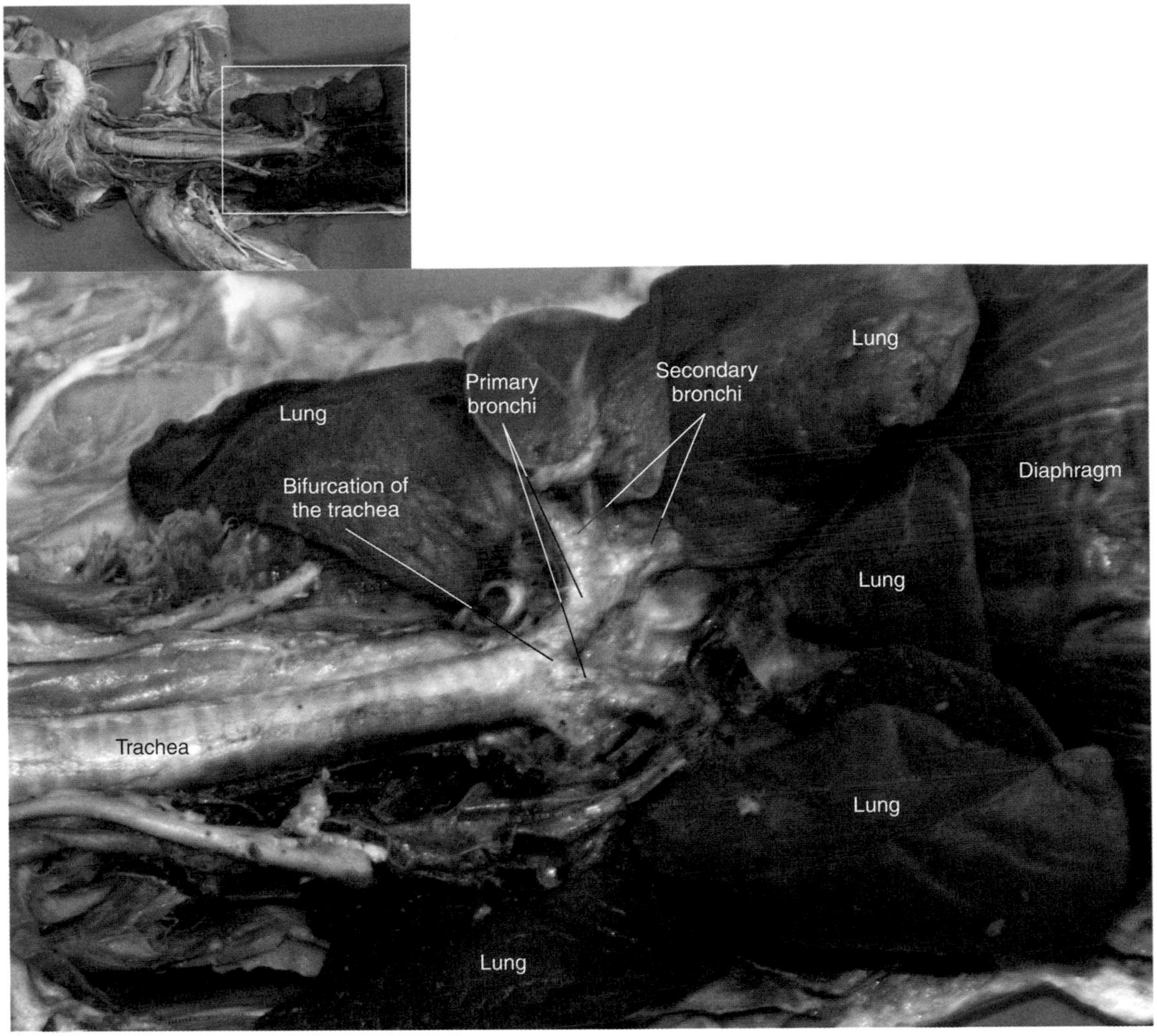

• **Fig. 13.16** Bifurcation of the trachea. With the heart removed, the bifurcation of the trachea is visible as it divides into primary bronchi. The primary bronchi then divide into secondary bronchi.

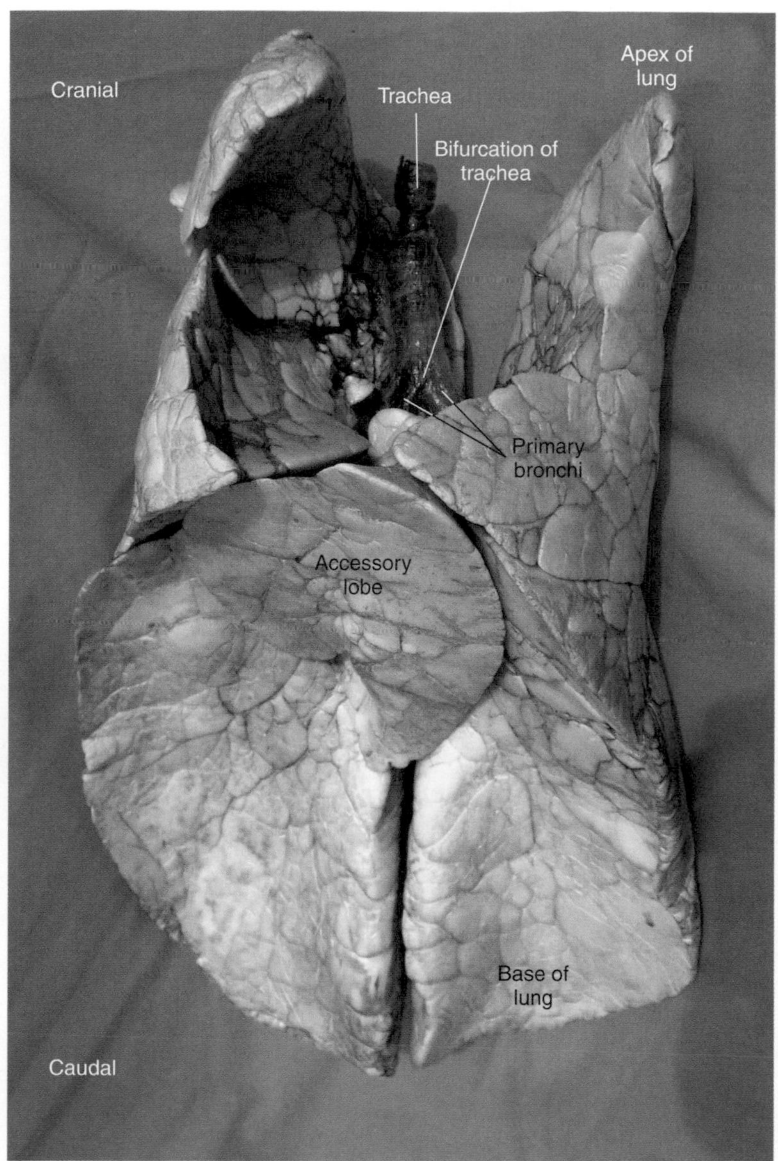

• **Fig. 13.17** Plasticized pig lungs. Ventral view with heart removed.

• **Fig. 13.18** Chest radiograph of a dog in lateral recumbency. The dark, air-filled trachea is seen as it travels to the lungs. The bifurcation of the trachea is visible as a dark circle at the termination of the trachea. The heart and some of its related blood vessels are also visible.

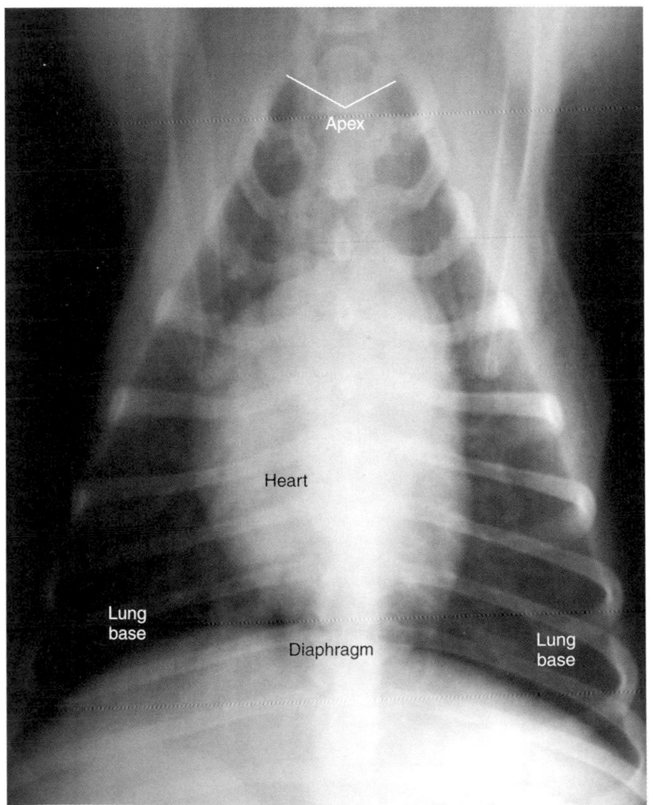

• **Fig. 13.19** Chest radiograph of a dog in sternal recumbency. The apex and the base of each lung are shown. The diaphragm separates the abdominal cavity from the thoracic cavity. The trachea is not visible on this view because it is obscured by the thoracic vertebrae and sternum.

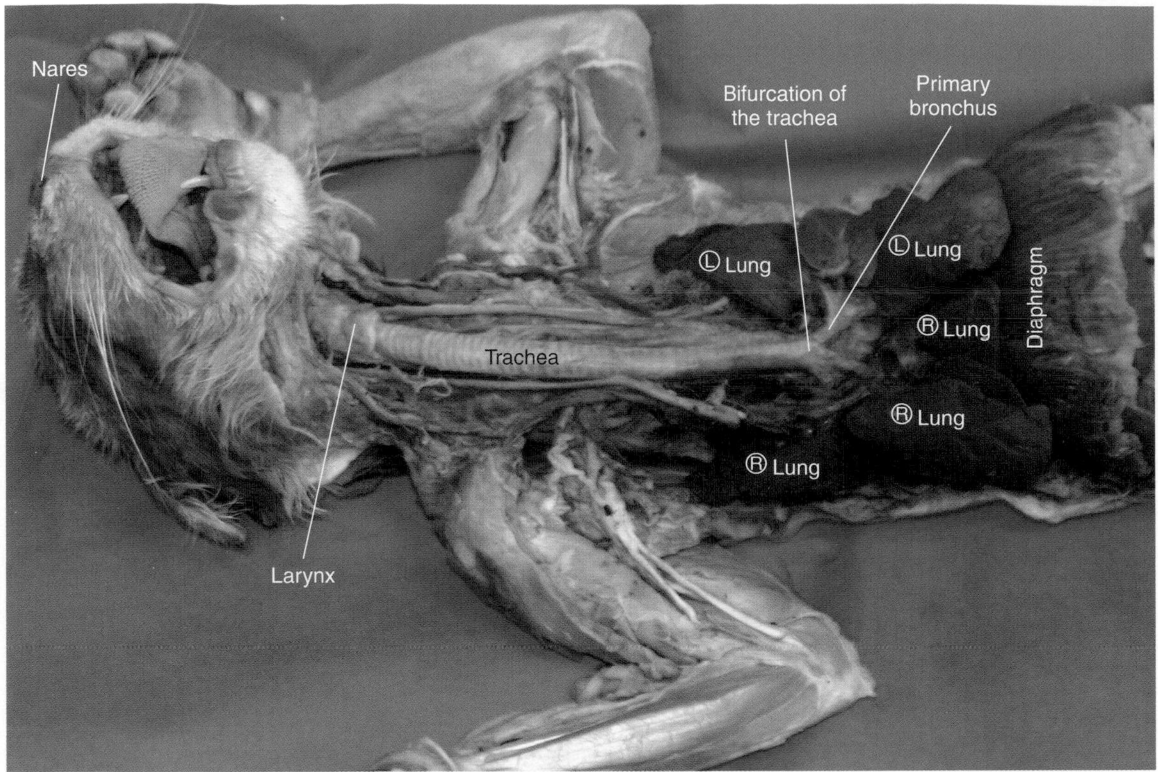

• **Fig. 13.20** The respiratory tract of a cat. (Heart removed.)

Suggested In-class Activities

Watch the Nares on Live Animals

Materials Needed

Live animals.

Procedure

Examine the snouts of as many animals as you can. Notice what happens to the nares and chest wall as the animal breathes. The nares of different species of animals differ in pliability and ability to dilate. Is the snout warm or cool? Is it moist or dry? Are the nares large and pliable or small and rigid? What happens to the nares when an animal pants?

Clinical Significance

By becoming familiar with what a healthy animal's snout looks and feels like, you will be able to detect abnormalities when you see them.

Palpate the Neck of an Animal

Materials Needed

Live animals and a restrainer (partner).

Procedure

Feel the rigid structure on the midline of the ventral surface of the neck. This is the trachea. Can you feel the cartilaginous rings?

Clinical Significance

When placing a breathing (endotracheal) tube in an animal, you should not be able to see or feel it slide down the neck from the outside because it is contained within the trachea. If you can feel the tube sliding down the neck outside the trachea, it is in the esophagus.

Auscultate (Listen to) the Breath Sounds and Lungs

Materials Needed

Live animals, a stethoscope, and a restrainer (partner).

Procedure

Place the stethoscope on the ventral neck surface (over the cranial trachea) and listen for breath sounds. These should be fairly loud because you're listening through thin tissues. Move the stethoscope to the chest wall of a standing animal just above the elbow and caudal to the scapula. Listen for the same breath sound you heard in the neck. This is the sound of air moving in the trachea and at the bifurcation. Gradually move the stethoscope to the ventral surface of the chest, listening at various points along the way for more breath sounds. These are the breath sounds of the lobes of the lungs. These sounds will be softer because they are traveling through lung tissue. Make sure you move your stethoscope around to listen to all the lung lobes.

Test to see how large or small an area can be auscultated for breath sounds. Do the lungs sound clear? Do you hear air smoothly moving or do you hear crackles and pops? Can you hear the respiratory sounds more easily on one side of the animal than the other? What happens when the animal pants? Listen to as many species of animals as possible.

With a stethoscope, listen to the animal's breathing. Count the number of breaths for 15 seconds then multiply that number by four to get the animal's respiratory rate per minute. Do you get the same number of breaths when you watch the animal's chest move as it breathes?

Clinical Significance

Know the normal breath sounds in a healthy animal so you can recognize abnormal sounds when you hear them. Listen to all lung lobes, as one lobe can be abnormal and the others not.

Peek Inside the Living Animal

(Fig. 13.21.)

Materials Needed

Radiographs of the thoracic cavity of various animals.

Procedure

View as many lateral and dorsoventral (DV) or ventrodorsal (VD) radiographs of the thoracic cavity as possible. Look at radiographs from a variety of species to identify the larynx, trachea, and lungs. Is the width of the trachea even all the way from the larynx to the lungs or does it narrow and widen? Are the lungs clear and black or do they have fuzzy areas of gray?

Clinical Significance

Knowing the normal appearance of structures will enable you to evaluate the quality of the radiographs you produce.

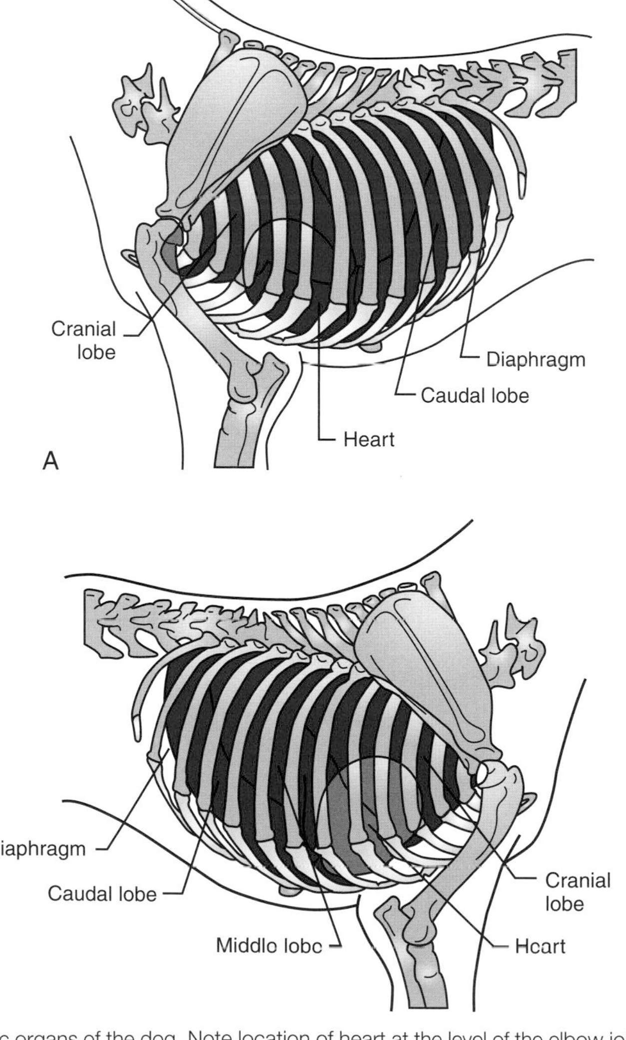

• Fig. 13.21 Thoracic organs of the dog. Note location of heart at the level of the elbow joint. (A) Left side. (B) Right side.

EXERCISES

The Skull and Neck

Exercise 1

Label the Structures in the Skull and Neck

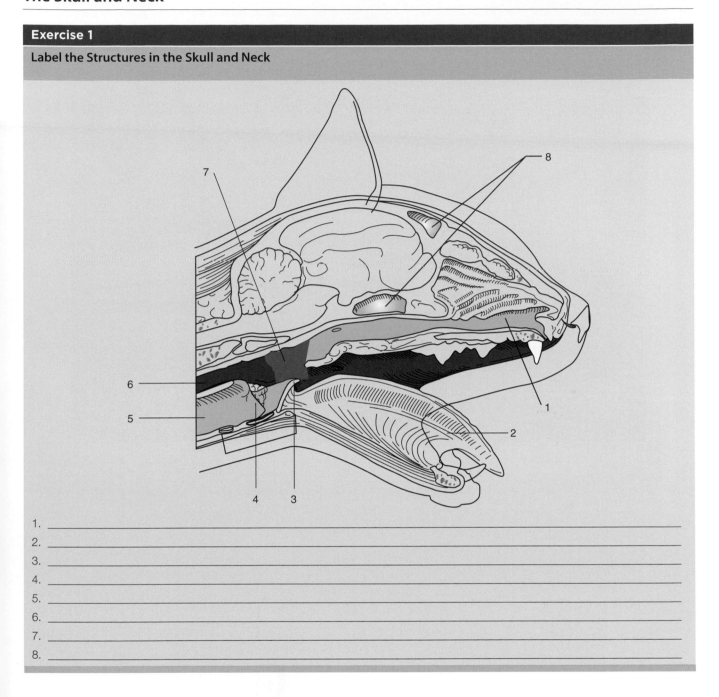

1. ______
2. ______
3. ______
4. ______
5. ______
6. ______
7. ______
8. ______

The Larynx and Trachea

Exercise 2

Label the Indicated Structures

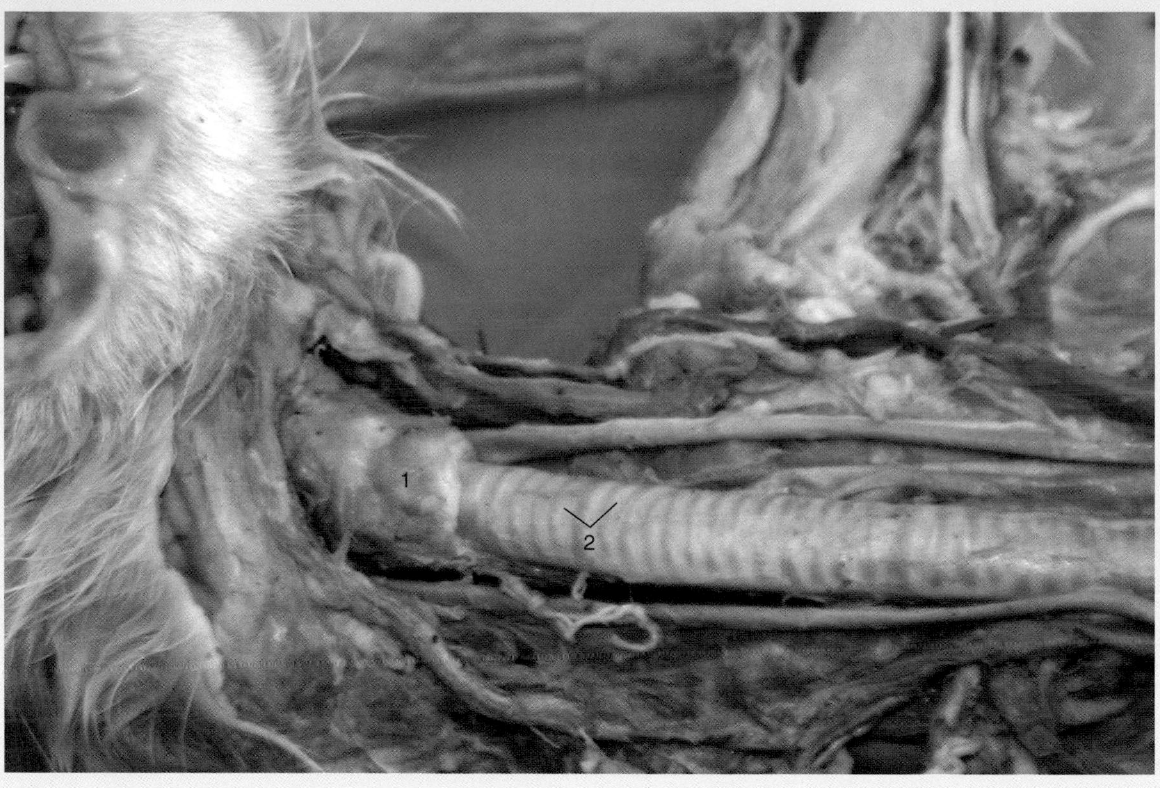

1. ______________________________

2. ______________________________ (be specific)

Structures of the Lower Respiratory Tract in the Thoracic Cavity

Exercise 3

Label the Structures of the Respiratory Tract

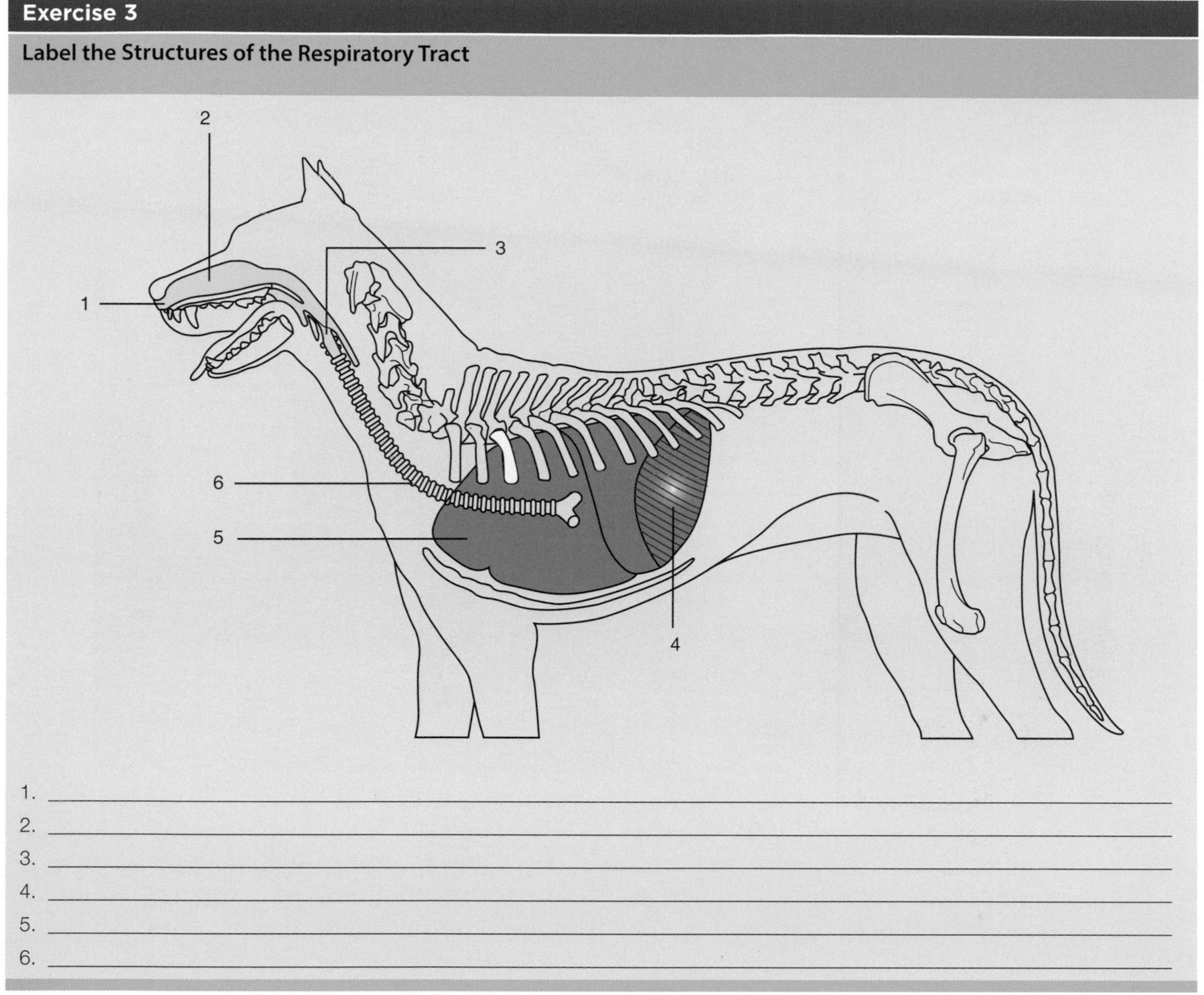

1. ______________________________
2. ______________________________
3. ______________________________
4. ______________________________
5. ______________________________
6. ______________________________

Exercise 4

Label the Structures in the Thorax of the Cat

Indicate right or left where applicable.

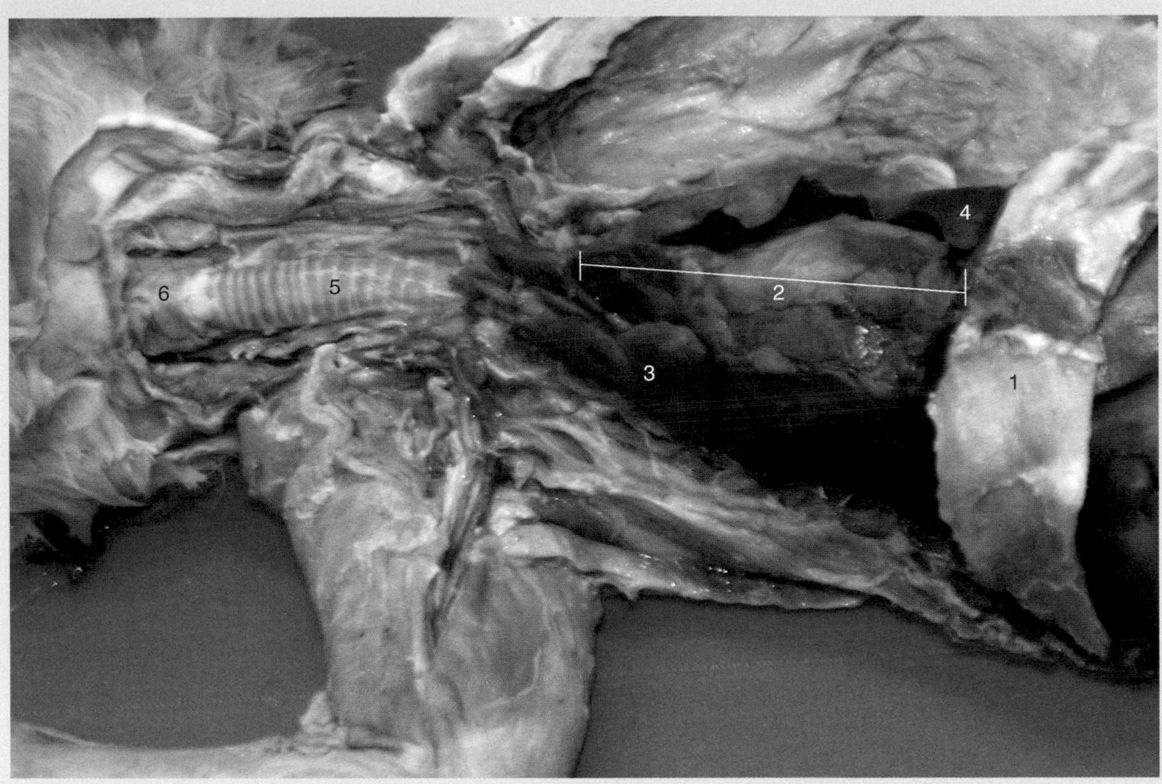

1. ______________________
2. ______________________
3. ______________________
4. ______________________
5. ______________________
6. ______________________

Exercise 5

Label the Structures in the Respiratory Tract of the Cat

Heart removed; indicate right or left where applicable.

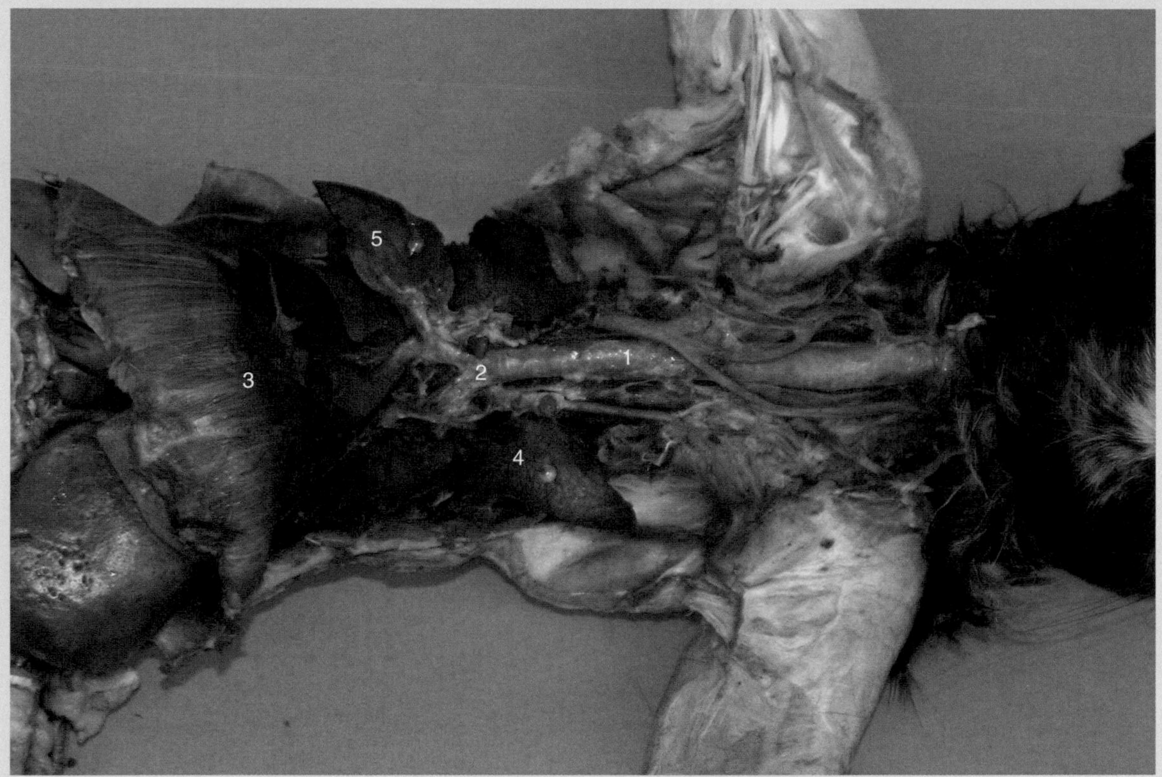

1. ______________________________
2. ______________________________
3. ______________________________
4. ______________________________
5. ______________________________

Exercise 6

Identify the Structures of the Lower Respiratory Tract of Cat

Identify the structures. Indicate right, left, and names of lung lobes where applicable.

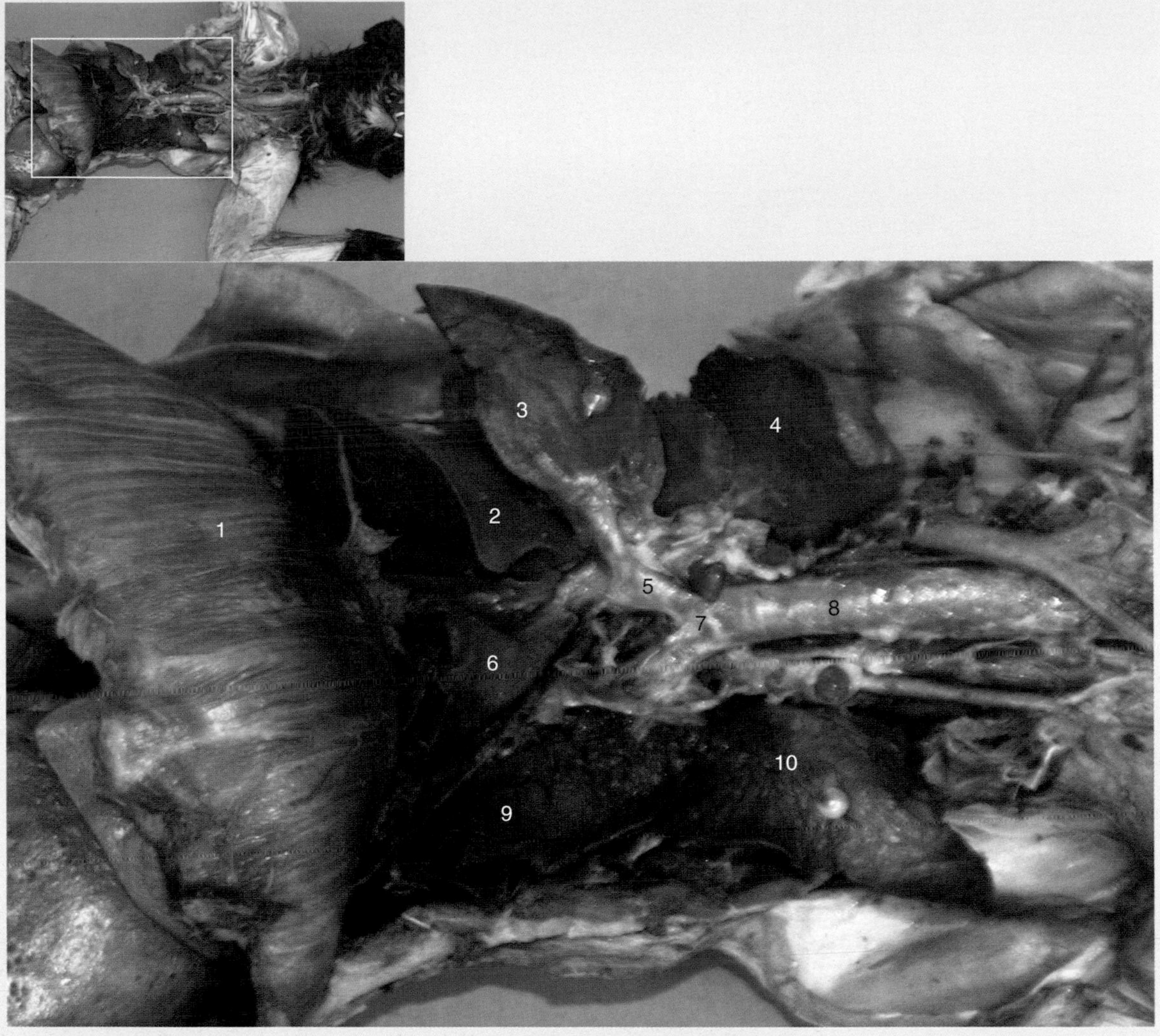

1. ______________________
2. ______________________
3. ______________________
4. ______________________
5. ______________________
6. ______________________
7. ______________________
8. ______________________
9. ______________________
10. ______________________

Exercise 7

Is This the Right or Left Side of the Cat? Why?

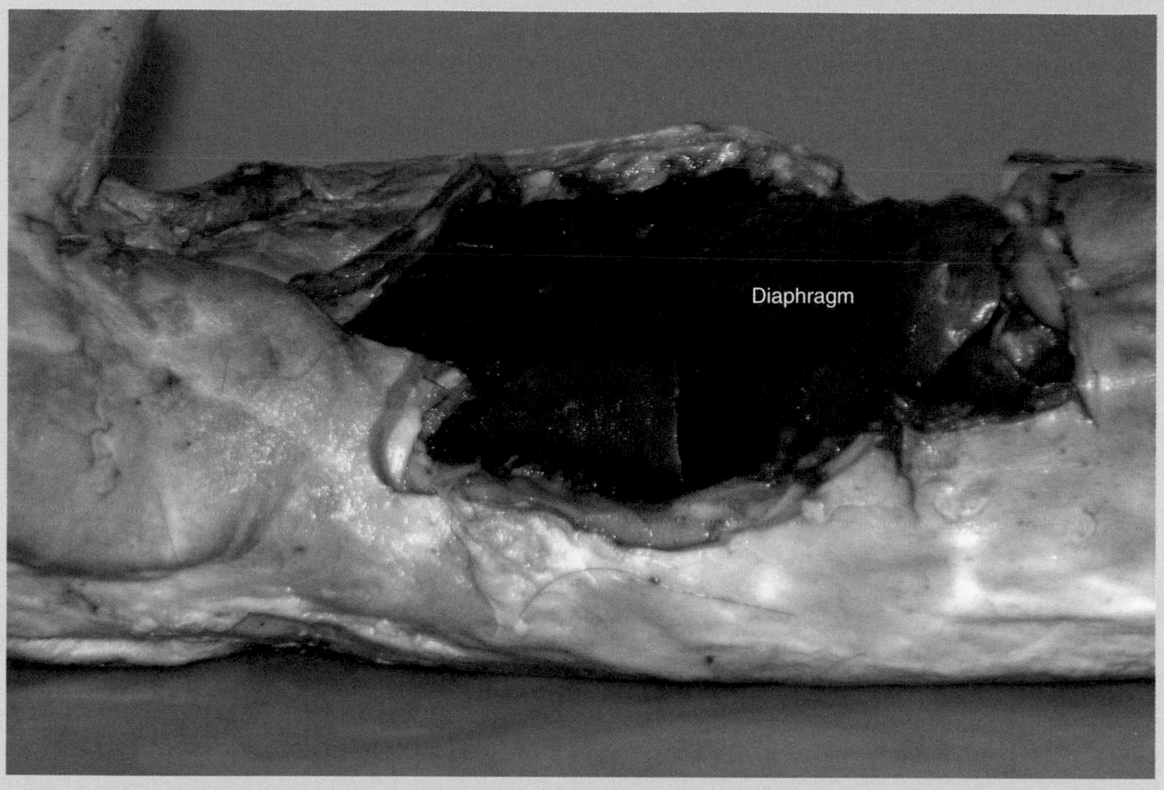

Exercise 8

Identify the Lobes of the Lung

Identify the structures. Indicate right, left, and lung lobe names where applicable.

1. ______________________
2. ______________________
3. ______________________
4. ______________________
5. ______________________
6. ______________________

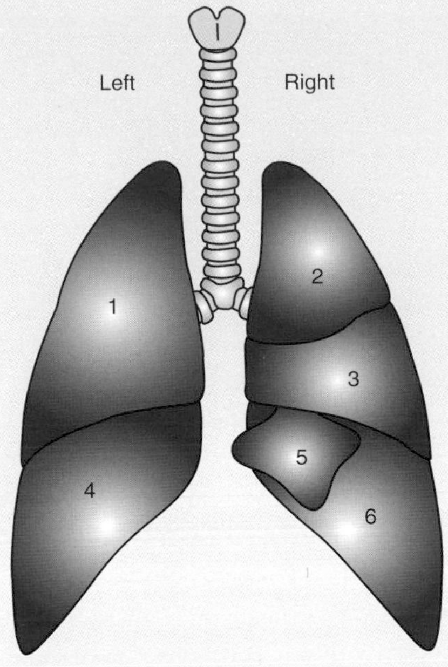

Critical and Clinical Thinking

Exercise 9

Name That Nose—Common Animals

Write the name of the animal species that owns each nose. These animals are commonly seen in veterinary practice.

a. ______________

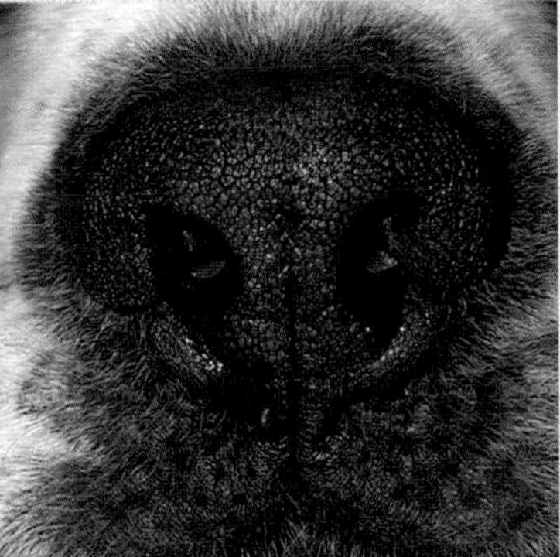

c. ______________

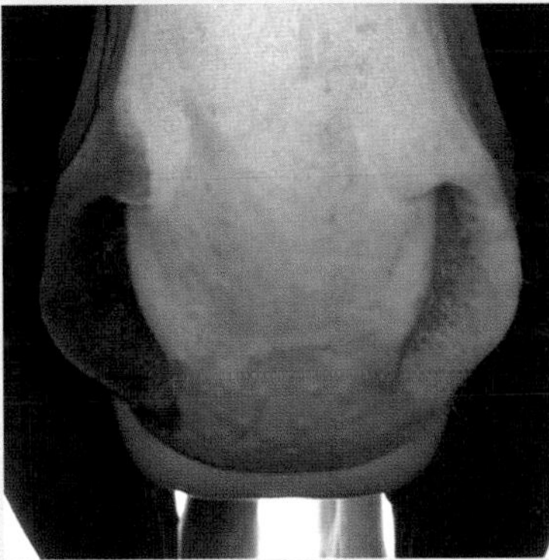

b. ______________

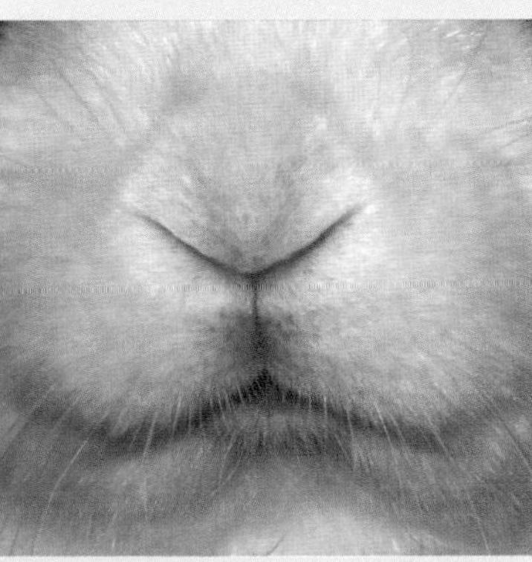

d. ______________

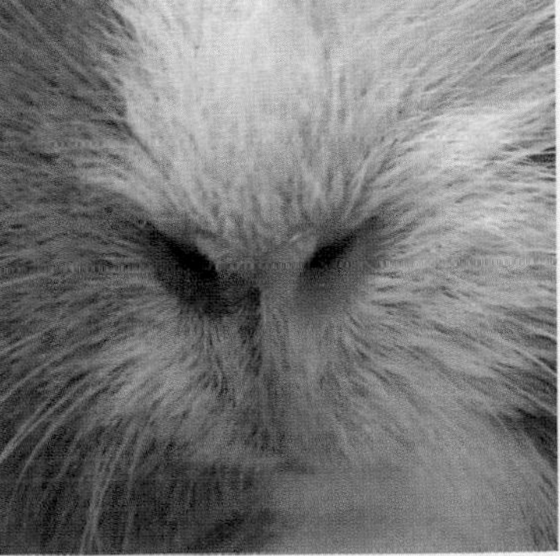

Exercise 9—cont'd

Name That Nose—Common Animals

e. ______________

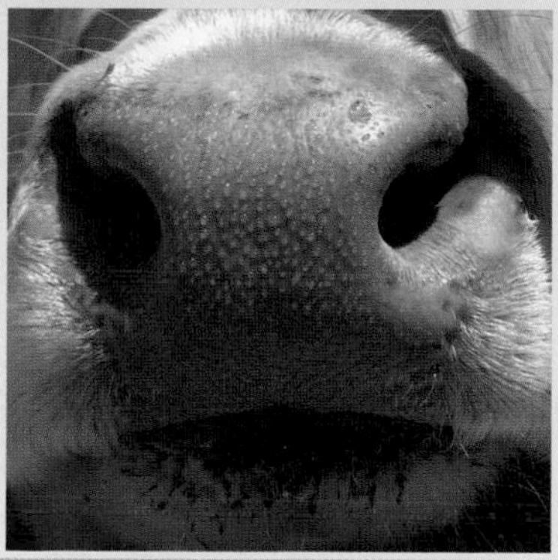

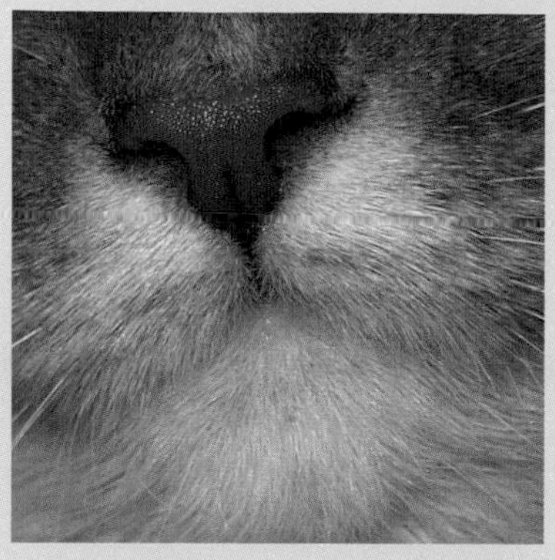

i. ______________

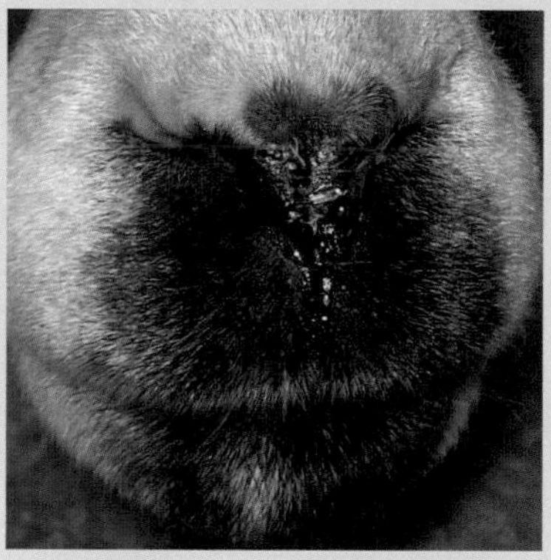

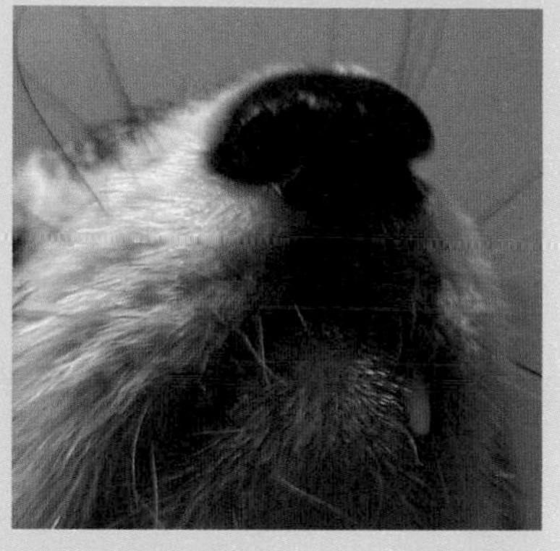

f. ______________

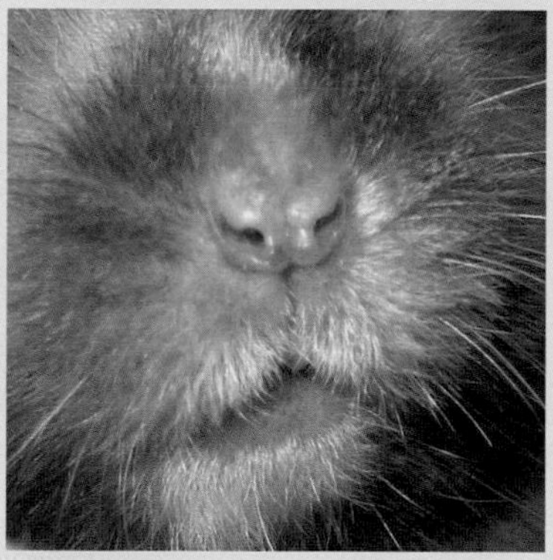

j. ______________

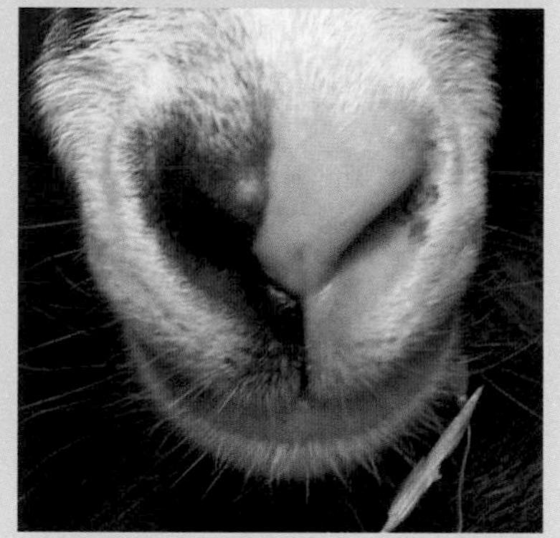

k. ______________

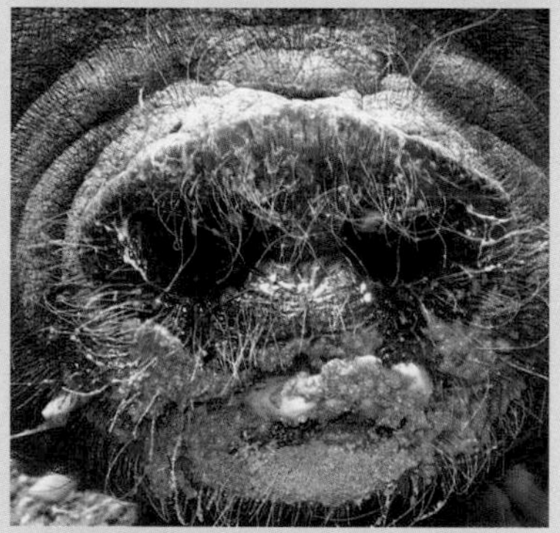

g. ______________

l. ______________

h. ______________

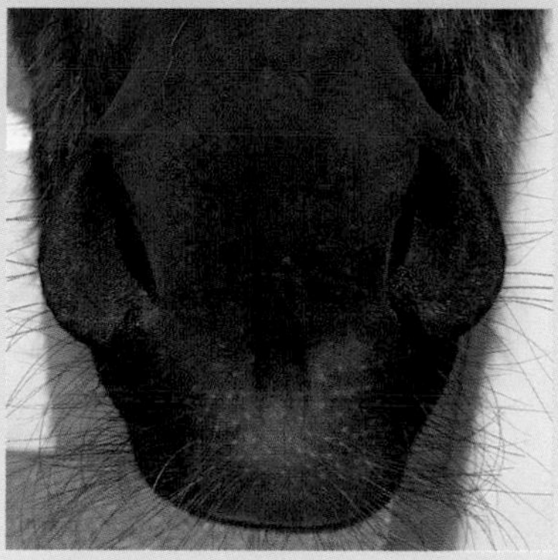

Exercise 10

Name That Nose—Exotic Animals

Select the name of the animal that owns each nose from the list.

Antelope (eland)	Camel	Chinchilla	Chinese red panda	Hedgehog
Llama	Patagonian cavy	Porcupine	Water buffalo	Zebra

a. ______________

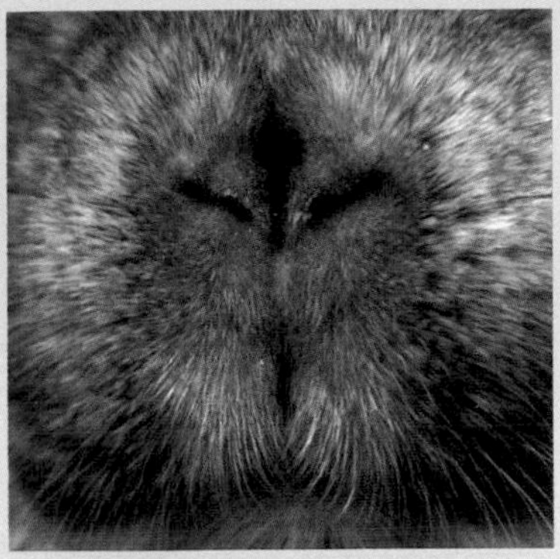

e. ______________

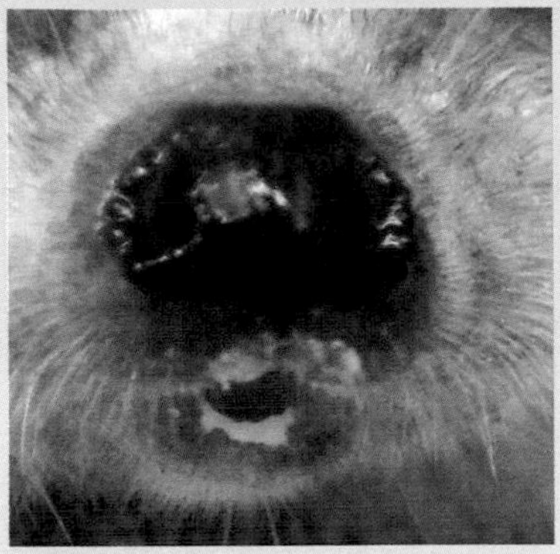

b. ______________

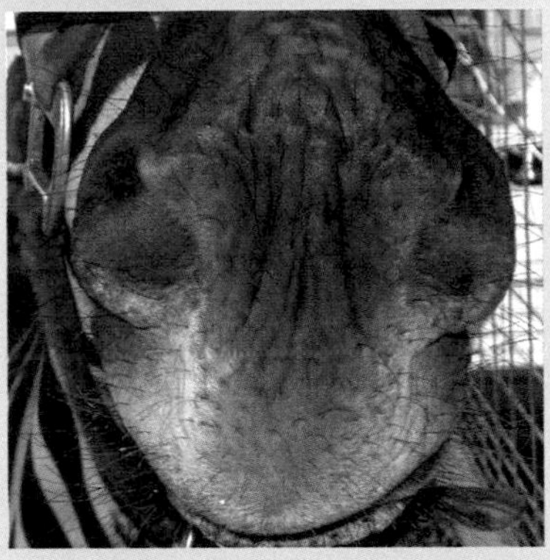

f. ______________

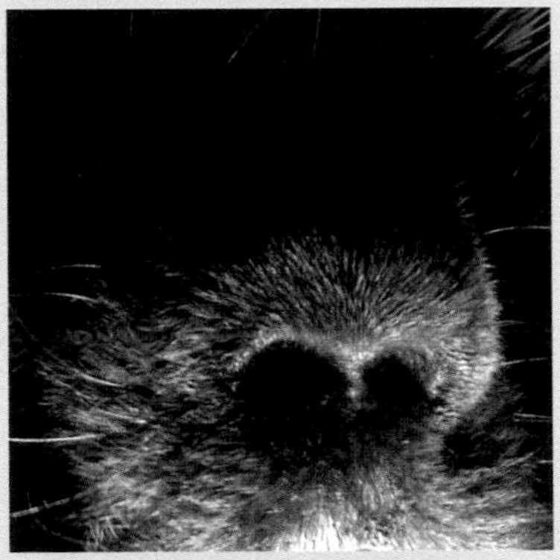

c. ______________

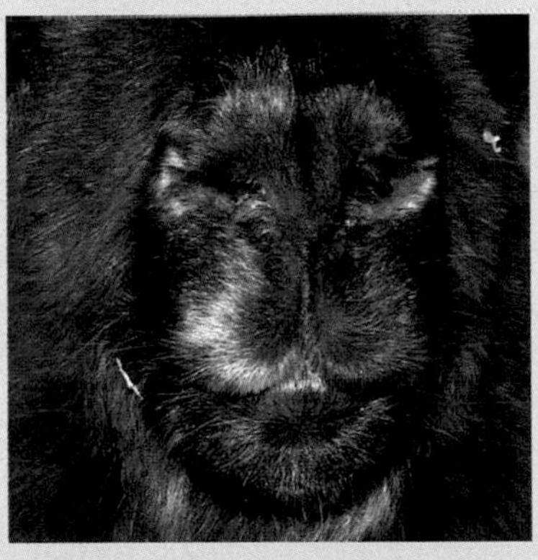

g. ______________

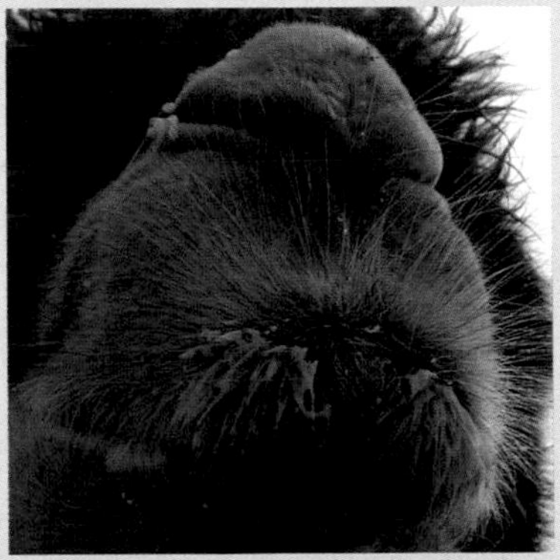

d. ______________

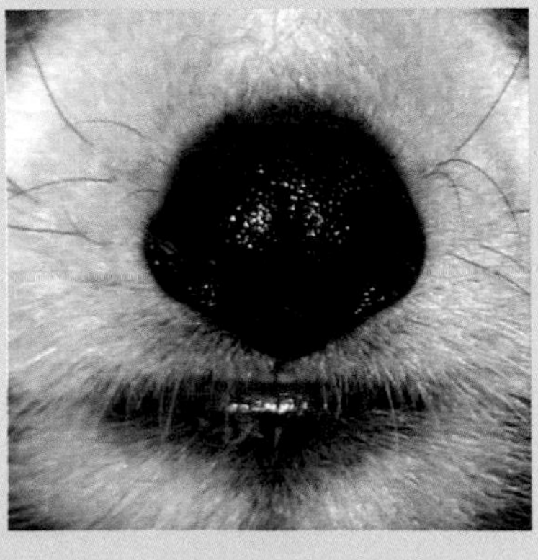

h. ______________

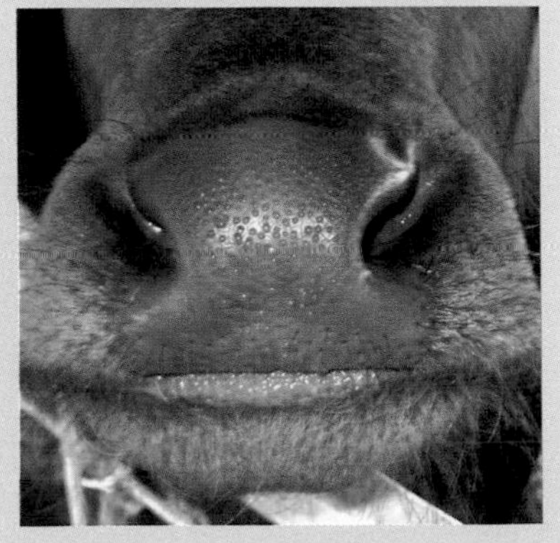

Exercise 10—cont'd

Name That Nose—Exotic Animals

i. ______________

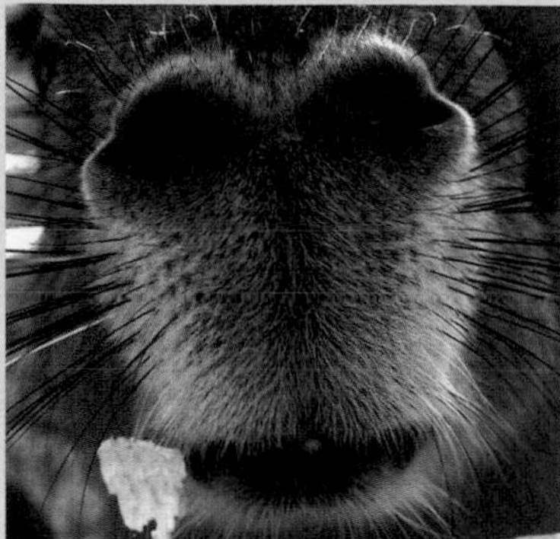

j. ______________

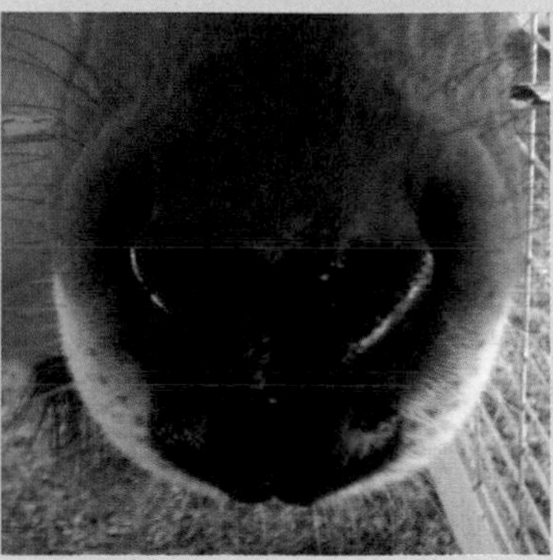

Exercise 11

Connect the Anatomic Dots

1. The two of us make up the upper respiratory tract: ______ ______________________________________
2. I make up the lower respiratory tract: ______________ ______________________________________
3. What are the three main things the nasal lining does to inhaled air to condition it before it passes down to the lungs? ______________________________________ ______________________________________
4. What is a paranasal sinus? ______________________ ______________________________________
5. ___________ is the thin dome-shaped muscular partition between the thoracic and abdominal cavities that aids the process of inspiration when it contracts.
6. What are the three main functions of the larynx? ________ ______________________________________
7. How does the epiglottis prevent interference between breathing and swallowing food? ________________ ______________________________________
8. ___________ is the tube leading from the pharynx to the stomach.
9. The ___________ is held open by hyaline cartilaginous structures that are (*complete* or *incomplete*) rings.
10. What are the largest respiratory branches of the trachea called? ______________________________ ______________________________________
11. What layers must oxygen and carbon dioxide pass through as they are exchanged between the blood in the alveolar capillaries and the air in the alveoli of the lungs? ______________________________________ ______________________________________

Exercise 12

Who Am I?

1. ______________ We are two fibrous connective tissue bands in the larynx that vibrate as air passes over us to produce sound. (Two words.)
2. ______________ I am also known as the windpipe.
3. ______________ As a thin dome-shaped muscle, I form the boundary between the thoracic and abdominal cavities.
4. ______________ I am a short, irregular tube of cartilage and muscle that connects the pharynx with the trachea.
5. ______________ I am the point at which the trachea divides into two primary bronchi.
6. ______________ I open into the larynx.
7. ______________ I am another name for nostrils.
8. ______________ I form the midline barrier that separates the left and right nasal passages.
9. ______________ I form the common passageway for the respiratory and digestive tracts.
10. ______________ I am made of cartilage; the vocal folds attach to me in the larynx.
11. ______________ As a convoluted air passageway in the nose, I conduct air between the nostrils and the pharynx.
12. ______________ We are thin, scroll-like bones that fill most of the space in the nasal cavity.
13. ______________ As microscopic, thin-walled sacs in the lung, we are surrounded by networks of capillaries.
14. ______________ I am an outpouching of the nasal passage that is housed within a space in a skull bone.
15. ______________ I am referred to also as a subdivision of the lung.

Exercise 13

Define Clinical Terms

1. Alveolar sacs ______
2. Alveoli ______
3. Arytenoid cartilage ______
4. Bifurcation of the trachea ______
5. Bronchioles ______
6. Bronchus ______
7. Diaphragm ______
8. Epiglottis ______
9. Esophagus ______
10. Glottis ______
11. Larynx ______
12. Lungs ______
13. Mediastinum ______
14. Nares ______
15. Nasal passages ______
16. Nasal septum ______
17. Paranasal sinus ______
18. Pharynx ______
19. Thoracic cavity ______
20. Trachea ______
21. Turbinates ______
22. Vocal cords ______

Exercise 14

Clinical Thinking Challenge

Support each of following correct statements with appropriate rationale, stating why or in what way each statement is correct.

1. Two steps are needed for respiration to take place in an animal's body, occurring in different anatomic structures.
2. Internal respiration is the real "business end" of respiration.
3. The respiratory system performs some secondary functions important to an animal's well-being.
4. Phonation is enhanced by structures additional to the larynx and vocal cords.
5. Acid–base balance is an important homeostatic mechanism in the body.
6. The respiratory system contributes to the process of acid–base control.
7. The nasal passages are not just simple tubes.
8. Two sets of scroll-like turbinates are found in each nasal passage.
9. The type of cells lining the nasal passages is critical to their function.
10. Sinuses can be clinically significant.
11. It is easy to choke if an animal tries to swallow and breathe at the same time.
12. The larynx has three main functions.
13. Coughing is a complex and often helpful and necessary function.
14. Techniques for passing ET tubes vary among species.

Exercise 14—cont'd

Clinical Thinking Challenge

15. Roaring (in horses) is actually due to a paralysis.

____

____

16. An anesthetized animal must be protected from aspiration of foreign material.

____

____

17. A thin layer of fluid lines each alveolus that contains a substance that prevents the alveoli from collapsing as air moves in and out during breathing.

____

____

18. The lungs of a fetus are nonfunctional but change dramatically at birth.

____

____

19. External intercostal muscles are responsible for inspiration.

____

____

20. Internal intercostal muscles and the abdominal muscles are responsible for expiration.

____

____

21. The quantity of air involved in respiration can be described by four standardized terms, each measuring something different.

____

____

22. The partial pressure of gases explains how and why respiratory gases diffuse.

____

____

23. Voluntary respiratory muscles carry out the seemingly automatic activity of breathing.

____

____

24. Coughs, sneezes, yawns, sighs, and hiccups, temporary interruptions in the normal breathing pattern, are triggered by different stimuli.

____

____

14

The Digestive System[a]

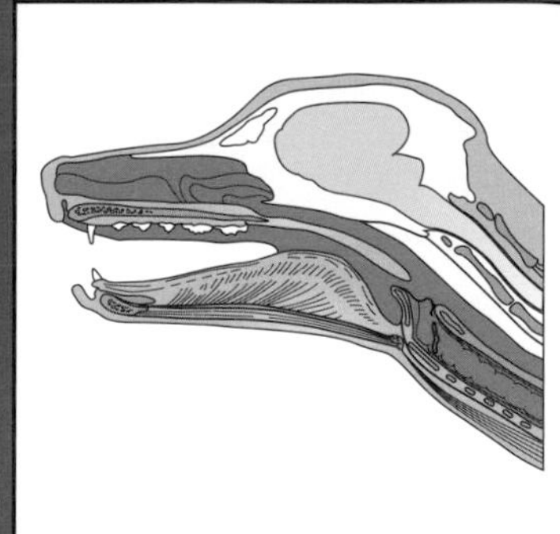

OVERVIEW AT A GLANCE

Salivary Glands 366

The Oral Cavity 367

The Esophagus and Stomach 369

The Intestinal Tract 373

Digestion-Related Organs 379

Exercises 379–397

The Oral Cavity 379–381

1. *Identify Tooth Structure 379*
2. *Label the Dentition in the Dog and Horse 380*
3. *Dental Charting 381*

Dental Formulas 381–382

4. *Dental Formula: Feline (Adult) 381*
5. *Dental Formula: Feline (Kitten) 381*
6. *Dental Formula: Bovine 381*
7. *Dental Formula: Porcine 382*

The Esophagus and Stomach 382–385

8. *Identify Structures on a Horse Stomach 382*
9. *Label and Define Anatomic and Physiologic Functions of Each Stomach Part 383*
10. *Student Lecture Presentation on Digestive Anatomy and Physiology 383*
11. *Compare and Contrast the Reticulum, Rumen, Omasum, and Absomasum for Student Lecture 385*

The Intestinal Tract 385–386

12. *Identify Polysaccharides 385*
13. *Identify Pancreatic Proteases 385*
14. *Explain Emulsification 385*
15. *Identify "Building Block" Molecules 386*
16. *Identify Structures in the Intestinal Tract and Trace Ingestion From Duodenum to Rectum 386*

Digestion-Related Organs 387–390

17. *Identify Digestion-Related Organs 387*
18. *Detail Liver Function 387*
19. *Identify Structures on the Feline Stomach, Duodenum, and Pancreas 388*
20. *Describe Exocrine and Endocrine Functions of the Pancreas 389*
21. *Clinical Application #1: Label the Digestive Tract of the Rabbit and Trace Hindgut Fermentation 389*
22. *Clinical Application #2: Client Consultation 390*

Review of Digestive Anatomy 390–393

23. *Identify Digestion-Related Feline Organs: Ventral Aspect 391*
24. *Identify Digestion-Related Feline Organs: Ventral Aspect, Omentum Removed 392*
25. *Identify Digestion-Related Feline Organs: Ventral Aspect, Jejunum Removed 393*

Review 394–395

26. *Label Stomach Structures 394*
27. *Label Anatomic Digestive Bovine Structures 395*

Critical and Clinical Thinking 396–397

28. *Critical Thinking: Label, Match, Fill In 396*
29. *Clinical Thinking Challenge 397*

LEARNING OBJECTIVES

- To identify and describe the anatomic layers that make up a tooth.
- To identify the four types of teeth: incisors, canines, premolars, and molars.
- To apply dental terminology to clinical situations.
- To calculate the total number of teeth for a species using the dental formula for that species.
- To identify the parts of the gastrointestinal tract.
- To understand the physiologic mechanism of each part of the gastrointestinal tract.
- To recognize and identify accessory digestive organs and to understand the function of these organs.
- To apply your understanding of the digestive system to a clinical scenario through both written and illustrated examples.

[a]The authors and publisher wish to acknowledge Andrea C. De Santis-Kerr for previous contributions to this chapter.

CLINICAL SIGNIFICANCE

To understand how an animal obtains and uses nutrient molecules from its food, we must examine the anatomy and physiology of the gastrointestinal tract and the related organs that comprise the digestive system. This knowledge is vital to veterinary technicians who regularly educate clients about nutrition and the plethora of disorders that may affect the health of their animal's digestive system. With a deeper understanding of these topics, you will be able to apply your knowledge to clinical situations on a daily basis.

Here are some key points to keep in mind as you work through this chapter:

1. Animals of different species are often classified according to the diets they consume.
   - Herbivore: An animal whose diet is primarily plants
   - Carnivore: An animal whose diet is primarily meat
   - Omnivore: An animal whose diet is a mixture of plants and meat
2. Animals may also be classified according to anatomic differences in their gastrointestinal tracts.
   - Monogastrics: Animals with a single stomach
   - Ruminants: Animals that do not have a single stomach, but instead a multichambered system comprising a reticulum, rumen, omasum, and abomasum
3. There are five key functions for which the gastrointestinal tract is responsible:
   - Prehension
   - Mechanical grinding or mastication (chewing)
   - Chemical digestion of food
   - Absorption of nutrients and water
   - Temporary storage and elimination of unabsorbed waste

INTRODUCTION

The purpose of this chapter is to reinforce the information about the digestive system contained in Chapter 16 of *Clinical Anatomy and Physiology for Veterinary Technicians.* Some topics covered in Chapter 17 (Nutrients and Metabolism) will also be visited. The various anatomic structures of the gastrointestinal tract and the physiologic function of each of these structures will be reinforced via interactive exercises as they relate to different species. Be sure to read Chapters 16 and 17 of *Clinical Anatomy and Physiology for Veterinary Technicians* before beginning this chapter.

MATERIALS NEEDED

Preserved cat for dissection
Dissection kit
Pieces of fresh rumen and reticulum (tripe) from the grocery store (if available)
Live cat or dog
Colored pencils

TERMS TO BE IDENTIFIED

- The digestive tract
  - Oral cavity
    - Hard palate
      - Rugae
      - Nasopalatine duct (incisive duct)
    - Soft palate
      - Palatine tonsils
    - Lips
      - Vestibule
      - Labial frenulum
    - Tongue
      - Lingual frenulum
      - Papillae
        - Filiform papilla
        - Fungiform papilla
        - Foliate papilla
      - Vallate papilla
    - Teeth
      - Crown and root
      - Dentine
      - Pulp
        - Enamel
      - Gingiva
  - Pharynx
    - Oropharynx
    - Nasopharynx
    - Laryngopharynx
  - Epiglottis
  - Esophagus
  - Monogastric stomach
    - Cardia (cardiac sphincter)
    - Fundus
    - Body
    - Antrum
    - Pylorus (pyloric sphincter)
  - Ruminant "stomach"
    - Reticulum
      - Ruminoreticular orifice
      - Reticulo-omasal orifice
      - Ruminoreticular fold
    - Rumen
      - Dorsal blind sac
      - Ventral blind sac
      - Dorsal sac
    - Ventral sac
    - Caudal groove
    - Omasum
    - Abomasum
  - Small intestine
    - Duodenum
    - Jejunum
    - Ileum
  - Large intestine
    - Cecum
    - Canine and feline:
      - ascending, transverse, and descending colon
    - Equine: ventral colon
      - (right and left halves), dorsal colon (left and right halves), and small colon. Colonic flexures in the horse: sternal, pelvic, and diaphragmatic flexures
  - Rectum
  - Anus
- Accessory digestive organs
- Salivary glands
  - Parotid gland
  - Mandibular gland
  - Sublingual gland
- Liver
  - Quadrate lobe
  - Left and right medial lobes
  - Left and right lateral lobes
  - Caudate lobe
- Gallbladder
- Bile ducts
  - Hepatic ducts
  - Cystic ducts
  - Common bile duct
- Pancreas
  - Common pancreatic duct and Vater's ampulla
  - Accessory pancreatic ducts

Salivary Glands

Before you begin your dissection of the digestive or alimentary tract, examine the salivary glands that assist in the mastication of food in the mouth. The largest and most prominent of these is the **parotid salivary gland,** which can be found encircling the ventral aspect of the ear. Using a scalpel, carefully remove the skin under the ear to reveal this gland. Ventral to the parotid salivary gland are the **mandibular** and **sublingual salivary glands.** Notice that the mandibular gland is slightly caudal to the sublingual gland (Fig. 14.1). The parotid, mandibular, and sublingual salivary glands have a textured, glandular consistency. Do not confuse the prominent but smooth mandibular lymph nodes with these salivary glands.

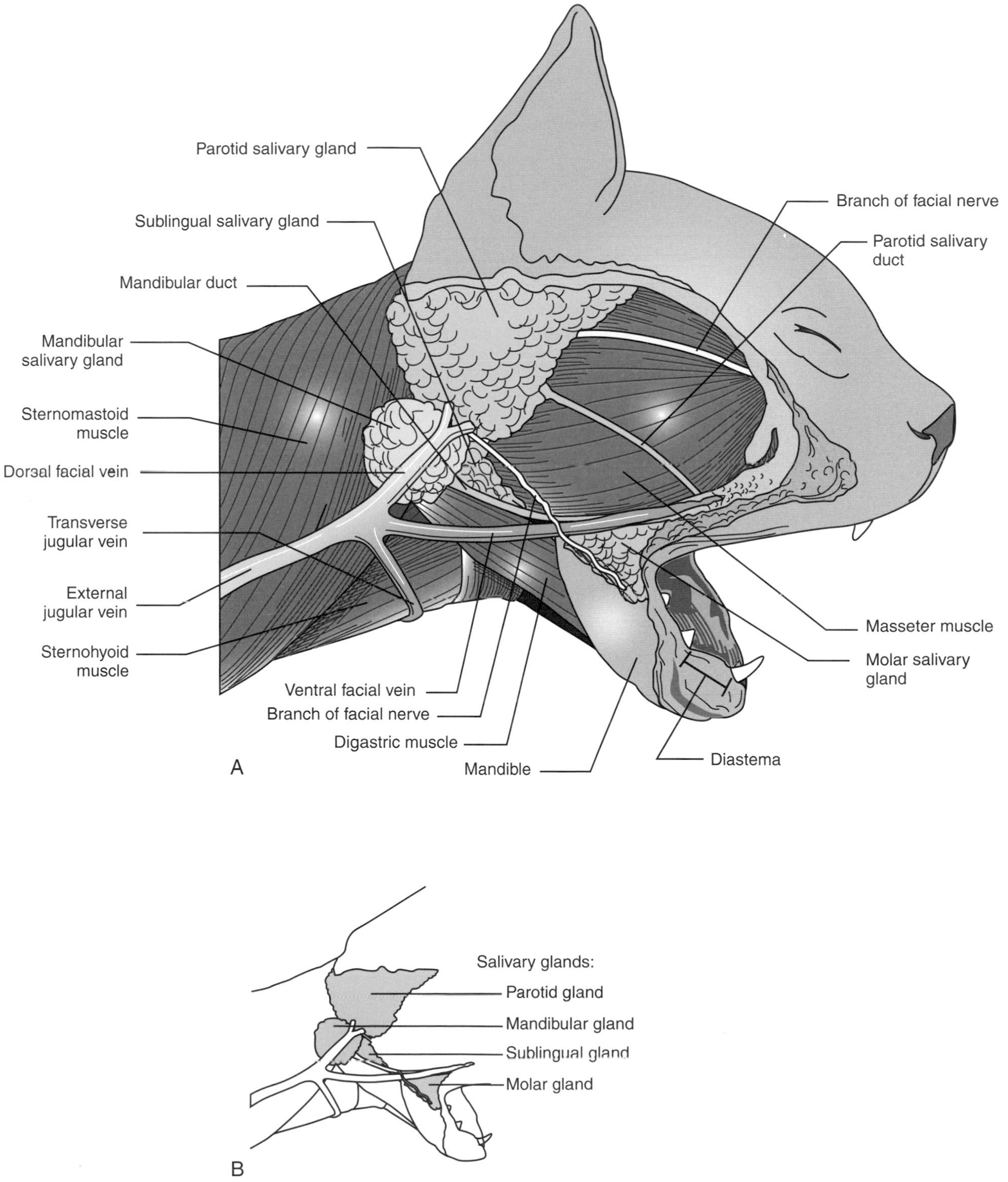

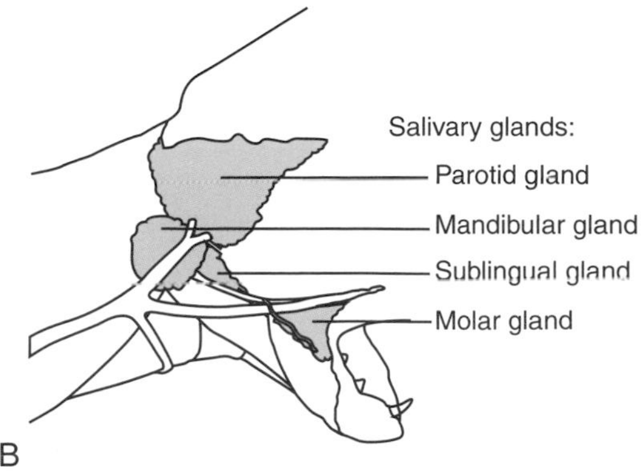

• **Fig. 14.1** (A) Lateral view of a cat's head with skin and adipose tissue removed. (B) Local region, ventral to the ear, showing the location of the parotid, mandibular, sublingual, and molar salivary glands.

Saliva is carried to the oral cavity by means of salivary ducts. Look for the **parotid duct,** which traverses the midsection of the masseter muscle and enters the mouth above the carnassial tooth (upper fourth premolar). The continuous deposition of saliva on the carnassial tooth accounts for its tendency to accumulate excessive amounts of tartar. The mandibular salivary gland provides saliva to the floor of the mouth near the lower incisors. The sublingual gland is the smallest of the three salivary glands and is located in the "V" formed by the dorsal and ventral branches of the facial vein.

The cat has two additional salivary glands, which are difficult to locate; the molar salivary gland is located in the corner of the mouth and the infraorbital salivary gland, as its name implies, is located on the floor of the orbit beneath the eye.

The Oral Cavity

Begin your dissection by examining the oral cavity of your cat. Some preserved cats are quite stiff and opening the mouth is difficult. Use a scalpel, scissors, and bone cutting forceps to cut through the masseter muscles and the ramus of the mandible on one side of the face. This will take some assertiveness. Place the cat in dorsal recumbency and reflect one half of the lower mandible to reveal the inside of the oral cavity. Be sure to cut through the vertical ramus.

Examine the exposed oral cavity (Figs. 14.2 and 14.3). Directly behind the incisors is a small nodule, which some pet owners have mistakenly thought to be a small oral tumor. This is the **incisive or nasopalatine duct** and forms a connection between the oral cavity and the nasal passage above it. Explore the rest of the oral cavity and locate the following structures:

1. The **hard and soft palates** separate the oral and nasal cavities. Notice the **rugae** that cover the hard palate (see Figs. 14.2 and 14.3).
2. To locate the **nasopharynx,** you will need to slice through the soft palate. The **oropharynx** is located ventral to the soft palate. The **laryngopharynx** is located cranial to the openings of the **esophagus** and trachea (larynx) (see Fig. 14.3).
3. The **labial frenulum** is the mucosal attachment to each lip along the upper and lower midlines (see Fig. 14.2).
4. In contrast, the **lingual frenulum** is located along the midline under the tongue (see Fig. 14.3).
5. The **vestibule** is the space between the teeth and the **lips** (see Fig. 14.2).
6. Note the smoothness of the soft palate and the **palatine tonsils** that are located on the lateral edges of the soft palate (see Figs. 14.2 and 14.3).

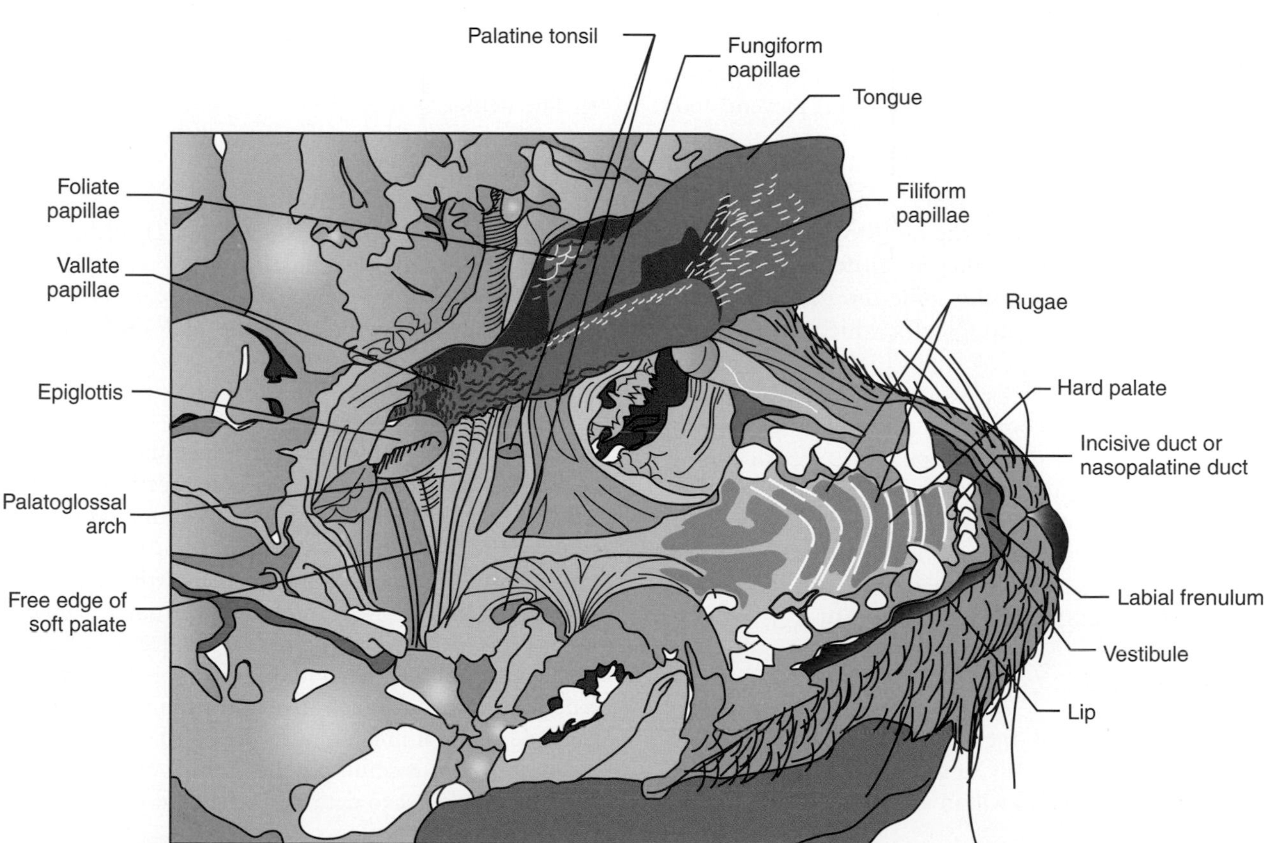

• **Fig. 14.2** A dorsoventrally dissected cat head showing the oral cavity, including the upper arcade, hard and soft palates, and surrounding structures.

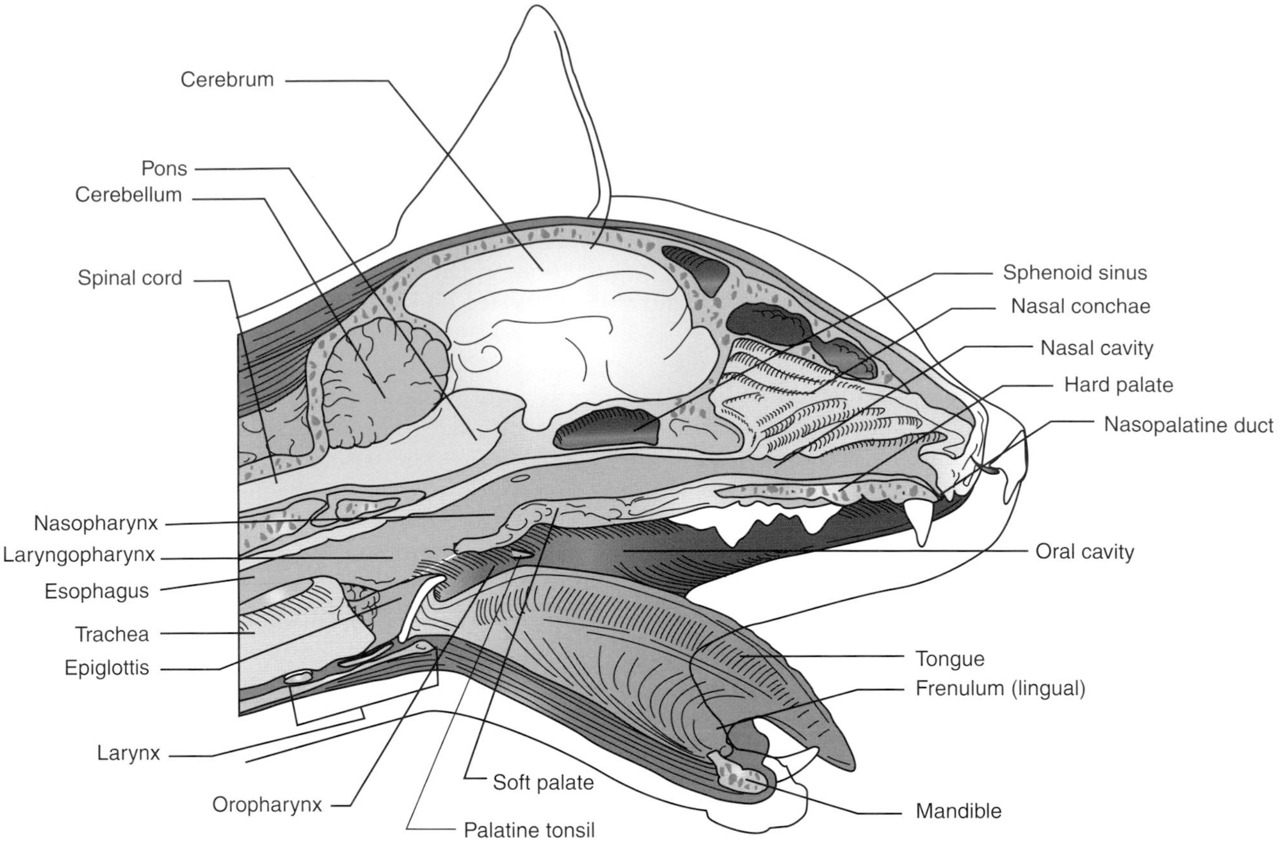

• **Fig. 14.3** Sagittal section of the head and neck of a cat.

7. Locate the **epiglottis,** which is an extension of the larynx and bends over the opening of the trachea (the **glottis**) when the animal is swallowing food. This prevents food from entering the trachea (and lungs) (see Figs. 14.2 and 14.3).
8. Examine the many **papillae** that cover the **tongue**. There are four types of papillae in the cat. Moving from the tip to the base of the tongue, they are **filiform, fungiform, foliate,** and **vallate papillae.** The filiform papillae are best known for their sharp spicules, which enable the cat to groom itself (see Figs. 14.2 and 14.3).

Because technicians play a key role in helping to maintain the oral health of companion animals by performing oral examinations and dental prophylactic teeth cleaning, pay particular attention to the teeth of your cat (Fig. 14.4). Understanding the structures of the tooth, the dental arcade, and dental formulas is important for the veterinary technician because supporting good oral veterinary health has become increasingly important in practice.

Tooth Structure

Review the anatomy of the tooth and dental arcade in Chapter 16 of the textbook. Complete Exercise 1. Questions relating to dental formulas will involve calculations.

Types of Teeth

Each species has a dental formula that indicates the number of incisor, canine, premolar, and molar teeth of that species. The formula is written with letters and numbers. The letters indicate the following: *I* for incisor, *C* for canine, *P* for premolar, and *M* for molar. The letters are written in lowercase for puppy and kitten formulas. Two numbers follow the letters: the first number represents the teeth in half of the upper arcade and the second number represents the teeth in half of the lower arcade. Because the numbers only represent one side of the animal's mouth (half of the upper and lower arcades), you must multiply the number of teeth in the formula by 2 in order to determine the total number of teeth.

Example: Adult dog

- The dental formula is $I\frac{3}{3}\ C\frac{1}{1}\ P\frac{4}{4}\ M\frac{2}{3}$ OR $\frac{3142}{3143}$. The slash mark separates the upper arcade number from the lower arcade number.
- Add the numbers together:
  - $3 + 3 + 1 + 1 + 4 + 4 + 2 + 3 = 21$ teeth, representing half of the total number
- Multiply the number by 2:
  - $21 \times 2 = 42$ total teeth in the adult dog's mouth

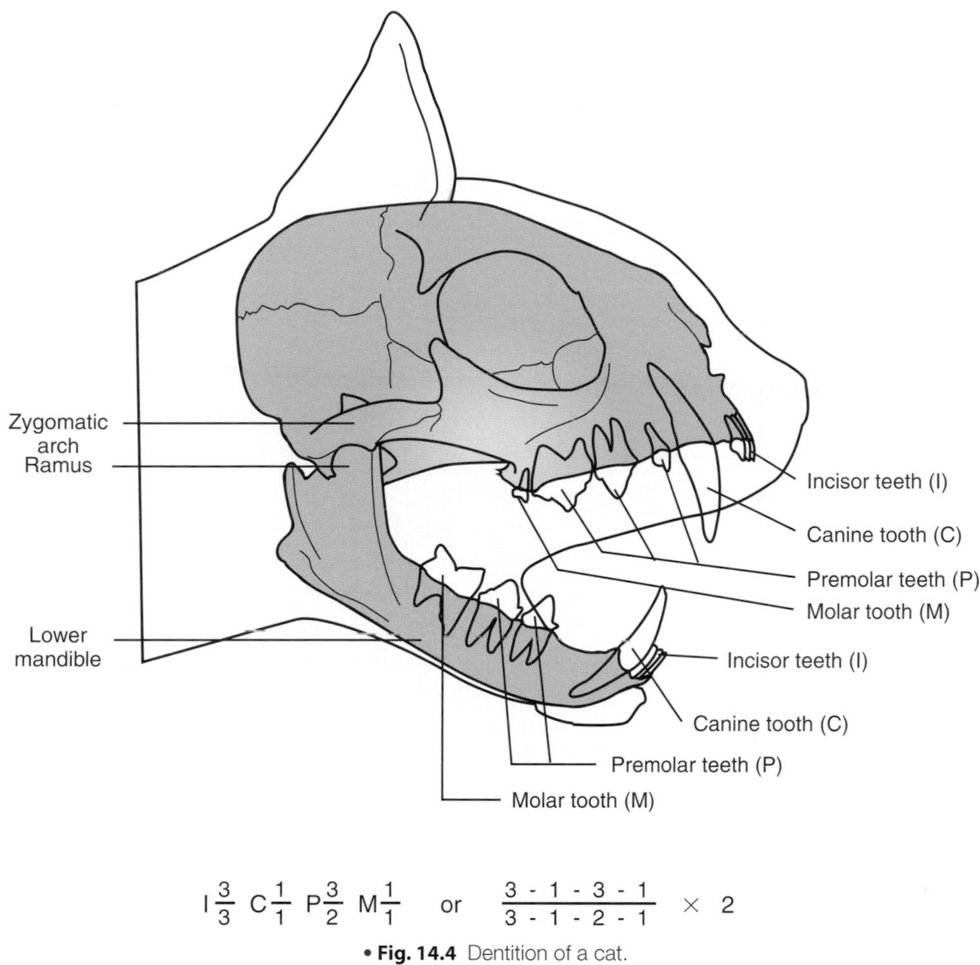

$$I\frac{3}{3}\ C\frac{1}{1}\ P\frac{3}{2}\ M\frac{1}{1} \quad \text{or} \quad \frac{3-1-3-1}{3-1-2-1} \times 2$$

• **Fig. 14.4** Dentition of a cat.

In-class Activity

Examine the oral cavity of a live cat or dog. What is the dental formula of the species you are examining? Do you see the accumulation of dental calculus or tartar? Are some teeth more affected than others? Which teeth are these? Why do you think these teeth are more affected than the others? Are any teeth missing? If so, which ones?

The Esophagus and Stomach

Dissection of the Esophagus and Stomach

After examination of the oral cavity in your dissection, lay your cat in dorsal recumbency and make a ventral midline incision in the neck of your cat, if needed, to locate the esophagus, which carries food from the oral cavity to the stomach. The esophagus can be found dorsal (underneath, in this position) the trachea. Note that it does not have cartilaginous rings to maintain an open lumen and therefore is less obvious than the trachea. Follow the esophagus through the thoracic cavity and note its passage through the diaphragm before it joins the stomach. In the abdominal cavity, palpate the thickening where the esophagus joins the stomach. This is the **cardiac sphincter** and is important in preventing the reflux of ingesta into the esophagus, which could cause discomfort and esophageal ulceration.

Carnivorous mammals such as cats, omnivores such as pigs, and some herbivores such as rabbits and horses are **monogastrics,** meaning that they have a single stomach to break down food. Conversely, many herbivores, such as deer, cattle, goats, and sheep, have multiple "stomachs" that help to break down plant matter before it enters the small intestine. These latter species are called **ruminants.**

Examine the stomach of your cat (Fig. 14.5A). Note its shape and position in situ. You will notice that the greater omentum originates from the greater curvature of the stomach and the lesser omentum originates from the lesser curvature of the stomach to attach to the abdominal wall. Also take note of the mesenteric connections between the stomach and the spleen. Consider that when a dog's stomach fills with air and turns, as in a gastric dilatation–volvulus (GDV, or "bloat"), the spleen often moves with the stomach as it rotates around the axis of the esophagus.

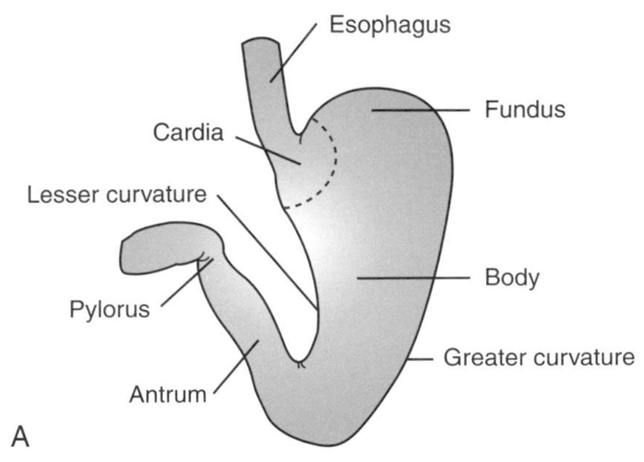

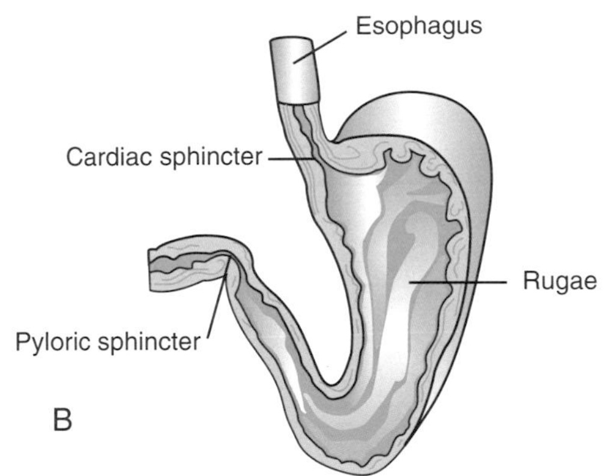

• **Fig. 14.5** Anatomy of the monogastric stomach. (A) External view. (B) Internal perspective.

The Monogastric Stomach

There are five components that make up the monogastric stomach (see Fig. 14.5), each with a specific and important function. These are the cardia, fundus, body, antrum, and pylorus. The **cardia** is located at the upper portion of the stomach where the esophagus enters. It acts as a muscular source of protection against reflux of stomach contents back into the esophagus. The fundus and body are expandable portions of the stomach that distend as ingesta accumulates. The **fundus** is referred to as a "blind pouch" and is located dorsal to the cardia. The **body** is considered the "middle" portion of the stomach. Both the fundus and the body contain gastric glands with parietal cells, chief cells, and mucous cells. The parietal cells are responsible for producing hydrochloric acid, the chief cells produce pepsinogen, and the mucous cells produce mucus. The distal portion of the stomach is the **antrum,** which functions to break down ingesta and aids in hydrochloric acid regulation through the release of the hormone gastrin. The "end" portion of the stomach is the **pylorus,** a muscular sphincter. The pylorus allows digested material to enter the small intestine at the duodenum while preventing any retrograde movement of these contents back into the stomach.

Using your scalpel, make a longitudinal incision along the greater curvature of the stomach and examine the stomach contents and the lining of each part of the stomach. Locate the **cardiac and pyloric sphincters** and examine them from the inside of the stomach (see Fig. 14.5B). Also, make note of the prominent rugae, wavelike undulations in the lining of the stomach, which increase surface area and which are evident in radiographs (x-rays) of air-filled stomachs.

The Ruminant Stomach

Ruminants, such as cows, sheep, and goats, do not have a single stomach like dogs, cats, horses, and humans, but instead have a four-chambered organ composed of a "forestomach," containing the reticulum, rumen, and omasum, and the "true stomach," which is called the abomasum. These fascinating compartmentalizations allow for maximum digestion and use of an herbivorous diet rich in cellulose, a tough and difficult nutrient to digest. The **rumen** and **reticulum** form the **reticulorumen** (Fig. 14.6A–C), which is located on the *left* side of the animal. Internally, the reticulum is lined with a characteristic hexagonal honeycomb appearance. Take a moment to examine the fresh pieces of reticulum, called tripe, which can be found in most grocery stores. The "honeycomb" lining of the reticulum increases its surface area, allowing for more absorption to take place. The rumen is the largest compartment of the forestomach and acts as a fermentation vat. It is lined with papillae and is separated into compartments by internal muscular walls called pillars, which allow selective regions of the rumen to mix and stir its contents as needed. Microbes within the rumen convert carbohydrate sources such as cellulose into volatile fatty acids (VFA) via an anaerobic biochemical process called fermentation. The VFAs are readily absorbed by the animal and converted into usable glucose. Contractions within the reticulum and rumen are called reticuloruminal contractions. These contractions are responsible for mixing ingesta, aiding in regurgitation of cud (partially digested food), and eructation (burping up excess carbon dioxide, which is a by-product of fermentation). As outlined in the textbook, each of these processes plays an important role in maintaining digestive equilibrium.

The **omasum** is the third compartment of the forestomach and aids in mechanical breakdown of ingesta and in the absorption of VFAs. Subsequently, the **abomasum** acts as the "true stomach" in the ruminant with functions comparable to those of the monogastric stomach. It contains glands that secrete acids and enzymes necessary for digestion to occur. Both the omasum and the abomasum are located on the right side of the ruminant (see Fig. 14.6D and E).

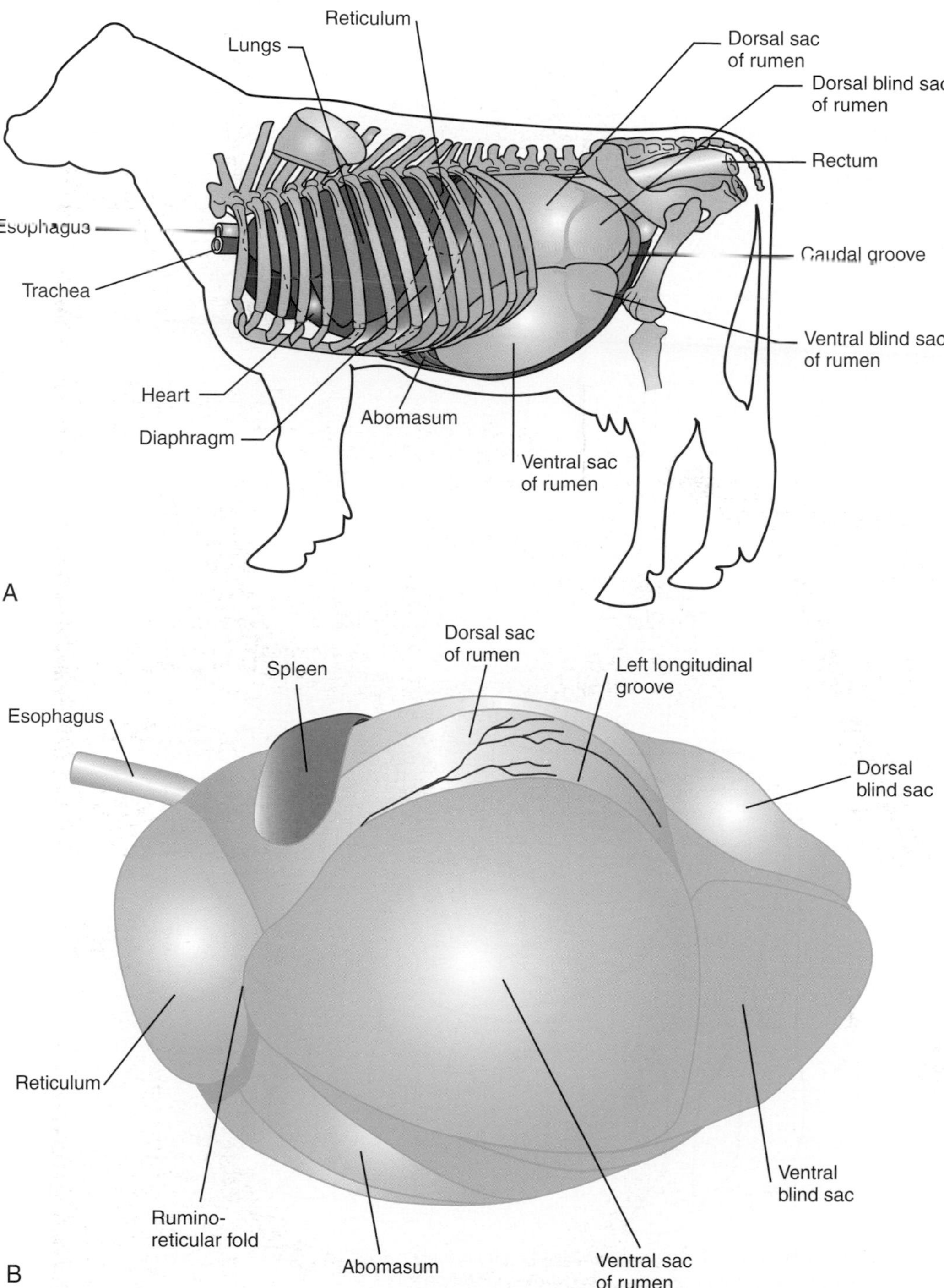

• **Fig. 14.6** (A) View from the left side of a cow showing the anatomic positions of the organs of the thorax and abdomen in situ. (B) The left side of the ruminant digestive tract.

Continued

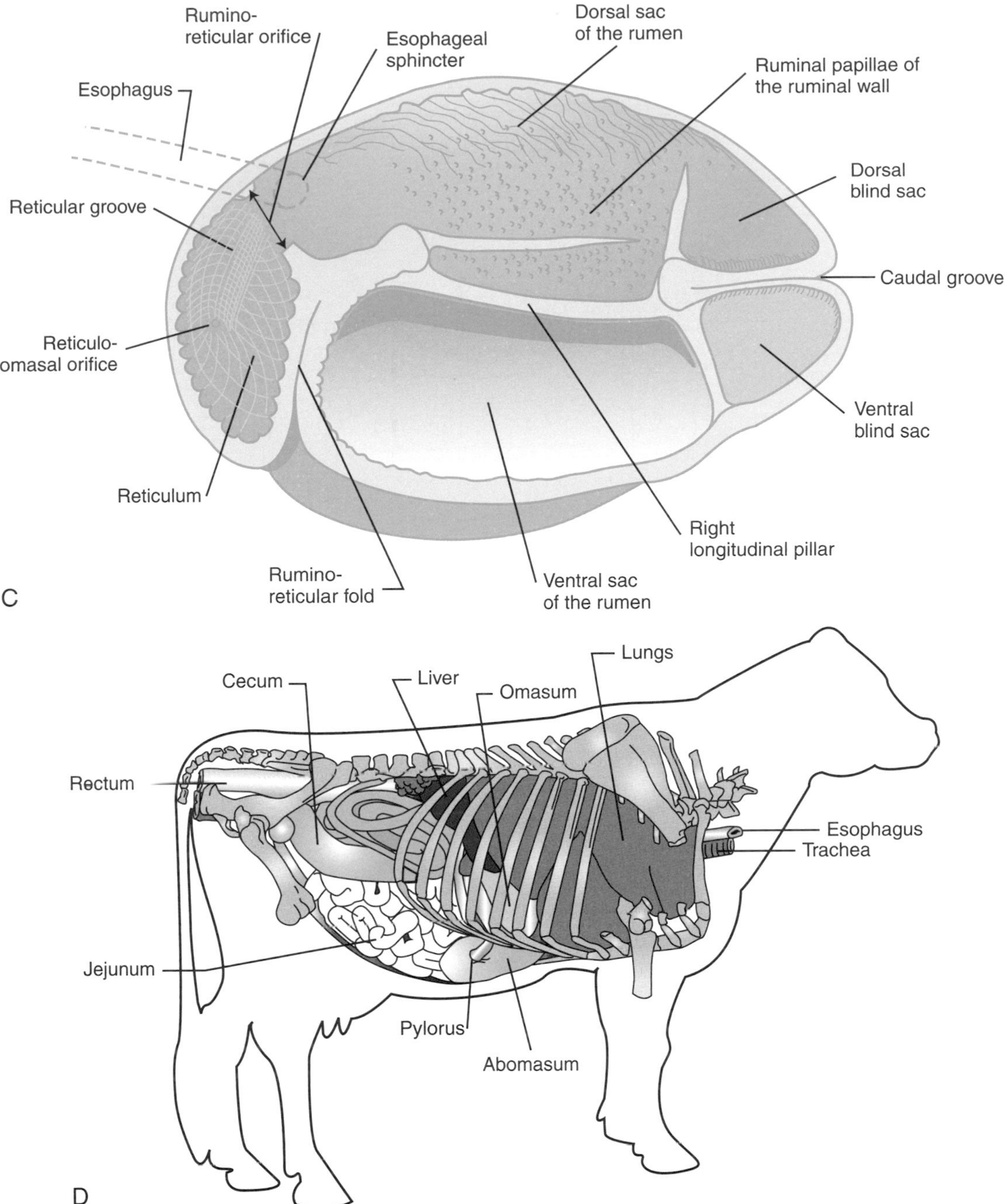

• Fig. 14.6, cont'd (C) Interior view of the rumen and reticulum. (D) View from the right side of a cow showing the anatomic positions of the organs of the thorax and abdomen in situ.

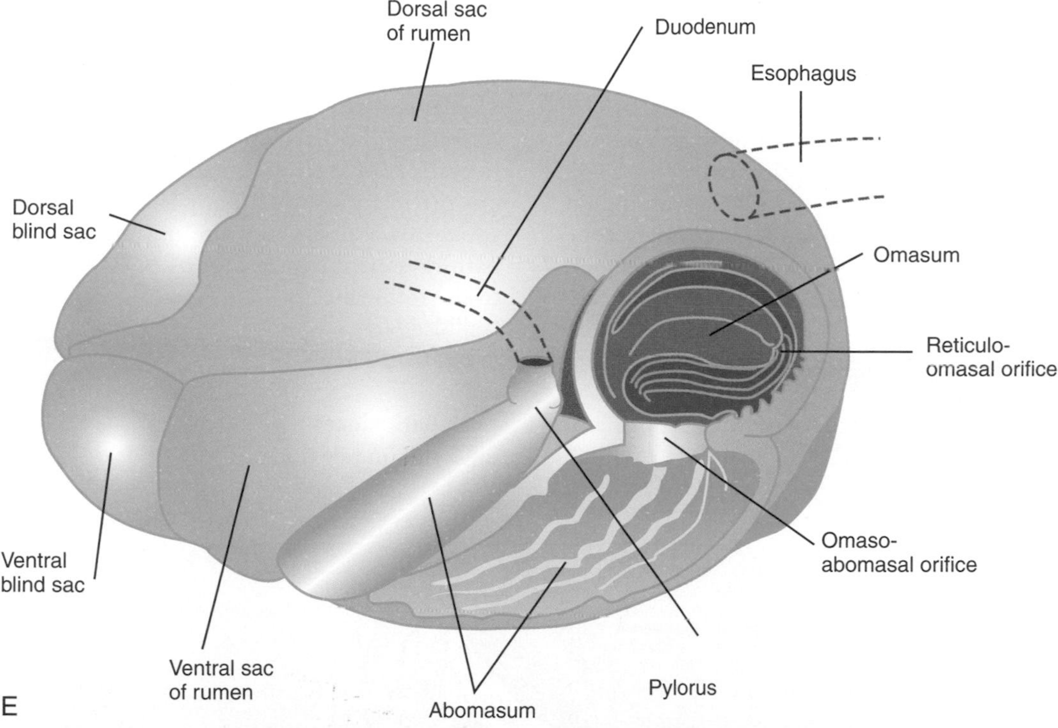

• **Fig. 14.6, cont'd** (E) The right side of the ruminant digestive tract.

CLINICAL APPLICATION 14.1

Traumatic Reticulitis in a Goat

Ruminants may sometimes eat heavy metallic objects, such as pieces of wire or nails. These objects either fall directly into the reticulum or are carried there by ruminal contractions. Heavy objects will settle at the bottom of the reticulum and sharp objects can be trapped by the honeycomb lining of the reticulum. Reticuloruminal contractions can cause a piece of wire or a nail to penetrate the wall of the reticulum. This penetration allows some of the contents of the reticulum, such as ingesta and bacteria, to leak out into the peritoneal cavity, causing peritonitis (inflammation of the peritoneum). In some cases, the object may penetrate the diaphragm and pierce the pericardial sac surrounding the heart. This results in a serious condition known as pericarditis (inflammation of the pericardium, the sac surrounding the heart). Fig. 14.7 shows a goat with traumatic reticulitis. Can you identify the wire penetrating the reticulum?

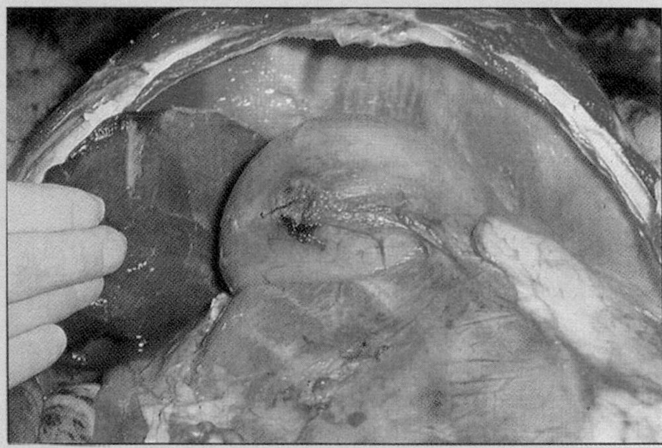

• **Fig. 14.7** Traumatic reticulitis or "hardware disease" in a goat, caused by wire penetration. (From Linklater KA, Smith MC: Color atlas of diseases and disorders of the sheep and goat, St Louis, 1993, Mosby.)

The Intestinal Tract

Small Intestine

The duodenum, jejunum, and ileum make up the small intestine. The **duodenum** is the first part of the small intestine. Extending from the pyloric region of the stomach, it forms a "U" shape around the head of the pancreas before connecting to the jejunum. It receives digestive enzymes directly from the pancreas through multiple ducts and also receives bile acids from the liver and gallbladder via the **common bile duct.** The **jejunum** is the longest portion of the small intestine and, not surprisingly, absorbs the bulk of the nutrients derived from food. The **ileum** is the shortest portion of the small intestine and forms a transitory link between the lengthy jejunum and the beginning of the large intestine.

All three sections of the small intestine perform peristaltic waves and segmental contractions to ensure the passage of digesta from one section to another. The three primary food groups—proteins, carbohydrates, and fat—are all broken down and absorbed in the small intestine. Carbohydrates, which are lengthy polysaccharide molecules, are broken down by enzymes in the duodenum into shorter disaccharides and monosaccharides. Protein digestion uses pancreatic enzymes known as proteases to break down proteins into amino acids. Fat digestion is accomplished via emulsification, with the aid of bile acids from the liver or **gallbladder,** into triglyceride molecules. These smaller molecules are moved to the jejunum, where they are absorbed by absorptive cells that line its lumen.

Dissection of the Small Intestine

Examine the small intestine in situ (Fig. 14.8). Notice the position of the pancreas relative to the duodenum and the connections between them. Also make note of the position of the gallbladder and liver, and the ductal connections between them and the duodenum (Fig. 14.9). These connections are critical in enabling the movement of enzymes from the pancreas to the duodenum and of bile from the liver and gallbladder to the duodenum. Digestion of nutrients could not be carried out without the relationships among these four organs. Carefully tweeze away tissue surrounding the ducts to uncover the pathways exhibited in Fig. 14.9. Pay particular attention to the following:

Gallbladder
- **Cystic duct**

Liver
- **Hepatic ducts**
- Common bile ducts

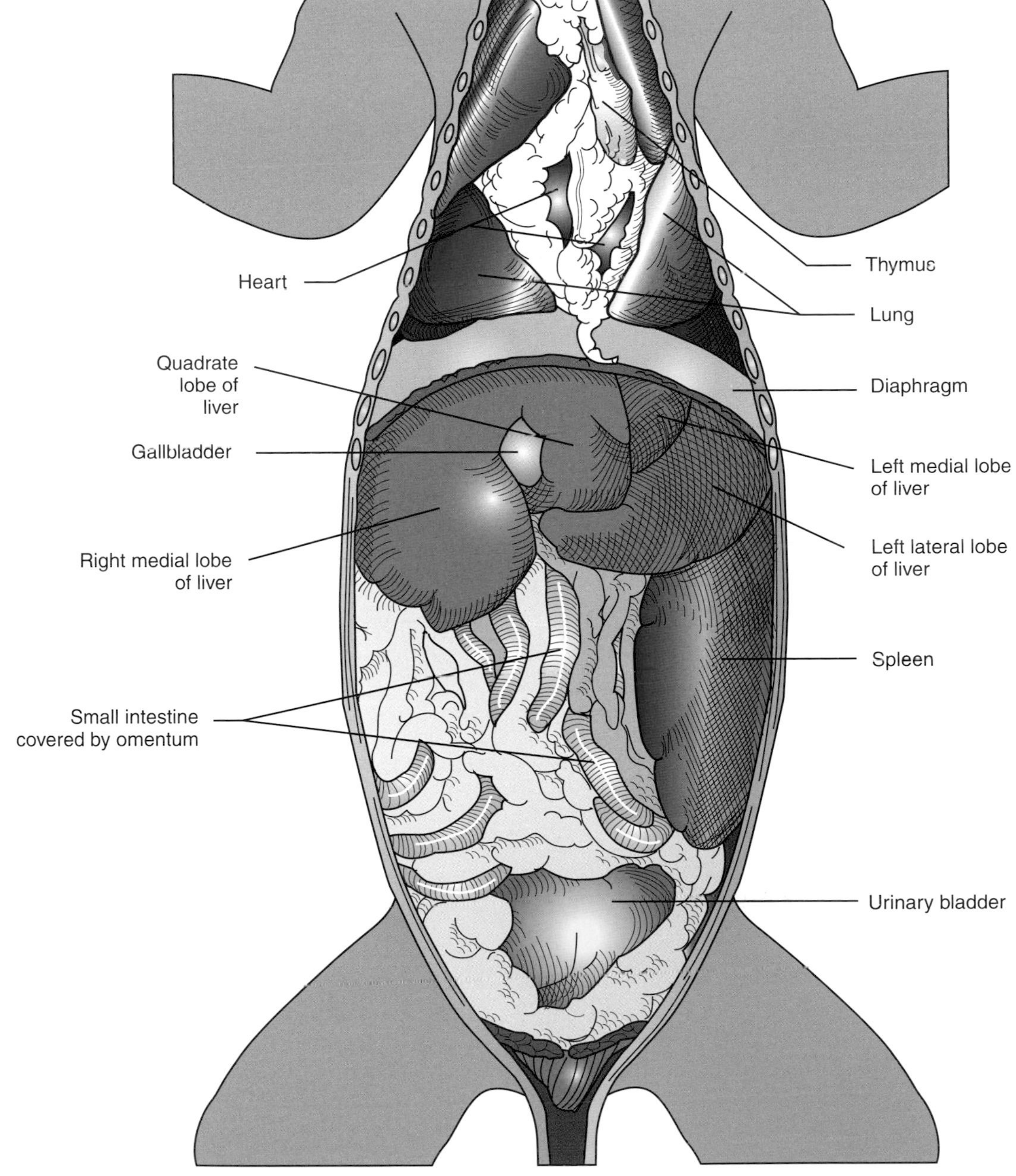

• **Fig. 14.8** The abdominal and thoracic viscera of a cat in situ.

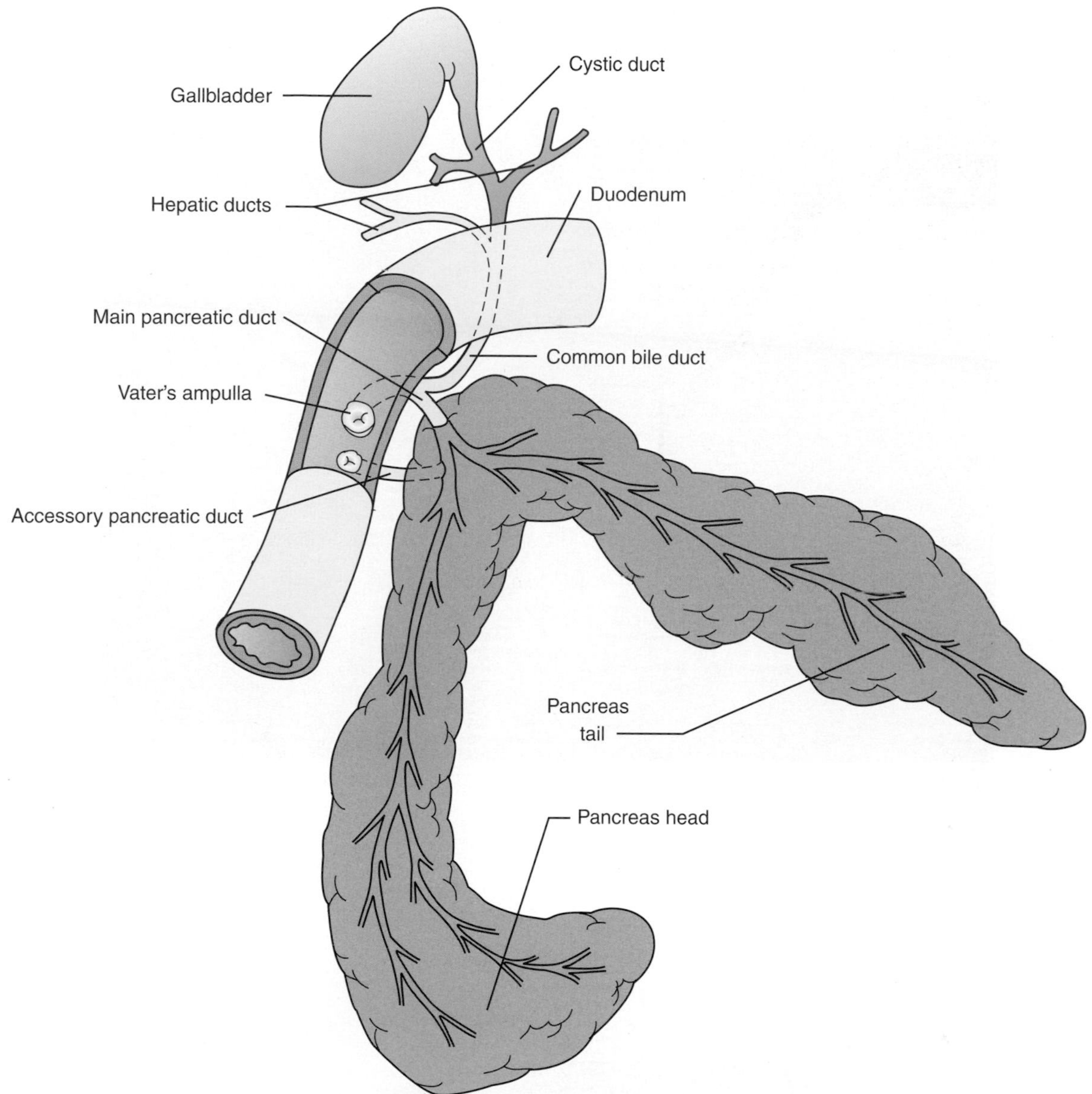

• **Fig. 14.9** Relative positions of the duodenum, pancreas, and gallbladder in a cat.

Pancreas
- Head of pancreas
- Tail of pancreas
- Main pancreatic duct
- **Accessory pancreatic duct**

Away from the pancreas, the small intestine transforms into a nutrient-absorbing machine called the jejunum before connecting to the ileum. Using your scissors, continue the longitudinal incision from the greater curvature of the stomach into the duodenum and down the length of the jejunum and ileum. Try to locate **Vater's ampulla** in the duodenum, which is the main port through which bile and pancreatic enzymes are delivered to the duodenum. Notice the contents of the small intestine and the texture of the lining of the small intestine. The velvety look of the jejunum, for example, is due to the presence of microvilli, which enhance the absorption of nutrients.

Fig. 14.10 is a picture of the small intestine of a foal. Examine the figure and use the identifiers to help you orient yourself to the location of the duodenum, jejunum, and ileum.

Based on the textbook readings and your knowledge of small intestinal physiology, please complete Exercises 12 through 15 related to small intestine digestion.

Large Intestine

In companion animals, the large intestine is composed of the cecum and the ascending, transverse, and descending colon. The **cecum** is a blind-ended pouch from which the ascending colon arises. It is located in the caudal right quadrant of the abdomen, and in humans and rabbits it has an added extension attached to it called the appendix. Refer to Figs. 14.11 and 14.12. Cut into the wall of the ileum and along its length. Continue cutting into the cecum and

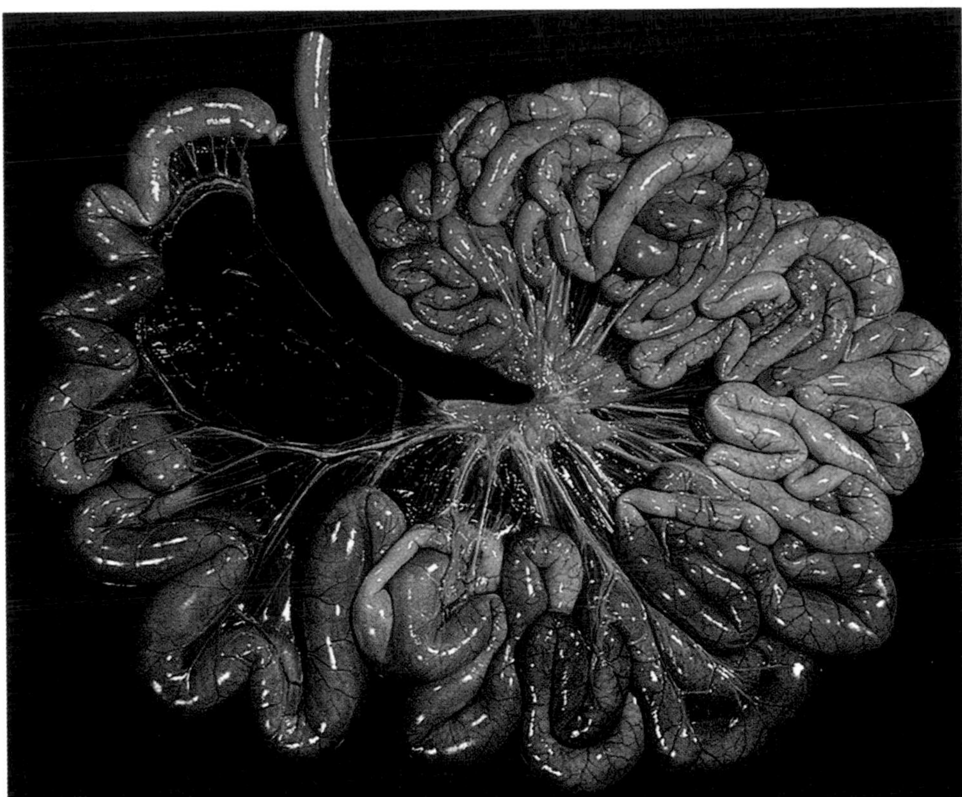

• Fig. 14.10 The small intestine of a foal. (From Clayton HM, Flood PF, Rosenstein DS: Clinical anatomy of the horse, St Louis, 2005, Mosby/Elsevier.)

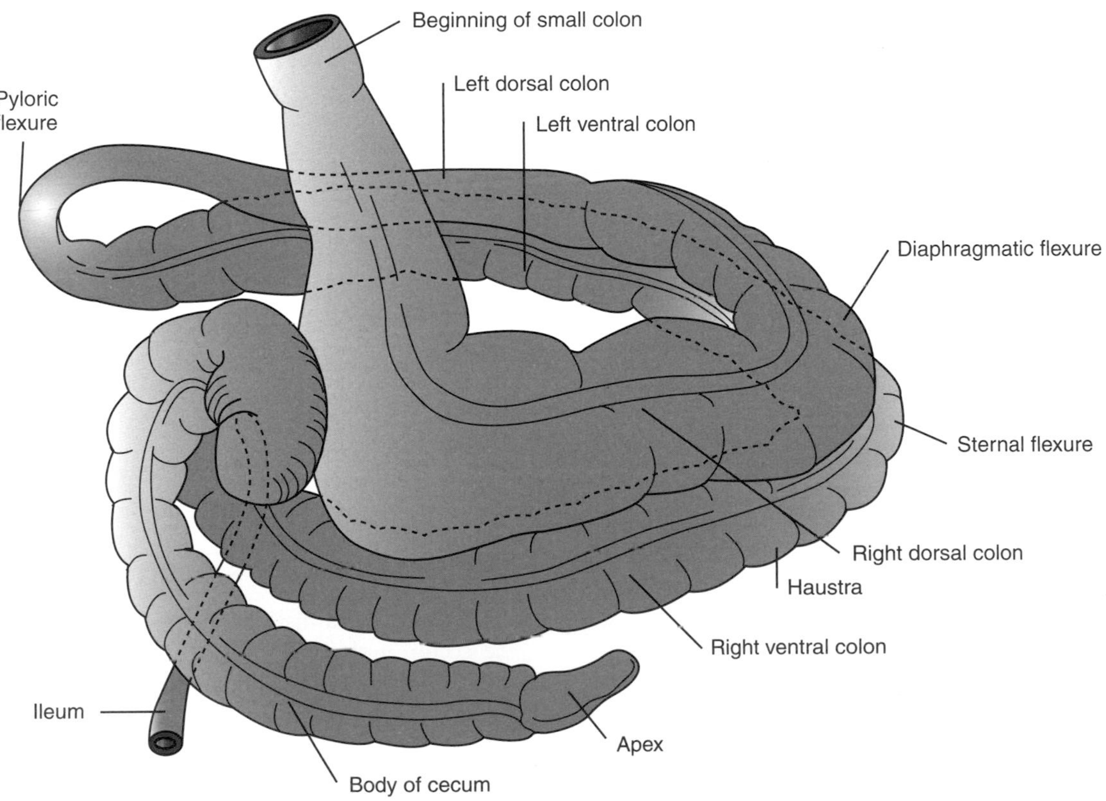

• Fig. 14.11 Topographic anatomy of colon and cecum of the horse. The head would be to the right of the figure.

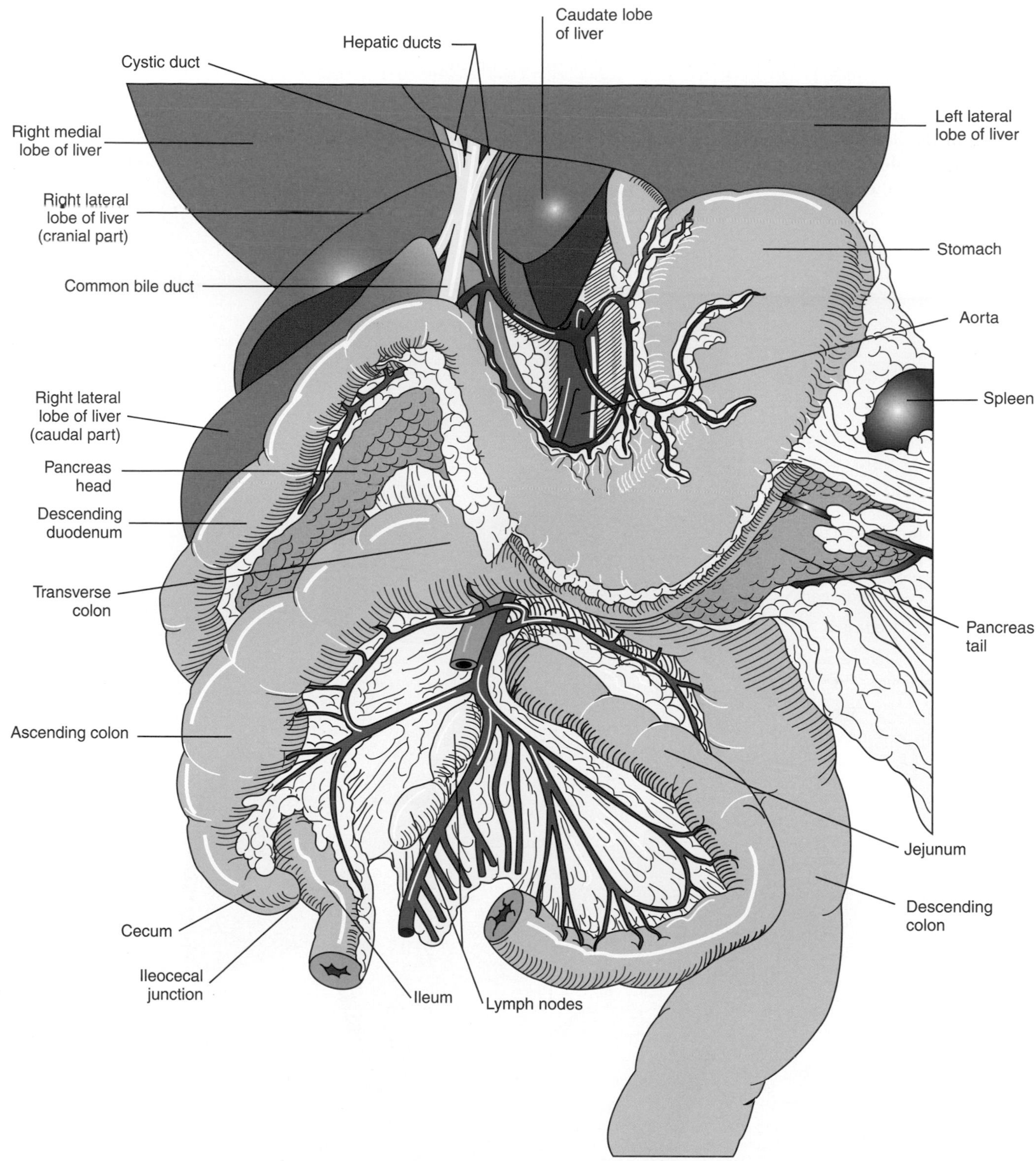

• **Fig. 14.12** Position of the ileum, cecum, and colon relative to the stomach and duodenum in a cat. The jejunum and ileum have been removed.

locate the sphincter muscle between the small and large intestines at the ileocecal junction. This is a common location for obstructions and intussusception in companion animals.

The **ascending, transverse,** and **descending colon** bear the important job of absorbing water and electrolytes from the ingesta; in this way, a solid stool or feces is formed. If progression through the colon is slowed, excessive amounts of water may be absorbed and the stool may be hard and pebbly. Under these circumstances, the animal is constipated. Conversely, if peristalsis through the colon is increased, there is little time for water absorption and the stool may therefore be excessively watery.

In herbivores, such as the horse and rabbit, fermentation takes place in the hindgut, resulting in a greater ability of the cecum and colon to digest ingesta. This is in sharp contrast to carnivorous species, such as the dog and cat, in which the cecum and colon are less well developed. The hindgut of the horse is divided into four sections: the **cecum, ventral colon, dorsal colon,** and **small colon.** The regions in which the large intestines curve or turn are called flexures. Three important flexures in the equine hindgut are the **sternal flexure, pelvic flexure,** and **diaphragmatic flexure.** It is essential to understand the anatomy of the equine hindgut, and particularly the locations of the flexures, because they are associated with impactions and are frequently the site of serious types of colic in horses.

The descending colon merges with the **rectum**, where feces are stored until defecation (Fig. 14.13).)

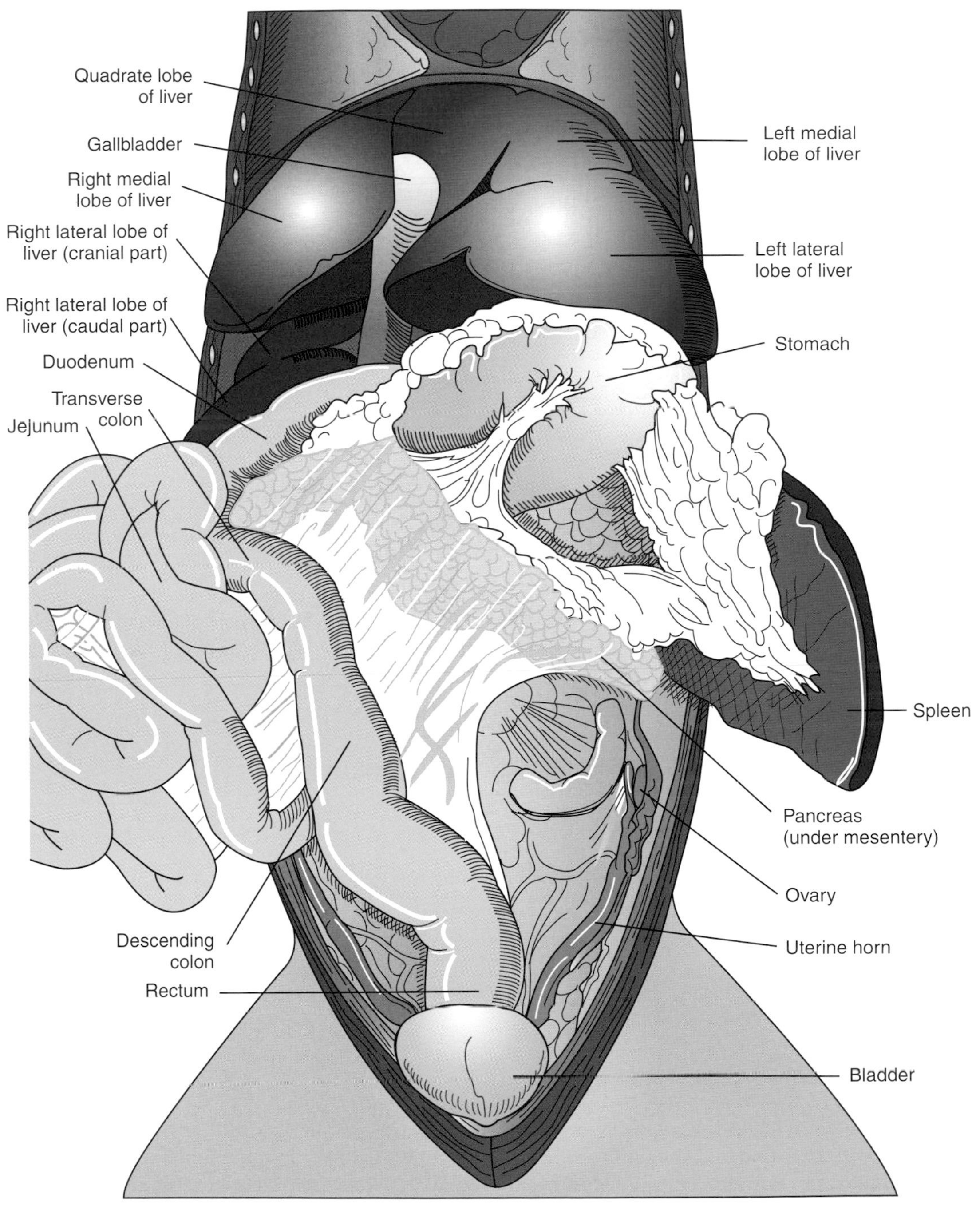

• **Fig. 14.13** Ventral view of the abdominal viscera in a cat. The jejunum and stomach are reflected to show the descending colon and rectum.

Digestion-Related Organs

Liver

Examine the liver in your dissected cat (see Figs. 14.12 and 14.13). Notice that it is the largest organ in the abdominal cavity and covers much of the stomach (see Fig. 14.13). The liver is a vital organ in the body and has many functions. The hepatic portal system delivers newly absorbed nutrients from the intestines directly to the liver. The liver uses the nutrients to build new molecules, such as the protein albumin, which is needed by the body to maintain colloid osmotic pressure in the blood vessels. It also detoxifies substances absorbed in the digestive tract (such as alcohol in humans) before these substances gain access to the systemic circulation. Huge volumes of blood circulate through the liver, making it ideally suited to remove bacteria, viruses, and damaged cells. The liver is also responsible for glycogen storage, bile production and excretion, lipid metabolism, and the production of numerous coagulation factors.

Pancreas

The pancreas is a gland with both endocrine and exocrine functions (see Figs. 14.12 and 14.13). The endocrine function of the pancreas includes the secretion of hormones, such as glucagon and insulin, directly into the bloodstream. These hormones are extremely important in maintaining the body's blood glucose levels.

The exocrine function of the pancreas involves the secretion of digestive enzymes, such as amylase, lipase, and numerous proteases, into the small intestines. These enzymes aid in the digestion of carbohydrates, proteins, and fat. The pancreas is also responsible for secreting bicarbonate into the duodenum. The bicarbonate, an alkaline substance, acts to neutralize the acidic contents from the stomach that enter the duodenum.

Endocrine alert: The pancreas is more than just a digestive organ. Turn to Chapter 11 to learn about its endocrine function!

EXERCISES

The Oral Cavity

Exercise 1

Identify Tooth Structure

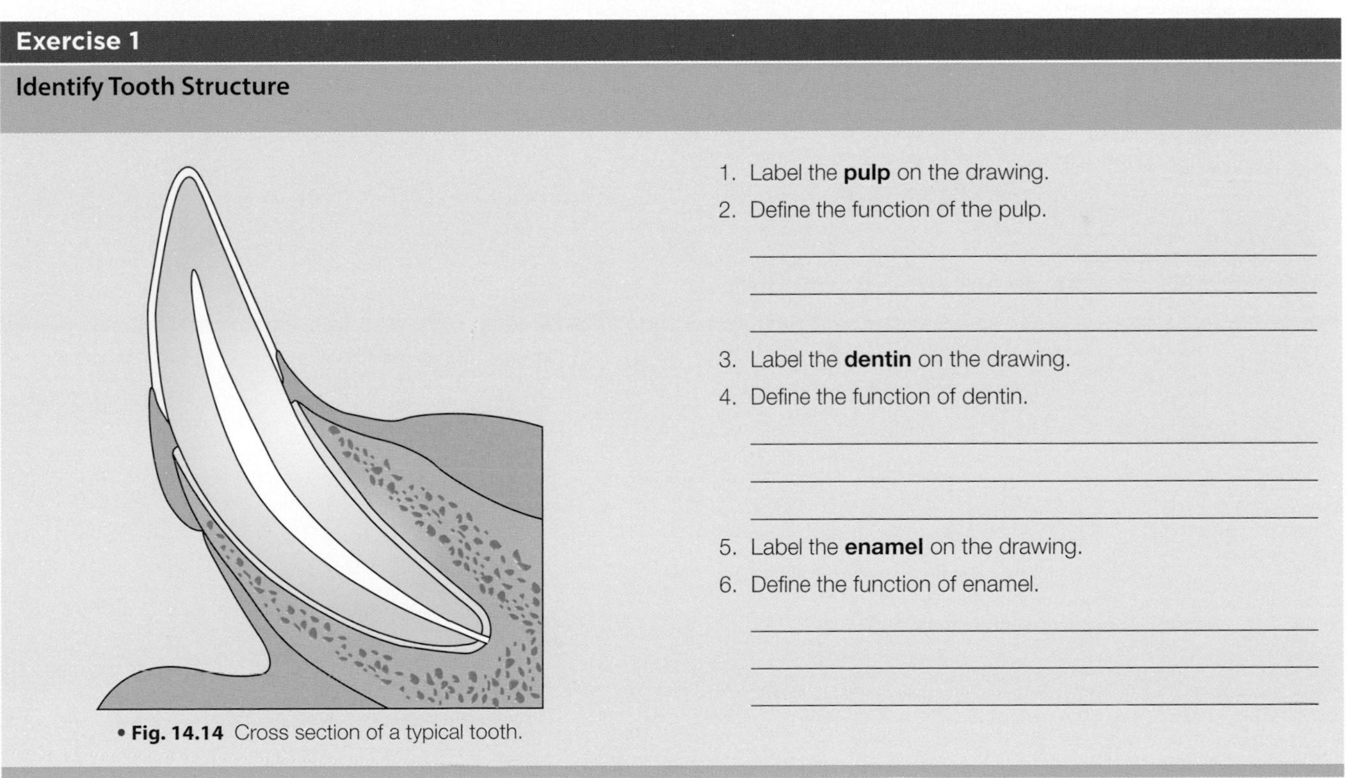

• **Fig. 14.14** Cross section of a typical tooth.

1. Label the **pulp** on the drawing.
2. Define the function of the pulp.

____

____

____

3. Label the **dentin** on the drawing.
4. Define the function of dentin.

____

____

____

5. Label the **enamel** on the drawing.
6. Define the function of enamel.

____

____

____

Exercise 2

Label the Dentition in the Dog and Horse

Dental Formulas for Several Domestic Species

Species	Dental Formula
Canine—puppy	$i\frac{3}{3}\,c\frac{1}{1}\,p\frac{3}{3}$
Canine—adult	$I\frac{3}{3}\,C\frac{1}{1}\,P\frac{4}{4}\,M\frac{2}{3}$
Feline—kitten	$i\frac{3}{3}\,c\frac{1}{1}\,p\frac{3}{2}$
Feline—adult	$I\frac{3}{3}\,C\frac{1}{1}\,P\frac{3}{2}\,M\frac{1}{1}$
Equine—adult	$I\frac{3}{3}\,C\frac{1}{1}\,P\frac{3-4}{3}\,M\frac{3}{3}$
Porcine—adult	$I\frac{3}{3}\,C\frac{1}{1}\,P\frac{4}{4}\,M\frac{3}{3}$
Bovine—adult	$I\frac{0}{3}\,C\frac{0}{1}\,P\frac{3}{3}\,M\frac{3}{3}$

Using the dental formulas, label the following structures on the diagrams of the dog (Fig. 14.15) and the horse (Fig. 14.16):

Incisor teeth (label with an I)

Canine teeth (label with a C)

Premolar teeth (label with a P)

Molar teeth (label with an M)

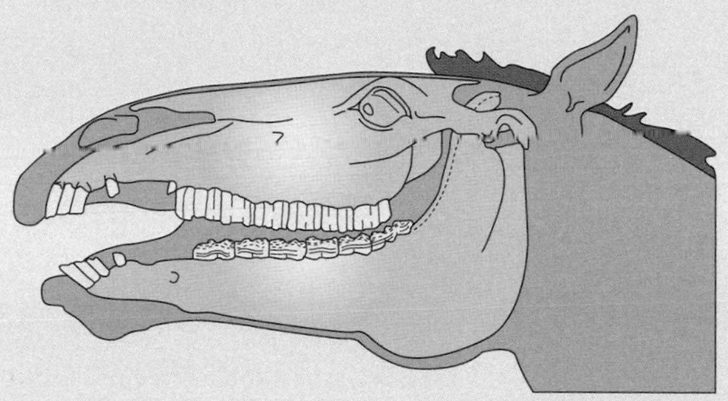

• **Fig. 14.16** Lateral view of normal equine dentition. (Adapted from Allen T, King C, Sperry-Allen D: Manual of equine dentistry, St Louis, 2003, Mosby.)

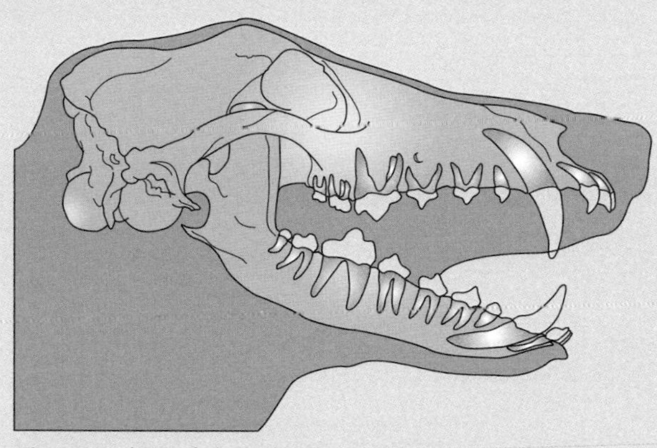

• **Fig. 14.15** Lateral view of a canine skull showing types of teeth.

Exercise 3

Dental Charting

"Max" Carr is a 9-year-old neutered male Golden Retriever. He comes to the All Creatures Animal Clinic to have his teeth cleaned. You are the veterinary technician responsible for Max's dental procedure.

Max's dental cleaning was successful, but Dr. Brown, the veterinarian, had to extract several of Max's diseased teeth. Dr. Brown asks you to update Mr. Carr on Max's dental procedure when it is time for Max to be discharged from the hospital.

You explain to Mr. Carr that two of Max's lower incisors were already missing before his dental procedure and the remaining four incisors had to be extracted because of decay. Use the diagram below to label the lower incisors on the *rostral* view in red.

Max had moderate gingivitis, an inflammation of the **gingiva** (gums), in the area of his upper premolars on both his right and left side. Please label Max's area of gingivitis on Fig. 14.17 in blue.

Lastly, you tell Mr. Carr that Max had a fracture on the crown of his upper right canine tooth. The fracture appeared as an area where the tooth had been "chipped" away, but there was no pulp exposure so it was not serious. You ask Mr. Carr what Max likes to chew on and he says that Max's favorite treat is a cow femur from the butcher. You explain to Mr. Carr that Max should not be given any more cow femurs as they could cause a more serious fracture in the future. Please label the area of Max's fracture in Fig. 14.17 in green.

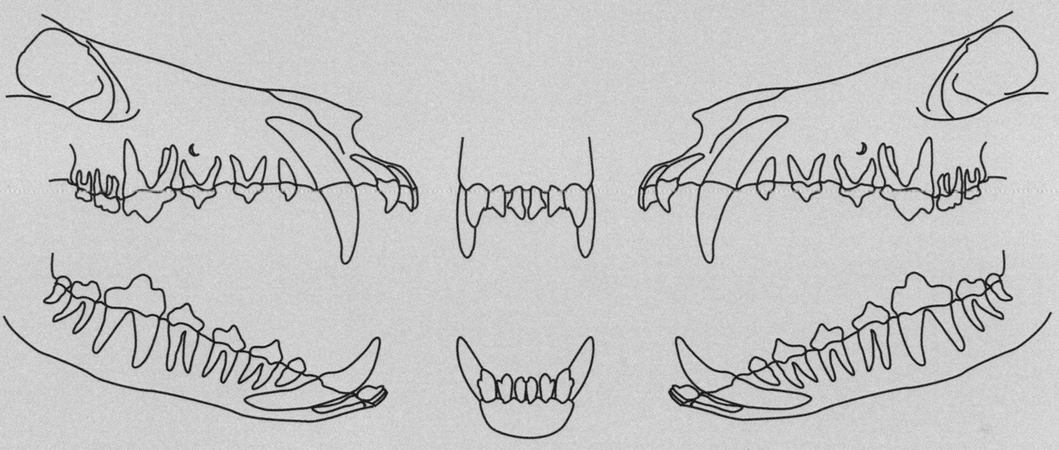

• **Fig. 14.17** Right and left lateral, and rostral views of canine dentition. (Adapted from Gorrel C, Derbyshire S: Veterinary dentistry for the nurse and technician, Oxford, 2005, Elsevier.)

Dental Formulas

Using the dental formulas presented in Exercise 2, determine the total number of teeth in each of the following species:

Exercise 4

Dental Formula: Feline (Adult)

- Dental formula = ____________________
- Total number of teeth = ____________________

Exercise 5

Dental Formula: Feline (Kitten)

- Dental formula = ____________________
- Total number of teeth = ____________________

Exercise 6

Dental Formula: Bovine

- Dental formula = ____________________
- Total number of teeth = ____________________

Exercise 7

Dental Formula: Porcine

- Dental formula = ____________________
- Total number of teeth = ____________________

The Esophagus and Stomach

Exercise 8

Identify Structures on a Horse Stomach

Match the following terms with the corresponding location in Fig. 14.18A. Enter the correct number on the line next to the term.

No.	Term
________	Greater curvature
________	Fundus
________	Pylorus
________	Esophagus
________	Lesser curvature
________	Antrum
________	Body of stomach
________	Cardia
________	Duodenum

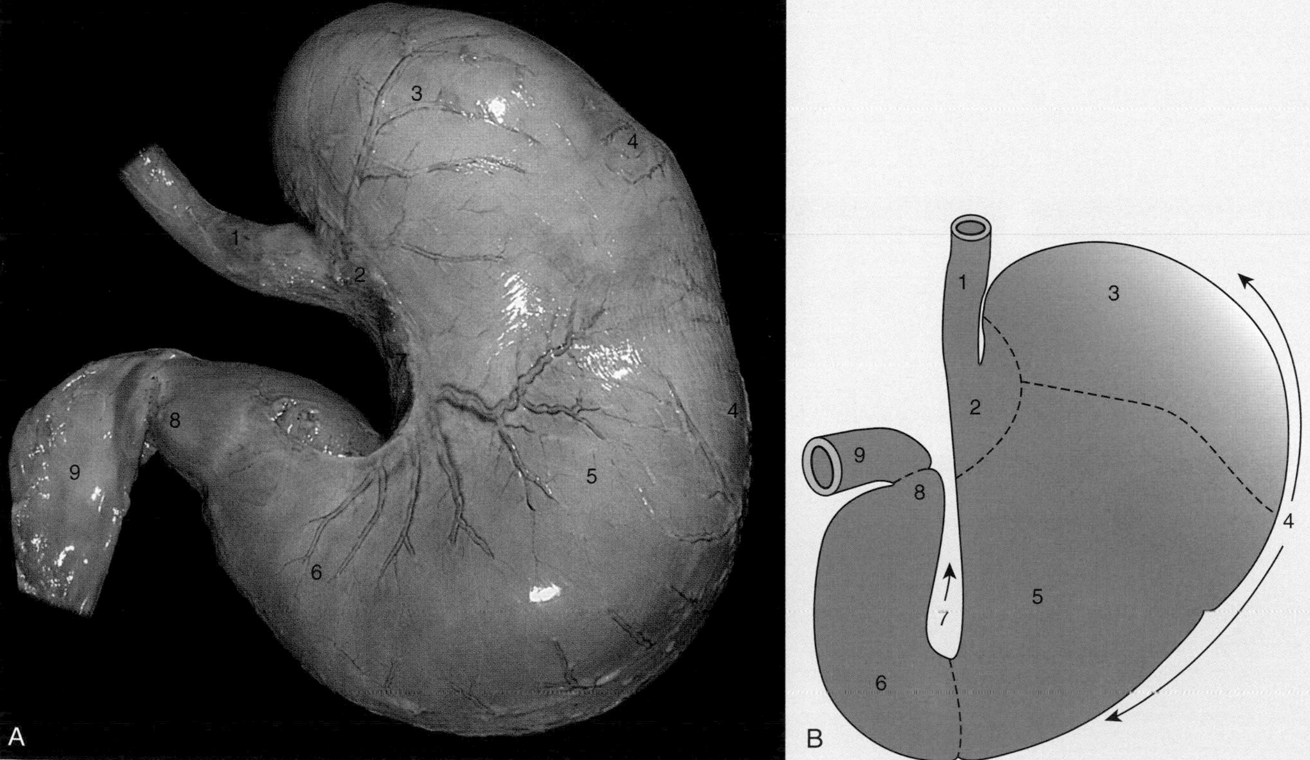

• **Fig. 14.18** Stomach of a horse. (A) Photograph of the stomach of a horse. (B) Illustration of the stomach of a horse. (A, From Clayton HM, Flood PF, Rosenstein DS: Clinical anatomy of the horse, St Louis, 2005, Mosby/Elsevier.)

Exercise 9

Label and Define Anatomic and Physiologic Functions of Each Stomach Part

Study the photograph of the stomach of a horse in Fig. 14.18A and then label the parts on the corresponding illustration Fig. 14.18B. In the space below, provide a detailed description of the anatomic and physiologic function of each part of the stomach.

Cardia: ______________________________

____

____

____

Fundus: ______________________________

____

____

____

Body: ______________________________

____

____

____

Antrum: ______________________________

____

____

____

Pylorus: ______________________________

____

____

____

Exercise 10

Student Lecture Presentation on Digestive Anatomy and Physiology

Ms. Davis, the animal science teacher from Northwest High School, calls the mixed animal practice at which you are currently employed and asks if you would like to be a guest lecturer during a series of presentations on digestive anatomy and physiology. She would like to have a veterinary professional talk to the students about the ruminant digestive tract. Because digestive anatomy and physiology has always been a favorite topic of yours, you agree to present the lecture.

On the day of the presentation, you come prepared with visual aids to enhance the students' understanding of ruminant digestive anatomy. Fig. 14.6A and B shows images of the rumen from the left side of the animal.

As you discuss each aspect of the anatomy and physiology of the ruminant digestive tract with the high school class, you will label each part of the figures in your presentation. Label the following structures in the figures where appropriate.

- Esophagus
  - Esophageal sphincter
- Reticulum
  - Ruminoreticular orifice
  - Reticulo-omasal orifice
  - Ruminoreticular fold
- Rumen
  - Dorsal blind sac
  - Ventral blind sac
  - Dorsal sac
  - Ventral sac
  - Caudal groove
- Abomasum

Continued

Exercise 10—cont'd

Student Lecture Presentation on Digestive Anatomy and Physiology

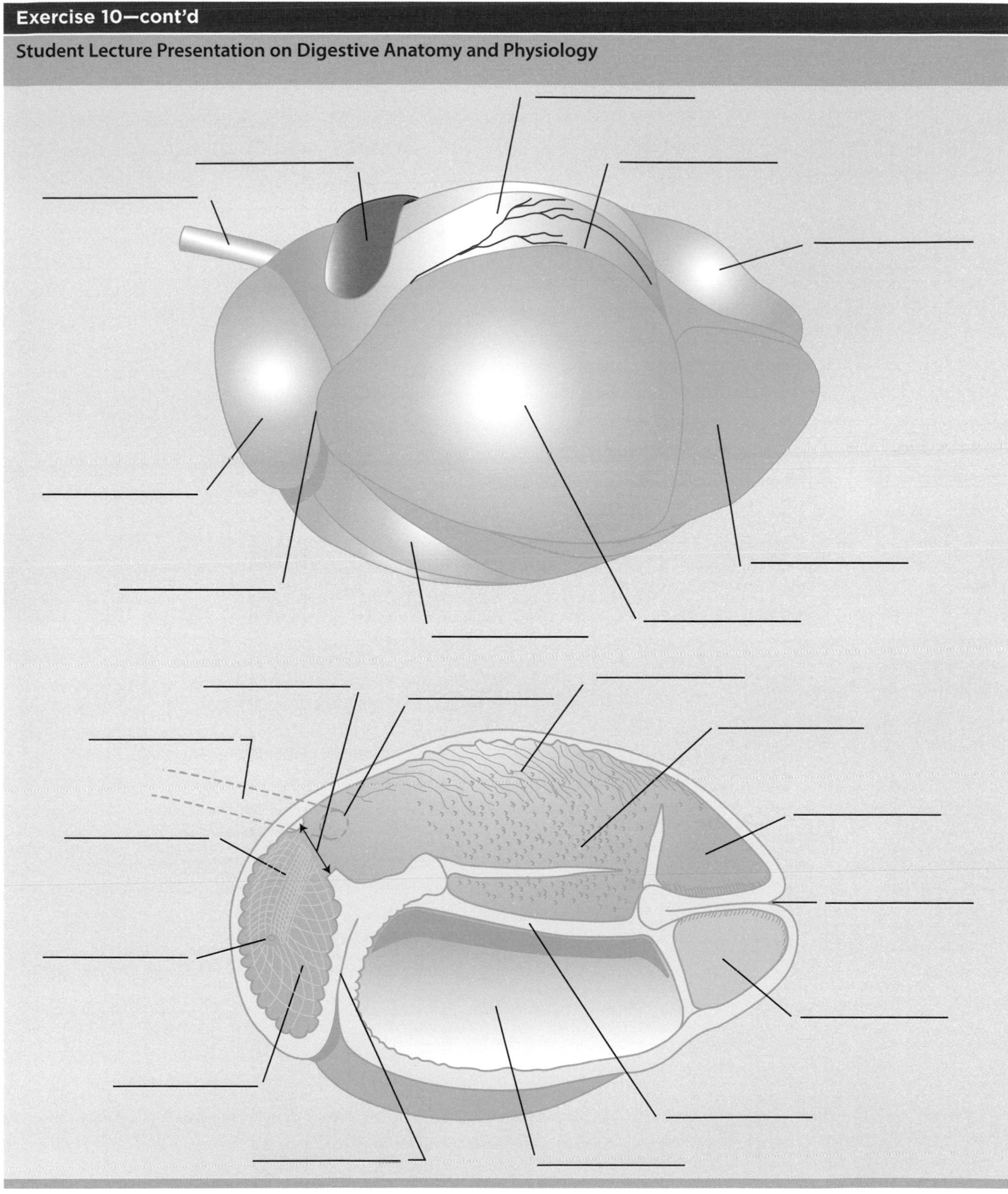

Exercise 11

Compare and Contrast the Reticulum, Rumen, Omasum, and Abomasum for Student Lecture

Now that you have identified the location of the reticulum, rumen, omasum, and abomasum, please explain to the students the anatomic and physiologic function of each of these structures. Provide a detailed description in the spaces below.

Reticulum: ______________________________

____

____

____

Rumen: ______________________________

____

____

____

Omasum: ______________________________

____

____

____

Abomasum: ______________________________

____

____

____

The Intestinal Tract

Exercise 12

Identify Polysaccharides

Name several "complex carbohydrates" or polysaccharides.

____

____

____

Exercise 13

Identify Pancreatic Proteases

Proteins must be broken down by proteases before they can be absorbed. The pancreas is responsible for producing five basic proteases. Name the five pancreatic proteases that aid in protein digestion:

a. ______________________________

b. ______________________________

c. ______________________________

d. ______________________________

e. ______________________________

Exercise 14

Explain Emulsification

Explain the process of emulsification. How do bile acids from the liver aid in fat digestion?

____

____

Exercise 15

Identify "Building Block" Molecules

What are the "building block" molecules derived from the digestion of fat?

____

____

Exercise 16

Identify Structures in the Intestinal Tract and Trace Ingestion From Duodenum to Rectum

Fig. 14.19 represents the intestinal tract of a horse. Using your knowledge of gastrointestinal anatomy, match the number in the illustration with the corresponding anatomic part below:

________ Transverse colon

________ Right dorsal colon

________ Sternal flexure of the colon

________ Pelvic flexure

________ Body of the cecum

________ Right ventral colon

________ Small colon

________ Left dorsal colon

________ Diaphragmatic flexure

________ Rectum

________ Left ventral colon

________ Apex of the cecum

The stomach, pylorus, and small intestinal structures (duodenum, jejunum, and ileum) are labeled for orientation.

Once you have completed the matching exercise, use a colored pencil or marker to trace the path that ingesta would follow from the start of the intestinal tract (duodenum) to the end of the intestinal tract (rectum). Use a dotted line if the path travels behind another part in the illustration.

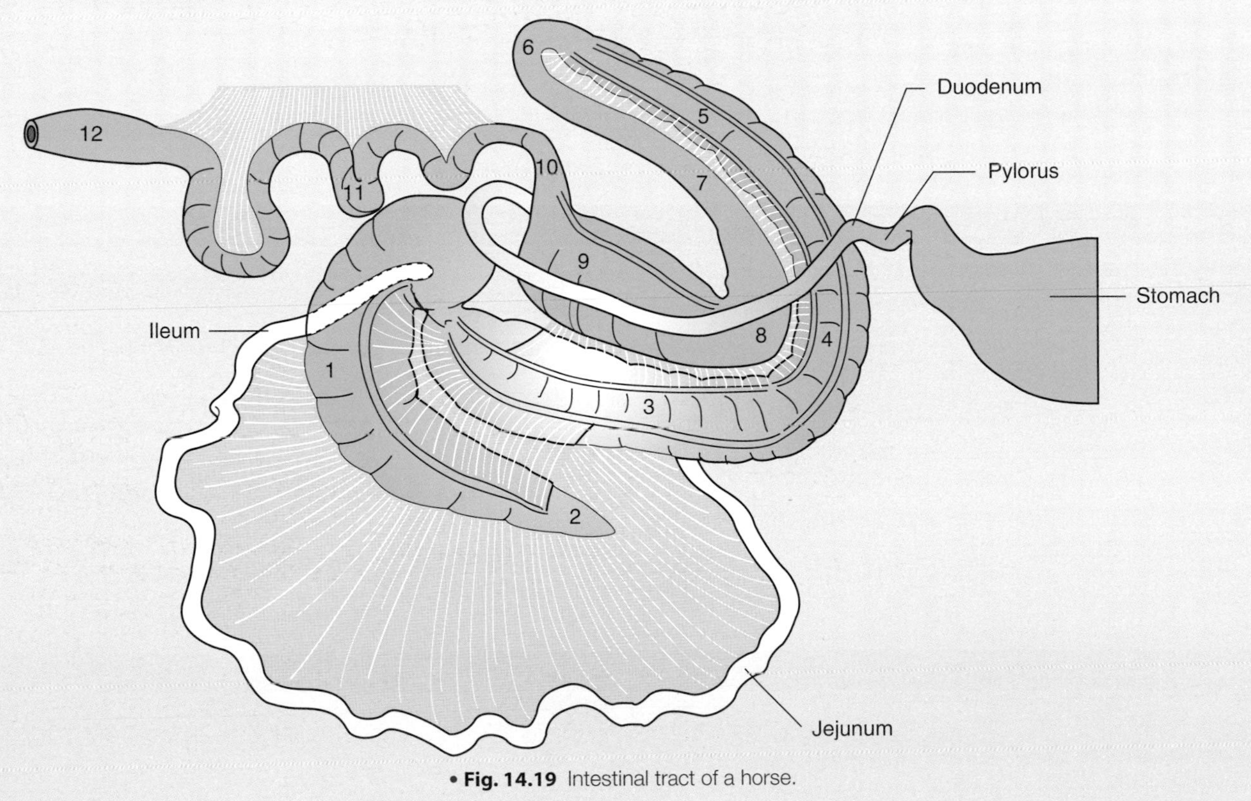

• **Fig. 14.19** Intestinal tract of a horse.

Digestion-Related Organs

Exercise 17

Identify Digestion-Related Organs

Label the structures indicated in Fig. 14.20.

_______ Gallbladder

_______ Left lateral lobe

_______ Quadrate lobe

_______ Left medial lobe

_______ Right lateral lobe (cranial and caudal parts)

_______ Right medial lobe

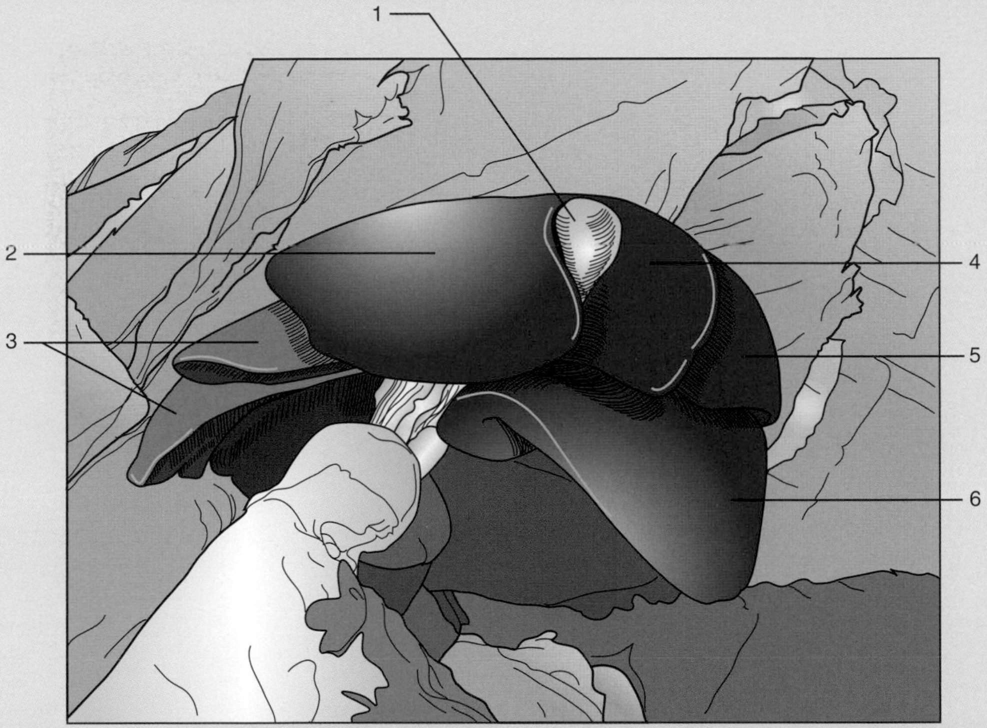

1
2
3
4
5
6

• **Fig. 14.20** Lobes of the liver in a cat.

Exercise 18

Detail Liver Function

Explain in as much detail as possible the various functions of the liver.

____

____

____

____

____

____

____

____

____

____

Exercise 19

Identify Structures on the Feline Stomach, Duodenum, and Pancreas

Fig. 14.21 is a photograph of the stomach, duodenum, and pancreas of a cat. Assign the correct number from the photo to the corresponding term below:

_________ Esophagus

_________ Jejunum (cut)

_________ Pylorus

_________ Tail of pancreas

_________ Antrum of stomach

_________ Ascending duodenum

_________ Head of pancreas

_________ Body of stomach

_________ Greater curvature of stomach

_________ Fundus of stomach

_________ Descending duodenum

_________ Lesser curvature of stomach

_________ Cardia of stomach

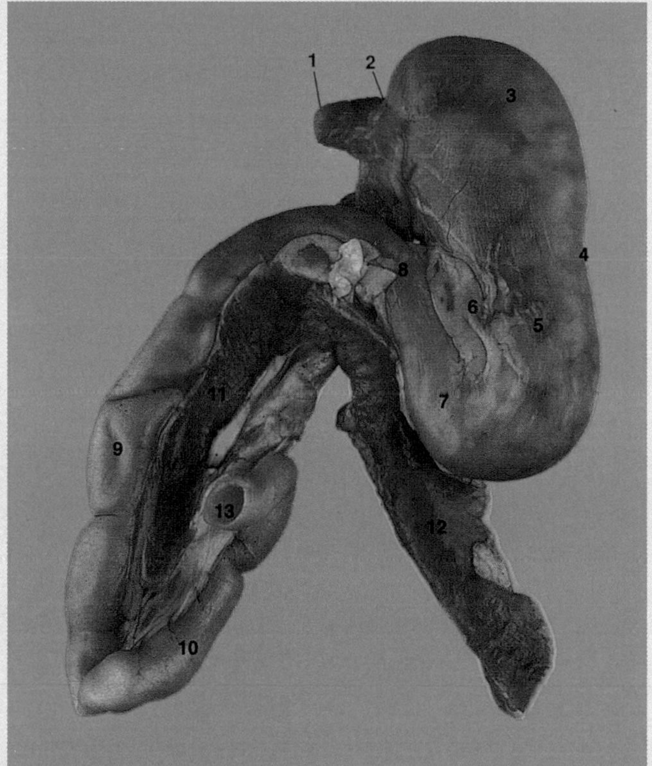

• **Fig. 14.21** The stomach, pancreas, and duodenum of a cat. (From Boyd JS, Paterson C, May AH: Color atlas of clinical anatomy of the dog and cat, ed. 2, St Louis, 2001, Mosby.)

Exercise 20

Describe Exocrine and Endocrine Functions of the Pancreas

Based on the textbook readings and your knowledge of pancreatic physiology, describe the exocrine and endocrine functions of the pancreas.

Exocrine: ____
____
____
____

Endocrine: ____
____
____
____

Exercise 21

Clinical Application #1: Label the Digestive Tract of the Rabbit and Trace Hindgut Fermentation

You are employed at a veterinary practice where birds, ferrets, rabbits, guinea pigs, iguanas, and many other exotic pets are seen. "Fluffy" Walters, a 3-year-old lop-eared rabbit, arrives for her annual examination. You take Mrs. Walters and Fluffy into an examination room to obtain some information from Mrs. Walters on Fluffy's health and behavior this past year and to take Fluffy's temperature, pulse, and respiration.

Mrs. Walters tells you that Fluffy has been active and is eating and drinking well. She says her only concern is that she noticed Fluffy eating her own feces very late at night. Mrs. Walters observed this behavior several times, each time late at night. She wants to know why Fluffy is doing this and if her diet is insufficient.

You explain to Mrs. Walters that this is natural rabbit behavior and that rabbits produce two types of feces. A rabbit's digestive system is adapted for hindgut fermentation, meaning that the cecum and colon of hindgut fermentators, such as the horse and guinea pig, have modifications specific to the dietary needs of that species. The cecum of the rabbit contains microbes that break down plant material, allowing starches and fiber to be digested. Cyclic contractions of the cecum move dietary contents rapidly through the gut, resulting in "soft" feces also referred to as "night feces" or "cecotrophs." The rabbit consumes the cecotrophs directly from the anus. This process is known as coprophagia. The cecotrophs are high in protein and vitamins B and K. This process allows the rabbit to benefit from valuable undigested nutrients the second time around. "Hard" feces are excreted during the day and are not ingested by the rabbit.

Fig. 14.22 is a figure of the gastrointestinal tract of the rabbit. Using the word bank, fill in the lines provided and label each part of the rabbit's digestive tract. Then, using colored pencils, shade in only those areas involved in hindgut fermentation.

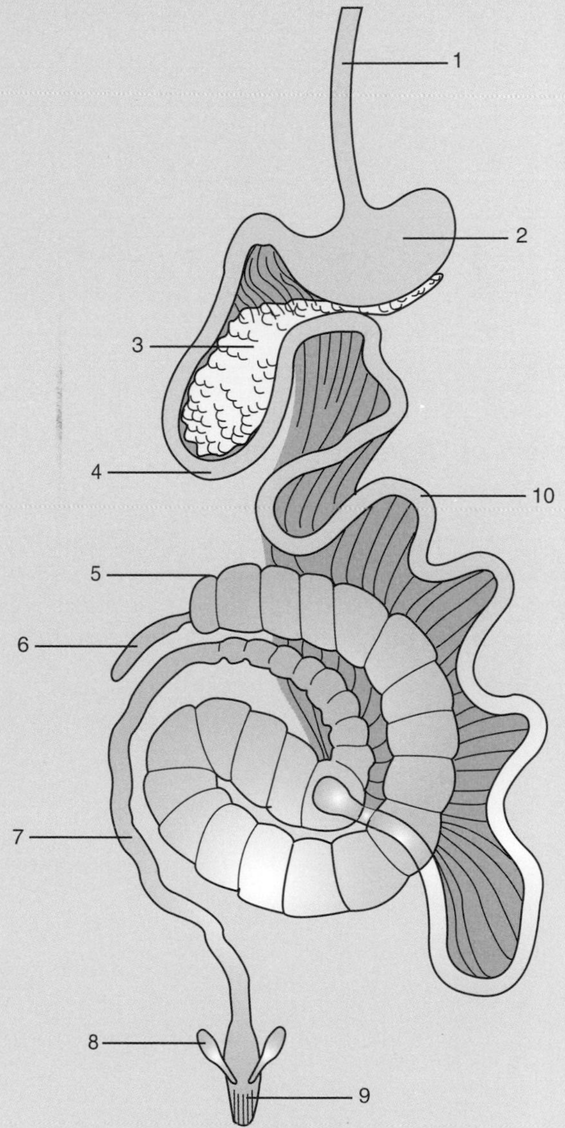

• **Fig. 14.22** The gastrointestinal tract of a rabbit.

Word Bank

_______ Esophagus
_______ Anal glands
_______ Jejunum
_______ Pancreas
_______ Appendix
_______ Colon
_______ Cecum
_______ Rectum
_______ Duodenum
_______ Stomach

Exercise 22

Clinical Application #2: Client Consultation

The receptionist at Critter Care Small Animal Clinic receives a phone call from Mrs. Clarke, a regular client of Critter Care. The receptionist asks you to talk to Mrs. Clarke because she has a medical question concerning her dog "Skittles." Skittles is a 14-year-old spayed female Dachshund. Mrs. Clarke informs you that Skittles has been having diarrhea for the past day and a half. You ask her if there has been any change in diet and Mrs. Clarke confirms she has indeed altered Skittles' diet. Skittles was receiving a high-quality adult dry dog food when Mrs. Clarke decided that she was at the age that she should eat a "senior" diet, so 2 days ago she began giving Skittles a high-quality senior canned food diet. She thought canned food would be easier for Skittles to chew since she has some dental disease. Please explain to Mrs. Clarke why you believe Skittles developed diarrhea. Also discuss with her what dietary changes you would implement right away to address the diarrhea problem. Finally, inform Mrs. Clarke about how she can introduce a new food into her dog's diet, in the future, without inducing diarrhea.

____

____

____

____

____

____

____

____

____

____

____

____

____

____

Review of Digestive Anatomy

The following feline dissection (Figs. 14.23–14.25) will allow you to review your digestive anatomy and apply your knowledge of the location of various anatomic structures. The pictures were taken with the cat in dorsal recumbency (on its back). Use the figures as a guide to help you "visualize" how the digestive structures are positioned in the abdomen. The series of photographs represents a dissection in progress. Each photo shows a different stage in the dissection with various structures removed.

Exercise 23

Identify Digestion-Related Feline Organs: Ventral Aspect

Match the correct number from Fig. 14.23 to the corresponding anatomic structure.

________ Gallbladder

________ Greater omentum

________ Jejunum

________ Left lateral lobe of liver

________ Descending duodenum

________ Right medial lobe of liver

________ Quadrate lobe of liver

________ Urinary bladder

________ Stomach

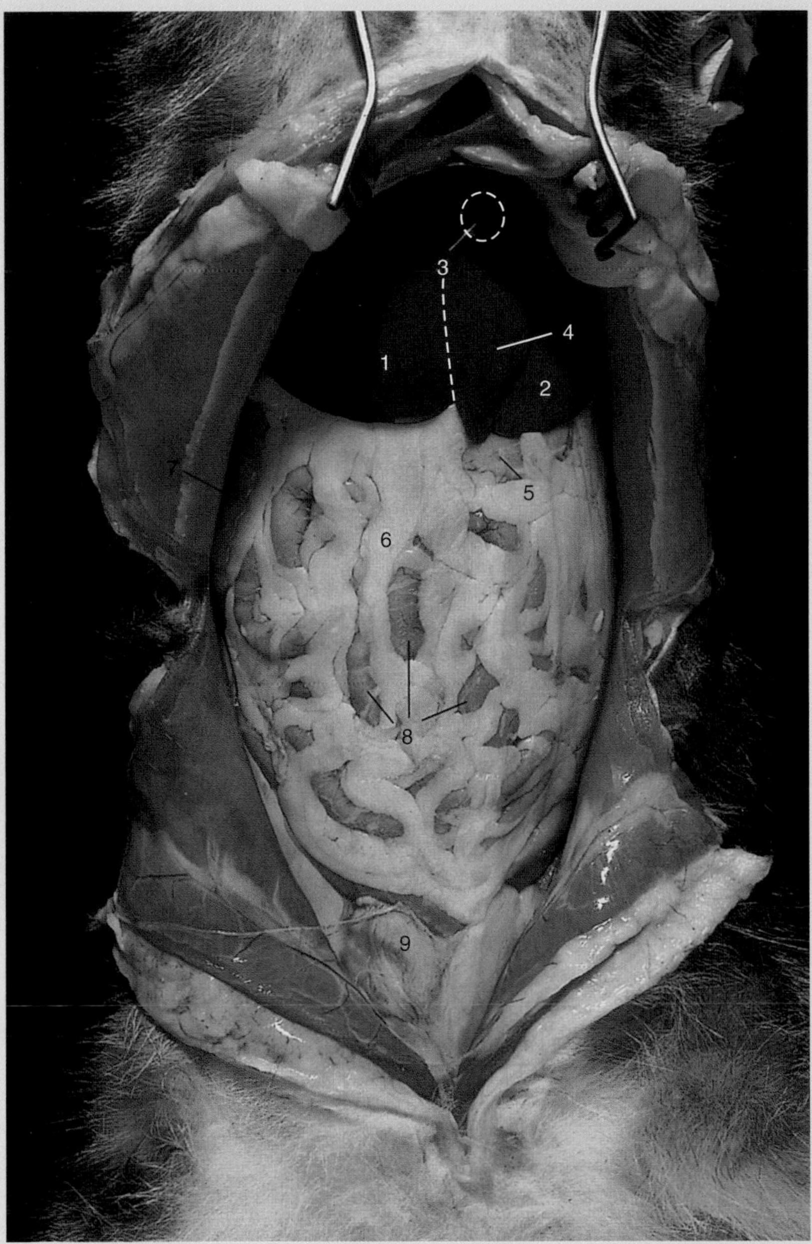

• **Fig. 14.23** Ventral aspect of the opened abdomen of a cat. (From Boyd JS, Paterson C, May AH: Color atlas of clinical anatomy of the dog and cat, ed. 2, St Louis, 2001, Mosby.)

Exercise 24

Identify Digestion-Related Feline Organs: Ventral Aspect, Omentum Removed

Match the correct number from Fig. 14.24 with the corresponding anatomic structure.

__________ Spleen	__________ Descending duodenum
__________ Urinary bladder	__________ Left lateral lobe of the liver
__________ Jejunum	__________ Greater curvature of the stomach
__________ Right lateral lobe of the liver	__________ Descending colon
__________ Gallbladder	__________ Right medial lobe of the liver
__________ Quadrate lobe of the liver	

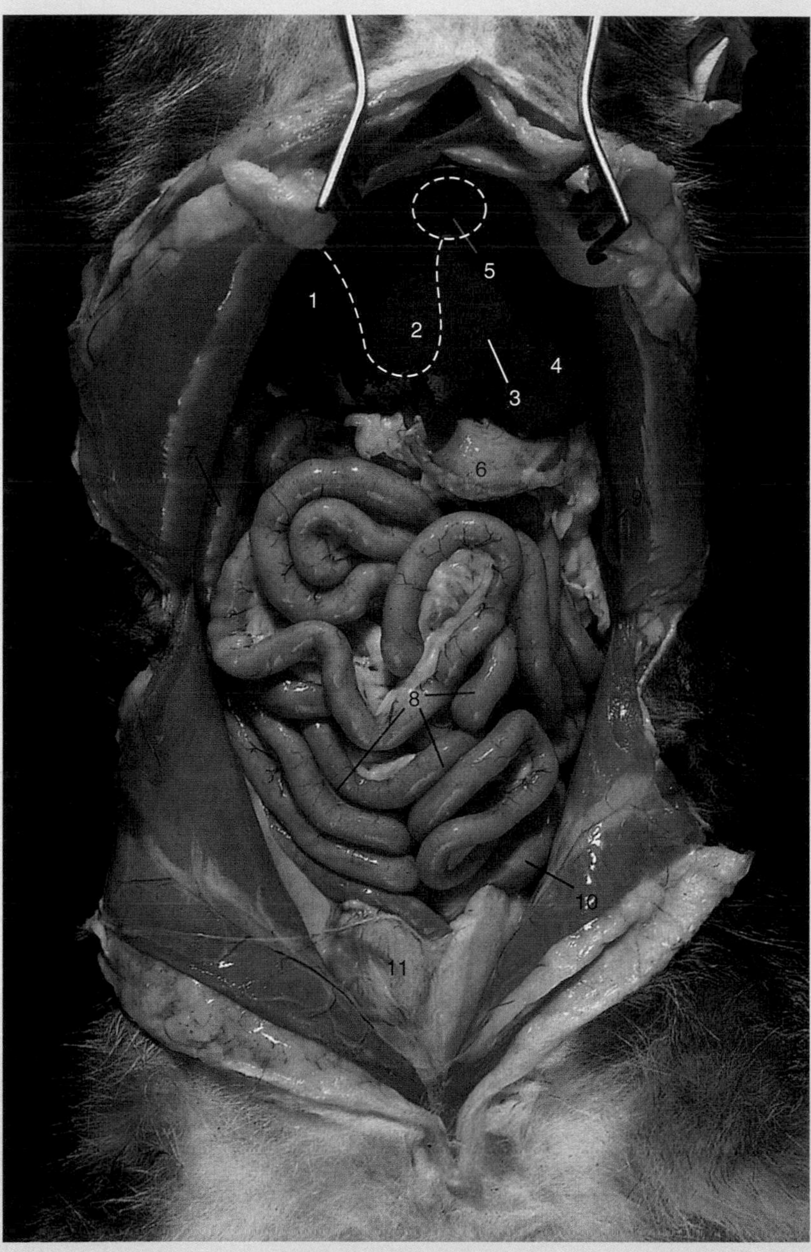

• **Fig. 14.24** Ventral aspect of the feline abdomen. The greater omentum has been removed. (From Boyd JS, Paterson C, May AH: Color atlas of clinical anatomy of the dog and cat, ed. 2, St Louis, 2001, Mosby.)

Exercise 25

Identify Digestion-Related Feline Organs: Ventral Aspect, Jejunum Removed

Match the correct number from Fig. 14.25 with the corresponding structure.

________ Spleen	________ Stomach
________ Urinary bladder	________ Ascending colon
________ Ileum	________ Descending colon
________ Ileocolic junction	________ Transverse colon
________ Liver	________ Cecum
________ Caudate lobe of the liver	________ Right ovary
________ Duodenum	________ Right uterine horn

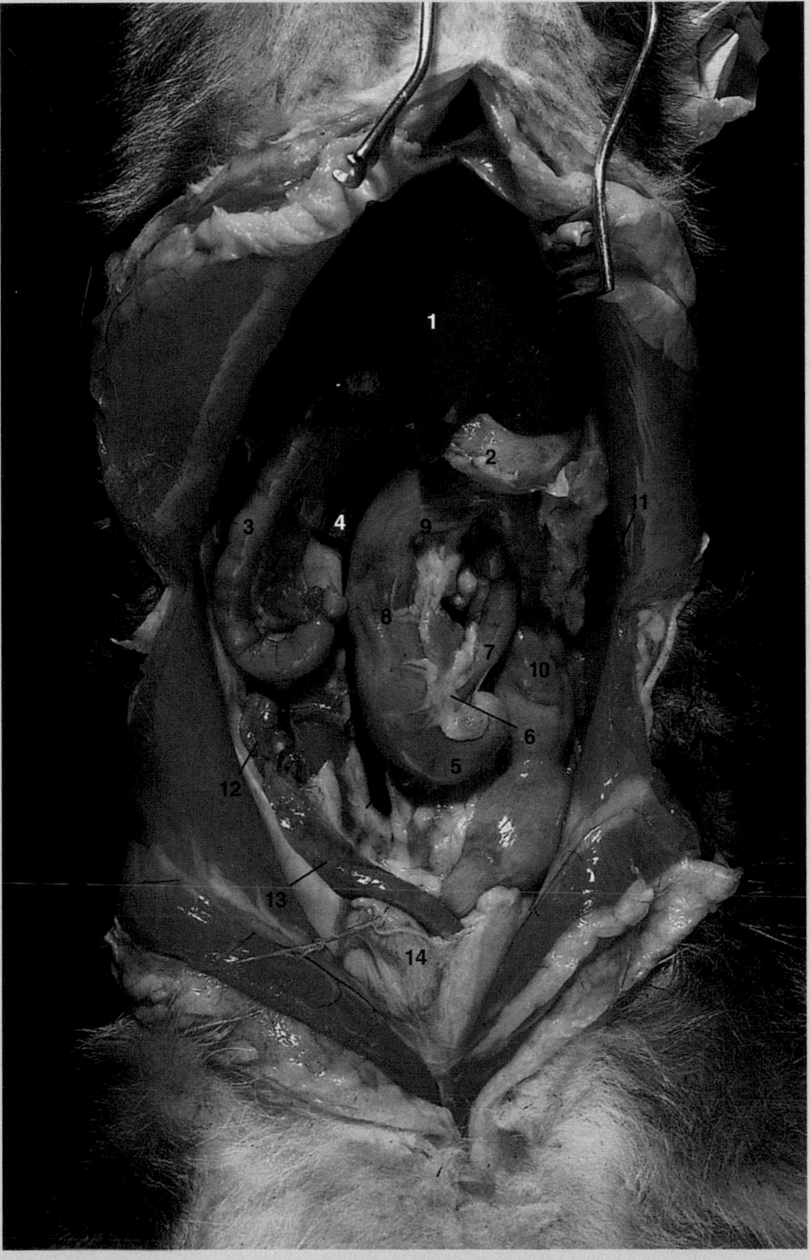

• **Fig. 14.25** Ventral aspect of the feline abdomen. The jejunum has been removed. (From Boyd JS, Paterson C, May AH: Color atlas of clinical anatomy of the dog and cat, ed. 2, St Louis, 2001, Mosby.)

Review

Exercise 26

Label Stomach Structures

Without looking up the answers, test your knowledge by filling in the blanks below:

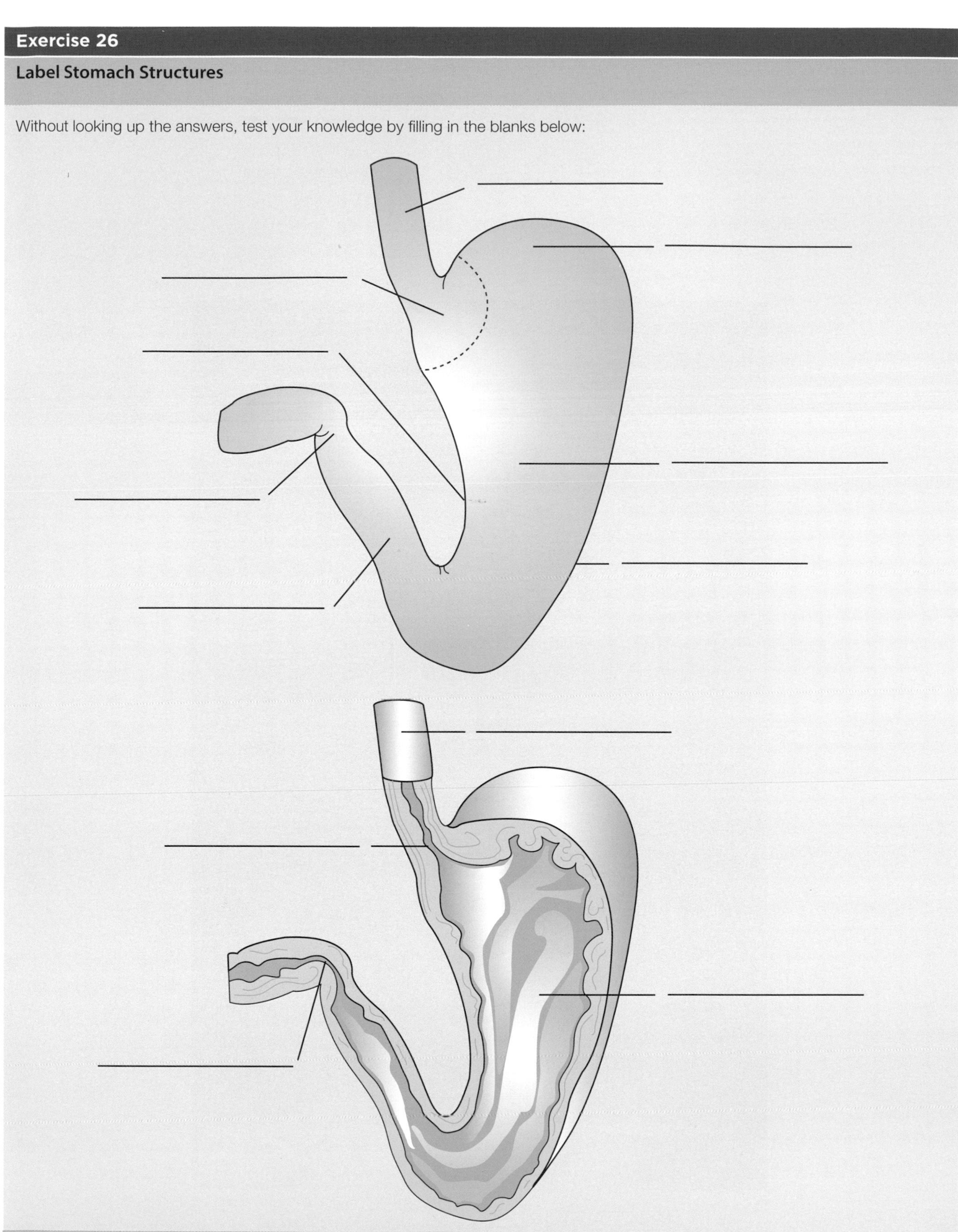

Exercise 27

Label Anatomic Digestive Bovine Structures

Label the anatomic parts below:

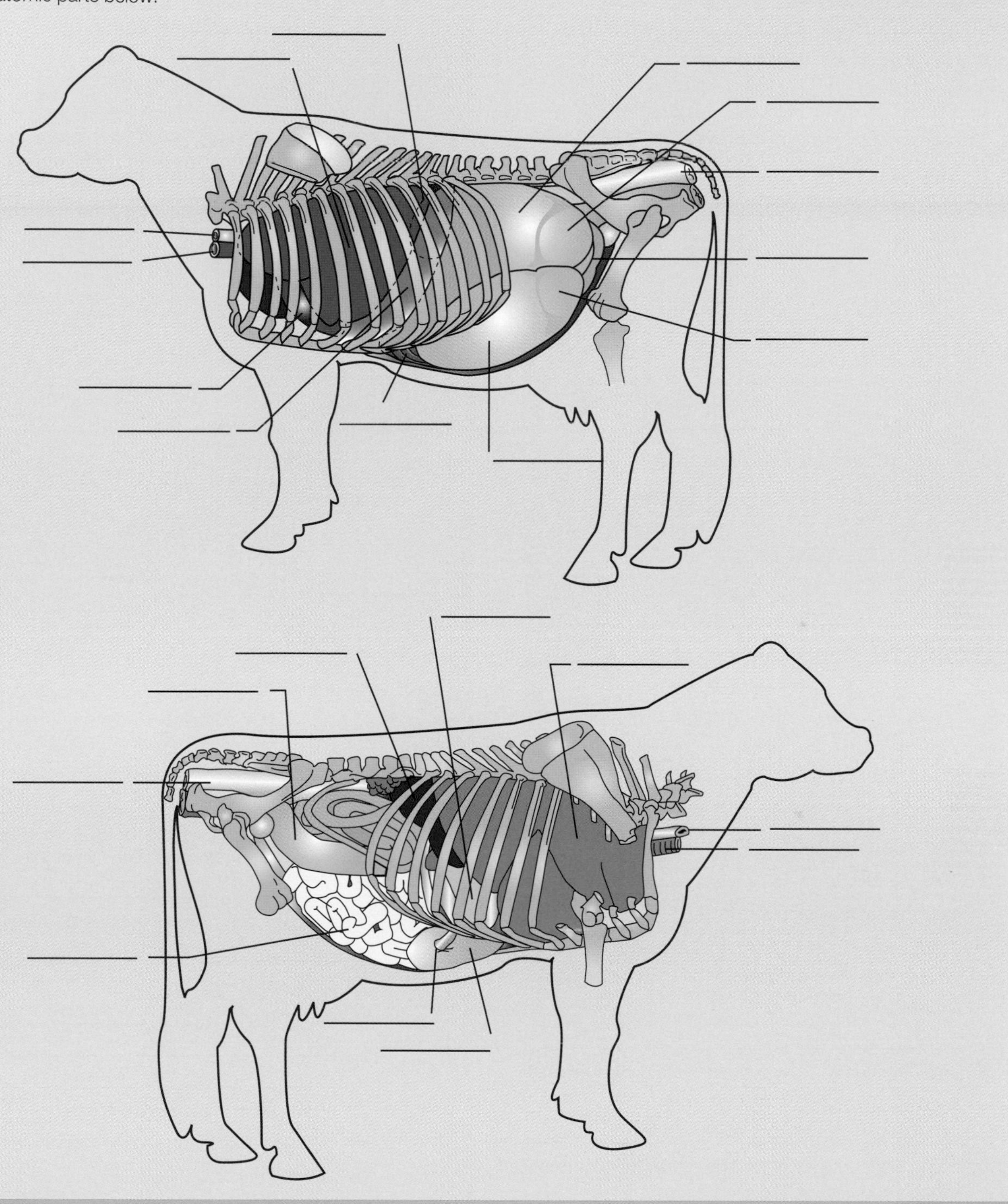

Critical and Clinical Thinking

Exercise 28

Critical Thinking: Label, Match, Fill in

Label the blank lines in this image.

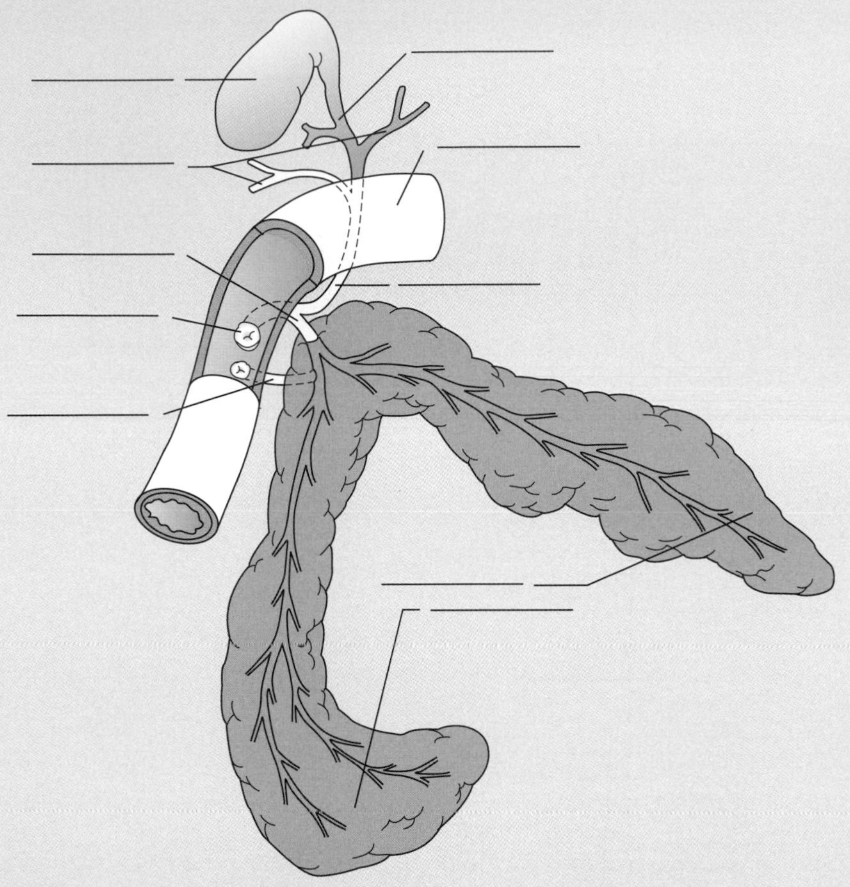

Fill in the blanks below:

1. Describe the difference between an herbivore, a carnivore, and an omnivore. ______________________________
____
2. What is the difference between a monogastric animal and a ruminant? ______________________________
____
3. What are the five key functions of the gastrointestinal tract? ______________________________
____
4. Name the four types of teeth and how they are classified in the dental formula. ______________________________
____
5. Which part of the ruminant digestive system most closely resembles the monogastric stomach?
____
6. What are the components of the small intestine? ________
____
7. What are the components of the large intestine? ________
____
8. Which digestion-related organs have both exocrine and endocrine function? ______________________________
____
____
9. An inflammation of the gingiva is called ______________.
10. The parotid salivary glands, the mandibular salivary glands, and the ______________ salivary glands are found in most domestic animals.
11. The esophagus is a tubular organ and contains the following layers: mucosa, submucosa, muscular layer, and ______________________________.

Exercise 28—cont'd

Critical Thinking: Label, Match, Fill in

12. An animal with a single stomach is referred to as a ________________________.
13. The equine hindgut is composed of the cecum, ventral colon, dorsal colon, and ________________________.
14. An animal whose diet consists of plants and meat is a ________________________.
15. The alimentary canal is another term used to describe the ________________________.
16. The muscular folds that divide the sacs of the rumen are called ________________________.

Match the words with the correct definition:

________ Eructation
________ Mastication
________ Regurgitation
________ Peristalsis
________ Prehension
________ Coprophagia
________ Emulsification
________ Defecation

a. The act of grasping food with the mouth.
b. The process of breaking down fat globules.
c. The consumption of feces.
d. The process of expelling gases orally—"burping."
e. The movement of *undigested* food back up the esophagus toward the mouth.
f. The act of chewing.
g. The process of expelling feces.
h. A wavelike motion that progressively moves through a tubular organ such as the small intestines.

Exercise 29

Clinical Thinking Challenge

Support each of following correct statements with appropriate rationale, stating why or in what way each statement is correct.

1. Herbivores are heavily dependent on microbial fermentation.
____
____
2. Carnivores have an inconspicuous and small cecum.
____
____
3. There are two types of digestion.
____
____
4. The gastrointestinal tract is regulated by two different control systems.
____
____
5. Lips help animals eat.
____
____
6. The soft palate forms a critical function during eating and swallowing.
____
____
7. Dentin plays a significant role in oral comfort.
____
____

Continued

Exercise 29 —cont'd

Clinical Thinking Challenge

8. Saliva has many functions.

9. The TMJ has three basic movements.

10. Animals with megaesophagus are fed in a position with the head elevated.

11. Once the swallowing reflex begins it cannot be stopped.

12. The glandular portion of the stomach can be divided into three basic regions.

13. Emesis is a protective mechanism.

14. Chemical digestion is divided into two phases.

15. The reticulorumen must maintain the proper bacterial balance.

16. Peyer's patches, found throughout the small intestine, help protect an animal.

17. Enzymes derived from the exocrine pancreas are vital to digestion.

18. All of the proteolytic enzymes are secreted by the pancreas in an inactive form called a proenzyme (or zymogen) and are activated in the lumen of the intestines.

19. Micelles are important to the process of digestion.

20. The horse has the largest and most complicated colon of the domestic species, and this is often referred to as the great colon.

21. Motility patterns in the large intestine in general consist of four different types.

15 The Urinary System[a]

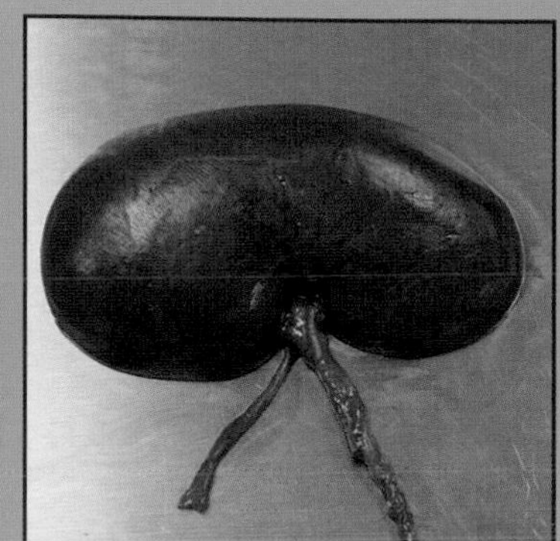

OVERVIEW AT A GLANCE

Blood Flow to and From the Kidneys 400

Nephron Notables 401

Urinary System Location 401

Kidney 402

Ureters 405

Urinary Bladder 406

Urethra 407

The Urinary System on Radiographs 408

Suggested In-Class Activities 409

Exercises 409–420

Blood Flow to and from the Kidneys 409

1. *Locate and Describe the Functions of Elements of the Kidney Blood Supply 409*

Nephron Notables 410

2. *Label the Indicated Structures on the Nephron 410*

Urinary System Location 411–414

3. *Label the Indicated Structures in the Female Canine Urinary System 411*
4. *Label the Indicated Structures on this Ventral View of the Male Feline Urinary System 412*
5. *Label the Indicated Structures in This View of the Canine Urinary System 413*
6. *Label the Indicated Structures of the Feline Urinary System 414*

Kidney—External 414

7. *Label the Indicated Structures on the Sheep Kidney 414*

Kidney—Internal 415

8. *Label the Indicated Structures on the Inside View of the Equine Kidney 415*
9. *Label the Indicated Structures on the Inside of the Sheep Kidney 415*

Clinical and Critical Thinking 416–420

10. *Define Clinical Terms 416*
11. *Define the Following Terms 416*
12. *Identify Renal Components 417*
13. *Anatomic Connections 418*
14. *Matching 419*
15. *Urinalysis 419*
16. *Terms and Conditions 419*
17. *Label the Indicated Structures in This Ventral View of the Canine Urinary System 420*

LEARNING OBJECTIVES

The objectives of this chapter are to describe and identify the location, appearance, and function of the structures of the urinary system. Read Chapter 18 in *Clinical Anatomy and Physiology for Veterinary Technicians,* for detailed descriptions of these structures.

CLINICAL SIGNIFICANCE

In clinical pathology classes, you will learn that signs often show up in both urine and blood when there is a disease in the urinary system. The urine and blood analyses often point to what part of the urinary system is involved. It is important that you understand the anatomy and physiology of the urinary system so you can correctly identify which part(s) of the system is affected by a disease condition and what the overall effects on the body might be.

INTRODUCTION

The urinary system is responsible for removing soluble waste material from the body. It does this by passing the blood through the kidneys, where the waste materials are removed along with any excess water the body needs to eliminate. Most of this work

[a]The authors and publisher wish to acknowledge Joann Colville and Amy Ellwein for previous contributions to this chapter.

INTRODUCTION—cont'd

occurs at the microscopic level in the nephrons. Here the waste materials and water are filtered out of the blood and processed in the tubules to become urine. The urine produced in each of the millions of nephrons is collected and passed from the kidney to the urinary bladder via the ureters. It is stored in the urinary bladder until it is passed from the body via the urethra.

TERMS TO BE IDENTIFIED

Nephron
- Afferent glomerular arterioles
- Bowman's capsule
- Collecting ducts
- Distal convoluted tubule
- Efferent glomerular arterioles
- Glomerulus
- Loop of Henle
- Peritubular capillaries
- Proximal convoluted tubule

Kidney
- Hilus
- Capsule
- Cortex
- Medulla
- Pelvis

Other structures
- Ureters
- Urethra
- Urinary bladder
- Suspensory ligament of the urinary bladder

MEDICAL WORD PARTS

Renal pertains to the kidney
Nephr/o pertains to a nephron or the entire kidney
Ureter/o pertains to the ureters
Cyst/o pertains to any bladder, including the urinary bladder
Urethr/o pertains to the urethra
Ur/o pertains to urine

Blood Flow to and From the Kidneys

Each kidney has a vast blood supply. Up to 25% of the blood pumped by the heart goes to the kidneys. In fact, every 4 or 5 minutes, all the circulating blood in the body passes through the kidneys.

- The renal artery branches directly off the abdominal aorta and brings blood to the kidney (Fig.15.1).
- The renal vein takes purified blood from the kidney and brings it to the caudal vena cava.

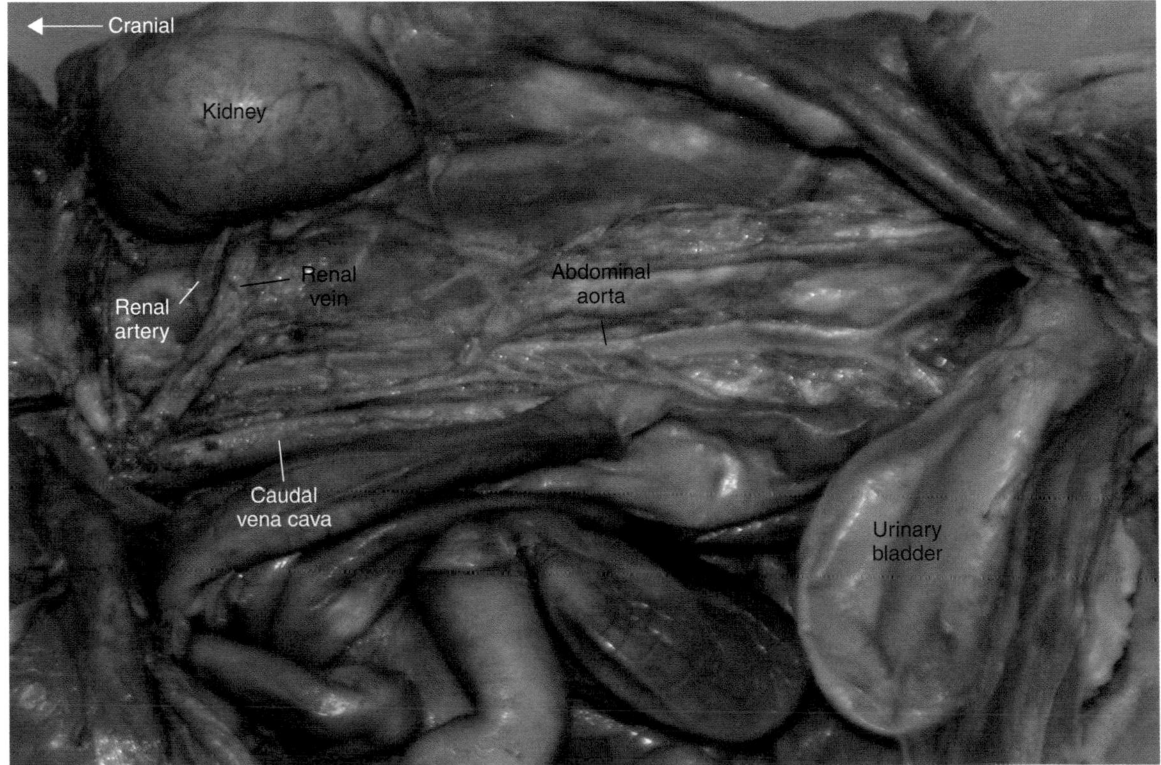

• **Fig. 15.1** Cat abdomen. The blood flow to and from the kidney is substantial.

Nephron Notables

Within the cortex and medulla of the kidney are packed hundreds of thousands of microscopic filtering, reabsorbing, and secreting units called *nephrons.*

- The **nephron** is the basic functional unit of the kidney.
- The afferent arterioles carry blood to the renal corpuscles.
- The **renal corpuscle** is located in the cortex of the kidney. It is made up of the glomerulus and Bowman's capsule.
- The **glomerulus** is a tuft of glomerular capillaries. **Bowman's capsule** is a double-walled capsule that surrounds the glomerulus.
- The space between the visceral and parietal layers is the capsular space.
- The **proximal convoluted tubule (PCT)** is a continuation of the capsular space of Bowman's capsule. It is the longest part of the tubular system of the nephron.
- The **loop of Henle** continues from the PCT, descends into the medulla of the kidney, makes a U-turn, and heads back up into the cortex.
- The **distal convoluted tubule (DCT)** is a continuation of the ascending part of the loop of Henle. The DCT follows a twisting path through the cortex. Even though it is also called a *convoluted tubule,* the DCT is not as twisted as the PCT.
- Parts of the loop of Henle and the collecting duct extend down into the renal medulla.
- The glomerular filtrate is changed to urine in the nephron tubules.
- The **collecting ducts** carry urine to the renal pelvis.

Urinary System Location

- Most of the structures of the urinary system are located within the abdominal cavity of the animal. The kidneys, however, are located outside the parietal layer of the peritoneum that lines the abdominal cavity (Figs. 15.2 and 15.3).
- The kidneys are located on the dorsal wall of the abdominal cavity outside of the parietal peritoneum. This position is called retroperitoneal.

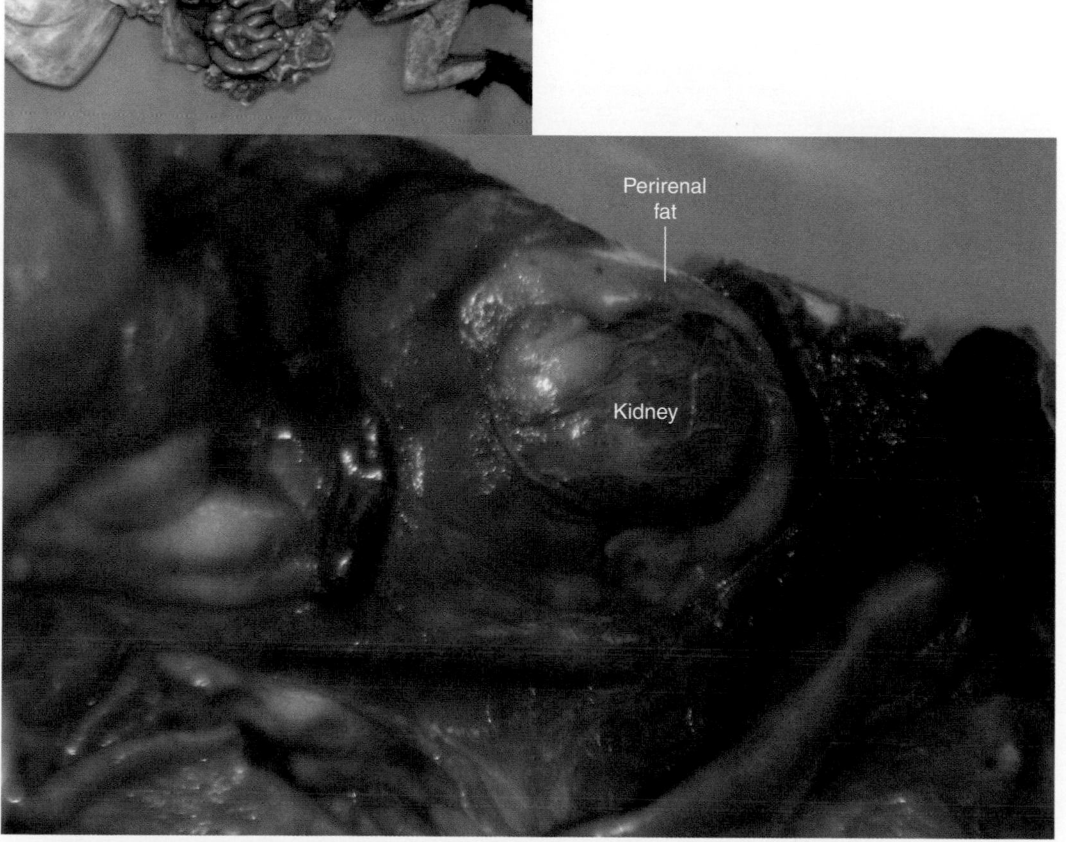

• **Fig. 15.2** Cat kidney. In this photograph, the kidney is covered with peritoneum (the wrinkled-appearing tissue on the kidney) and padded with perirenal fat.

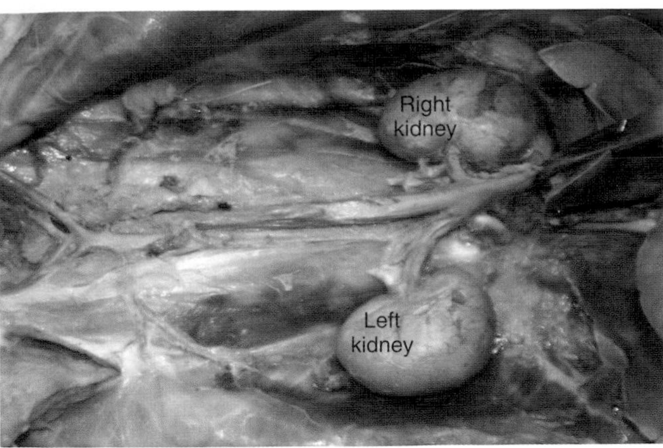

• **Fig. 15.3** Cat abdomen. The digestive system has been removed to allow a better view of the locations of the kidneys.

- The right kidney is located more cranial than the left kidney.
- The right kidney is nestled in a depression in the liver, and the left kidney sits just caudal to the stomach.

Kidney

External Kidney Features

- The kidney is covered with a thick, fibrous **capsule** (Fig.15.4).
- The **hilus** is the indented area of the kidney where the ureter, renal artery, renal vein, and nerves enter and leave the organ (Figs. 15.5–15.7).

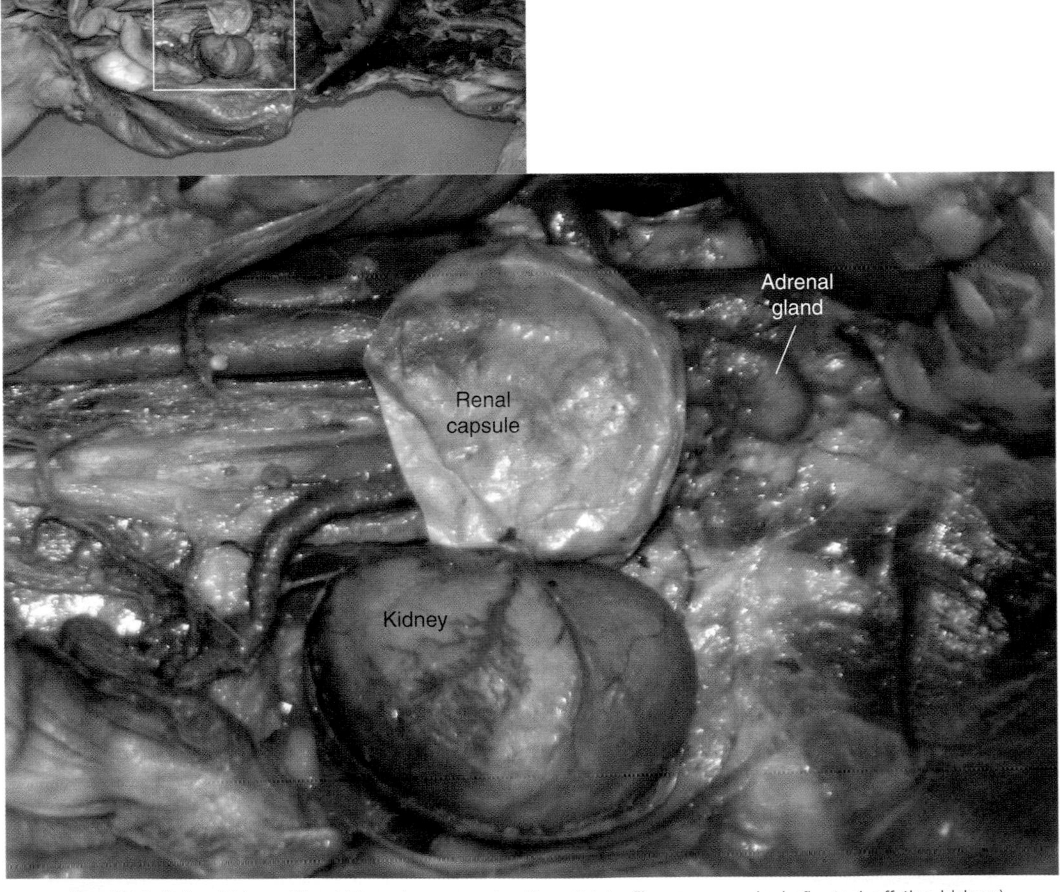

• **Fig. 15.4** Feline kidney. The kidney is covered with a thick, fibrous capsule (reflected off the kidney). The little bean-shaped structure wrapped around the vein, slightly cranial and medial to the kidney, is the adrenal gland.

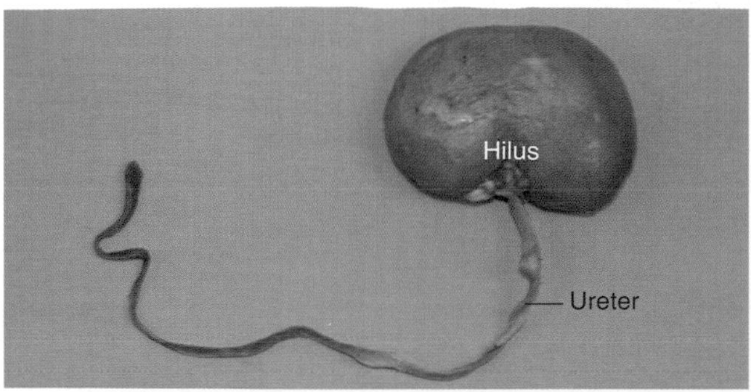

• **Fig. 15.5** Sheep kidney with the ureter. The kidneys of sheep, and those of most other animals, are shaped like a kidney bean.

Internal Kidney Features

- The interior of the kidney is divided into the renal cortex, the renal medulla, and the renal pelvis (Figs. 15.8–15.11).
- The renal **cortex** is the outer layer that is lighter in color and has a rough granular appearance.
- The renal **medulla** is the inner layer that is darker in color and has a smooth, striated appearance.
- The renal **pelvis** is the area where all the collecting ducts converge.
- The renal pelvis narrows at the hilus to become the ureter.

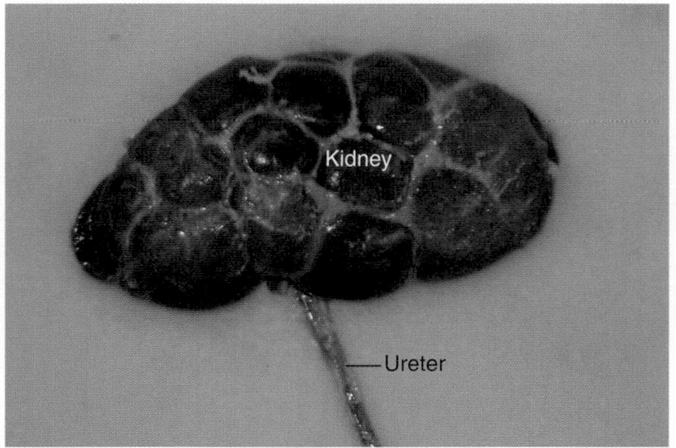

• **Fig. 15.6** Cow kidney with the ureter. The cow kidney is divided into lobes and has a "lumpy" appearance.

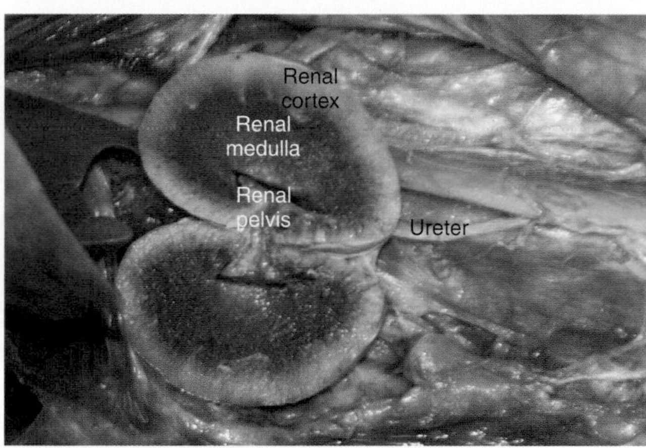

• **Fig. 15.8** Interior of the feline kidney.

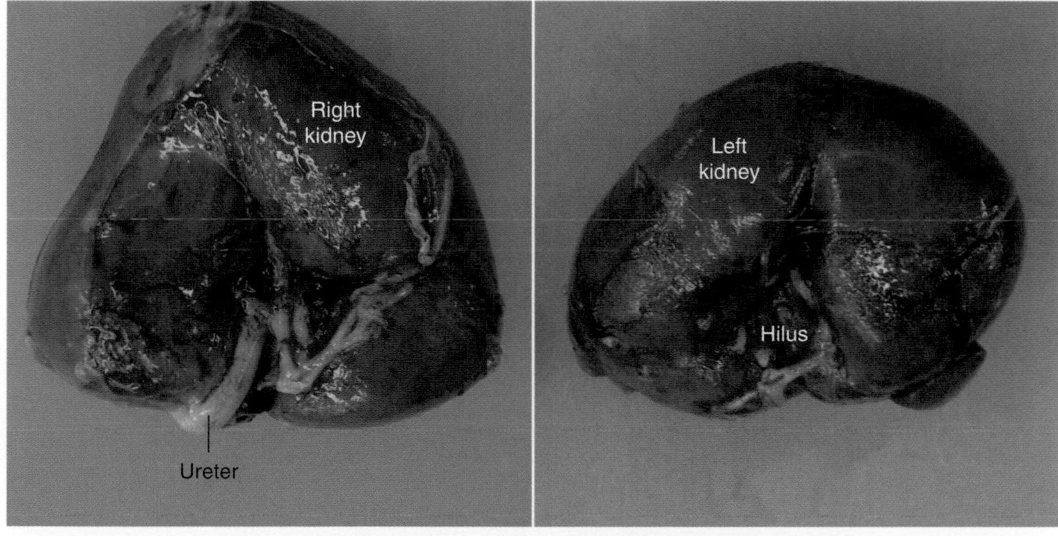

• **Fig. 15.7** Horse kidneys. The right kidney of a horse is heart-shaped, and the left kidney is bean-shaped.

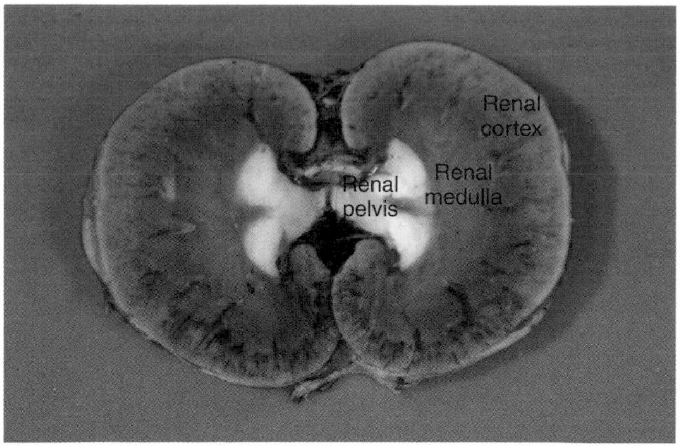

• **Fig. 15.9** Interior of a latex-injected sheep kidney. The arteries are injected with red latex and the veins with blue. Notice how vascular the cortex of the kidney is.

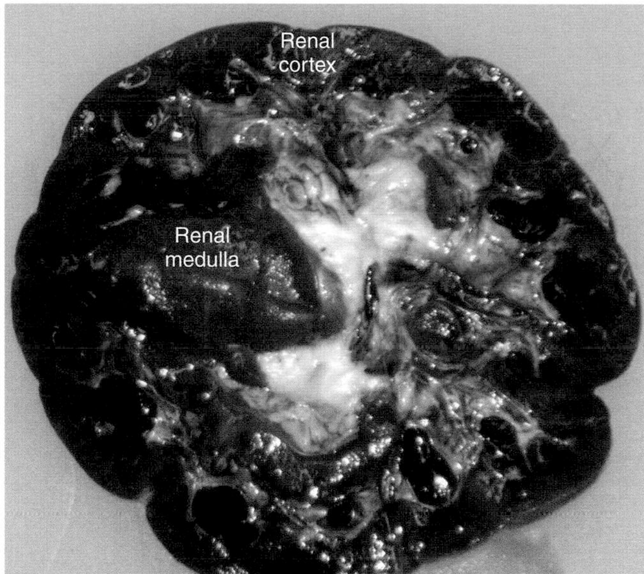

• **Fig. 15.10** Interior of both halves of a cow kidney. Cattle kidneys do not have renal pelvises. The newly formed urine travels directly from the collecting ducts into the ureters.

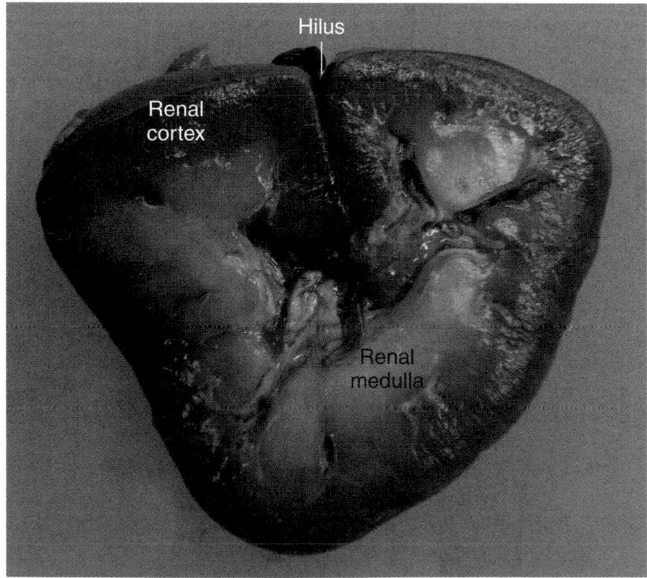

• **Fig. 15.11** Interior of the right kidney of a horse.

Ureters

- A **ureter** is a tube that carries urine from the kidney to the urinary bladder (Figs. 15.12 and 15.13).
- There is one ureter attached to each kidney.
- The ureter leaves the kidney at the hilus, travels caudally, then enters the urinary bladder on its dorsolateral surface, just cranial to the neck.
- The openings from the ureters into the bladder and the opening from the bladder into the urethra, if connected, form an inverted triangle, referred to as the trigone of the bladder.

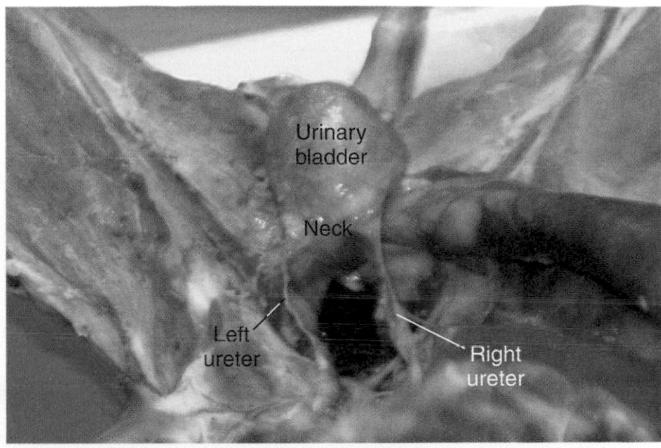

• **Fig. 15.13** Feline ureters and urinary bladder. Note where the ureters enter the urinary bladder.

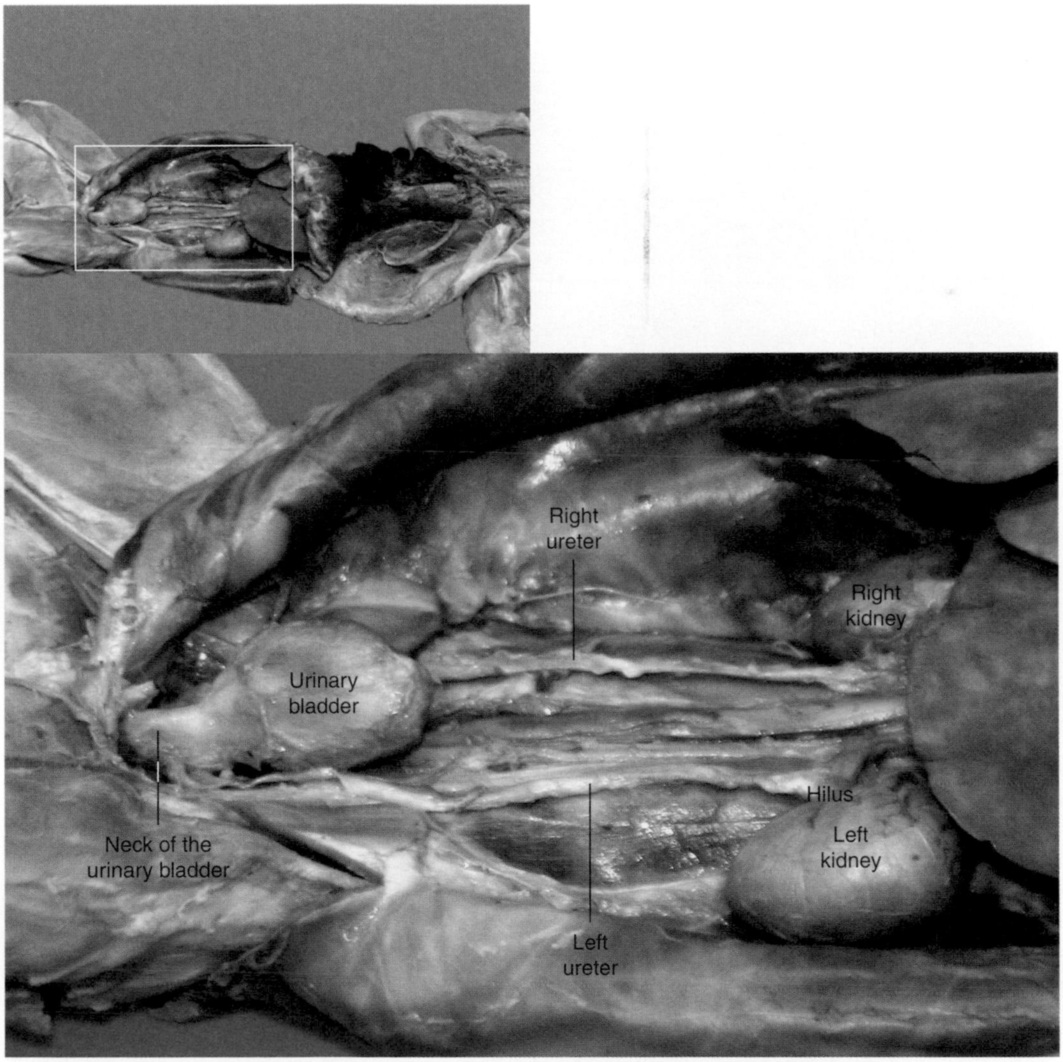

• **Fig. 15.12** Cat abdomen. The digestive tract has been removed to show the urinary structures.

Urinary Bladder

- The **urinary bladder** is a sac that functions as a reservoir for urine (Fig.15.14).
- The urinary bladder is supported by a **suspensory ligament** that attaches to the abdominal wall.
- The urachus is a tube in the fetus that runs from the cranial tip of the urinary bladder to the umbilical cord. It carries fluid from the urinary bladder to the allantoic sac of the placenta. This tube closes up when the animal is born. The remnant of the urachus is located on the cranial surface of the suspensory ligament.

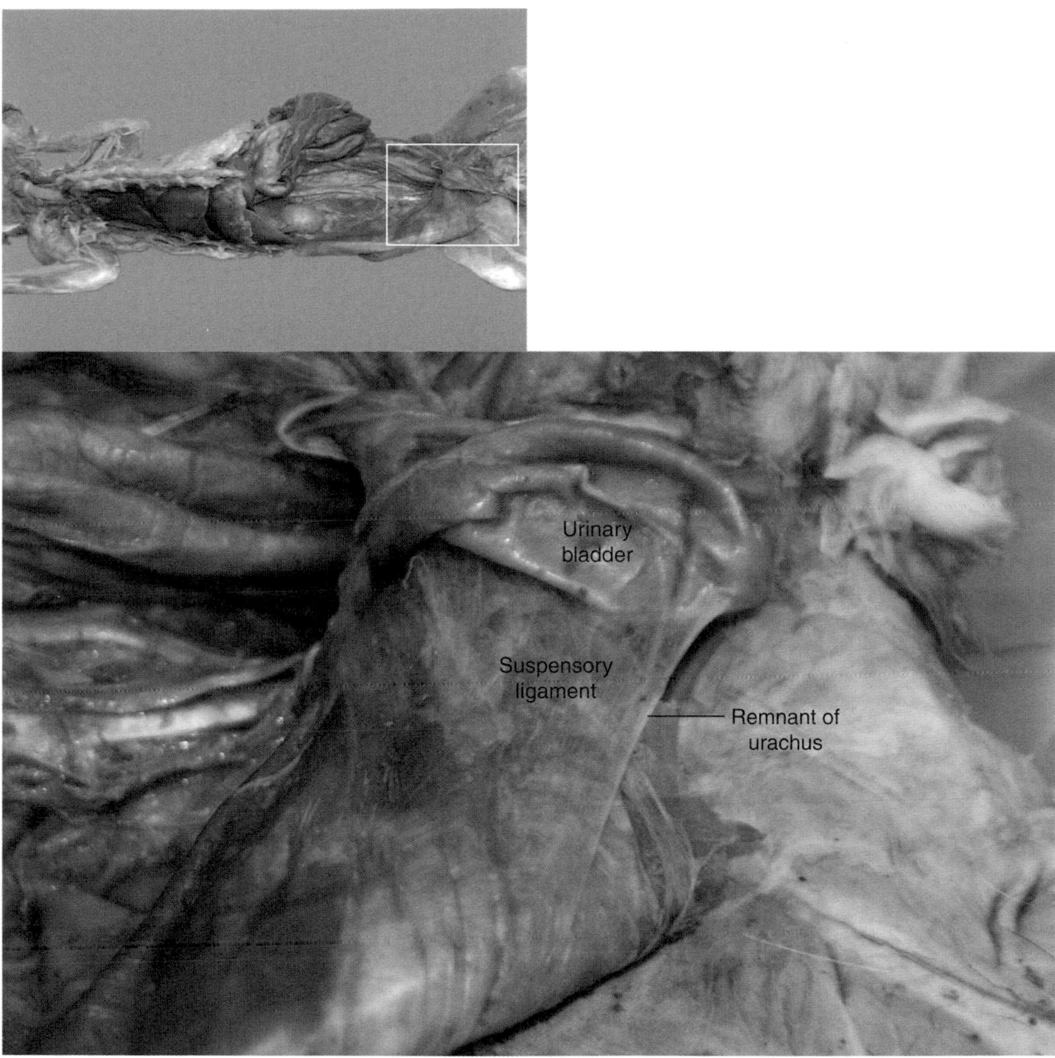

• **Fig. 15.14** Cat urinary bladder (reflected caudally). Notice how far caudal the urinary bladder is positioned in the abdomen.

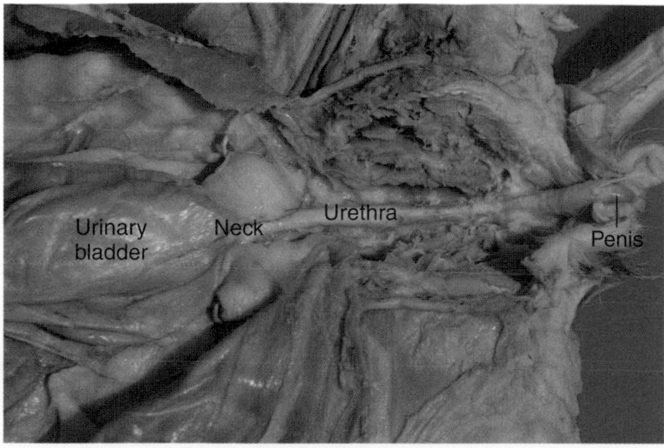

• **Fig. 15.15** Male **feline** urethra.

Urethra

- The **urethra** is a tube that carries urine from the urinary bladder to the outside of the body (Figs. 15.15–15.17).
- The urethra begins caudally to the sphincter muscle that controls the release of urine from the urinary bladder.

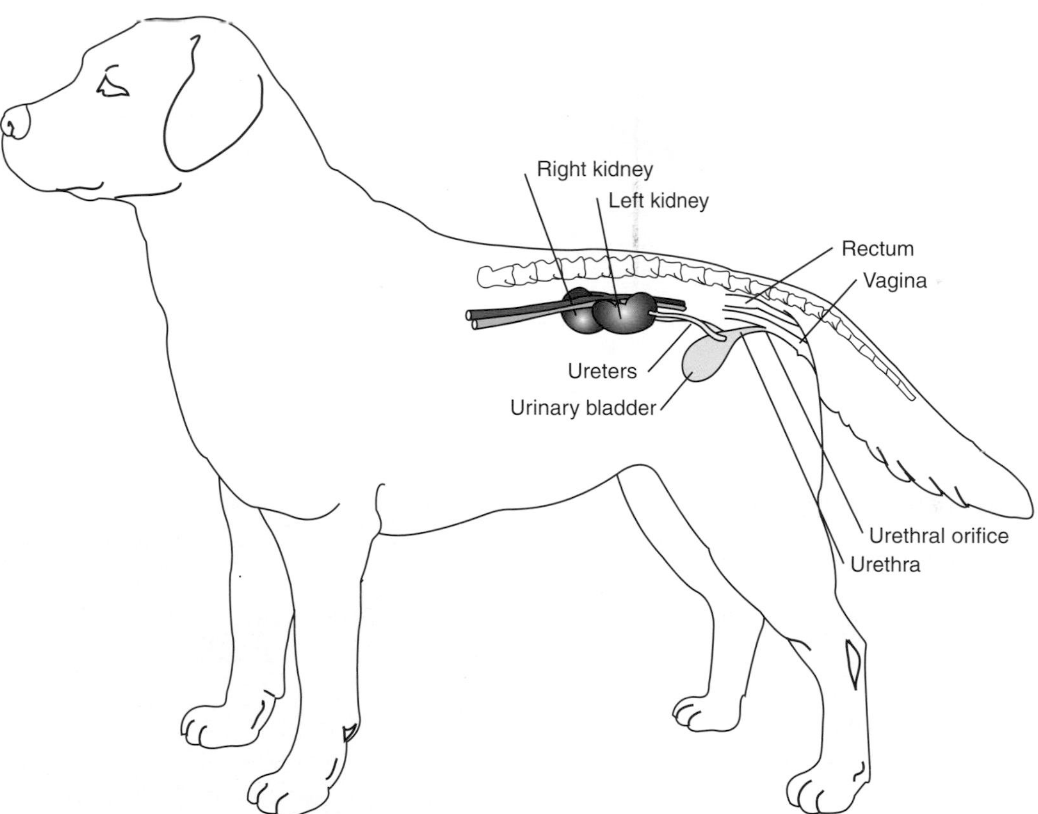

• **Fig. 15.16** In the female (in this case, a dog), the urethra opens onto the floor (ventral surface) of the vulva, not directly to the outside of the animal.

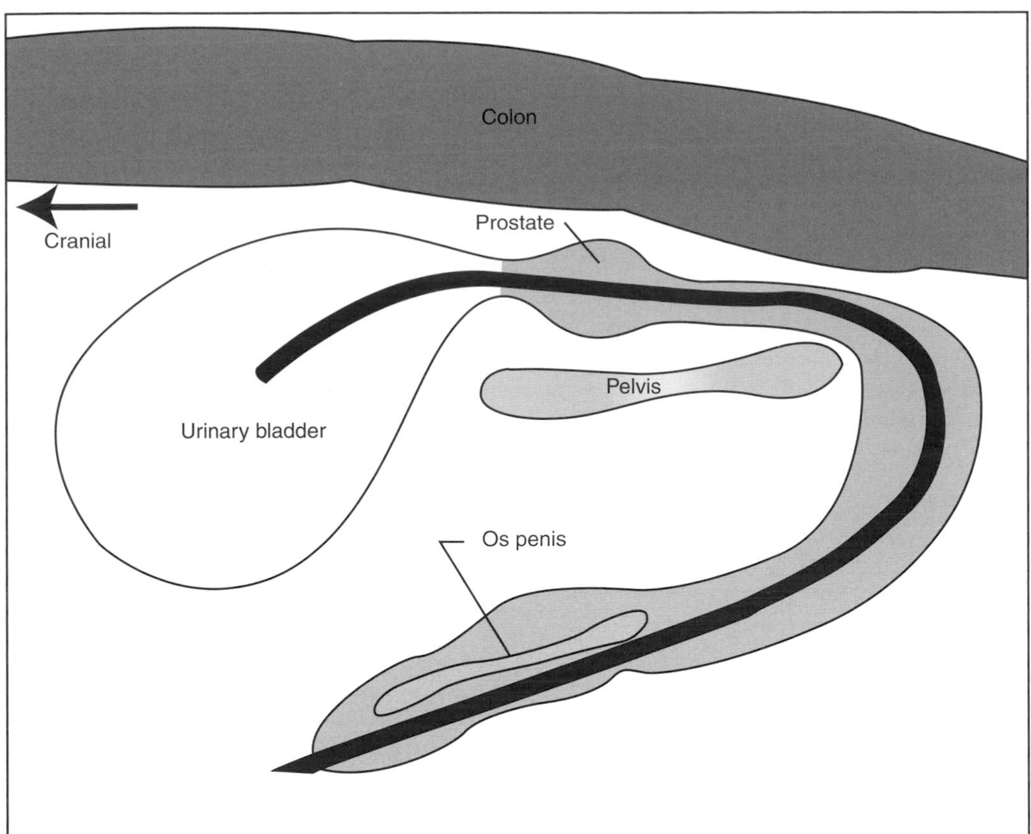

• **Fig. 15.17** In the male (in this case, a dog), the urethra is located in the penis and opens to the outside at the tip of the penis. In many animals, the urethra makes a U-turn after leaving the bladder to follow the penis to the ventral surface of the body. In some animals (cats, for example), the urethra and penis make no curve and open directly under the tail. In this illustration, a urinary catheter is inserted through the urethra into the urinary bladder.

The Urinary System on Radiographs

- A normal dog or cat kidney is about the same length as 2 to 2½ lumbar vertebrae (Fig. 15.18).
- The kidneys are located in the cranial-dorsal part of the abdomen.
- The kidneys stand out from the background because of the fat (perirenal fat) around them.
- The urinary bladder is located in the caudal-ventral part of the abdomen.

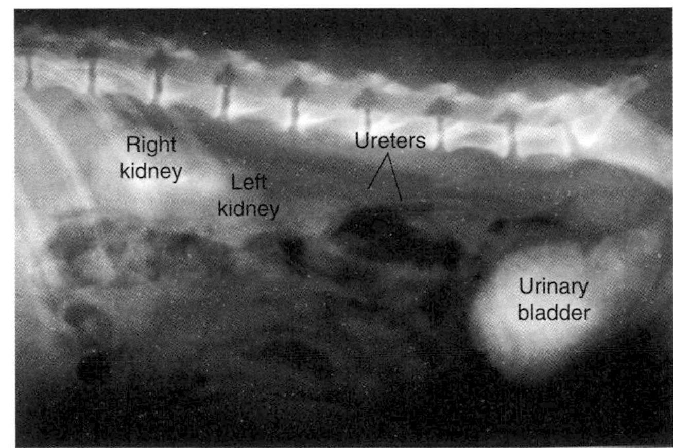

• **Fig. 15.18** Lateral contrast radiograph (excretory urogram) of a canine abdomen. A radiopaque dye was injected into the animal's bloodstream before the radiograph was taken. The kidneys have removed the dye from the blood and concentrated it in the urine, making urinary structures appear white on the radiograph.

Suggested In-Class Activities

Palpate the Urinary Bladder of an Animal

Materials Needed

Live animals and a restrainer (partner)

Palpate (feel) the urinary bladder in a dog or cat first thing in the morning when the bladder is most likely to be full. You should become familiar with the feel of the urinary bladder in a standing animal and in an animal in lateral recumbency.

Clinical Significance

If possible, the urinary bladder should always be palpated as part of a routine physical examination of a dog, cat, or other small animals. To be able to detect abnormalities, we must know how a normal urinary bladder feels. Without that knowledge, things such as a pregnant uterus, an abdominal tumor, or feces in the colon can be confused with the urinary bladder. Caution: a very distended bladder has fragile walls, so if you suspect something is blocking urine release from the bladder, you should palpate the area with extreme care, if at all. Overdistended bladders can be ruptured by vigorous palpation.

Peek Inside the Living Animal

Materials Needed

Radiographs of the abdominal cavity of various animals.

Find as many urinary system structures as you can on radiographs of the abdominal cavity.

Clinical Significance

Kidney and urinary bladder stones may be visible on radiographs. An abnormal size or shape of the kidneys can also be seen on a radiograph. It is important to be familiar with normal radiographic anatomy to be able to distinguish abnormal conditions from artifacts.

EXERCISES

Blood Flow to and from the Kidneys

Exercise 1

Locate and Describe the Functions of Elements of the Kidney Blood Supply

The main blood vessels responsible for the journey through the kidneys each have a unique function. List the function and anatomic positioning for kidney-related structures listed in the table.

Kidney Blood Supply	Location	Function
Renal artery	________________ ________________	________________ ________________
Afferent glomerular arterioles	________________ ________________	________________ ________________
Glomerular capillaries	________________ ________________	________________ ________________
Efferent glomerular arterioles	________________ ________________	________________ ________________
Peritubular capillaries	________________ ________________	________________ ________________
Renal vein	________________ ________________	________________ ________________

Nephron Notables

Exercise 2

Label the Indicated Structures on the Nephron

1. ______________________________
2. ______________________________
3. ______________________________
4. ______________________________
5. ______________________________
6. ______________________________
7. ______________________________
8. ______________________________
9. ______________________________

Urinary System Location

Exercise 3

Label the Indicated Structures in the Female Canine Urinary System

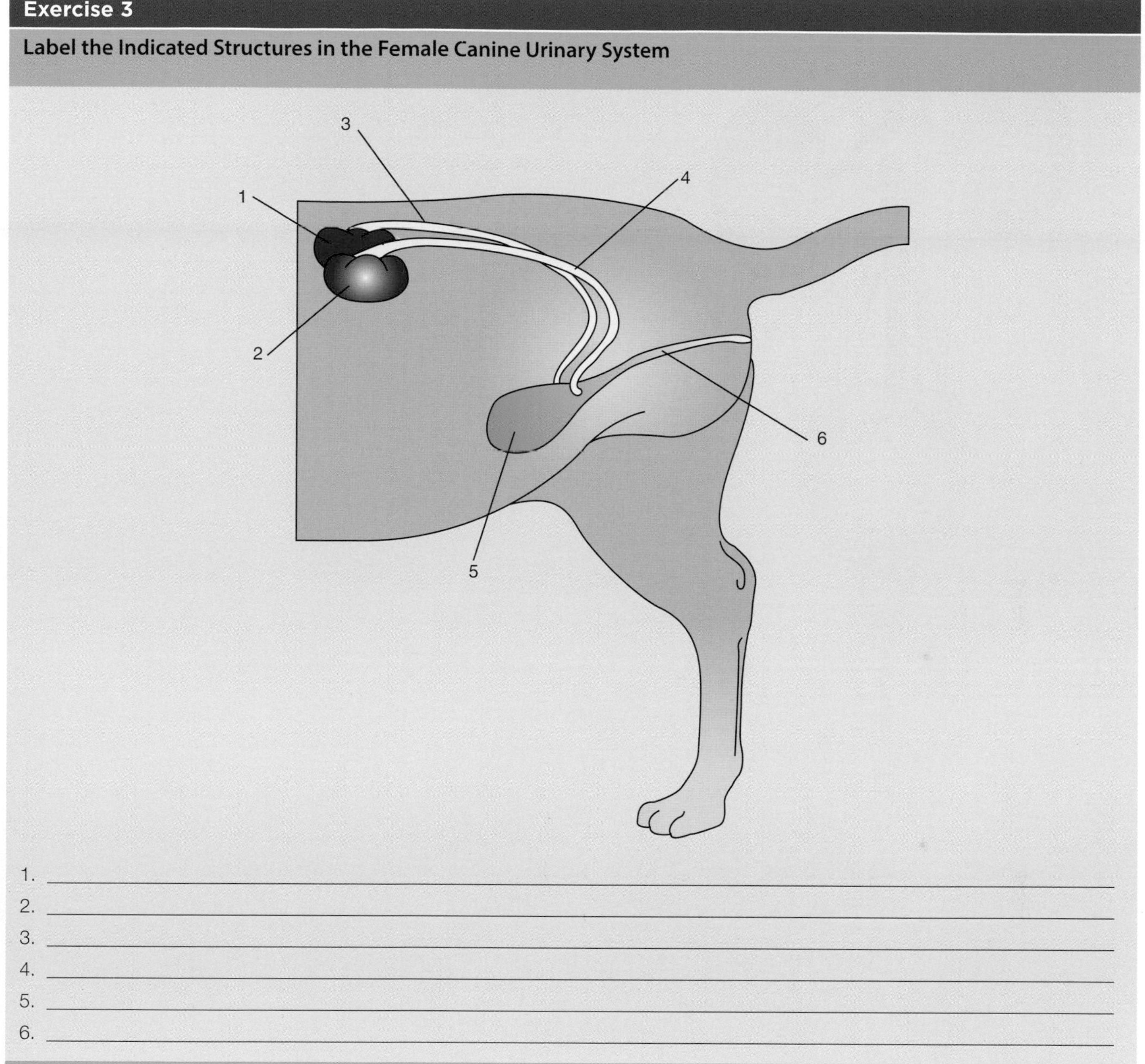

1. ____________________
2. ____________________
3. ____________________
4. ____________________
5. ____________________
6. ____________________

Exercise 4

Label the Indicated Structures on this Ventral View of the Male Feline Urinary System

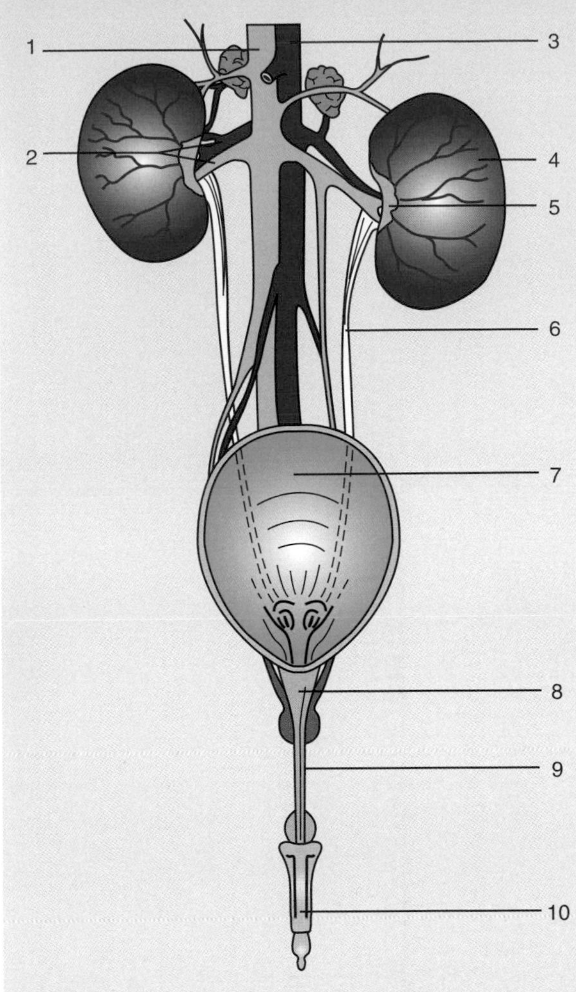

1. ______________________
2. ______________________
3. ______________________
4. ______________________
5. ______________________
6. ______________________
7. ______________________ (a part of the bladder)
8. ______________________
9. ______________________
10. ______________________

Exercise 5

Label the Indicated Structures in This View of the Canine Urinary System

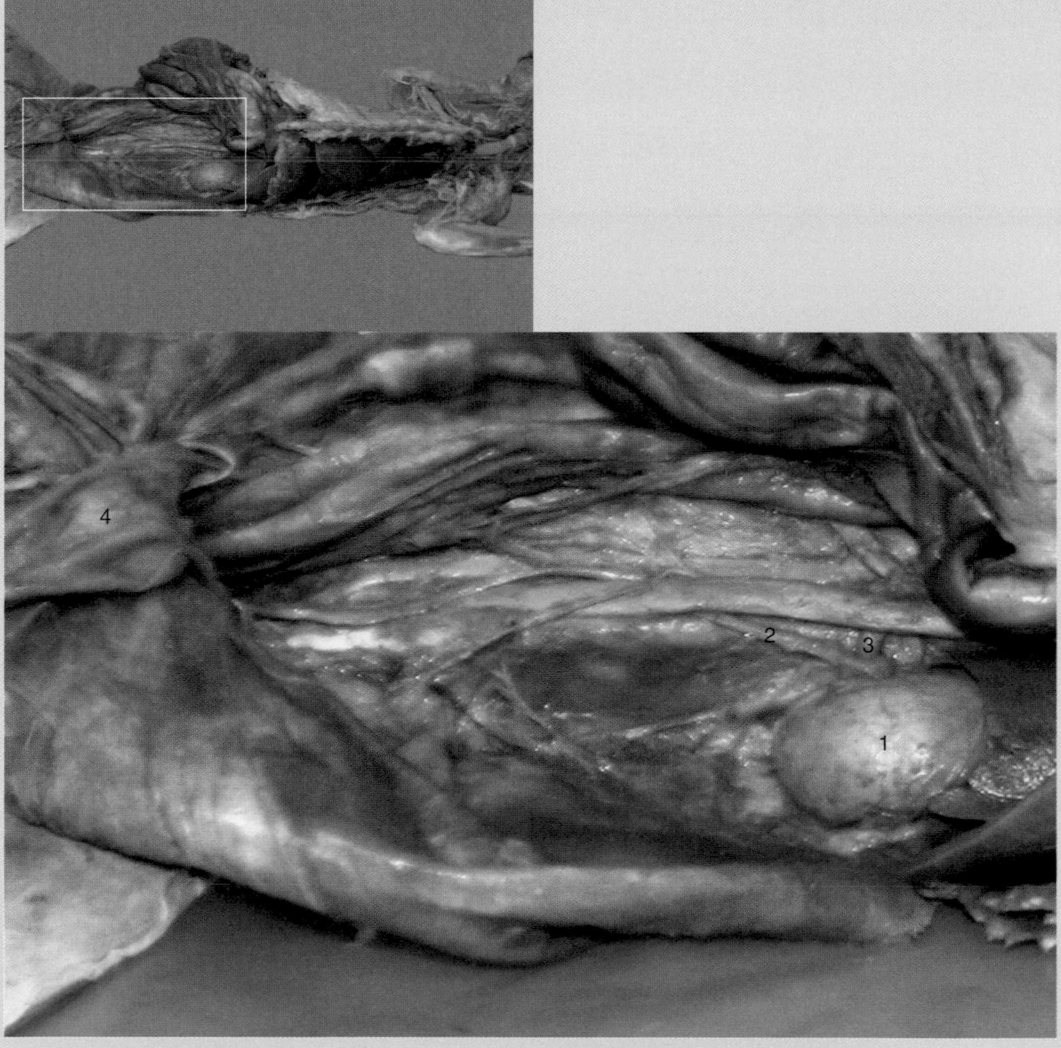

1. ______________________________
2. ______________________________
3. ______________________________
4. ______________________________

Exercise 6

Label the Indicated Structures of the Feline Urinary System

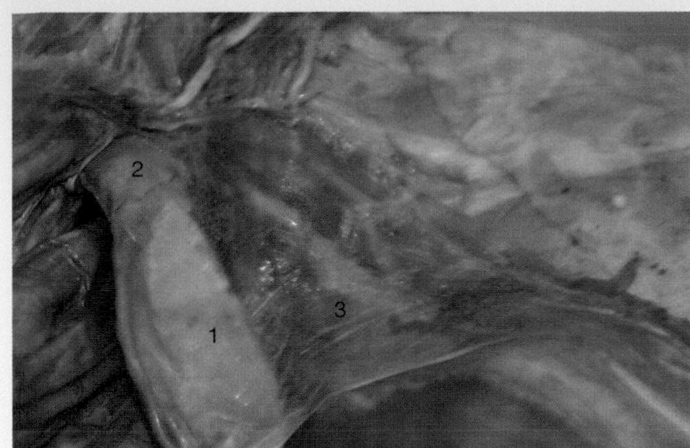

1. ______________________________
2. ______________________________
3. ______________________________

Kidney—External

Exercise 7

Label the Indicated Structures on the Sheep Kidney

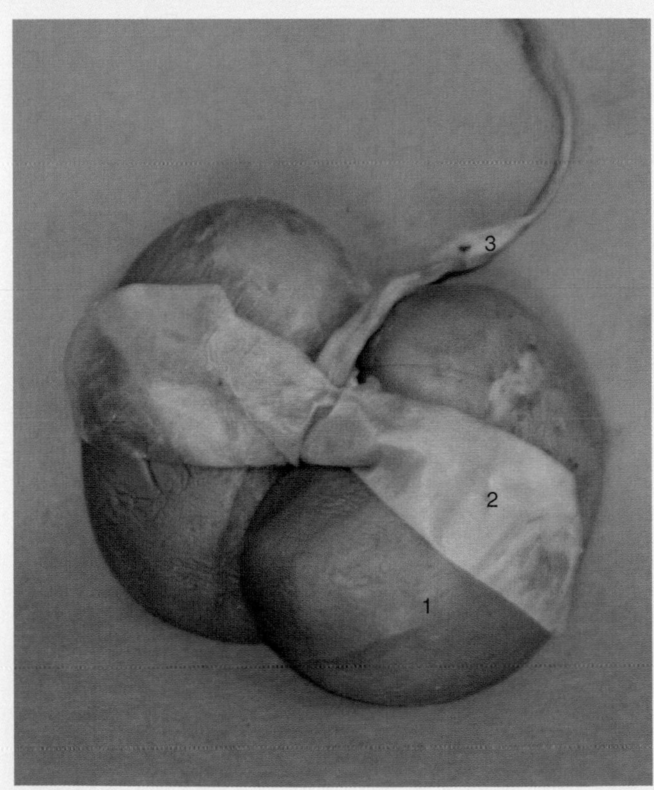

1. ______________________________
2. ______________________________
3. ______________________________

Kidney—Internal

Exercise 8

Label the Indicated Structures on the Inside View of the Equine Kidney

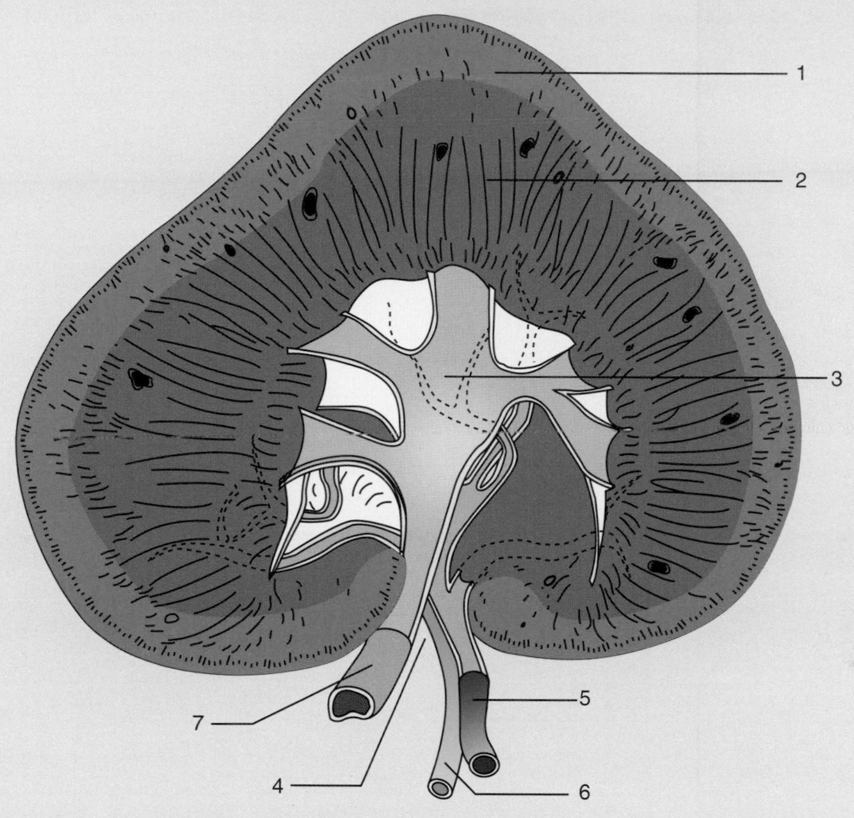

1. ______
2. ______
3. ______
4. ______ (an area)
5. ______
6. ______
7. ______

Exercise 9

Label the Indicated Structures on the Inside of the Sheep Kidney

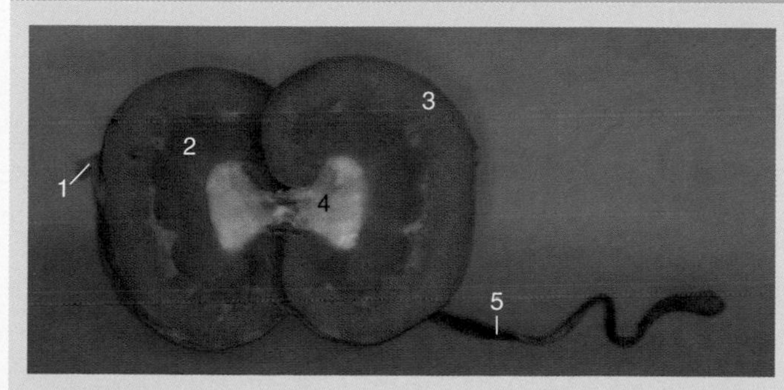

1. ______
2. ______
3. ______
4. ______
5. ______

Clinical and Critical Thinking

Exercise 10

Define Clinical Terms

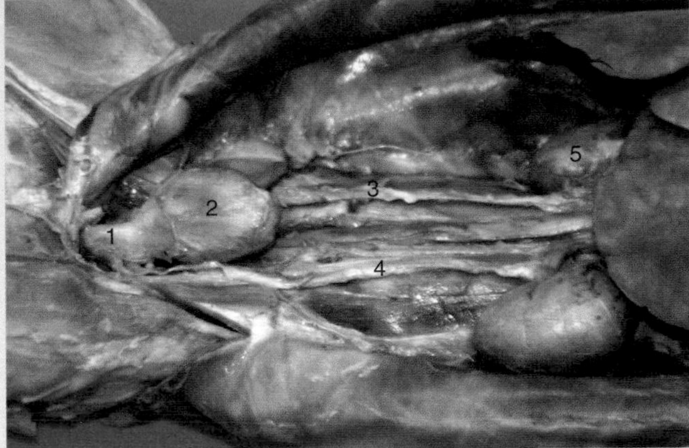

Identify the following anatomic terms in the image:

- Neck of the bladder
- Urinary bladder
- Right ureter
- Left ureter
- Right kidney

1. ______
2. ______
3. ______
4. ______
5. ______

Exercise 11

Define the Following Terms

1. Afferent glomerular arterioles ______
2. Bowman's capsule ______
3. Collecting ducts ______
4. Distal convoluted tubule ______
5. Efferent glomerular arterioles ______
6. Glomerular capillaries ______
7. Glomerulus ______
8. Hilus of the kidney ______
9. Kidney ______
10. Loop of Henle ______
11. Nephron ______
12. Peritubular capillaries ______

Exercise 11—cont'd

Define the Following Terms

13. Proximal convoluted tubule ________________________________
14. Renal artery ________________________________
15. Renal capsule ________________________________
16. Renal corpuscle ________________________________
17. Renal cortex ________________________________
18. Renal medulla ________________________________
19. Renal pelvis ________________________________
20. Renal vein ________________________________
21. Ureters ________________________________
22. Urethra ________________________________
23. Urinary bladder ________________________________

Exercise 12

Identify Renal Components

1. ____________ The tuft of capillaries found in the renal corpuscle.
2. ____________ The tubular structure that leaves the urinary bladder and carries urine out of the body.
3. ____________ The renal _____ is the first part of the nephron.
4. ____________ The process by which substances that the body needs to eliminate in greater amounts than were filtered in the renal corpuscle are moved from the blood in the peritubular capillaries into the tubules of the nephron.
5. ____________ The process by which some substances that were filtered out of the blood in the renal corpuscle, but are still needed in the body, are returned from the tubules of the nephron to the blood in the peritubular capillaries.
6. ____________ The outer portion of the kidney.
7. ____________ The muscular tube that moves urine from the kidney to the urinary bladder.
8. ____________ The _____ is the part of the nephron that dips into the renal medulla.
9. ____________ The inner part of the kidney.
10. ____________ The indented area of the kidney where blood and lymph vessels, nerves, and the ureter enter and leave the organ.

Continued

Exercise 12—cont'd

Identify Renal Components

11. ______________ The arteriole that carries blood into the glomerulus of the renal corpuscle.
12. ______________ The basic functional unit of the kidney.
13. ______________ The _____ vein carries purified blood out of the kidney.
14. ______________ The arteriole that carries blood out of the glomerulus of the renal corpuscle.
15. ______________ The _____ kidney is located more caudally in the abdomen than the other kidney.
16. ______________ The _____ ducts carry urine from nephrons to the renal pelvis.
17. ______________ The _____ convoluted tubule is the last tubular portion of the nephron.
18. ______________ The _____ convoluted tubule is the first part of the tubular nephron.
19. ______________ The _____ artery is the major arterial blood supply to the kidney.

Exercise 13

Anatomic Connections

1. What is the basic functional unit of the kidney? ______________________________
2. Which kidney is usually located more cranially than the other? ______________________________
3. What tubes take the newly formed urine from the kidneys to the urinary bladder? ______________________________
4. Is the glomerulus located in the renal *cortex* or *medulla?* ______________________________
5. Is the distal convoluted tubule located in the renal *cortex* or *medulla?* ______________________________
6. Are the renal corpuscle and the proximal convoluted tubule located in the renal *cortex* or *medulla*? ______________________________
7. Are the loops of Henle located in the renal *cortex* or *medulla?* ______________________________
8. How many ureters are found in a normal urinary system? ______________________________
9. What urinary system structure is located retroperitoneally? ______________________________
10. Are the blood vessels that carry blood into the glomeruli *afferent* or *efferent* arterioles? ______________________________
11. Is the hilus of a kidney in the body located on the *lateral* or *medial* side of the kidney? ______________________________

Exercise 14

Matching

____________ Heart-shaped kidney	a. Cat
____________ Lumpy or lobed kidney	b. Cow
____________ Bean-shaped kidney	c. Horse

Exercise 15

Urinalysis

A urinalysis ("UA") is the laboratory analysis of a urine sample. It can be performed by commercial laboratory or veterinary personnel within a veterinary clinic. Follow these steps to fill in the table.

1. In Column B, list what each type of exam evaluates.
2. In Column C, indicate the method/equipment required.
3. List the norms associated with each analysis.

	Aspect examined	Method	Norms
Gross examination (physical exam)			
Chemical analysis			
Microscopic exam			

Exercise 16

Terms and Conditions

Identify each of the following terms and/or conditions by the description given.

1. ________________ The presence of urinary stones.
2. ________________ The easiest waste material to evaluate.
3. ________________ Urinary aggregates seen in dogs, cattle, sheep, and goats, uncommon in horses.
4. ________________ Associated with an obstruction preventing urine being expelled from the body.
5. ________________ Associated with an inability of the kidney to regulate urine production adequately because of damaged nephrons.
6. ________________ Associated with decreased blood flow to the kidneys, and may be caused by dehydration, congestive heart failure, or shock.

Exercise 17

Label the Indicated Structures in This Ventral View of the Canine Urinary System

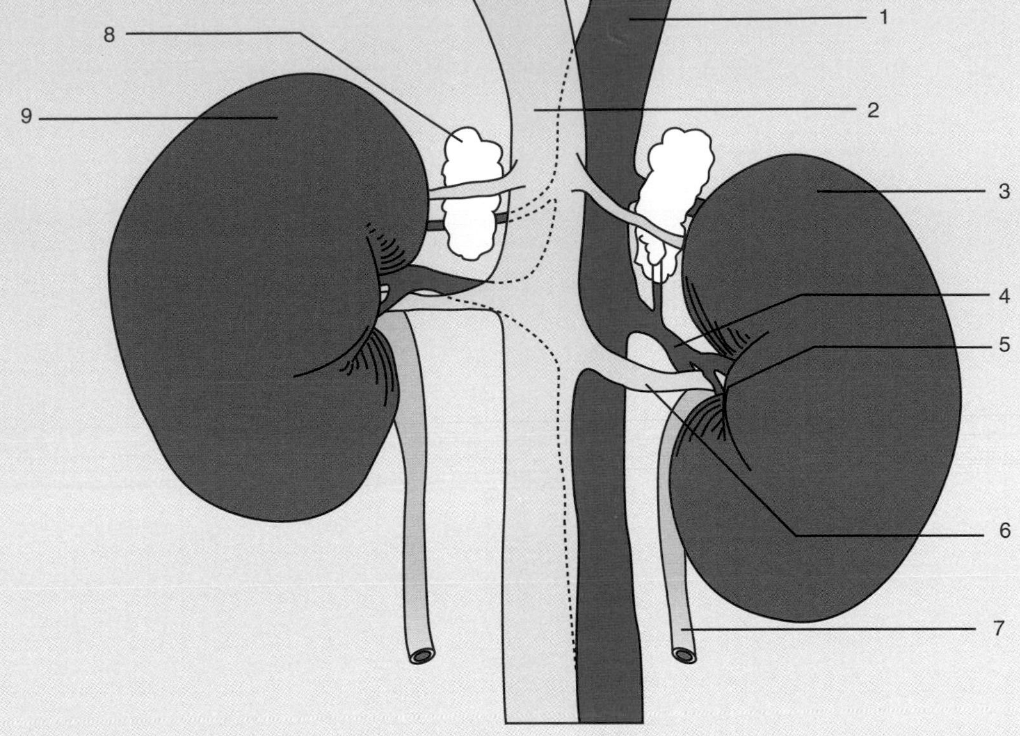

1. ______
2. ______
3. ______
4. ______
5. ______
6. ______
7. ______
8. ______
9. ______

16

The Reproductive System[a]

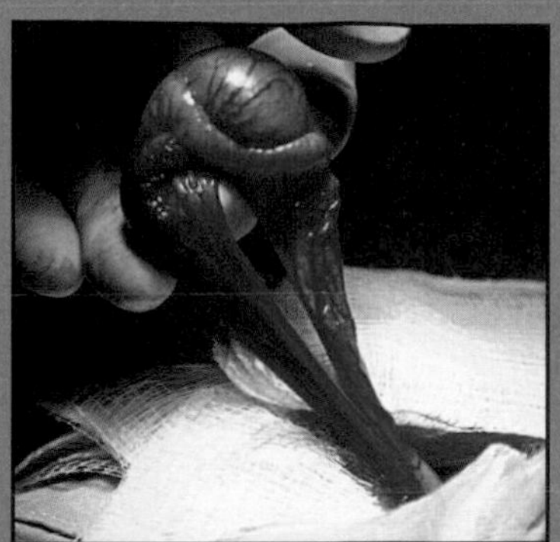

OVERVIEW AT A GLANCE

The Male Reproductive System 422

The Female Reproductive System 431

Exercises 440–448

Male Reproductive System 440–443

1. *Label the Parts of the Male Reproductive Tract (Bull) 440*
2. *Identify the Layers of the Vaginal Tunic of a Testicle 441*
3. *Identify the Structures of the Male Reproductive Tract (Cat) 442*
4. *Identify the Structures of the Male Reproductive Tract (Dog) 443*

Female Reproductive System 444–445

5. *Label the Parts of the Female Reproductive System 444*
6. *Identify the Female Reproductive System Structures (Cat) 445*

Critical and Clinical Thinking 445–448

7. *Identify Clinical Terms 445*
8. *Who Am I? 447*
9. *Clinical Thinking Challenge #1 448*
10. *Clinical Thinking Challenge #2 448*

LEARNING OBJECTIVES

The objectives of this chapter are to describe and/or identify the location and function of the structures of the male and female reproductive systems. For more information, read Chapters 19 and 20 in *Clinical Anatomy and Physiology for Veterinary Technicians*.

CLINICAL SIGNIFICANCE

Veterinary clients generally fall into one of two groups when it comes to reproduction: those who want their animals to reproduce and those who want to prevent them from reproducing. It is important for us to understand the male and female reproductive organs and structures so we can be of help to both groups.

INTRODUCTION

The reproductive system's sole purpose is to produce offspring. It affects other parts of the body, including behavior, but all those influences are focused on promoting breeding and pregnancy. For the reproductive system to carry out its mission, the physical and behavioral characteristics of a female animal and a male animal must be prepared and coordinated. So, the reproductive system really includes the reproductive structures and processes of both male and female animals.

For convenience, we will divide the content into the male and female reproductive systems.

The Male Reproductive System

- Produces male sex hormones (principally testosterone)
- Produces and stores the male reproductive cells (spermatozoa)
- Delivers them to the female reproductive tract at the time of breeding

The Female Reproductive System

- Produces the female sex hormones (principally estrogen)
- Produces the female reproductive cells (ova)
- Receives the spermatozoa-containing semen at the time of breeding
- Produces pregnancy-promoting hormones (principally progesterone)
- Houses and nourishes the developing offspring after fertilization of the ovum has taken place

At the end of the gestation (pregnancy) period, contractions of the uterus and abdominal muscles push the fully developed offspring out into the world. The birth process is called parturition.

[a]The authors and publisher wish to acknowledge Joann Colville and Amy Ellwein for previous contributions to this chapter.

TERMS TO BE IDENTIFIED

Male reproductive structures
- Accessory reproductive glands
- Bulb of the glans (in dogs)
- Bulbourethral glands
- Corpus cavernosum penis
- Corpus cavernosum urethrae
- Cremaster muscle
- Efferent duct
- Epididymis (head, body, tail)
- Interstitial cells
- Os penis
- Parietal vaginal tunic
- Pelvic urethra
- Penile urethra
- Penis (root, body, glans)
- Prepuce
- Prostate
- Retractor penis muscle
- Scrotum
- Seminal vesicles
- Seminiferous tubules
- Sigmoid flexure
- Spermatic cord
- Testes (testicles)
- Testicular capsule (tunica albuginea)
- Vas deferens
- Visceral vaginal tunic

Female reproductive structures
- Body of the uterus
- Broad ligament
- Cervix
- Clitoris
- Fimbriae
- Infundibulum
- Labia
- Ovarian blood vessels
- Ovary
- Oviducts
- Placenta
- Round ligament
- Suspensory ligament of the ovary
- Uterine blood vessels
- Uterine horns
- Uterus
- Vagina
- Vestibule
- Vulva

MATERIALS NEEDED

Preserved specimens: intact male and intact female.

Live animals, male and female.

MEDICAL WORD PARTS

Orchi/orchido/orchio = testis
Sperma-/spermato-/spermo = semen, spermatozoa
Vas-/vaso = duct, blood vessel
Oo = egg, ovary
Oophor/oophoro = ovary
Ovari/ovario/ovi/ovo = ovary
Hyster/hystero = uterus
Mast/masto = breast
Salping/salpingo = oviduct

The Male Reproductive System

The Scrotum

- The **scrotum** is a sac of skin that holds the testes and helps regulate their temperature (Figs. 16.1–16.3).
- The testes must be kept slightly cooler than the core body temperature for spermatozoa production (spermatogenesis) to proceed normally.
- The scrotum regulates the temperature of the testes by pulling them closer to or letting them hang farther away from the body as the environmental temperature varies.
  - The **cremaster muscle** is attached to the tip of the scrotum and, by contracting or relaxing, allows the testes to be brought closer to the body or to hang farther away from the body.
  - When environmental temperatures are cool, the cremaster muscle contracts, pulling the scrotum and testes up closer to the warm body.
  - In warmer temperatures, the cremaster muscle relaxes and the scrotum and testes hang farther away from the warm body.

The Testes

- The **testes** are the male gonads (Fig. 16.4).
- They are housed outside the abdomen in the scrotum.
- The testes develop before birth in the abdominal cavity and descend into the scrotum at, or soon after, birth.
- They produce spermatozoa in the microscopic **seminiferous tubules**.
  - The seminiferous tubules are connected to a complex duct system that will eventually carry the spermatozoa to the **efferent ducts**, epididymis, and vas deferens.
- They produce male hormones or androgens in the microscopic interstitial cells located between the seminiferous tubules.
  - Hormone production is under the influence of luteinizing hormone (LH), which is produced in the anterior pituitary gland.
- The primary androgen produced by the interstitial cells is testosterone.

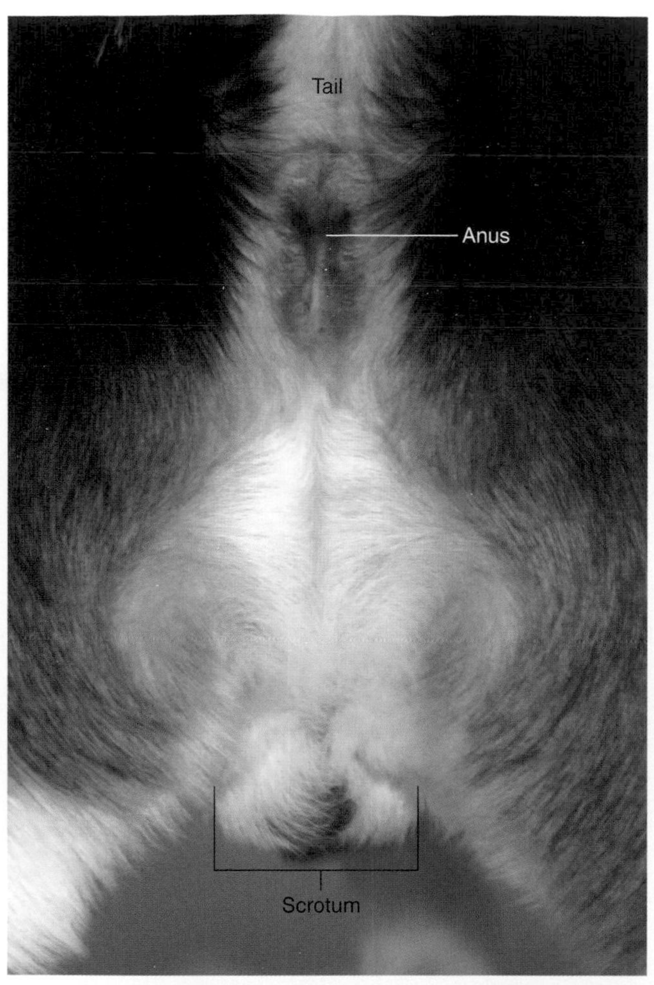

• **Fig. 16.1** Canine scrotum. Caudal view of a male Beagle.

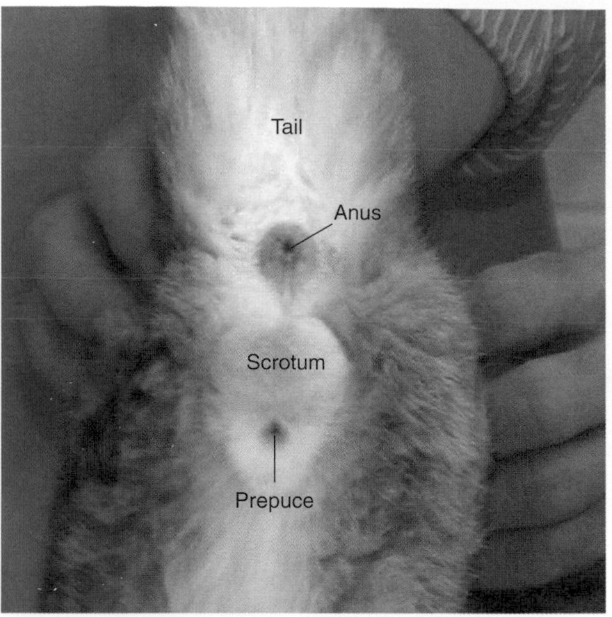

• **Fig. 16.3** Feline scrotum. Caudal view of a male cat.

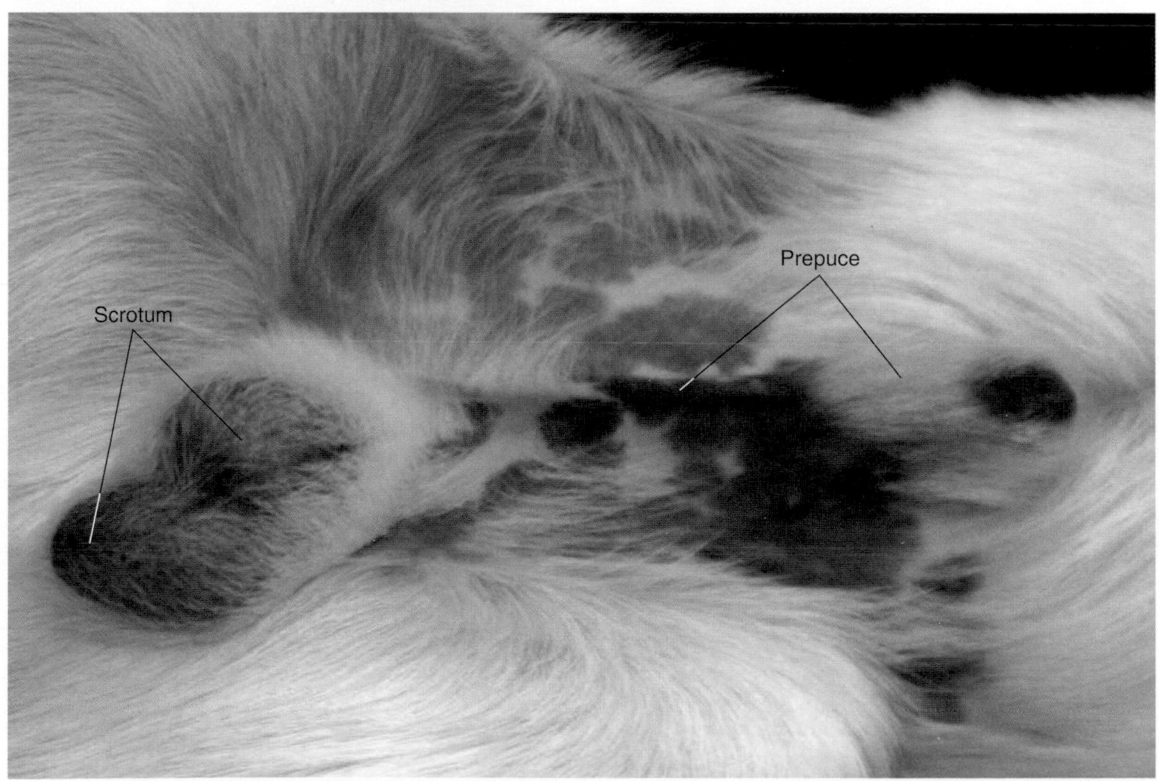

• **Fig. 16.2** Canine scrotum. Ventral view of a male Beagle.

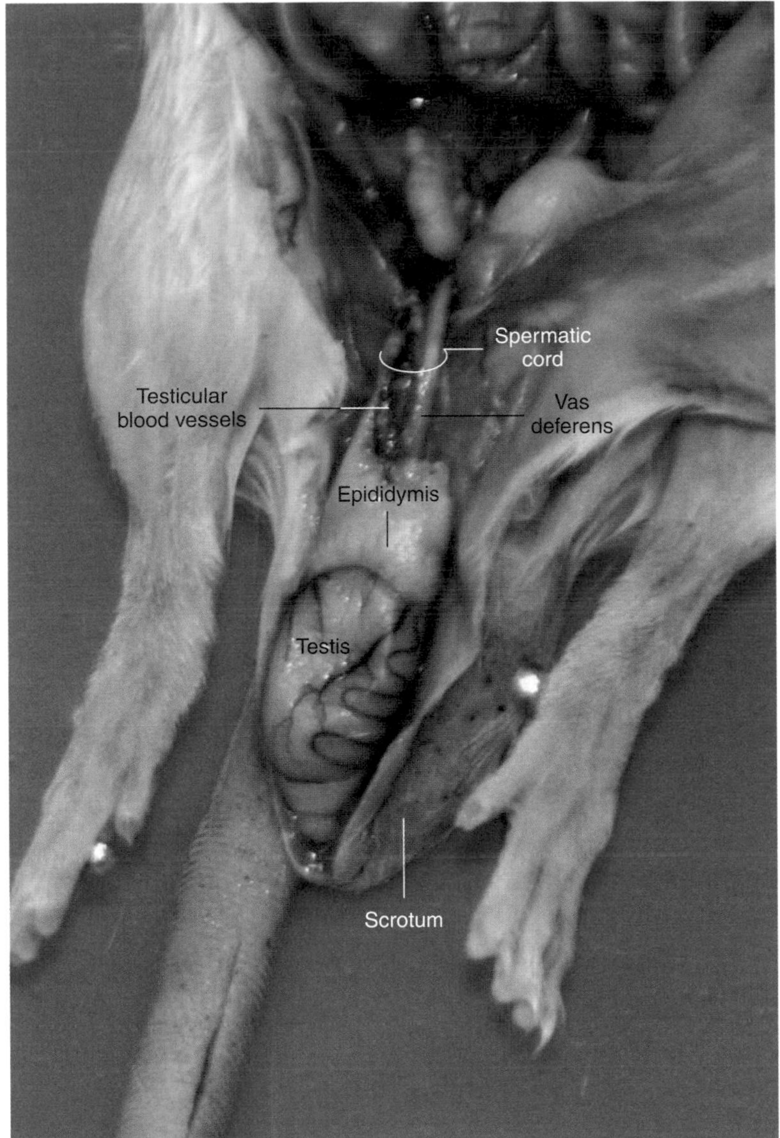

• **Fig. 16.4** Rat scrotum with testis exposed. Ventral view of preserved specimen.

Vaginal Tunics and Testis Capsule

- The tunics are derived from the abdominal peritoneum (Fig. 16.5).
- The **parietal vaginal tunic** forms a grossly visible fibrous sac around each testis and spermatic cord (Fig. 16.6).
- The **visceral vaginal tunic** tightly adheres to the testes—it is not grossly visible.
- The **testis capsule**:
  - Is located beneath the vaginal tunics.
  - Is also known as the tunica albuginea.
  - Is composed of dense fibrous connective tissue.
  - Provides support and protection for the testis.
  - Sends branches (called septa) into the testis that divide it into microscopic lobules, each containing seminiferous tubules and **interstitial cells**.

Epididymis

- A "ribbon-like" structure that lies along the surface of the testis (Fig. 16.7).
- Spermatozoa mature and are stored in the **epididymis** until ejaculation.
- Spermatozoa enter the epididymis from the efferent ducts of the testis and exit into the vas deferens.
- The epididymis has three parts:
  - The head of the epididymis is where spermatozoa enter from the efferent ducts.
  - The body of the epididymis is the main portion of the epididymis that lies along the side of the testis.
  - The tail of the epididymis continues on as the vas deferens.

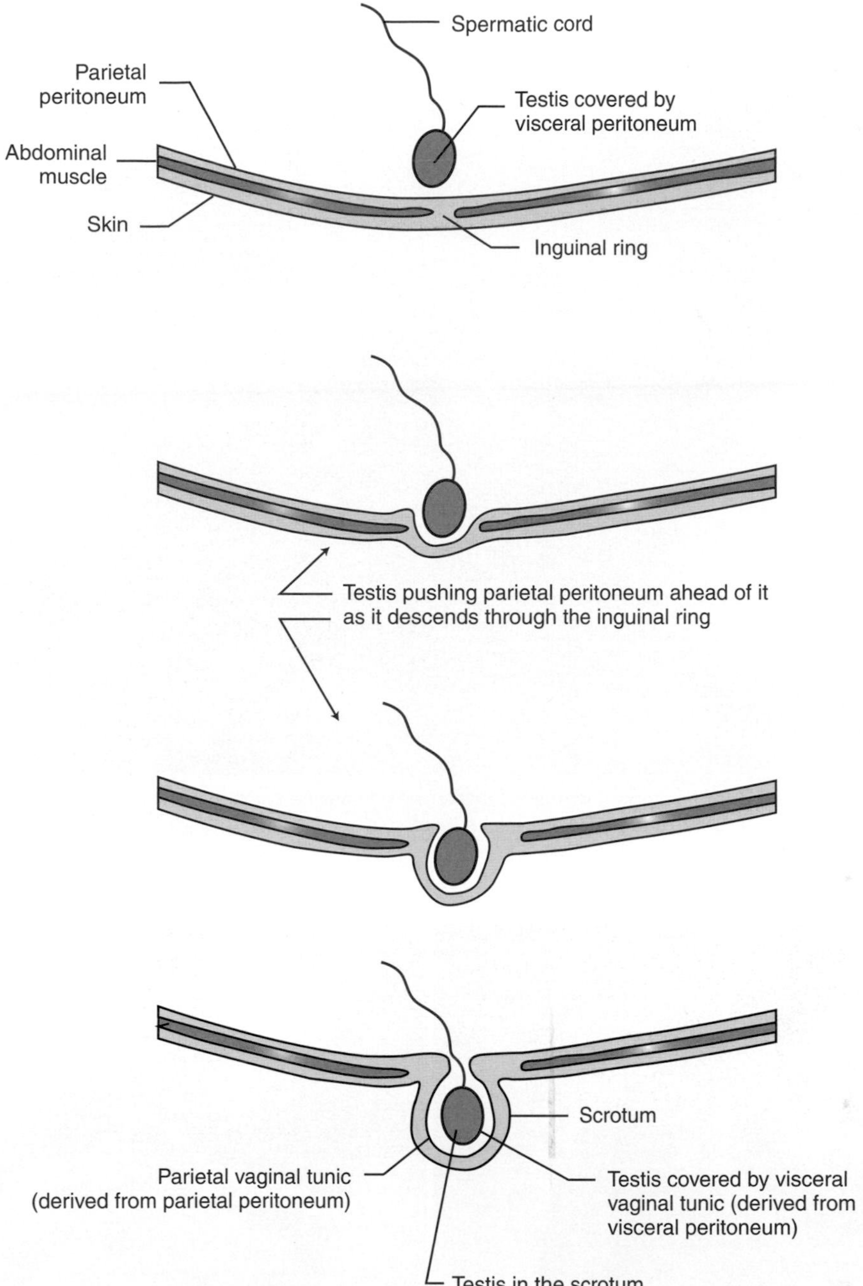

• **Fig. 16.5** Formation of the vaginal tunics.

Vas Deferens

- The **vas deferens** is also known as the ductus deferens.
- It is a thick muscular tube composed mainly of smooth muscle.
- It extends from the tail of the epididymis to the pelvic portion of the urethra.
- It makes up part of the spermatic cord.
- It passes from the scrotum through the inguinal ring to the abdomen.
- In the abdomen, it leaves the rest of the spermatic cord and loops caudally to join the urethra just caudal to the neck of the urinary bladder.
- Its function is to propel the spermatozoa and the fluid they are suspended in into the urethra during ejaculation.

Spermatic Cord

- The **spermatic cord** links the testes with the rest of the body.
- It is made up of tubular layers of connective tissue that enclose blood vessels, nerves, lymph vessels, and the vas deferens (see Fig. 16.7).
- The testicular artery runs down the center of the spermatic cord to carry blood to the testes.

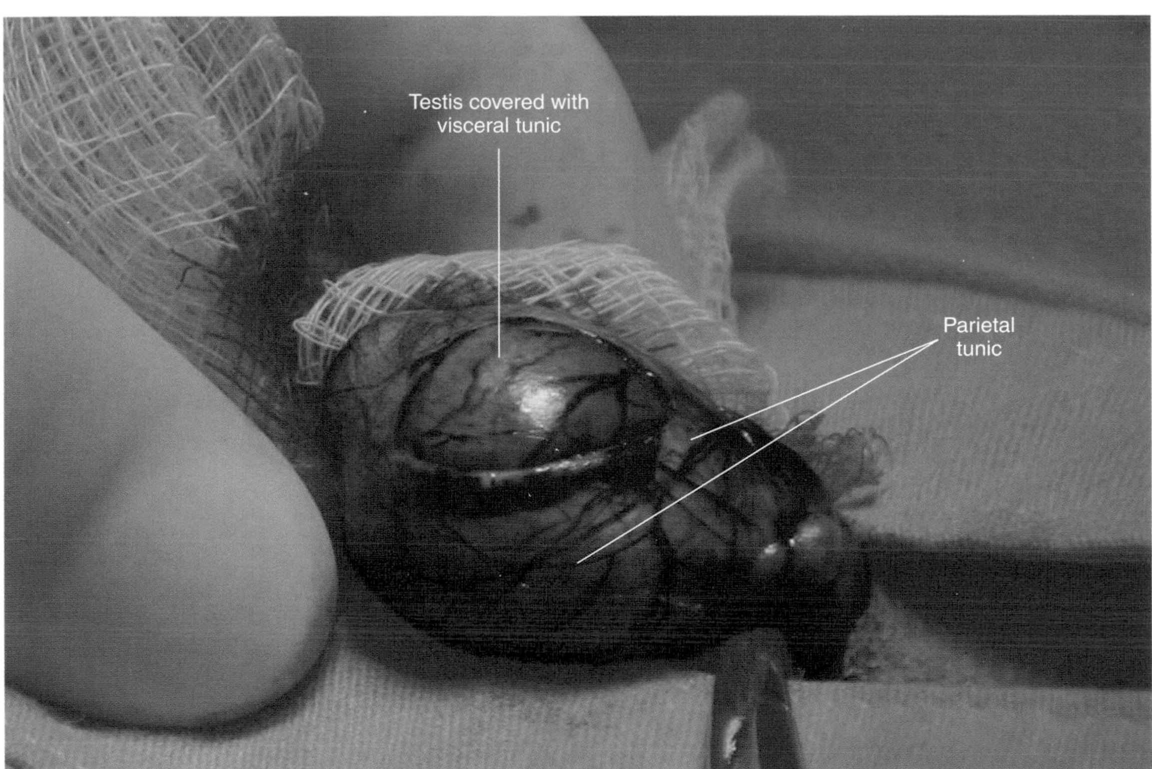

• **Fig. 16.6** Canine testis removed from scrotum. An incision has been made in the parietal vaginal tunic, exposing the visceral vaginal tunic-covered testis beneath it.

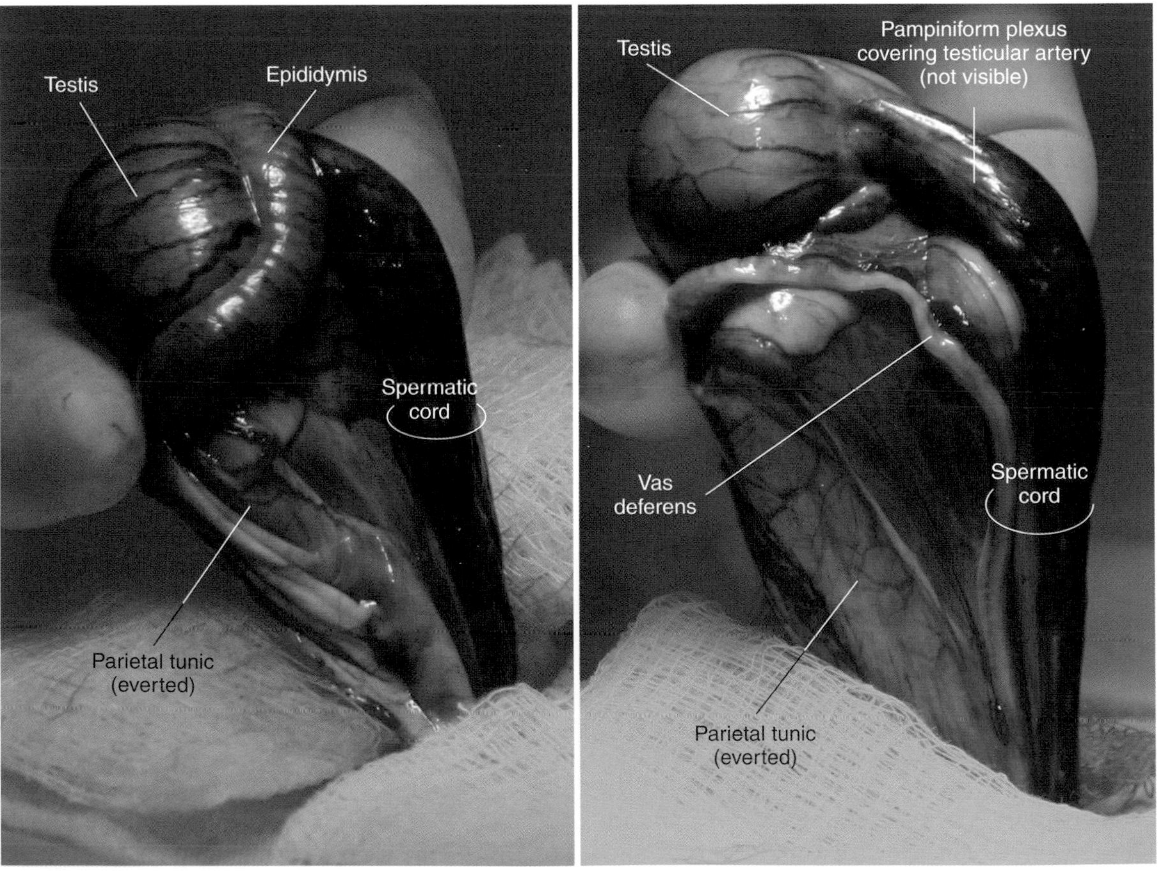

• **Fig. 16.7** Canine testis, epididymis, vas deferens, and spermatic cord removed from scrotum.

- The testicular artery is surrounded by a dense network of tiny veins called the pampiniform plexus that forms from the testicular vein (see Fig. 16.7).
- The combination of the testicular artery and the pampiniform plexus acts as a heat-exchange system to help maintain the temperature of the testes slightly cooler than body temperature.
  - The blood in the testicular artery starts out at body temperature as it enters the spermatic cord.
  - The blood returning from the testis in the pampiniform plexus is cooler than body temperature.
  - The blood in the testicular artery is cooled by the blood in the pampiniform plexus as it passes down the spermatic cord.
  - The blood in the pampiniform plexus is warmed by the blood in the testicular artery as it passes up in the spermatic cord.
  - This heat exchange keeps the testes cooler than the body and rewarms the blood from the testes before it enters the body again.

The Urethra

The urethra carries urine from the urinary bladder outside the body, but it also has reproductive roles (Fig. 16.8).

- The **pelvic urethra** is the part of the urethra that lies within the pelvic cavity.
- The **penile urethra** runs the length of the penis.
- The vas deferens and the accessory reproductive glands enter the pelvic urethra.
- At ejaculation, spermatozoa and fluids from the accessory reproductive glands are mixed in the urethra to form semen.
- Urine flow is blocked when ejaculation occurs, and semen is pumped out by rhythmic contractions of muscles around the urethra.

The Accessory Reproductive Glands

- The **accessory reproductive glands provide** most of the total liquid volume of semen.
- They include the **prostate gland**, **seminal vesicles**, and **bulbourethral glands**.
- Their secretions enter the pelvic portion of the urethra.
- Which accessory reproductive glands are present depends on the species of animal (Table 16.1).
- The single prostate gland surrounds the urethra and has multiple ducts that enter the urethra.
  - This is the only accessory reproductive gland present in dogs.
- The paired seminal vesicles are also known as the vesicular glands.
  - They are not found in dogs and cats.
- The paired bulbourethral glands are also known as Cowper's glands.
  - They are not found in dogs.

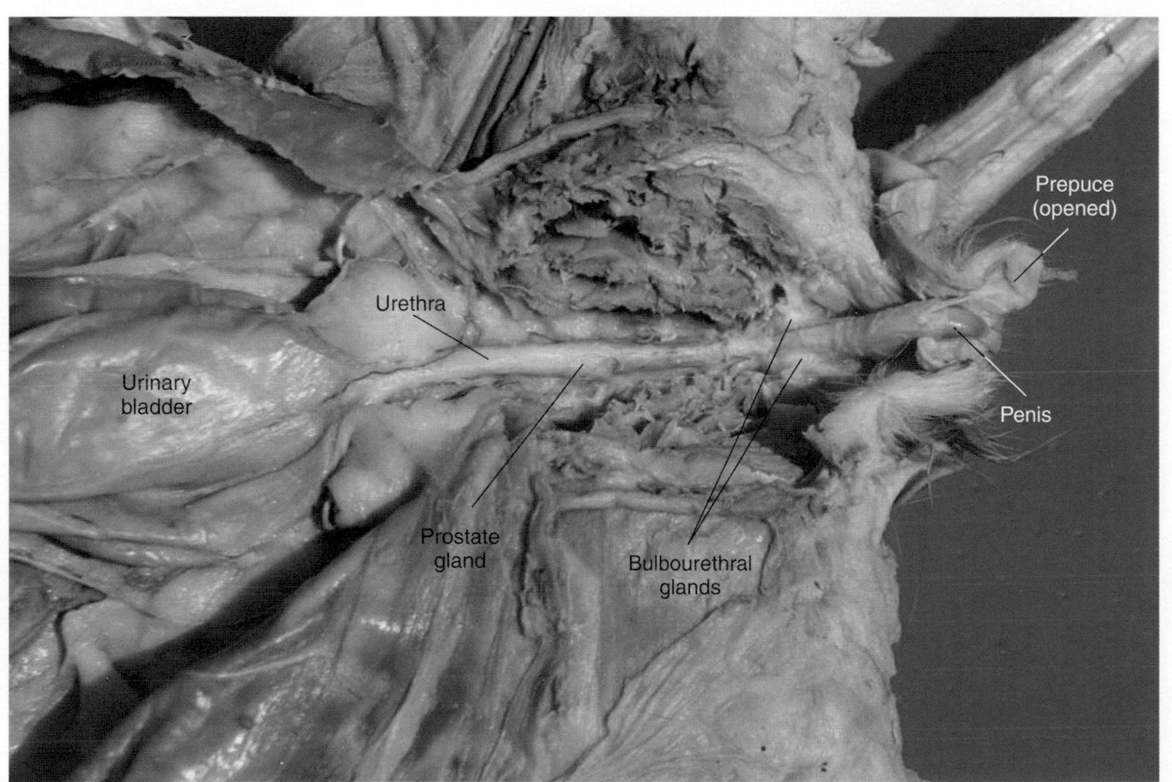

• **Fig. 16.8** Feline urethra, prostate, bulbourethral glands, and penis. Ventral view of preserved specimen.

- They are the most caudal of the reproductive accessory glands, located near the caudal brim of the pelvis.
- They produce a mucus-containing fluid that clears and lubricates the urethra before ejaculation.

The Penis

- The **penis** is the male breeding organ (Fig. 16.9).
- It is composed of muscle, erectile tissue, and connective tissue.
- It has a large blood supply and many sensory nerve endings.

TABLE 16.1 Male Accessory Reproductive Glands

Animal	Prostate Gland	Seminal Vesicles	Bulbourethral Glands
Boar	+	+	+
Bull	+	+	+
Cat	+	–	+
Dog	+	–	–
Human	+	+	+
Ram	+	+	+
Stallion	+	+	+

+, Indicates the presence of a gland; -, indicates the gland is absent.

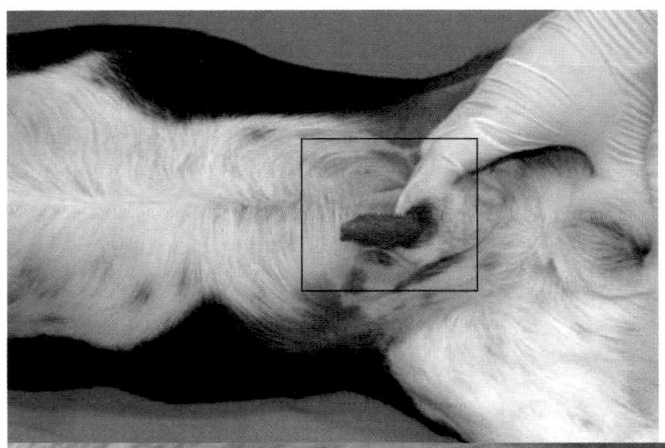

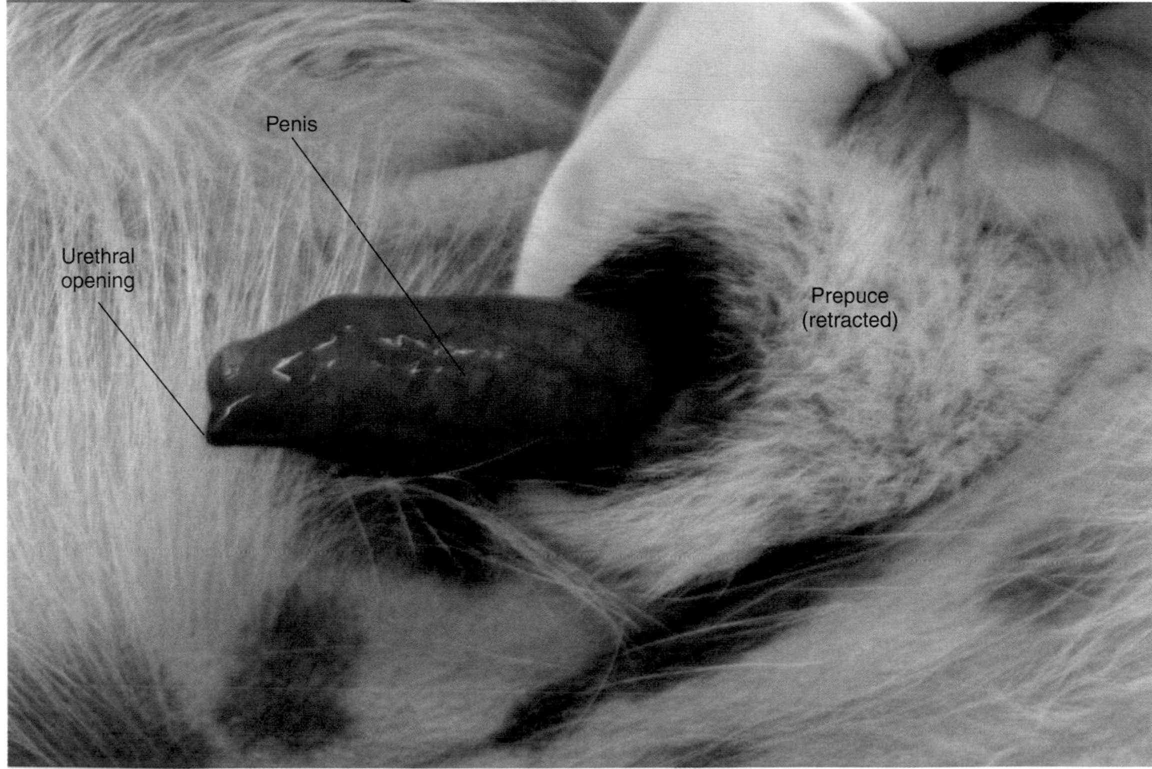

• **Fig. 16.9** Canine penis.

- When stimulated, the erectile tissue becomes engorged with blood, which causes the penis to enlarge and stiffen.
- The penis is composed of three parts.
  - The **roots** attach the penis to the brim of the pelvis with two connective tissue bands covered with muscle.
  - The **body** is the largest part of the penis and contains the erectile tissue.
  - Erectile tissue is a spongy network of tiny blood-filled sinuses that are surrounded by fibrous connective tissue.
  - There are two main erectile tissue structures in the penis.
  - The corpus cavernosum urethrae, also known as the corpus spongiosum, is erectile tissue that forms a sleeve around the urethra as it passes through the body of the penis.
  - The corpus cavernosum penis is a larger mass of erectile tissue that lies mainly dorsal to the urethra.
  - In the nonerect state, blood flow into and out of the erectile tissue is equal.
  - When an erection occurs, the flow of blood into the erectile tissue exceeds the flow out. The blood-filled sinuses swell, enlarging and stiffening the penis.
  - The erectile tissue sinuses are prevented from overfilling by the nonelastic fibrous connective tissue surrounding them.
- The **glans** of the penis is the most distal part of the penis.
  - The glans makes up the free tip of the penis.
  - Its size, extent, and shape vary among species.
  - It contains many sensory nerve endings.

The Prepuce

- The **prepuce** is the sheath of skin that encloses the penis when it is not erect.
- It is composed of skin on the outside and mucous membrane on the inside, where it comes into contact with the penis.

The Os Penis

- This bone (part of the visceral skeleton) is found in the canine penis (Fig. 16.10).
- It is located dorsal and lateral to the penile urethra.
- It usually has little clinical significance unless it is fractured or urinary stones get lodged in the urethra below and proximal to it.

The Bulb of the Glans

- This is also called the bulbus glandis (Figs. 16.11 and 16.12).
- It is found in dogs.
- It is erectile tissue derived from the corpus cavernosum urethrae that enlarges during breeding after ejaculation has occurred.
- After ejaculation, swelling of the **bulb of the glans** and contractions of muscles around the vagina of the female cause the male and female to "tie" together for 15 to 20 minutes. The male dismounts and turns, so the animals are "butt-to-butt." Injury can occur if the animals are forcibly separated prematurely.

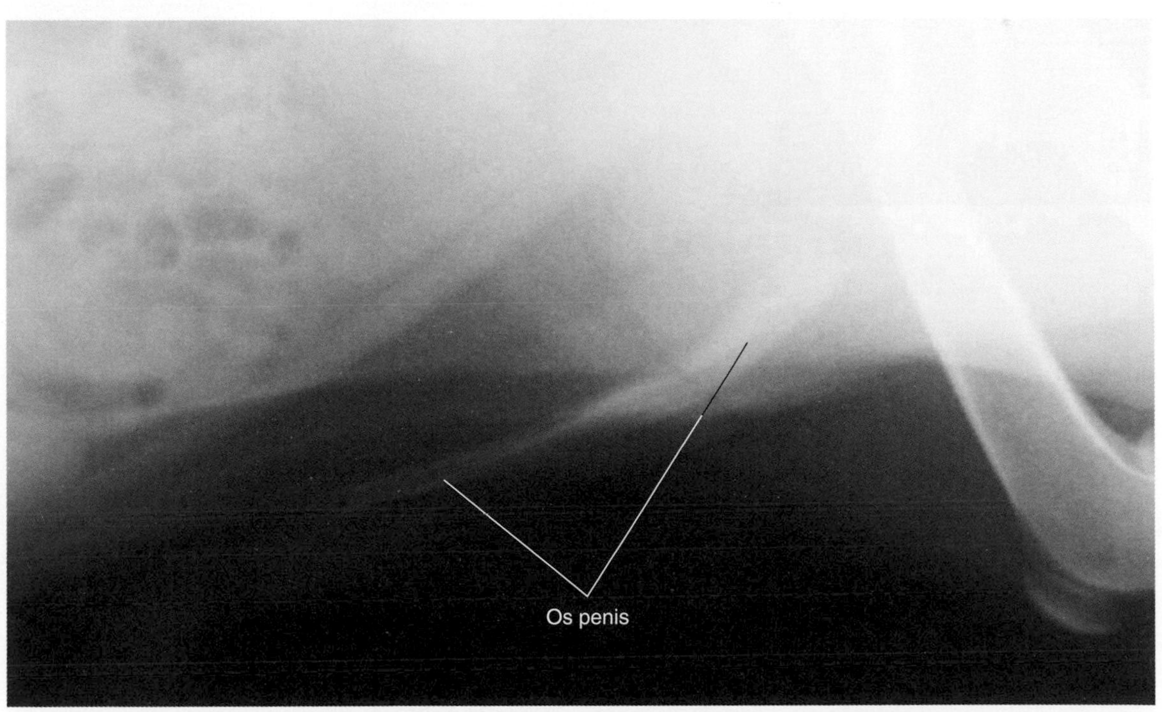

• **Fig. 16.10** Canine os penis.

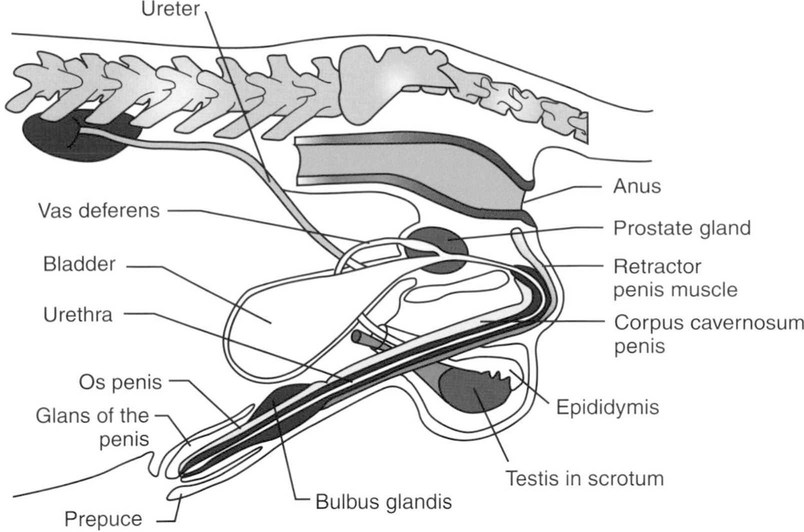

• **Fig. 16.11** Reproductive tract of a male dog.

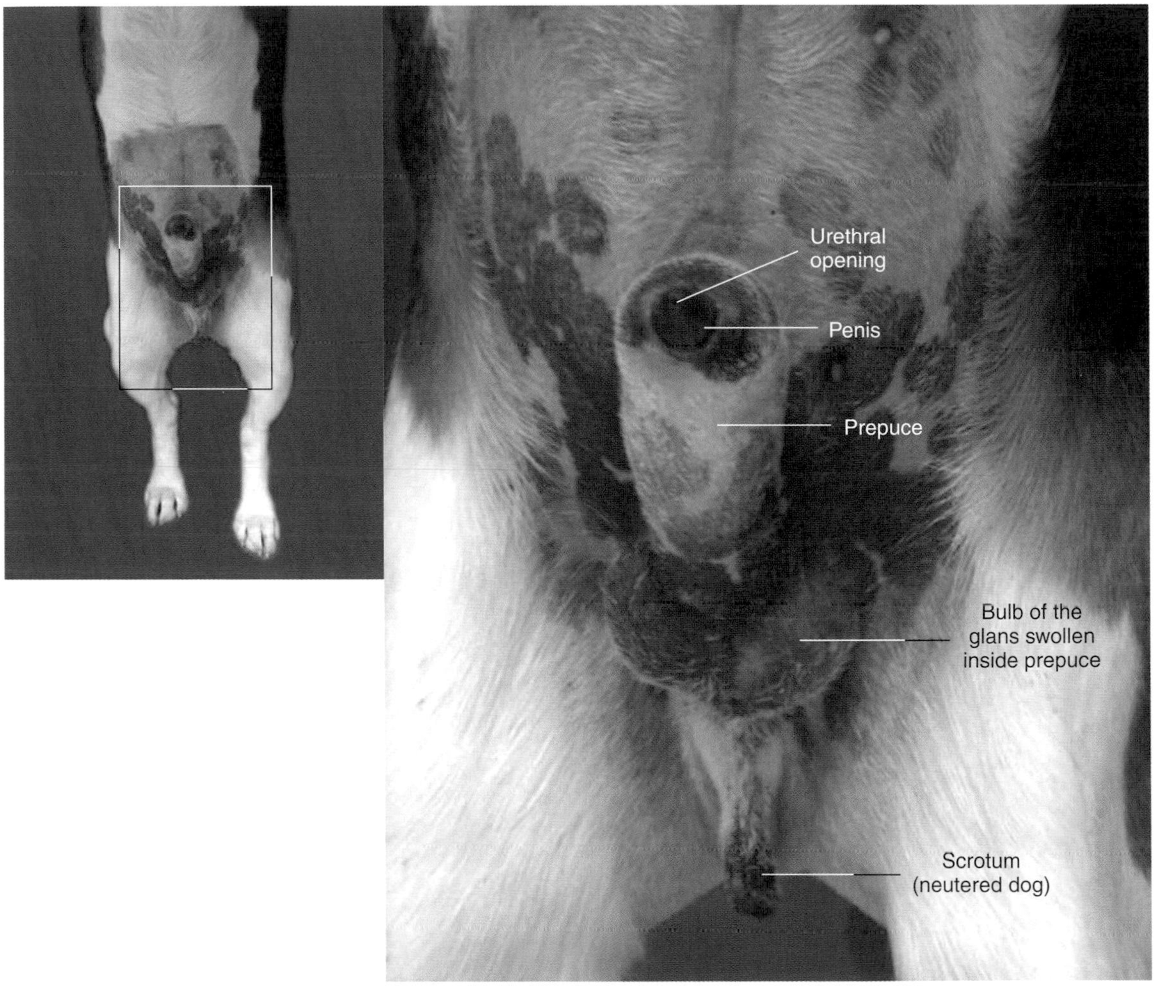

• **Fig. 16.12** Canine bulb of the glans.

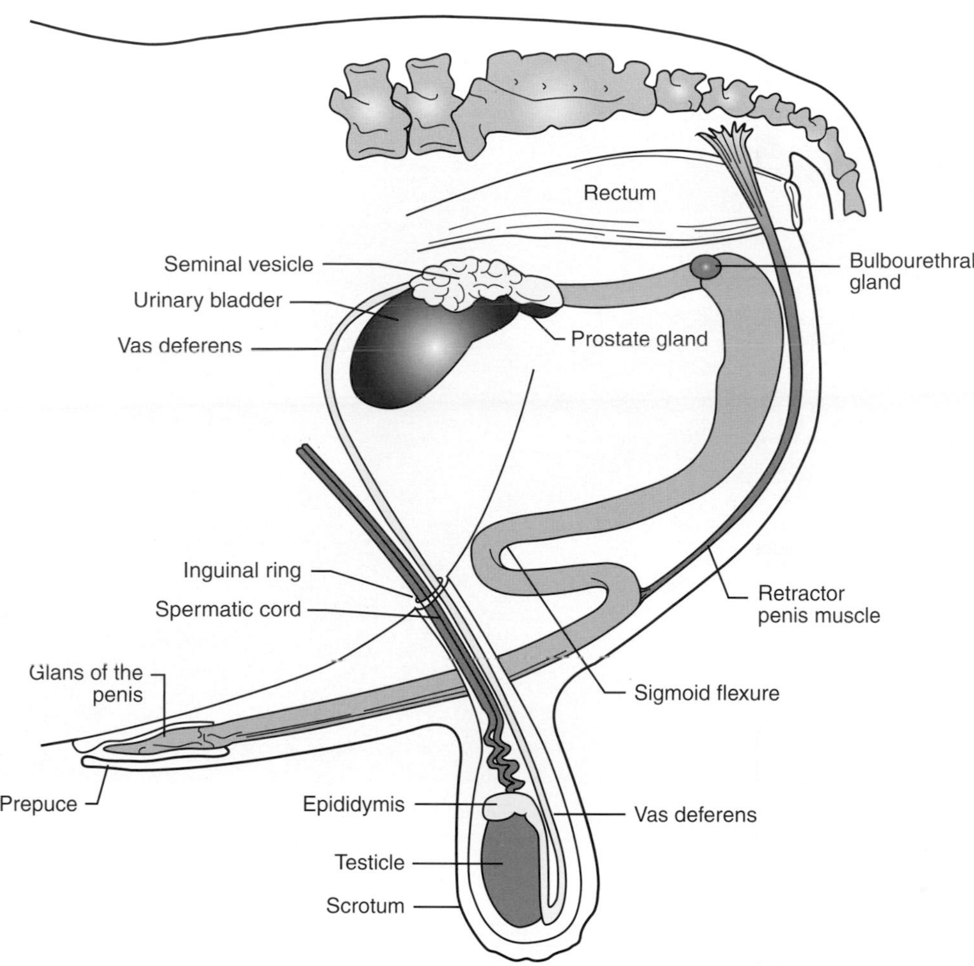

• **Fig. 16.13** Reproductive tract of a bull.

The Sigmoid Flexure

- The **sigmoid flexure** is an S-shaped bend in the nonerect penis of bulls, rams, and boars (Fig. 16.13).
- Erection of the penis straightens the sigmoid flexure.
- It is held in place by the **retractor penis muscle**.
  - The retractor penis muscle pulls the nonerect penis back into the S-shaped sigmoid flexure.
  - When the penis becomes erect, the retractor penis muscle stretches, and the penis straightens.
  - When the erection subsides, the retractor penis muscle pulls the penis back into the nonerect S-shape.

The Female Reproductive System

The Ovaries

- The ovaries are the female gonads (Fig. 16.14).
- They are homologous (have the same embryologic origin) to the male testes.
- Located in the abdomen near the kidneys, they are suspended from the dorsal part of the abdomen by the **suspensory ligament** of the ovary (see Fig. 16.18).
- Their shape varies among species; most are almond-shaped, but the horse's is kidney bean-shaped, and the pig's look like a grape cluster.
- Their function is to produce the reproductive cell (ovum) and hormones (estrogens and progestins).
- The ovaries undergo cyclical changes under the stimulation of follicle-stimulating hormone (FSH) and luteinizing hormone (LH) from the pituitary gland.
  - Each ovum develops in a fluid-filled, blister-like follicle, which produces estrogen hormones that prepare the reproductive tract for breeding.
  - After ovulation (release of a mature ovum), the empty follicle develops into the solid corpus luteum, which produces progestin hormones that help maintain pregnancy if the ovum has been successfully fertilized (Fig. 16.15).

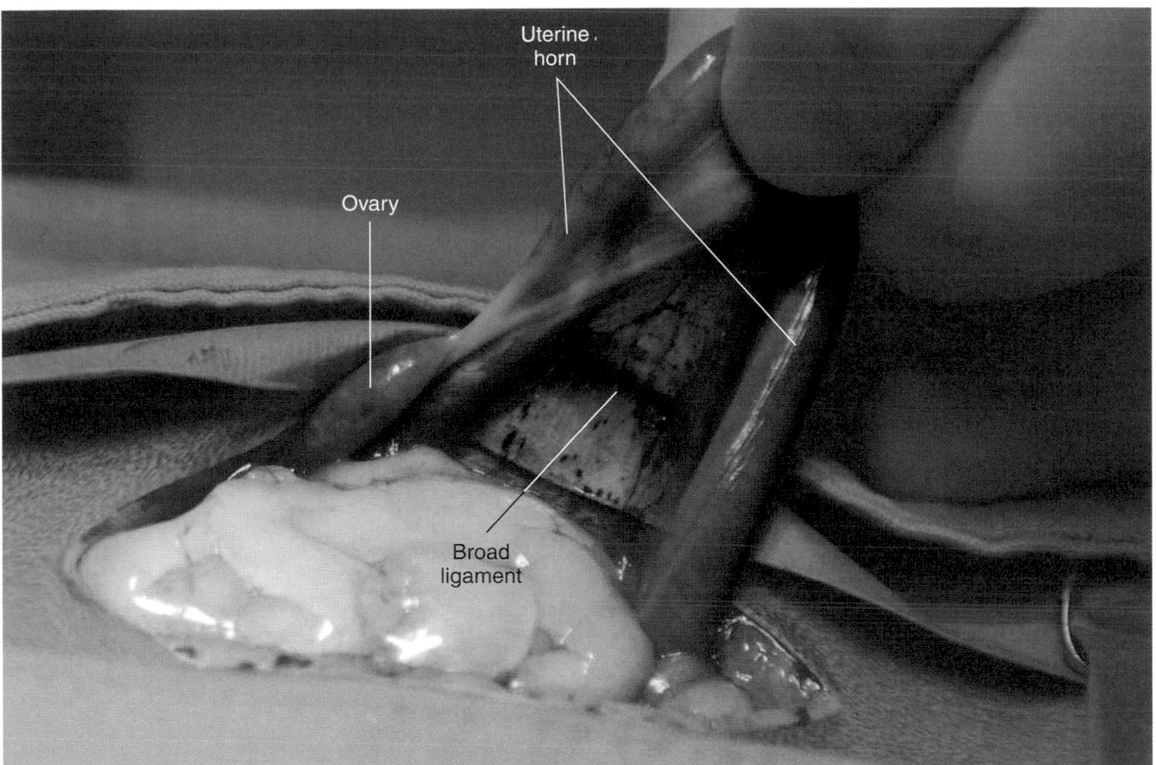

• **Fig. 16.14** "Quiet" feline ovary during the anestrus period.

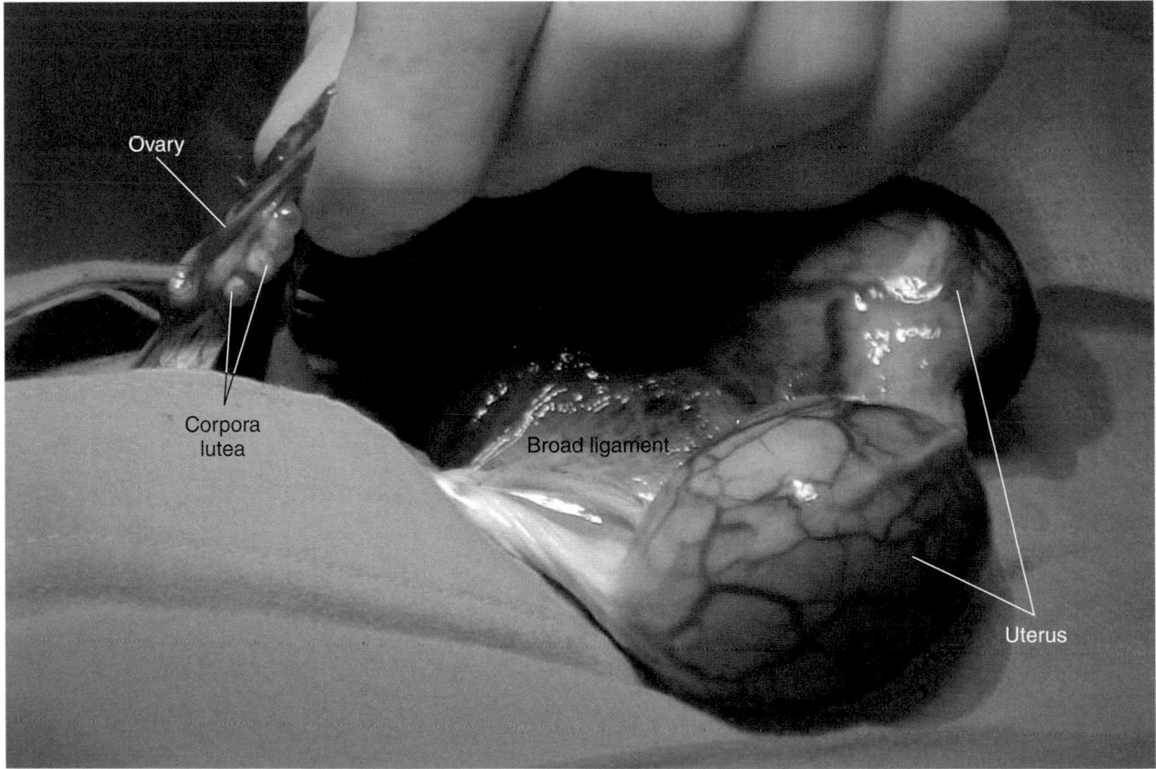

• **Fig. 16.15** Ovary of a pregnant cat showing corpora lutea.

The Oviducts

- The **oviduct** is a small, convoluted tube that extends from the tip of the uterine horn toward the ovary (Fig. 16.16).
- It is also known as the Fallopian tube or uterine tube.
- It "catches" the ovum when ovulation occurs and conducts it to the uterus.
- The **infundibulum** is the funnel-like expansion at the ovarian end of the oviduct. It contains smooth muscle and is lined with cilia, which beat rhythmically to conduct an ovum into the oviduct.
  - The infundibulum has finger-like extensions on its free edge called **fimbriae**, which seek out and cover a developing follicle so it can catch the ovum when it is released.
- The oviduct is the usual site of fertilization of the ovum by a spermatozoon.
- The oviduct is not physically attached to the ovary.

The Uterus

- The **uterus** is the hollow, muscular organ where pregnancy is maintained (Fig. 16.17).
- It is composed of a caudal **body** and two **horns** that extend cranially toward the ovaries.
- It is Y-shaped in domestic animals—the horns of the uterus are represented by the arms of the Y. The body of the uterus is the stem of the Y.
- The cervix is located at the most caudal portion of the uterine body, between the uterus and the vagina (see below).
- The uterus is suspended from the dorsal part of the abdomen by the broad ligament.
- A fertilized ovum enters the uterus from the oviduct and implants in the uterine wall.
- During parturition (the birth process), the muscle of the uterus contracts in the early part of labor and presses the fetus against the cervix, which causes the cervix to dilate. Then, assisted by abdominal muscle contractions, the

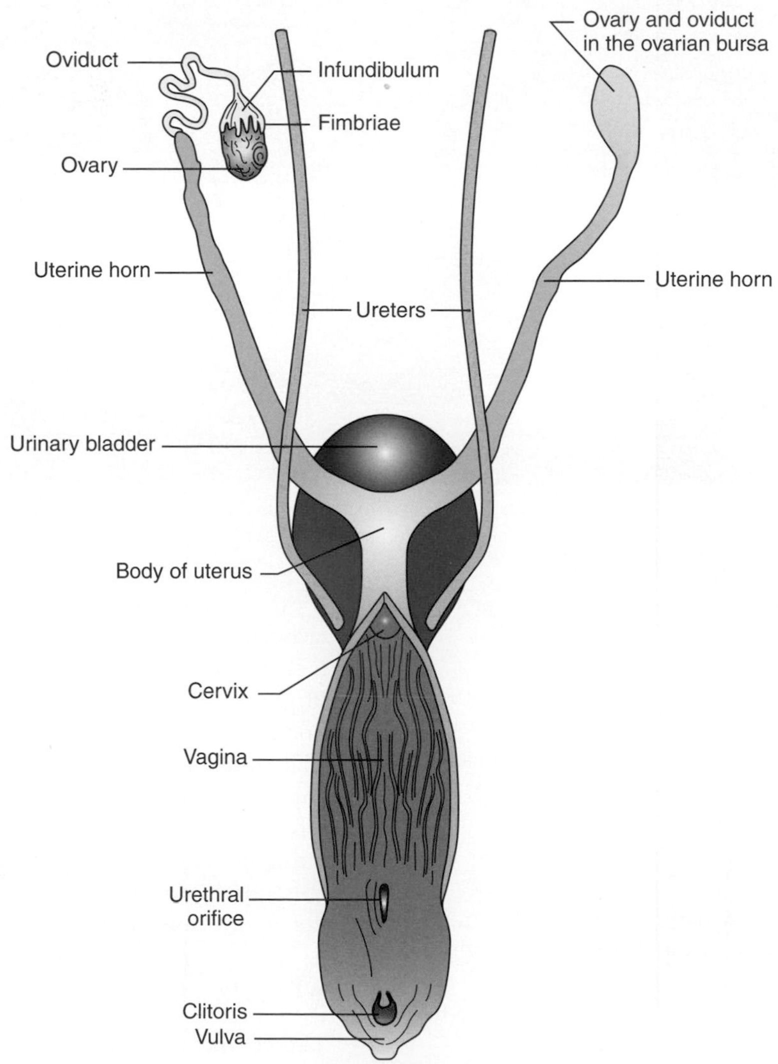

• **Fig. 16.16** The reproductive system of a bitch. Dorsal view.

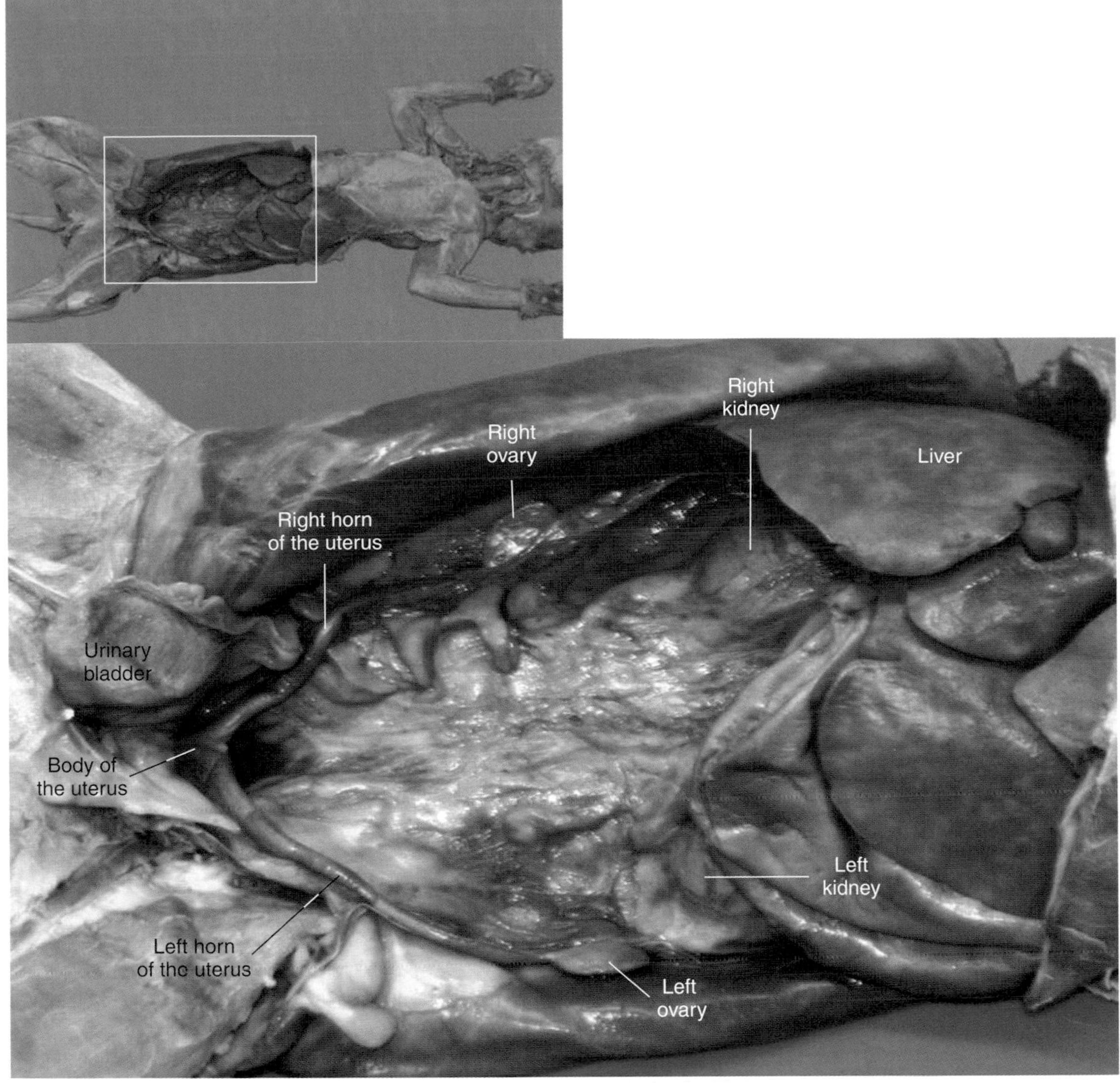

• **Fig. 16.17** Organs of the female reproductive system in the cat. Ventral view with the intestines removed. Note the dorsal location of the uterus and ovaries and the proximity of the ovaries to the kidneys.

uterus pushes the newborn, followed by its placenta, out into the world.

Suspensory Ligaments

Three connective tissue ligaments suspend the abdominal female reproductive organs from the dorsal body wall (Fig. 16.18).

The **broad ligament** is the largest of the three.

- It is a broad sheet of connective tissue that supports the ovary, oviduct, and uterus.
- It is formed from the peritoneum of the dorsal abdomen.
- There are two broad ligaments supporting the reproductive organs on each side.
- The broad ligament contains blood vessels and nerve fibers that supply the reproductive organs.
- It is transected during ovariohysterectomy (spay) surgery to allow the uterine horns to be removed.

The suspensory ligament of the ovary forms the cranial end of the broad ligament.

- It extends cranially and dorsally from the ovary and attaches to the dorsal body wall near the last rib.
- It is usually stretched or cut during ovariohysterectomy surgery to allow the ovary to be brought up into the incision so its blood vessels can be ligated (tied off).

The **round ligament** of the uterus is a lateral fold of the broad ligament made up of fibrous tissue and blood vessels.

- It runs from the uterine horn to the area of the inguinal ring.
- It is transected during an ovariohysterectomy to allow the uterine horns to be removed.

The Cervix

- The **cervix** is located at the caudal end of the uterine body between the uterus and the vagina (Fig. 16.19).
- It serves as a muscular "valve" that keeps the uterus sealed off from the vagina most of the time.
  - It opens during estrus to allow spermatozoa to enter.

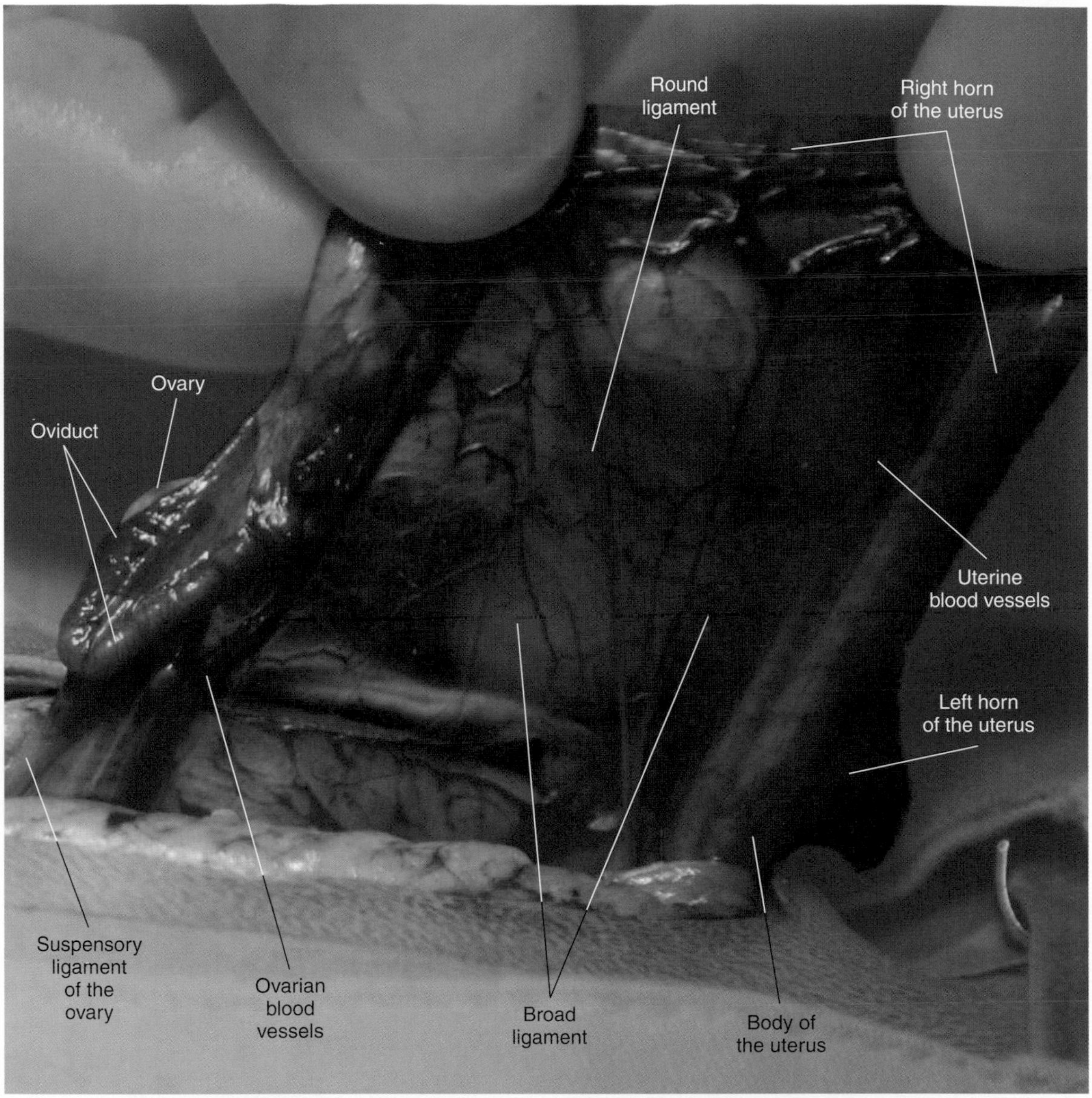

Round ligament
Right horn of the uterus
Ovary
Oviduct
Uterine blood vessels
Left horn of the uterus
Suspensory ligament of the ovary
Ovarian blood vessels
Broad ligament
Body of the uterus

• **Fig. 16.18** Suspensory ligaments of the feline female reproductive system.

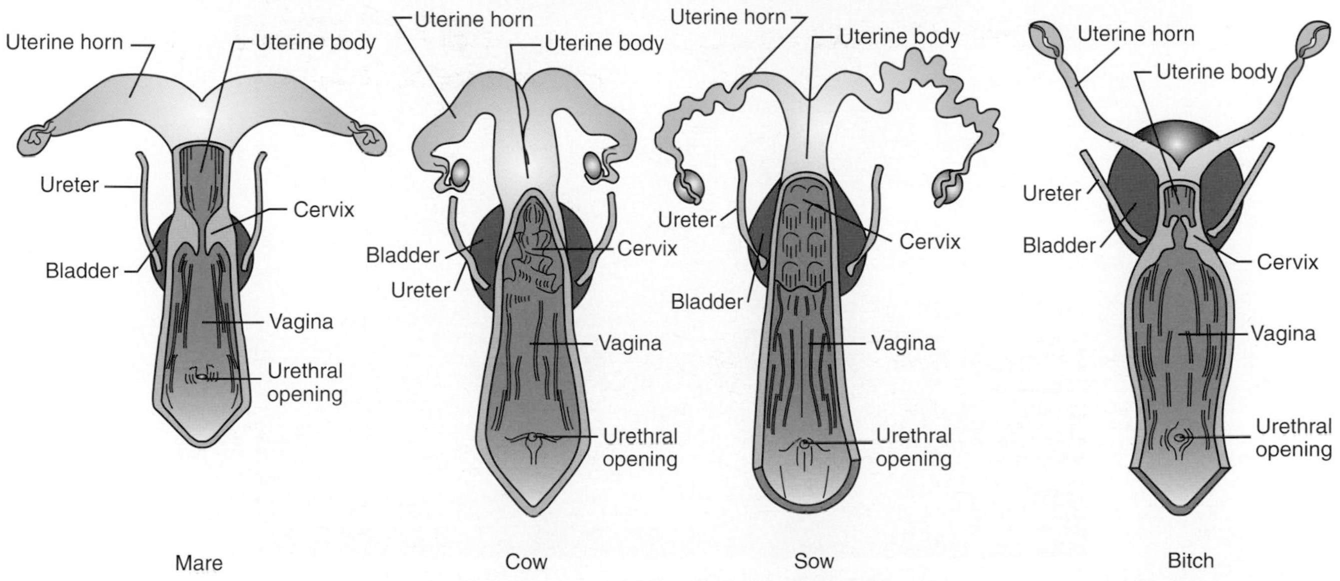

• **Fig. 16.19** Comparison of female reproductive tracts. Dorsal view.

- It opens again at the end of pregnancy to allow the fetus to pass into the vagina. Uterine contractions in early labor press the fetus against the cervix, causing it to open (dilate).

The Vagina

- The **vagina** is the tube between the cervix and vulva that has two main functions:
  - It receives the penis during breeding.
  - It is the birth canal.
- The vagina can stretch considerably to accommodate the penis or the fetus.
- The lumen is normally closed except during breeding and parturition (the birth process).
- It is lined with mucous glands that provide lubrication.

The Vulva

- The **vulva** is the only part of the female reproductive system visible externally (Fig. 16.20).
- It has three main parts:
  - The **labia** form the external boundary of the vulva (labia means lips).
  - The **vestibule** is the short space between the labia and the vagina. The urethra opens onto the floor (ventral surface) of the vestibule.
  - The **clitoris** (homologous to the male penis) is located caudal to the urethral opening on the vestibule floor.
  - The clitoris is composed of erectile tissue and a glans and is covered with many sensory nerve endings.
  - It is attached by two roots.

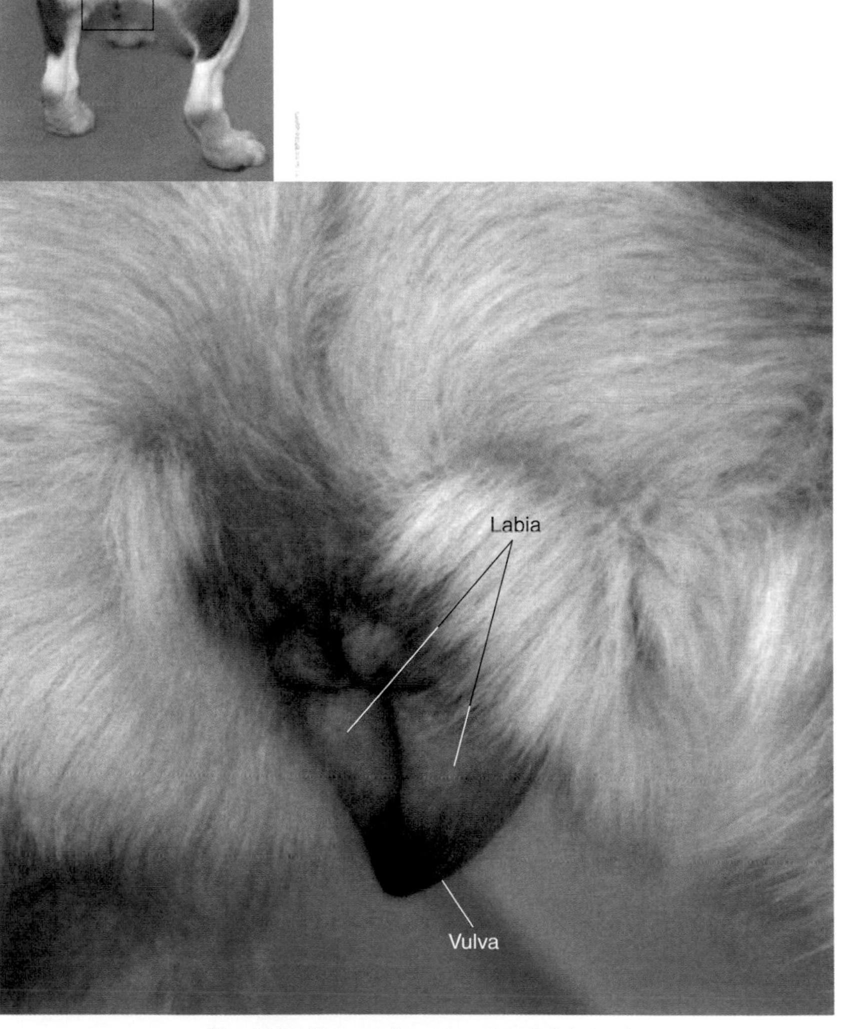

• **Fig. 16.20** The swollen vulva of a bitch in heat.

The Placenta

- The **placenta** is a developing fetus' life support system during pregnancy.
- It forms around the developing fetus and attaches to the uterine lining.
- Different species have different types of placental attachment to the lining of the uterus (Figs. 16.21–16.23).
- The placenta allows nutrients, waste materials, and respiratory gases to be exchanged between the fetal and maternal bloodstreams.
- The fetus is linked to the placenta by the umbilical cord (Figs. 16.24 and 16.25).

FUN FACT

Because each placentome must separate after birth for the placenta to be expelled, ruminant animals generally have the highest incidence of retained placenta of the common domestic species. This often requires veterinary intervention.

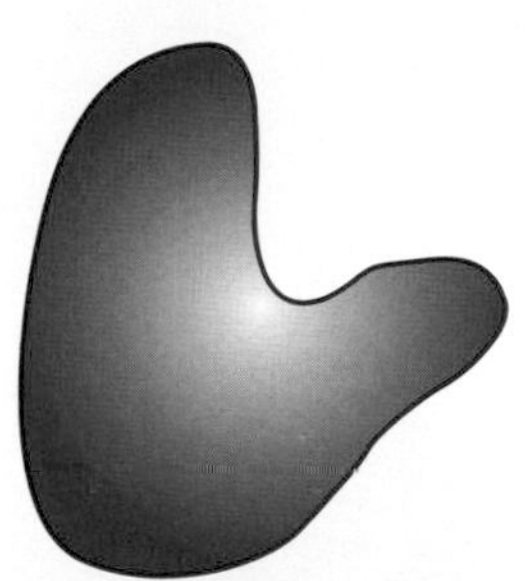

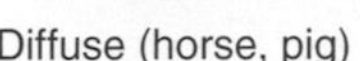

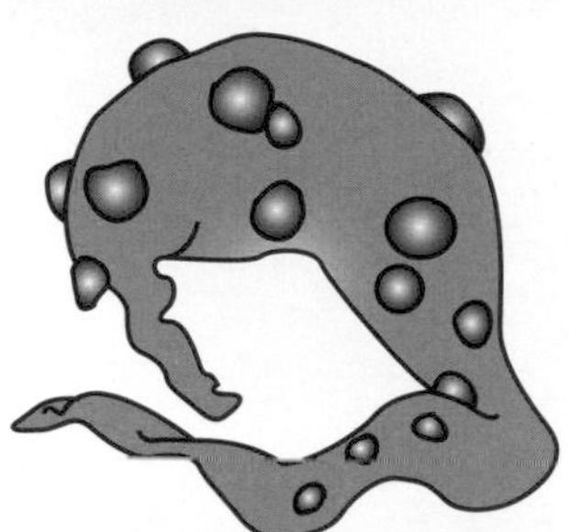

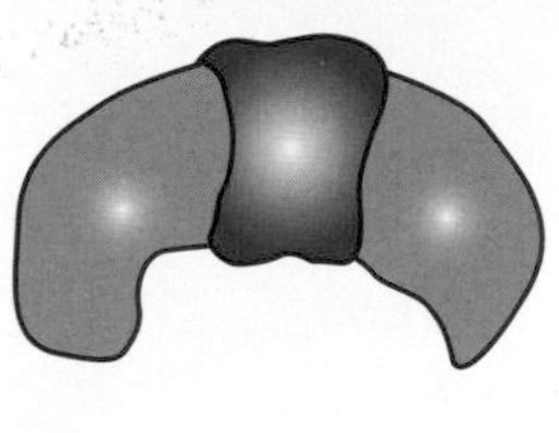

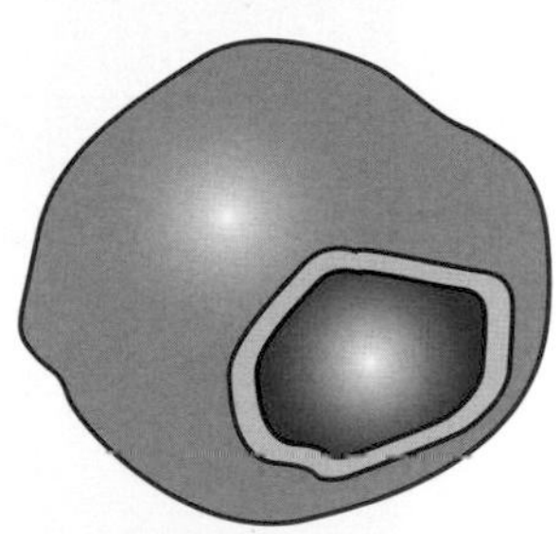

Diffuse (horse, pig) | Cotyledonary (ruminants) | Zonary (dogs, cats) | Discoid (primates, rodents, rabbits)

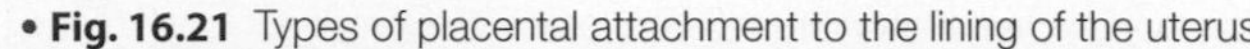

• **Fig. 16.21** Types of placental attachment to the lining of the uterus.

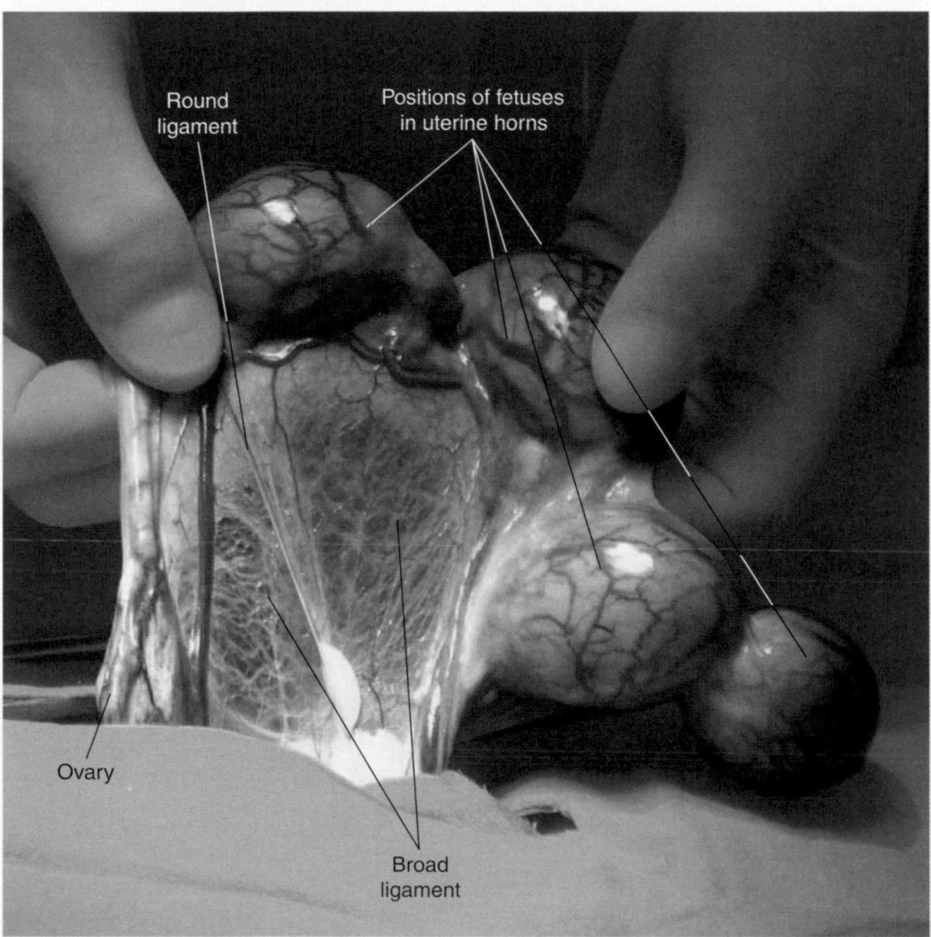

• **Fig. 16.22** Early pregnancy in a cat. Compare this figure to the nonpregnant uterus in Fig. 16.18. Note the enlarged blood vessels.

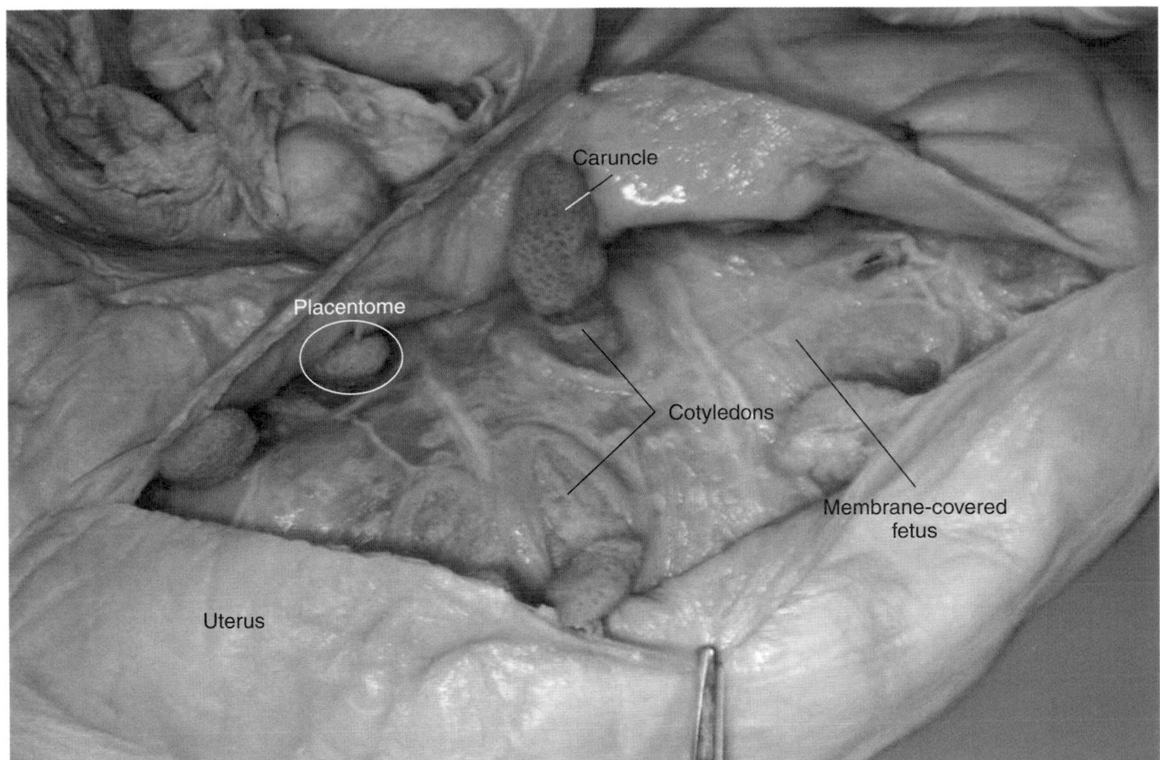

• **Fig. 16.23** Cotyledonary placental attachment in a preserved pregnant cow uterus. The many sites where the placenta and uterus are attached are called placentomes. Each consists of a cotyledon from the surface of the placenta that tightly attaches to a caruncle from the lining of the uterus.

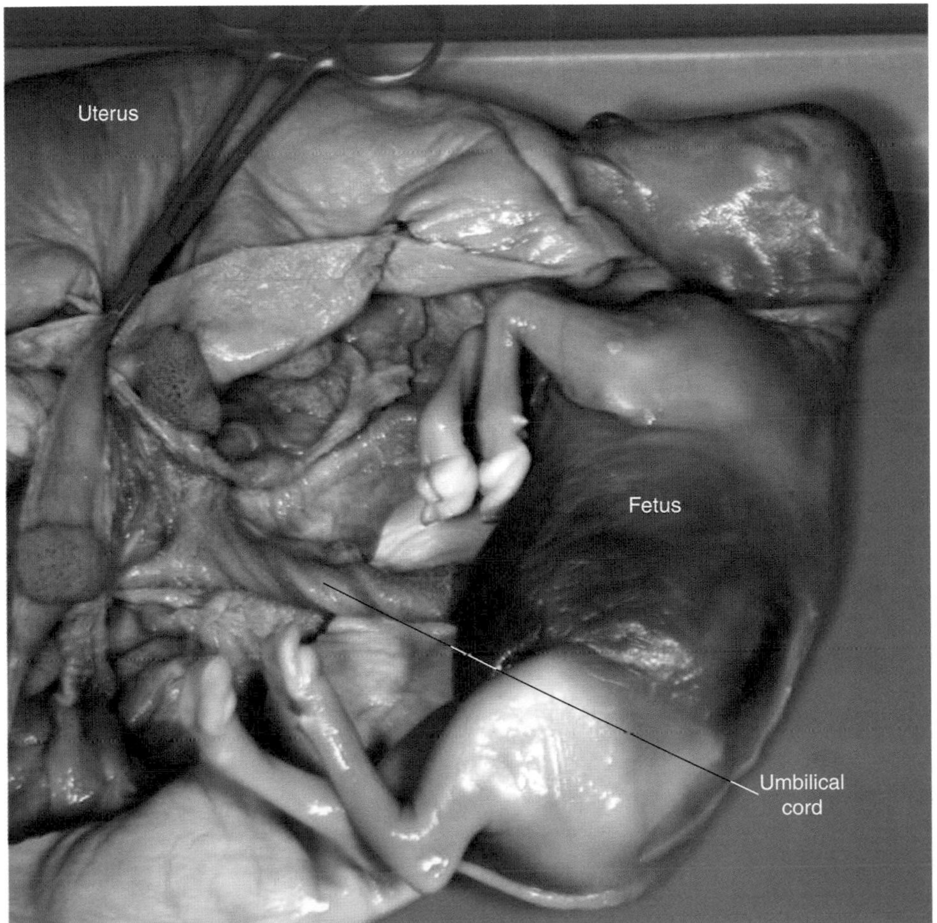

• **Fig. 16.24** Umbilical cord in preserved pregnant cow uterus. The umbilical cord links the fetus with the placenta. It contains arteries that bring waste-filled blood from the fetus to the placenta; a vein that brings nutrient and oxygen-rich blood back to the fetus from the placenta; and the urachus, a tube that runs from the urinary bladder of the fetus to one of the placental sacs around the fetus (the allantoic sac).

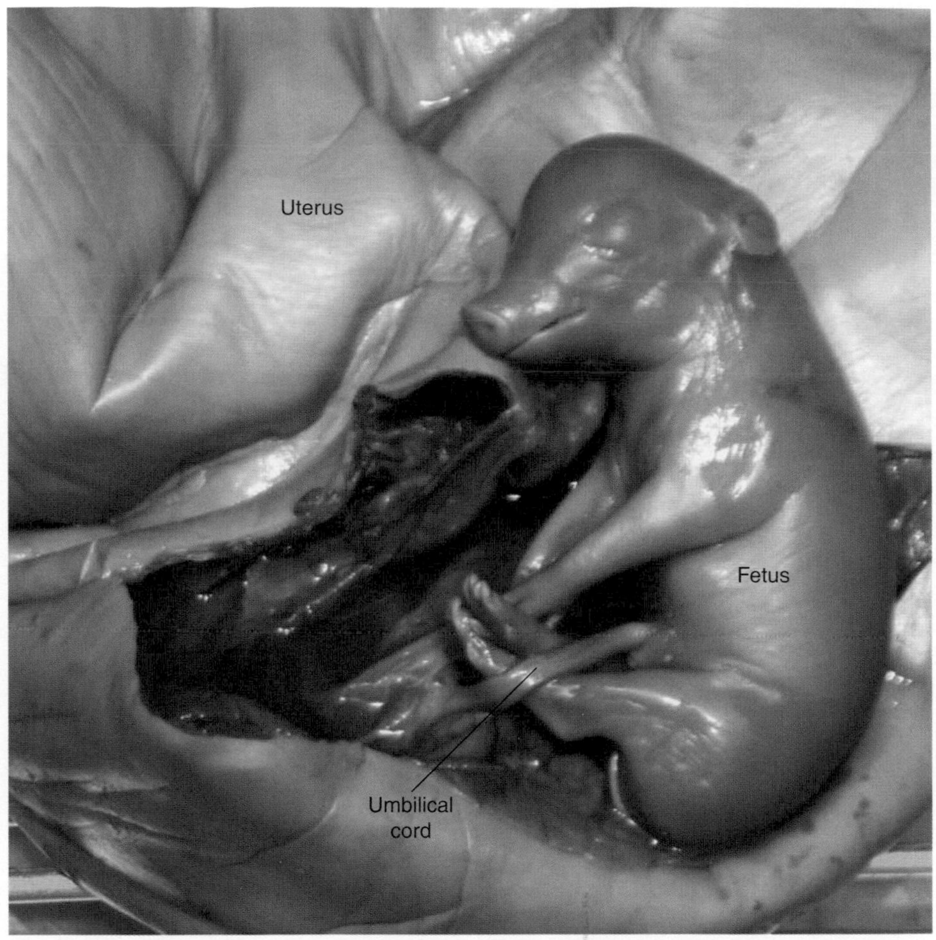

• **Fig. 16.25** Umbilical cord in preserved pregnant sow uterus.

EXERCISES

Male Reproductive System

Exercise 1

Label the Parts of the Male Reproductive Tract (Bull)

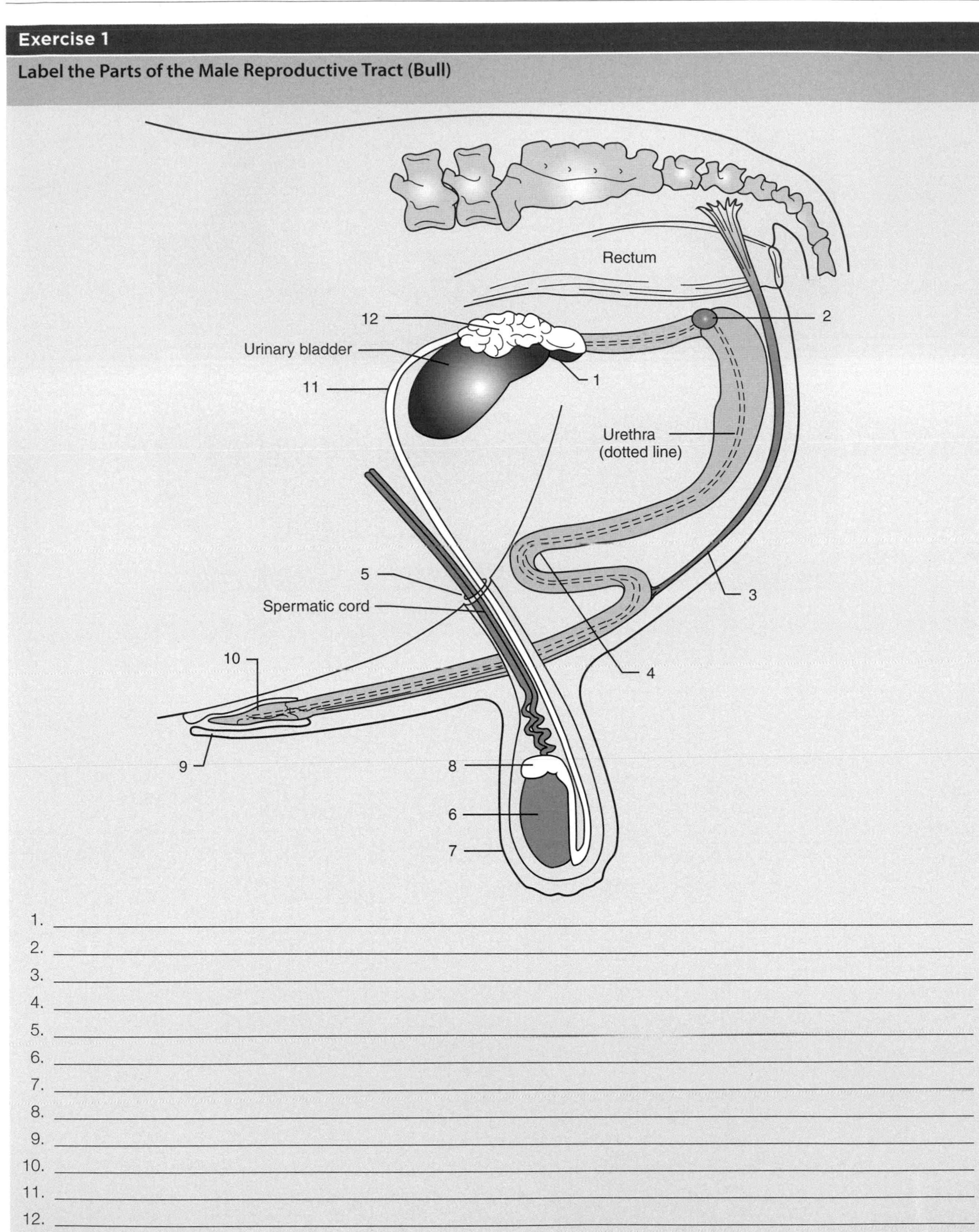

1. __________
2. __________
3. __________
4. __________
5. __________
6. __________
7. __________
8. __________
9. __________
10. __________
11. __________
12. __________

Exercise 2

Identify the Layers of the Vaginal Tunic of a Testicle

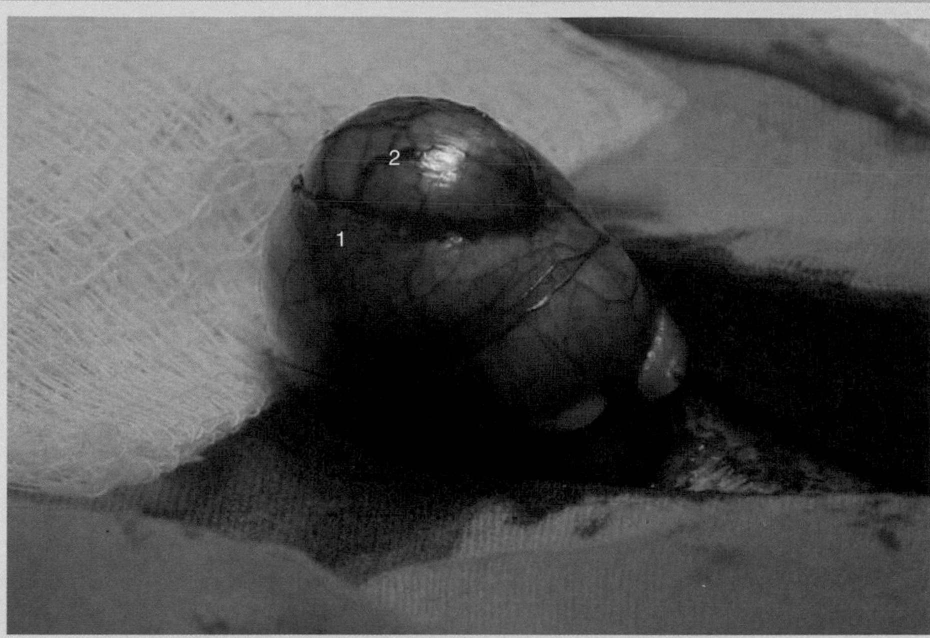

1. ____________________
2. ____________________

Exercise 3

Identify the Structures of the Male Reproductive Tract (Cat)

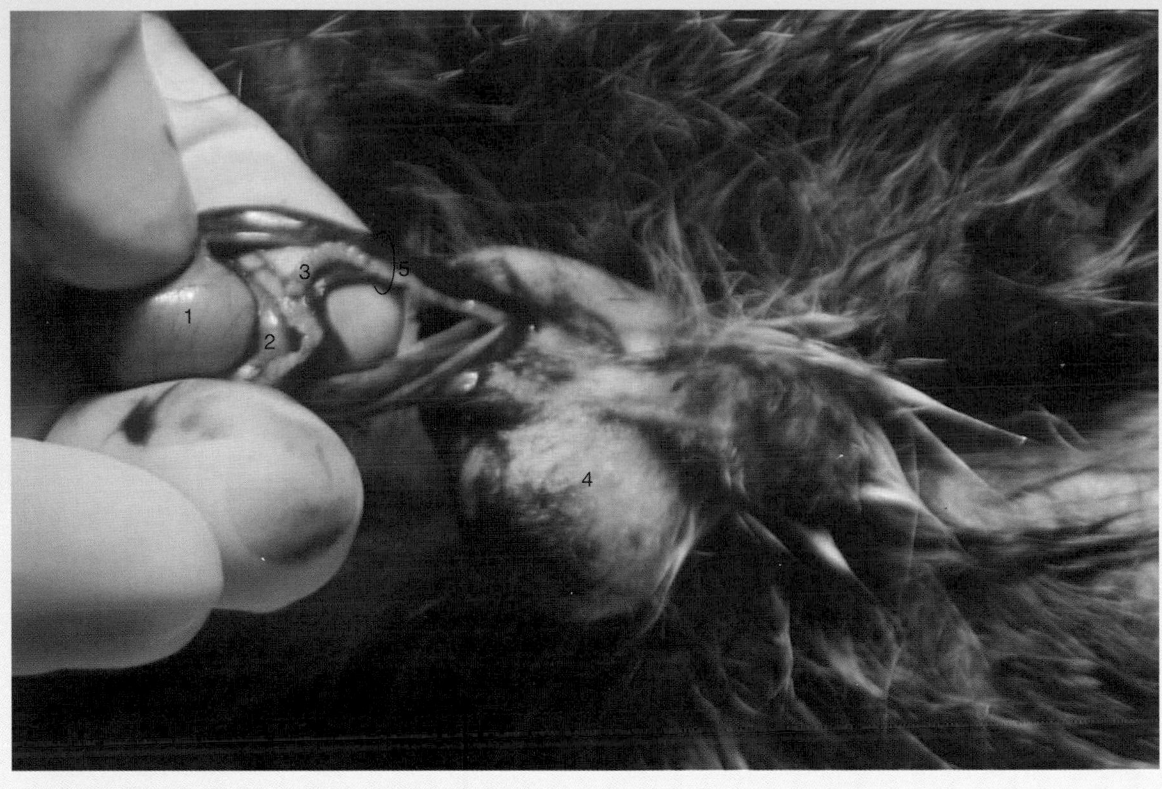

1. ______
2. ______
3. ______
4. ______
5. ______

Exercise 4

Identify the Structures of the Male Reproductive Tract (Dog)

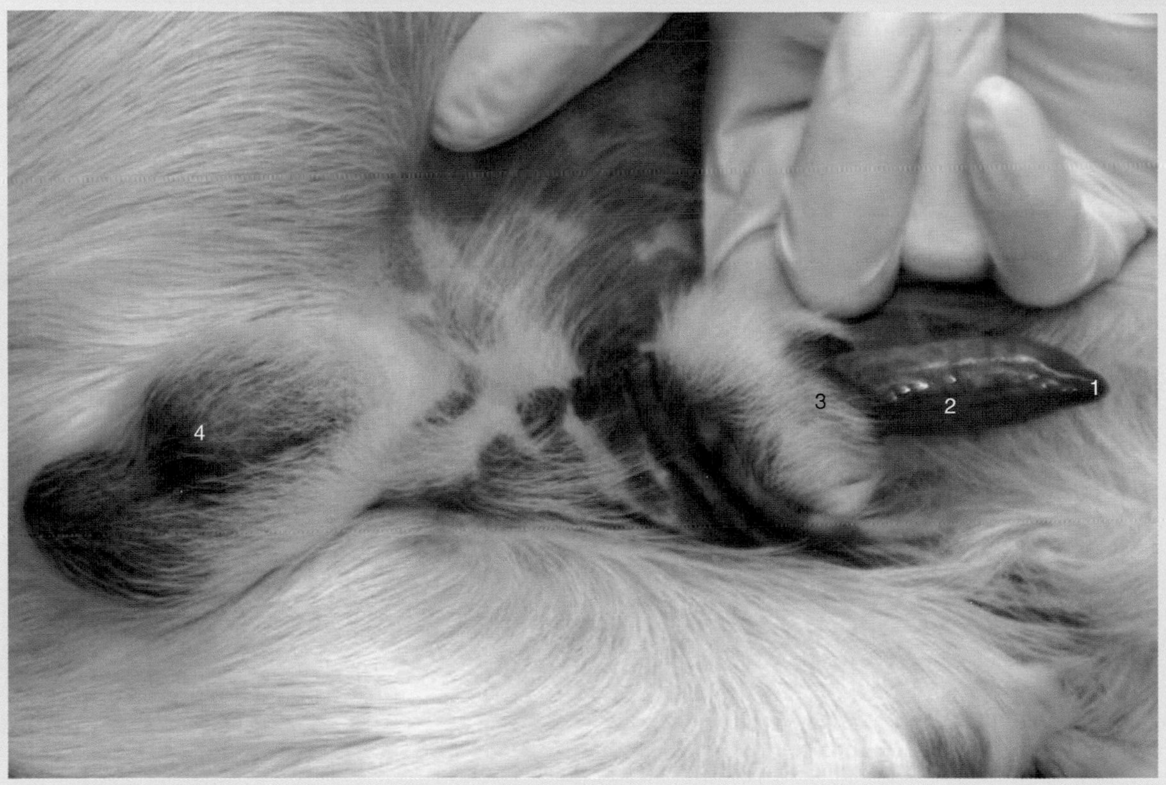

1. ______________________________
2. ______________________________
3. ______________________________
4. ______________________________

Female Reproductive System

Exercise 5

Label the Parts of the Female Reproductive System

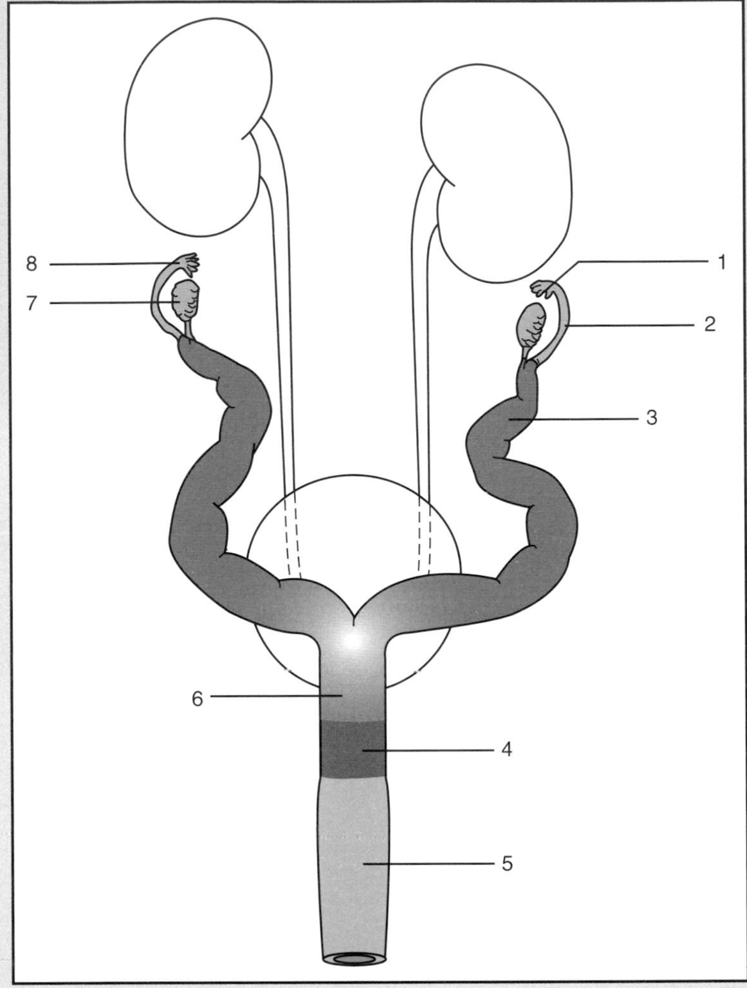

1. ______________________
2. ______________________
3. ______________________
4. ______________________
5. ______________________
6. ______________________
7. ______________________
8. ______________________

Exercise 6

Identify the Female Reproductive System Structures (Cat)

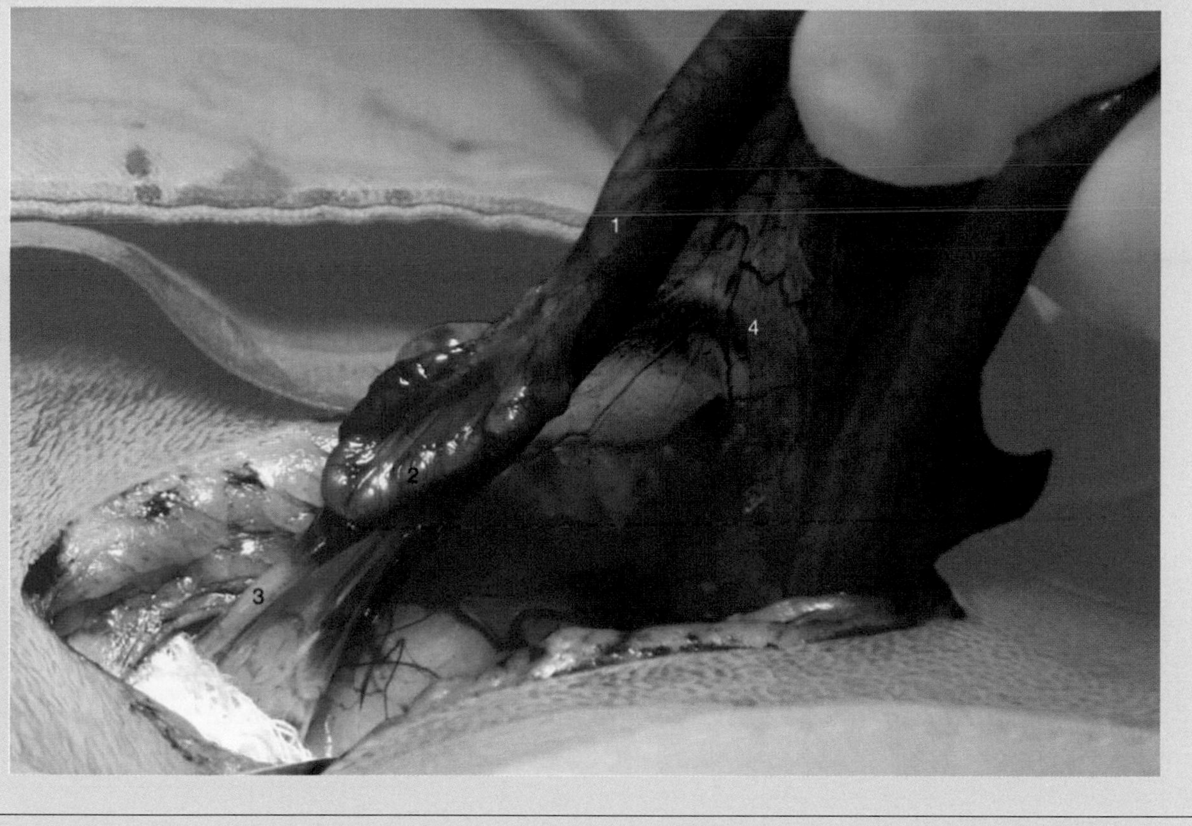

1. ______
2. ______
3. ______
4. ______

Critical and Clinical Thinking

Exercise 7

Identify Clinical Terms

1. Accessory reproductive glands ______
2. Body of the uterus ______
3. Broad ligament ______
4. Bulb of the glans ______
5. Bulbourethral glands ______
6. Cervix ______
7. Clitoris ______

Continued

Exercise 7—cont'd

Identify Clinical Terms

8. Corpus cavernosum penis
9. Corpus cavernosum urethrae
10. Cremaster muscle
11. Epididymis
12. Fimbriae
13. Infundibulum
14. Labia
15. Os penis
16. Ovarian suspensory ligament
17. Ovary
18. Oviducts
19. Parietal vaginal tunic
20. Pelvic urethra
21. Penile urethra
22. Penis
23. Placenta
24. Prepuce
25. Prostate
26. Retractor penis muscle
27. Scrotum
28. Seminal vesicles
29. Sigmoid flexure
30. Spermatic cord
31. Testes
32. Tunica albuginea
33. Uterine horns

Exercise 7—cont'd

Identify Clinical Terms

34. Uterus ____________________
____
____
____

35. Vagina ____________________
____
____
____

36. Vas deferens ____________________
____
____
____

37. Vestibule ____________________
____
____
____

38. Visceral vaginal tunic ____________________
____
____
____

39. Vulva ____________________
____
____
____

Exercise 8

Who Am I?

1. ____________ I am an enlarged area of the canine penis made up of erectile tissue that swells after ejaculation and allows the bitch and dog to "tie" to enhance conception.
2. ____________ As one of the male accessory reproductive glands, I secrete a mucus-containing fluid just before ejaculation to lubricate the urethra and clear it of urine.
3. ____________ We are paired sheets of connective tissue that suspend the uterus from the dorsal part of the abdominal cavity.
4. ____________ I am the sphincter muscle that functions as a valve between the uterus and the vagina.
5. ____________ As the smaller of the two erectile tissue structures in the body of the penis, I form a sleeve around the urethra.
6. ____________ I am the muscle that raises and lowers the testes in the scrotum to help control their temperature.
7. ____________ A ribbon-like structure, I lie along the surface of the testes and store spermatozoa before ejaculation.
8. ____________ We are the outer lips of the vulva.
9. ____________ I am the bone in the penis of a dog.
10. ____________ We are the female gonads.
11. ____________ I am the male copulatory (breeding) organ.
12. ____________ As a life-supporting system for a developing fetus, I am a multilayered fluid-filled sac that surrounds the fetus and links it to the blood supply of the uterus.
13. ____________ I am the skin-covered sheath around the free end of the penis.
14. ____________ I am the only accessory reproductive gland in dogs.
15. ____________ I am the muscle capable of pulling the nonerect penis of animals with a sigmoid flexure back into its S-shaped configuration.
16. ____________ A sac of skin, I house the testes.
17. ____________ I am a cord-like connective tissue structure that encloses blood vessels, nerves, lymphatic vessels, and the vas deferens as they pass between the testes and the abdominal cavity.
18. ____________ I am the womb (where pregnancy is maintained).
19. ____________ As the tube between the cervix and the vulva, I receive the penis at breeding and form the birth canal at parturition.
20. ____________ I am the muscular tube that carries spermatozoa and the fluid they are suspended in from the epididymis to the urethra.
21. ____________ I form the entrance to the vulva between the labia and the vagina.
22. ____________ I am the external portion of the female reproductive system.
23. ____________ I am a tough, fibrous connective tissue capsule that protects the testes.

Exercise 9

Clinical Thinking Challenge #1

1. ________________ The _____ is known as the "birth canal."
2. ________________ What structure "catches" the ovum as it is released from the ovary?
3. ________________ The smooth muscle sphincter between the vagina and the uterus is the _____.
4. ________________ The ovary produces _____ and _____ (hormones).
5. ________________ Is the oviduct attached to the ovary? (*Yes* or *no*.)
6. ________________ What structure keeps the ovary, oviduct, and uterus suspended in place?
7. ________________ The epididymis is where _____ are stored until ejaculation.
8. ________________ The testes must be kept *warmer* or *cooler* than core body temperature?
9. ________________ Spermatozoa are produced in the _____ tubules.
10. ________________ The cervix is *open* or *closed* in a female who is not pregnant or in heat?
11. ________________ The structure in the female that is homologous to the male penis is the _____.
12. ________________ What structure in the male penis causes dogs to "tie" after mating?
13. ________________ The _____ is the slit-like opening in the abdominal muscles through which the spermatic cord passes into the abdomen. (Two words)
14. ________________ Name one structure inside the scrotum of an animal.
15. ________________ What tube connects the epididymis with the urethra? (Two words)
16. ________________ What muscle helps regulate the temperature of the testes?
17. ________________ What two common domestic animals do not have seminal vesicles?
18. ________________ Two connective tissue layers that surround the testes. They were formed from layers of peritoneum.

Exercise 10

Clinical Thinking Challenge #2

Support each of the following correct statements with appropriate rationale, stating why or in what way each statement is correct.

1. The reproductive system is unusual and differs from other body systems.

   ____

   ____

2. The diploid chromosome number is always an even number.

   ____

   ____

3. A YY chromosome combination is not possible.

   ____

   ____

4. Meiosis is referred to as reduction division.

   ____

   ____

5. There are three main tasks of the male reproductive system.

   ____

   ____

6. The scrotum helps regulate body temperature.

   ____

   ____

7. It is important that Sertoli cells help shield the developing spermatozoa from the body's immune system.

   ____

   ____

Exercise 10—cont'd

Clinical Thinking Challenge #2

8. The urethra of the male has two functions and two portions.

9. There are three main parts of the penis.

10. There are three main reproductive organs in the female.

11. Ovaries have two main functions. The hormones produced fall into two categories.

12. The thick wall of the uterus is made up of three layers.

13. The estrous cycle can be divided into a series of four characteristic stages (and one that occurs in some animals between breeding seasons) that reflect what is going on in the ovary.

17 Pregnancy, Development, and Lactation

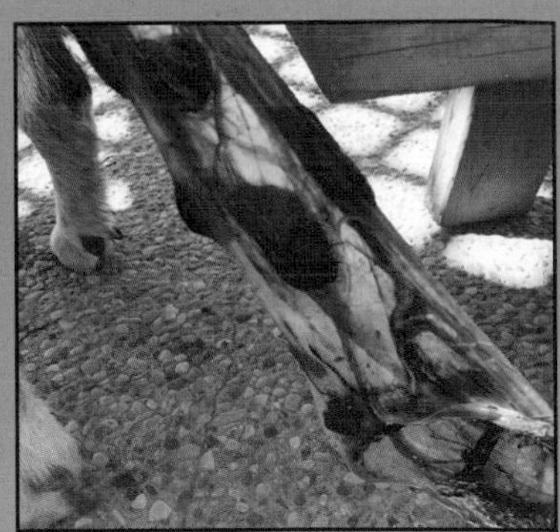

OVERVIEW AT A GLANCE

Pregnancy 451

Development 452

Lactation 452

Suggested In-Class Activities 453

Bibliography 453

Exercises 453–456

Pregnancy 453–455

1. *Identify the Ovarian Cycle 453*
2. *Identify the Uterine Layers 454*
3. *Match the Types of Placental Attachment 454*
4. *Identify the Type of Placental Attachment 455*

Development 455

5. *Clinical Thinking Challenge #1: Client Education 455*

Lactation 455

6. *Define Lactation Terms 455*

Clinical and Critical Thinking 456

7. *Identify Key Female Hormones of Breeding, Gestation, Parturition, and Lactation 456*
8. *Clinical Thinking Challenge #2: Name the Offspring 456*
9. *Clinical Thinking Challenge #3: Explain the Processes in the Reproductive Cycle 456*

LEARNING OBJECTIVES

The objectives for this chapter are to describe and/or identify the location and function of the structures related to pregnancy, development, and lactation. For more information, refer to Chapter 20 in *Clinical Anatomy and Physiology for Veterinary Technicians.*

CLINICAL SIGNIFICANCE

Fully understanding pregnancy and development will allow a technician to better assist with breeding, parturition, and reproductive surgeries.

INTRODUCTION

The scope of veterinary science includes all stages of animal life, including breeding, parturition, and reproductive surgery. The conception, and subsequent birth, of a new animal is not a static process but one full of dynamic sequences of events that must occur at just the right time and in just the right order. When the events do line up to produce a pregnant state, even more events must occur to support the new and growing life. A clear understanding of the processes of breeding, fertilization of the ovum, pregnancy, zygote/embryo/fetal development, birth, and lactation/nursing is instrumental to the practice and enjoyment of veterinary medicine.

TERMS TO BE IDENTIFIED

Allantoic sac
Blastocyst
Corpus luteum
Cotyledonary attachment
Diffuse attachment
Ectoderm
Endoderm
Endometrium
Mesoderm
Mesometrium
Multiparous
Myometrium
Oxytocin
Placenta
Progesterone
Prolactin
Relaxin hormone
Umbilical cord
Uniparous
Zonary attachment
Zygote

Pregnancy

The Ovaries

- The ovary is both an endocrine organ that produces estrogen and progestin hormones and a reproductive organ that produces ova (eggs). The ovaries are sensitive to the effects of the luteinizing hormone (LH) and follicle stimulating hormone (FSH), which are critical for the ovarian cycle and pregnancy.
- During the ovarian cycle, the primary follicle will grow into a mature follicle within the ovary. During ovulation, the follicle will rupture, releasing the ovum. The site on the ovary where the follicle ruptured will become the corpus luteum under the influence of LH.
- The ovaries of a pregnant animal will contain at least one **corpus luteum** (pl. corpora lutea), which is a temporary hormone-secreting tissue.
  - The corpus luteum (Latin for "yellow body") develops after ovulation and will secrete progestin hormones (including progesterone) to maintain the pregnancy.
    - A **uniparous** species (species that usually only gives birth to a single offspring) typically has only a single corpus luteum.
    - A **multiparous** species (species that usually gives birth to multiple offspring) typically has multiple corpora lutea (one per released follicle).
  - The corpus luteum will feel solid, whereas a follicle is a fluid-filled superficial sac.
  - If the ova are not fertilized, the corpus luteum will be reabsorbed.
- In sows and cows, the ovaries secrete **relaxin hormone** to assist in relaxation of the cervix in preparation for parturition.

The Uterus

- The uterus is a Y-shaped structure (except in primates) where the fetus develops and grows. The shape of the uterus is species specific. Dogs and cats have a Y-shaped uterus with long uterine horns, whereas a cow has a T-shaped uterus with relatively shorter horns.
- It contains three layers:
  - **Endometrium**: This inner layer contains mucous membranes and blood vessels that enlarge during pregnancy to support the embryo nutritionally until it implants. This layer is also important in placental development.
  - **Myometrium**: This layer consists of smooth muscle that will contract at the time of parturition to deliver the fetus. It is sensitive to the hormone oxytocin.
  - **Mesometrium**: This outer layer attaches the uterus to the dorsal abdominal wall.
- During pregnancy, the embryo(s) attach and develop in the uterine horns.
  - Embryos are distributed between both uterine horns.
- The uterus grows and expands throughout the pregnancy. Late in pregnancy, the uterine horns can bend back upon themselves to allow for more growth of the fetus and uterus. To supply the ever-growing uterus and fetus, the blood vessels that bring nutrients and remove metabolic waste enlarge significantly.
- The uterine blood vessels become tortuous in appearance (large and twisted) later in pregnancy.
- During the progression of the pregnancy, the uterus moves in a ventral direction due to the weight of the uterus and fetus.
  - After making a ventral midline incision, the uterus will be the first tissue you typically find in a female in late pregnancy, in contrast to a non-pregnant female.
- The cervix (a sphincter muscle at the caudal aspect of the body of the uterus) will be closed during pregnancy and relaxed during parturition to allow for the passage of the newborn. Since rabbits have two separate uterine horns, they have two cervices.

The Placenta

- This multilayer tissue forms around the fetus and attaches to the endometrium (the lining of the uterus) during the first trimester.
  - The attachment point is pink and rough in appearance.
  - The **allantoic sac** (also called the first water bag) is a fluid-filled sac connected to the fetal urinary bladder via the urachus. This contains the amniotic sac.
  - The amniotic sac (also called the second water bag) is a fluid filled sac that contains the fetus.
- The **placenta** is responsible for supplying nutrients and oxygen to, as well as clearing waste from, the fetus.
- The blood supplies of the pregnant female and the offspring are completely separate. The blood vessels are, however, in close proximity to allow the exchange of nutrients, oxygen, and waste without mixing fetal and maternal blood.
- There are four main types of placental attachment:
  - **Diffuse attachment** is seen in horses, camelids, and pigs, and allows the entire surface of the placenta to attach to the uterine lining.
  - **Cotyledonary attachment** is seen in ruminants and contains multiple smaller, round, raised attachment sites that resemble inverted mushroom caps.
    - The attachment sites increase in size throughout the pregnancy.
  - **Zonary attachment** is seen in carnivores and consists of a belt-like attachment band around the middle of the placenta.
  - **Discoid attachment** is found in primates, rodents, and rabbits, and it consists of one large disc-shaped attachment site.
- The **umbilical cord** is the only direct point of placental attachment to the fetus.
  - The umbilical cord contains multiple vessels in addition to the urachus.
    - The umbilical cord of the cat contains two arteries and two veins.

- The umbilical cord of the dog contains two arteries and one vein.
- Arteries bring blood that contains metabolic waste to the placenta to allow it to be deposited into the maternal blood stream and be eliminated by the mother.
- Veins take blood containing nutrients and oxygen from the placenta to the fetus.
- The urachus is a tube that empties the fetus' urinary bladder into the allantoic sac.

- In a bitch or mare, the placenta secretes relaxin hormone prior to parturition, which assists in relaxing the cervix.

Development

In the first trimester:

- A **zygote** becomes a **blastocyst** (hollow ball), arrives in the uterus, and attaches to the uterine wall (implantation).
  - This occurs approximately 2 weeks after ovulation in dogs and cats.
  - This occurs approximately 3 weeks after ovulation in horses and cattle.
- The average size of a Beagle fetus is 4 mm on day 20.

In the second trimester:

- Placental development occurs.
- The corpus luteum finishes developing.
- Differentiation of tissues occurs. There are originally three main types of cell/tissue:
  - **Endoderm** develops into mucous membranes, the respiratory system, and the digestive system.
  - **Mesoderm** develops into connective tissue, muscle, and the urinary, circulatory, and reproductive systems.
  - **Ectoderm** develops into the integumentary and nervous systems.
- Organ development occurs. This includes the differentiation of males and females based on external genitalia.
- The average size of a Beagle fetus is 65 mm on day 40.

In the third trimester:

- Organ growth occurs—the organs developed in the second trimester, and now during the third trimester they increase in size.
  - Because the organs are growing but not developing, we can now safely take radiographs to determine the number of offspring.
- The average size of a Beagle fetus is 165 mm on day 63.

Lactation

Mammary Glands

Location

- They are found from the axillary to inguinal regions in multiparous species.
- They are found in the inguinal regions of uniparous species (except for apes and elephants).

Microscopic Anatomy

- The mammary glands are modified sweat glands that contain ducts and secretory tissue.
  - The secretory parts are called alveoli (this is the same term used for lung tissue, but the tissues function differently).
    - Surrounding each alveolus are contractile cells to help with milk let-down.
  - The milk enters small ducts that empty into ever-larger ducts (similar to the arrangement of the bronchi in the lungs).
  - The milk empties from the large ducts into the gland sinus and then into the teat sinus, where milk is stored during milk let-down.
  - Each teat contains an opening called a papillary duct (streak canal).
    - Some species contain multiple openings per teat (e.g., dogs), whereas other species contain a single opening (e.g., ruminants).
    - A smooth sphincter muscle controls milk flow.
  - Each gland has an associated artery, vein, and lymphatic vessel.

Gross Anatomy

- When multiple glands are located on one side of the ventral midline, they are referred to as a mammary chain.
- Each chain is a separate structure, which allows for the surgical removal of one mammary chain without affecting the other side in cases of neoplasia.
- Species have different numbers of teats—they are typically arranged in staggered pairs.
- Supernumerary teats are extra teats that may be connected to the main teat or be independent. They are often removed from milking cows and does because they can interfere with automatic milking machines.

Species	Normal Number of Teats
Bovine	4
Swine	14
Equine	2
Ovine	2
Caprine	2
Feline	10
Canine	10

Hormones

- There are three main hormones responsible for lactation.
  - **Progesterone** is secreted from the corpus luteum throughout pregnancy and promotes mammary secretory gland development.
  - **Prolactin** is secreted from the anterior pituitary gland and results in milk/colostrum production.
  - **Oxytocin** is secreted from the posterior pituitary gland and results in milk let-down.

Suggested In-Class Activities

Dissection Questions

Perform a dissection of any pregnant mammal and address the following questions.

1. Do the number of corpora lutea match the number of fetuses? Why or why not?
2. Upon entering the abdomen of a non-pregnant female, you typically encounter the omentum or intestines first. What structure did you first encounter and why?
3. In swine breeding operations, fourteen teats is a desirable attribute. Why are sows with significantly fewer teats often eliminated from the breeding herd?
4. Examine the fetus. Which trimester was it in? What evidence points to your answer?
5. After making an incision into the uterus, are you able to identify the placenta attachment type? What other species would also have this attachment type? What is the function of the placenta?
6. When examining the ovaries, do you find any raised nodules? Do they feel solid or fluid-filled? Are they more likely corpora lutea or follicles?
7. Do multiparous species have relatively larger or smaller uterine horns? Why do you think this is?

Bibliography

Aspinall V, Cappello M: Introduction to veterinary anatomy and physiology, ed 2, New York, 2009, Elsevier.

Colville T, Bassert JM: Clinical anatomy and physiology for veterinary technicians, ed 3, St Louis, 2014, Mosby.

Evans HE, deLahunta A: Miller's anatomy of the dog, ed 4, St Louis, 2013, Elsevier.

Frandson RD, Wilke WL, Fails AD: Anatomy and physiology of farm animals, ed 7, Ames, IA, 2009, Wiley-Blackwell.

Kainer RA, McCracken TO: Dog anatomy: a coloring atlas. Jackson, WY, 2003, Teton NewMedia.

Pasquini C, Spurgeon T, Pasquini S: Anatomy of domestic animals, ed 8, Pilot Point, TX, 1997, Sudz.

EXERCISES

In addition to the material in this Laboratory Manual chapter, refer to textbook Chapter 20: Pregnancy, Development, and Lactation. Thoroughly read the chapters before performing these exercises and activities.

Pregnancy

Exercise 1

Identify the Ovarian Cycle

Order the following sequence of events of the ovarian cycle (acknowledgment: these stages would not all be present at one time in an ovary) beginning with #1 in the diagram.

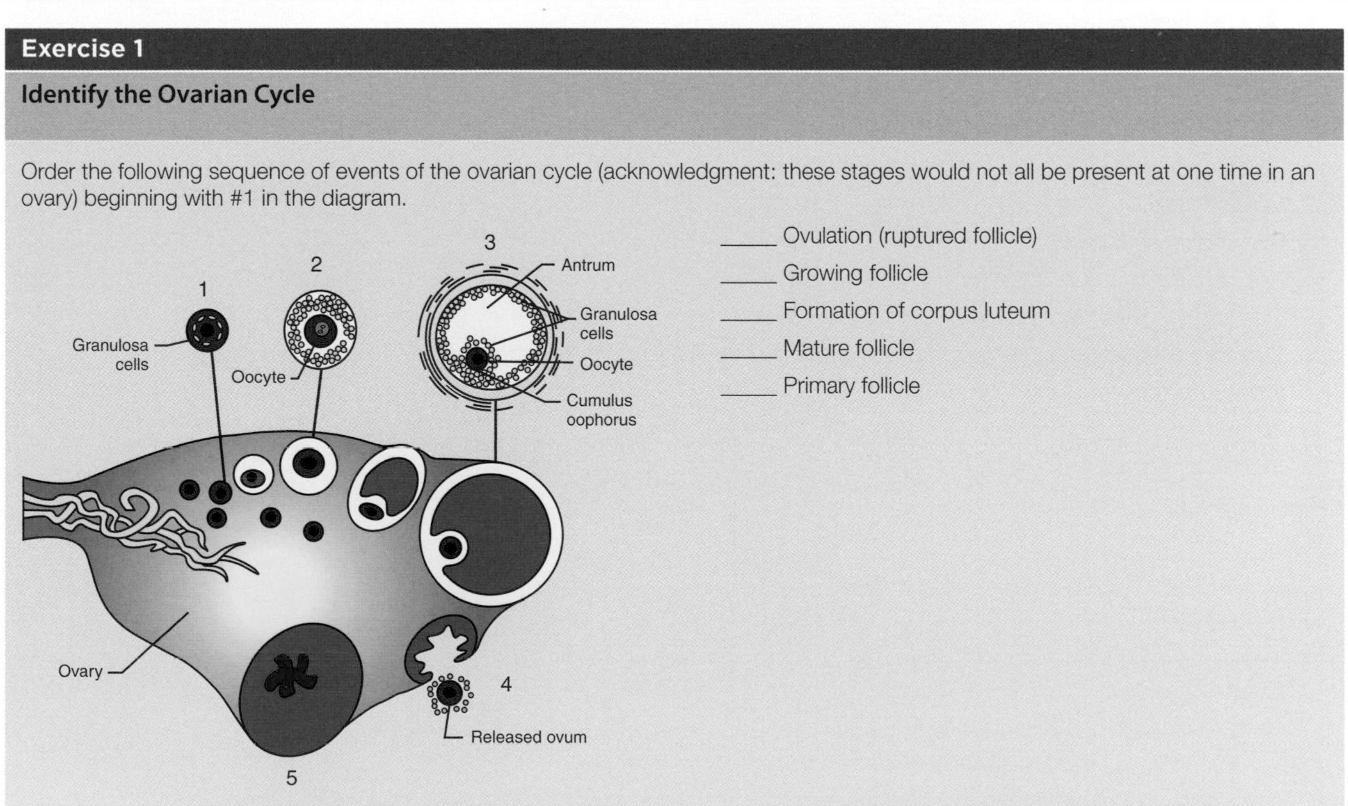

_____ Ovulation (ruptured follicle)
_____ Growing follicle
_____ Formation of corpus luteum
_____ Mature follicle
_____ Primary follicle

Exercise 2

Identify the Uterine Layers

Identify the layer of the uterus in each of the following descriptions.

1. Endometrium
2. Myometrium
3. Mesometrium

_____ High progesterone levels keep this layer quiet.
_____ The blastocyte embeds here.
_____ The mucous membranes and blood vessels of this layer enlarge during pregnancy.
_____ Contracts at time of parturition.
_____ Important to placental development.
_____ Attaches the uterus to the dorsal abdominal wall.
_____ Provides nutritional support prior to embryo implantation.
_____ The blastocyst dissolves this layer, making a small pit.
_____ Combined estrogen and prostaglandin levels increase this layer's sensitivity to oxytocin.

Exercise 3

Match the Types of Placental Attachment

Match the type of placental attachment to the descriptions. Indicate all that apply in the spaces below.

Type of Placental Attachment

Discoid ______________________________
Zonary ______________________________
Cotyledonary ______________________________
Diffuse ______________________________

1. Small, discrete, and numerous areas of attachment.
2. Seen in horses.
3. Found in rodents.
4. Seen in pigs.
5. Contains one large disc-shaped attachment site.
6. Detaches easily from the uterine lining and passed after the delivery of the newborn.
7. Increases in size throughout the pregnancy.
8. Allows entire surface of the placenta to attach to the uterine lining.
9. Seen in ruminants.
10. Seen in cattle.
11. Seen in sheep.
12. Found in rabbits.
13. Seen in goats.
14. Most complicated type of attachment.
15. Found in primates.
16. Seen in camelids.
17. Very important to ensure this type of placenta is completely delivered.
18. Contains a belt-like attachment band around the middle of the placenta.
19. Contains multiple smaller, round, raised attachment sites that resemble inverted mushroom caps.
20. Seen in carnivores.

Exercise 4

Identify the Type of Placental Attachment

Identify the type of placental attachment.

A ____________

B ____________

C ____________

D ____________

Development

Exercise 5

Clinical Thinking Challenge #1: Client Education

A client has brought her Cocker Spaniel in for a check-up. She suspects the bitch is pregnant. The 9-year-old daughter is very excited when you confirm the client's suspicion; the bitch is in the second trimester of pregnancy. The daughter asks many questions and wants to know what is going on with her dog and what they can expect as the pregnancy develops. Explain the stages of pregnancy in terms the daughter can understand.

Lactation

Exercise 6

Define Lactation Terms

Milk let-down

Involution of the mammary gland

Colostrum

Meconium

Lactation

Clinical and Critical Thinking

Exercise 7

Identify Key Female Hormones of Breeding, Gestation, Parturition, and Lactation

Complete the table by identifying the key hormone and source for each of the stages in the reproductive life of a female animal.

	Hormone	Source
Breeding	__________	__________
Gestation	__________	__________
Parturition	__________	__________
Lactation	__________	__________

Exercise 8

Clinical Thinking Challenge #2: Name the Offspring

For each of the species listed, correctly identify the name of the offspring.

Species	Offspring	Species	Offspring
Alpaca	__________	Horse	__________
Ass/donkey	__________	Llama	__________
Camel	__________	Monkey	__________
Cattle	__________	Mouse	__________
Cockroach	__________	Mule	__________
Elk	__________	Octopus	__________
Ferret	__________	Otter	__________
Fly	__________	Parrot	__________
Gerbil	__________	Rabbit	__________
Goat	__________	Rat	__________
Goose	__________	Snake	__________
Guinea pig	__________	Swan	__________
Hamster	__________	Wolf	__________
Hedgehog	__________	Worm	__________

Exercise 9

Clinical Thinking Challenge #3: Explain the Processes in the Reproductive Cycle

1. When is the full genetic map for the new animal established?

____

____

____

2. What happens during cleavage?

____

____

____

Exercise 9—cont'd

Clinical Thinking Challenge #3: Explain the Processes in the Reproductive Cycle

3. What is allantois, where is it found, and what purpose does it serve?

4. What actually happens when the "water breaks" during a pregnancy?

5. Why is it important to ensure complete placental delivery, especially in ruminant animals?

6. Precisely what triggers parturition?

7. What are the three distinct stages of parturition and what happens during each?

8. What is dystocia and what are the most common causes?

9. Describe involution of the uterus.

10. In what ways do cows' teats differ from those of other animals?

11. The udder of a high-producing dairy cow can weigh more than 100 lb at milking time. Describe the anatomic support system.

18 Avian Anatomy[a]

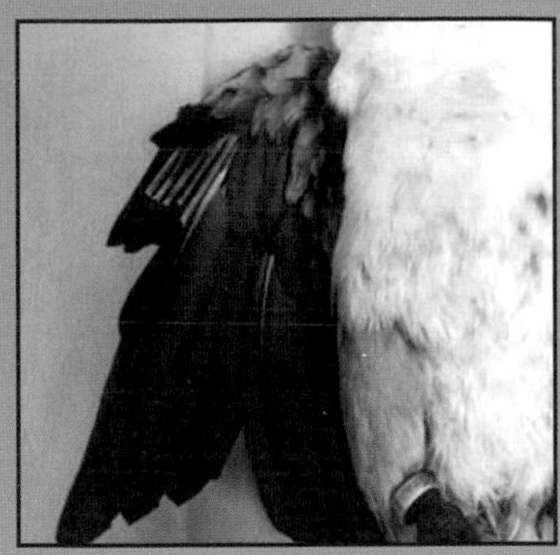

OVERVIEW AT A GLANCE

Feather Types and Structure 459

Skeletal Anatomy 460

Wing Anatomy 460

Ocular Anatomy 460

Beak Anatomy 460

Digestive Anatomy 460

Cardiac Anatomy 461

Respiratory Anatomy 461

Reproductive Anatomy 461

In-Class Necropsy Exercise 461

Exercises 466–477

Feather Types and Structure 466–468

1. *Label and Describe Feather Structure 466*
2. *Draw Feather Types 467*
3. *Feather Identification 468*

Skeletal Anatomy 469–470

4. *Explore the Avian Lightweight Skeletal Structure 469*
5. *Label an Avian Skeleton 470*

Wing Anatomy 471–472

6. *Explore an Avian Pectoralis Muscle 471*
7. *Clinical Application: Label an Avian Leg Skeleton 471*
8. *Clinical Application: Identify Avian Foot Type 472*

Ocular Anatomy 472–473

9. *Label an Avian Eye 472*
10. *Explore an Avian Eye 473*

Beak Anatomy 473

11. *Explore an Avian Beak 473*

Digestive Anatomy 474

12. *Label and Describe an Avian Digestive System 474*

Cardiac Anatomy 475

13. *Label an Avian Heart 475*

Respiratory Anatomy 475

14. *Label, Color, and Describe an Avian Respiratory System 475*

Reproductive Anatomy 476

15. *Label, Color, and Discuss an Avian Reproduction System 476*
16. *Describe Avian Ovulation 476*

Critical and Clinical Thinking 477

17. *Define the Term Necropsy 477*
18. *Explore the Anatomic Structure of the Avian Species 477*
19. *Clinical Thinking Challenge 477*

LEARNING OBJECTIVES

1. To become familiar with the anatomic structures of each body system of the bird.
2. To understand the physiologic function of each body system.
3. To identify and draw various anatomic structures.
4. To describe in detail the adaptations of various anatomic structures of the bird.
5. To apply anatomic and physiologic knowledge to clinical scenarios.

CLINICAL SIGNIFICANCE

Understanding the many unique anatomic and physiologic characteristics of the avian species, not found in mammals, is important to clinical practice. The importance of understanding these unique features and the relevance of that understanding to clinical practice can readily be noted in the following systems review.

- **The integumentary system** of the avian species is composed of the skin, glands, beaks, claws, and six types of feathers (contour, semiplume, down, filoplume, bristle, and powder down feathers).
- **The musculoskeletal system** contains the axial skeleton, appendicular skeleton, and associated muscles. The avian skeleton has several modifications that allow it to be lightweight yet strong. These are: reduction in the number of bones, fusion of bones, reduced bone density, and the loss of an internal bone matrix.
- **The senses** of birds include sight, sound, touch, taste, and smell.
- **The digestive system** of the bird is composed of the beak, mouth, esophagus, stomach, liver, pancreas, small intestines,

[a]The authors and publisher wish to acknowledge Andrea C. De Santis-Kerr for previous contributions to this chapter.

CLINICAL SIGNIFICANCE—cont'd

large intestines, and cloaca. The crop is a dilation of the esophagus in some species. It acts as a storage pouch for food. The stomach is divided into a glandular stomach, the proventriculus, and a muscular stomach, the gizzard. The cloaca is divided into three sections: the coprodeum, urodeum, and proctodeum.

- **The cardiovascular system** reveals the avian heart to consist of four chambers: the right atrium, left atrium, right ventricle, and left ventricle.
- **The respiratory system** is composed of the oral cavity, trachea, syrinx, bronchi, parabronchi, air sacs, and lungs. The syrinx is considered the "voice box" of birds. The parabronchi are connected to air capillaries and aid in gas exchange. There are a total of nine air sacs in the bird.
- **The urinary system** consists of the kidneys and ureters. Birds do not have urinary bladders.
- **The reproductive system** in males contains the testes, and in females the ovaries, infundibulum, magnum, isthmus, uterus, and vagina.

INTRODUCTION

The environmental and selective forces of our early planet sculpted birds from ancient terrestrial, reptilian-like creatures into magnificent animals capable of flight. Feathers are unique to birds, along with a specialized lightweight skeleton and an intricate series of air sacs, which are part of the avian respiratory system. These anatomic features are particularly important in enabling birds to fly. The diverse array of avian beaks or bills is also a reflection of adaptive forces, giving insight into the dietary preferences of each species. Other features of the bird include gastrointestinal structures, such as the **crop, proventriculus, gizzard,** and **cloaca. Reproductive gonads** enlarge and then shrink during the mating and nonmating seasons, respectively, to minimize weight during migration. These are some of the fascinating aspects of avian anatomy and physiology. (Read Chapter 21 from *Clinical Anatomy and Physiology for Veterinary Technicians,* before beginning this chapter.)

MATERIALS NEEDED

Preserved pigeon, for dissection
Pencil or pen
Colored pencils

TERMS TO BE IDENTIFIED

- Structures of the integumentary system
  - Feather types and feather structures
    - Contour
    - Semiplume
    - Down
    - Filoplume
    - Bristle
    - Powder down
- Structures of the axial and appendicular skeleton
  - Pectoralis muscle
- Structures of the avian eye
- Structures of the digestive system
  - Crop
  - Proventriculus
  - Gizzard
  - Cloaca
- Structures of the cardiac system
  - Right atrium
  - Left atrium
  - Left ventricle
  - Aorta
- Structures of the respiratory system
  - Syrinx
  - Lungs
  - Air sacs
- Structures of the female reproductive system
  - Ovary
  - Infundibulum
  - Magnum
  - Isthmus
  - Uterus
  - Vagina
- Necropsy images
  - Pectoral muscles
  - Heart
  - Liver
  - Spleen
  - Proventriculus
  - Gizzard
  - Cloaca

Feather Types and Structure

Feathers are unique structures associated with birds. They enable the bird to fly, but they also serve many other important functions, such as protection from environmental elements by repelling water, insulation by trapping air in the under plumage, and acting as a source of communication via seasonal and age-related plumage changes. There are six types of feathers: contour, semiplume, down, filoplume, bristle, and powder down.

Contour feathers are especially prominent on the wings and tail (see Exercise 1). Each contour feather is composed of numerous structures. The rachis is the main shaft of the feather, with the vane appearing as delicate branches along either side of the rachis. The vane consists of barbs, **barbules**, and **hooklets,** which create a weblike structure.

The degree of tightness or looseness of the "web" varies with species, resulting in differences in airflow through the feathers. The **inferior umbilicus** is located at the base of the feather and acts as a passage for blood vessels to nourish developing feathers. Other structures of the feather include the superior umbilicus, originating at the site of the webbed part of the feather, and the calamus or quill, which begins at the inferior umbilicus and concludes at the superior umbilicus.

Skeletal Anatomy

The avian skeleton has several modifications that create a lightweight structure, enabling the bird to take flight. A reduction in the number of bones and fusion of specific bones to create bony plates should be noted when studying the avian skeleton. Reduced bone density and loss of an internal bone matrix are also important evolutionary modifications that add to the bird's flying capability.

Structures of the avian skeleton can be classified as part of the axial skeleton or the appendicular skeleton. The axial skeleton consists of the skull, vertebral column, and sternum. The vertebral column is divided into five sections: cervical vertebrae, thoracic vertebrae, lumbar vertebrae, sacral vertebrae, and coccygeal vertebrae. The number of vertebrae in the bird differs considerably from that of mammals. One of the most notable areas of difference is the cervical vertebrae. Birds possess anywhere from 11 to 25 cervical vertebrae depending on the species. Mammals have seven cervical vertebrae. Another unique feature of the bird is the formation of a bony plate called the synsacrum. Several of the lumbar vertebrae, sacral vertebrae, and coccygeal vertebrae fuse to form the synsacrum. The most caudal coccygeal vertebrae in the bird are also fused to form the pygostyle, which supports the tail feathers. The cranial coccygeal vertebrae are mobile, allowing the bird to adjust feather movement and aid in flight. The sternum is also included in the framework of the axial skeleton. It is concave in shape and contains a bony ridge known as the keel in certain species of birds. The sternum acts as a place of attachment for several muscles, including the flight muscles.

The appendicular skeleton consists of the pectoral girdle, wings, pelvic girdle, legs, and feet—all of which aid the bird in movement, whether on the ground or in the air. The coracoids, scapulas, and clavicles form the pectoral girdle, also known as the shoulder. The humerus is an important bone extending from the shoulder to the elbow that acts as the site of attachment of the wing muscles. The radius and ulna form the forearm, extending from the elbow to the wrist. The pelvic girdle also consists of several bones: the ileum, ischium, and pubis. The ileum is fused to the synsacrum, and the ischium and pubis are fused to the ileum anteriorly. Four bones make up the avian leg. They are the femur, tibiotarsus, fibula, and tarsometatarsus.

Wing Anatomy

The **pectoralis muscle** and the supracoracoideus muscle are two essential muscular components that generate wing motion. Upon contraction, the pectoralis is responsible for creating the downstroke of the wing. Conversely, the supracoracoideus is responsible for creating the upstroke. Together, these muscles, along with the assistance of the skeletal system, provide the bird's ability to fly.

Ocular Anatomy

The avian eye is a highly developed structure. It consists of three layers: the fibrous tunic, uveal tunic, and neural tunic. The sclera, cornea, and sclerotic ring are the framework for the fibrous tunic. The cornea is the transparent portion of the outer anterior surface of the eye. It is protected by three eyelids: the upper eyelid, lower eyelid, and the nictitating membrane or "third eyelid." The uveal tunic consists of the choroids, iris, and ciliary muscles. The most inner tunic is the neural tunic in which the retina is located. Photoreceptor cells, such as rods and cones, are contained inside the retina. Cones are associated with daylight and color vision, whereas rods are responsible for aiding in night vision. The bird has a significantly increased number of photoreceptor cells compared with mammals, accounting for its excellent visual acuity.

Beak Anatomy

A bird's beak is an important structure that is used for eating, grooming, carrying items, and as a means of protection. The beak consists of an upper and a lower mandible. A keratin layer grows continuously over the mandible. In captive birds, whose environmental access is limited, the beak will often need to be trimmed because of the bird's inability to wear down the keratin.

Beaks are physically adapted to the variable dietary needs and foraging habits of different types of birds, such as seedeaters, woodpeckers, raptors, and shorebirds. A thick beak can act as a crushing device, whereas a blunt beak acts as a chisel. Meat eaters (raptors) have a sharp beak for tearing muscle, as opposed to many shorebirds, which have a long beak that is better adapted to foraging in sandy areas.

Digestive Anatomy

The avian digestive system is adapted to maximize energy from what is consumed, to meet a high metabolic rate. Many of the digestive organs have modifications from those seen in mammals. The digestive system is composed of the beak, mouth, esophagus, stomach, liver, pancreas, small intestine, large intestine, and **cloaca.** For purposes of this laboratory manual, we will focus on those structures unique to the avian species.

The esophagus assists in the movement of ingesta from the mouth into the stomach. In many species of birds, the esophagus has an area of dilation where food can be stored. This area is known as the **crop** and varies from a simple dilation or single pouch to a double pouch, depending on the species of bird.

The stomach of a bird can be divided into two sections: a glandular stomach known as the **proventriculus** and a muscular stomach known as the **gizzard**. The main function of the proventriculus is to initiate chemical digestion of ingesta through the use of mucosal and digestive glands. The gizzard functions to grind coarse ingesta.

The cloaca is the final structure of the digestive system and is found in both birds and reptiles. It is divided into three sections: the coprodeum (receives waste from the intestines), the urodeum (receives waste from the urogenital system), and the proctodeum (stores waste). The waste products are then expelled through an opening known as the vent.

Cardiac Anatomy

Birds have a four-chambered heart similar to those of mammals. The right ventricle receives deoxygenated blood from the **right atrium** and subsequently pumps the blood into the lungs where it becomes oxygenated. The **left atrium** receives the oxygenated blood from the lungs and transports it to the **left ventricle**, where it is pumped to the rest of the body through the **aorta**.

Respiratory Anatomy

The important structures of the avian respiratory system include the trachea, syrinx, bronchi, parabronchi, air sacs, and lungs. The trachea, or "windpipe," is made up of cartilaginous rings and receives air from the mouth and nasal structures. The air then passes into the bronchi, the area where the trachea bifurcates. The two bronchi are directed into each side of the lungs and terminate in the posterior air sacs. When the bronchi enter the **lungs** they are called mesobronchi and they lack their earlier cartilaginous structure. Secondary bronchi, called ventrobronchi, diverge from the mesobronchi and give rise to parabronchi. Gas exchange between air capillaries and blood capillaries occurs at the parabronchi level.

As detailed in the textbook, the **syrinx** is considered the sound-producing organ or "voice box" of a bird. It is a tracheal enlargement situated above the level of the sternum. Specialized vibrating membranes are contained within the syrinx. These membranes are stimulated when air is moved over them, creating sound. The vocal muscles then determine the sophistication of the vocalization. This is demonstrated in songbirds, who have much more developed vocal muscles than other avian species, allowing them to produce more elaborate vocalizations.

There are nine air sacs within the respiratory system. Eight of these are paired (cranial thoracic, caudal thoracic, cervical, and abdominal air sacs) and one is unpaired (interclavicular air sac). They serve to maintain air volume while providing warmth and humidification, aiding in thermoregulation, and providing buoyancy when necessary.

Reproductive Anatomy

The gonads are organs that produce reproductive cells called gametes. The gonads in the female bird consist of the **ovaries**, with the left ovary functional and the right ovary acting as a rudimentary structure. The testes are the gonads of a male bird.

During ovulation, an egg, or ovum, is released from the follicle of the ovary and passed into the oviduct. The oviduct consists of five sections: the **infundibulum**, **magnum**, **isthmus**, **uterus**, and **vagina**. Each structure has a specific function, such as grasping the ovum as it enters the oviduct (infundibulum), depositing the albumin or "egg white" (magnum), and forming the keratin shell membrane and hard exterior shell (isthmus).

In-class Necropsy Exercise

Description of Exercise

A necropsy is a postmortem examination of an animal cadaver. Participating in necropsy procedures is another important aspect of veterinary technology. This exercise will outline the initial basic steps of an avian necropsy. It can also be used to supplement an avian dissection laboratory.

Procedure

1. The first step in a necropsy is to wear the appropriate protective clothing, including a laboratory coat, disposable surgical gloves, and face mask or eye shield as needed.
2. Assemble your equipment, including instruments for dissection, a scale to weigh the carcass, and a camera to photograph any lesions found.
3. Weigh the carcass (note whether it is wet or dry) (Fig. 18.1).
4. Examine the external features of the carcass. Keep a systematic approach to ensure you examine all external structures. You may want to work from head to tail, starting with the oral cavity and beak (Fig. 18.2). Examine the external auditory meatuses. They will be covered by feathers known as ear coverts. Examine the eyelids and eyes (Fig. 18.3). Now examine the feathers, skin, feet, and cloaca.
5. For the internal examination, the feathers on the ventral surface of the body should be plucked (Fig. 18.4). The carcass is first moistened with disinfectant.
6. The carcass is positioned on its back with its ventral surface exposed. The carcass may need to be secured to the table with a suitable method such as rope restraints.

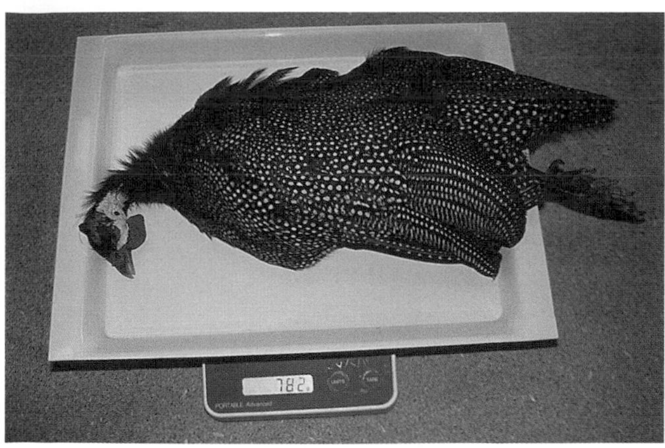

• **Fig. 18.1** Helmeted guinea fowl before examination. Collection of body weights of specimens is an integral part of a necropsy. (From Samour J: Avian medicine, London, 2000, Mosby.)

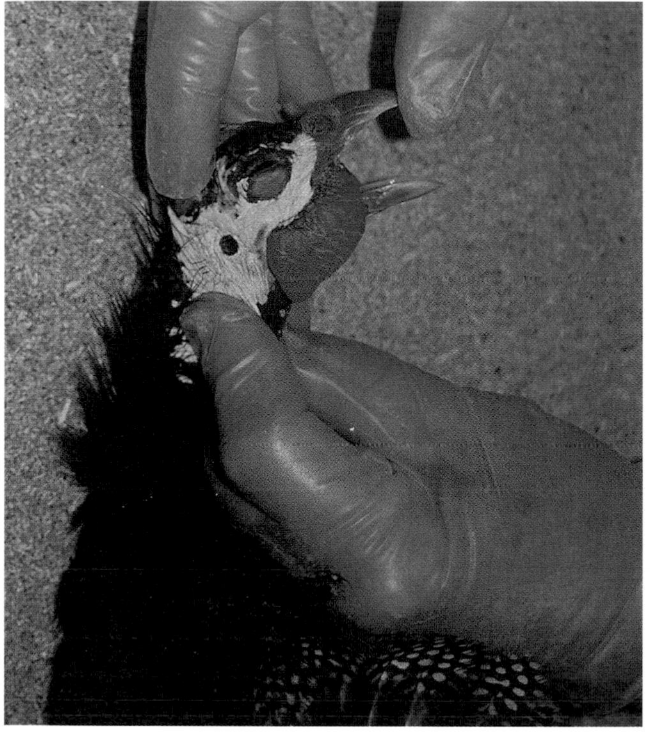

• **Fig. 18.2** Examination of the oral cavity and the beak. (From Samour J: Avian medicine, London, 2000, Mosby.)

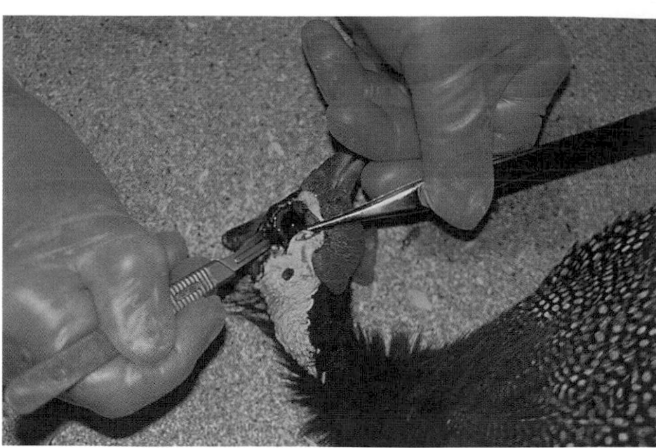

• **Fig. 18.3** Examine the eyes by deflecting the eyelids. (From Samour J: Avian medicine, London, 2000, Mosby.)

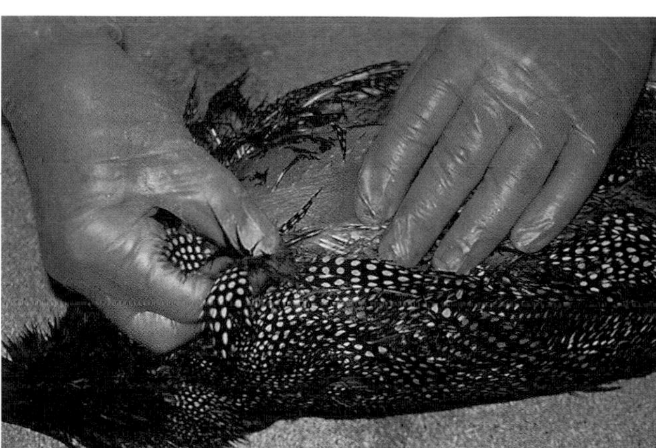

• **Fig. 18.4** Carefully pluck the feathers of the ventral surface of the body, using the other hand to tense the skin to avoid tearing. (From Samour J: Avian medicine, London, 2000, Mosby.)

7. The skin is removed to expose the ribs and the muscles of the thorax, abdomen, and legs. Identify the **pectoral muscles** (Fig. 18.5).

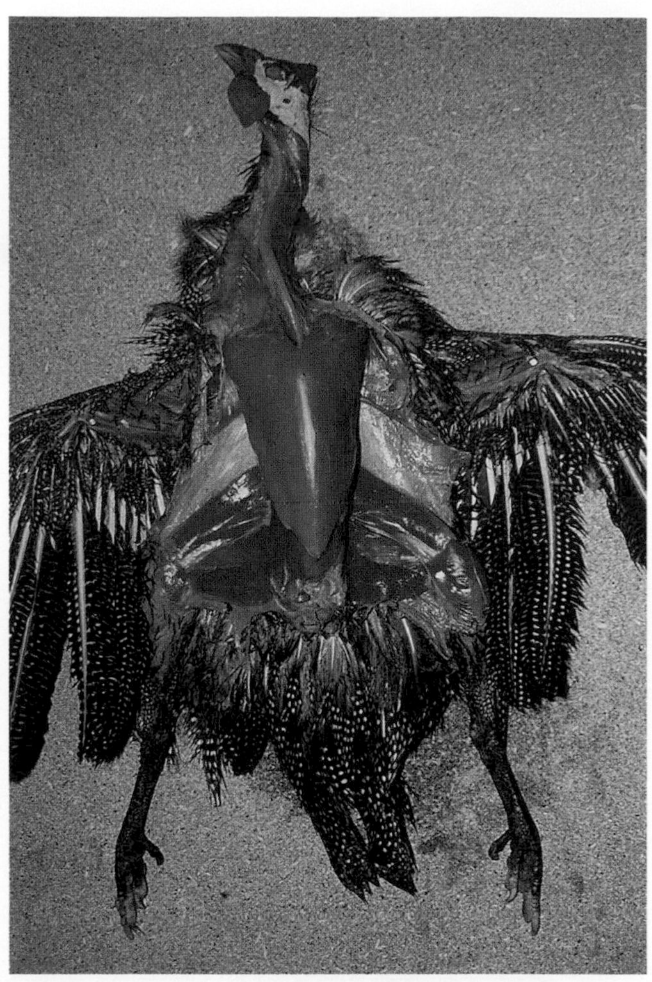

• **Fig. 18.5** Deflect the skin by blunt dissection to expose the subcutaneous tissues of the neck, pectoral muscles, rib cage, and abdominal and leg muscles. (From Samour J: Avian medicine, London, 2000, Mosby.)

8. Make a small incision near the cloaca and extend it cranially to the sternum. This exposes the organs in the abdominal cavity. Identify the **cloaca** (Fig. 18.6).

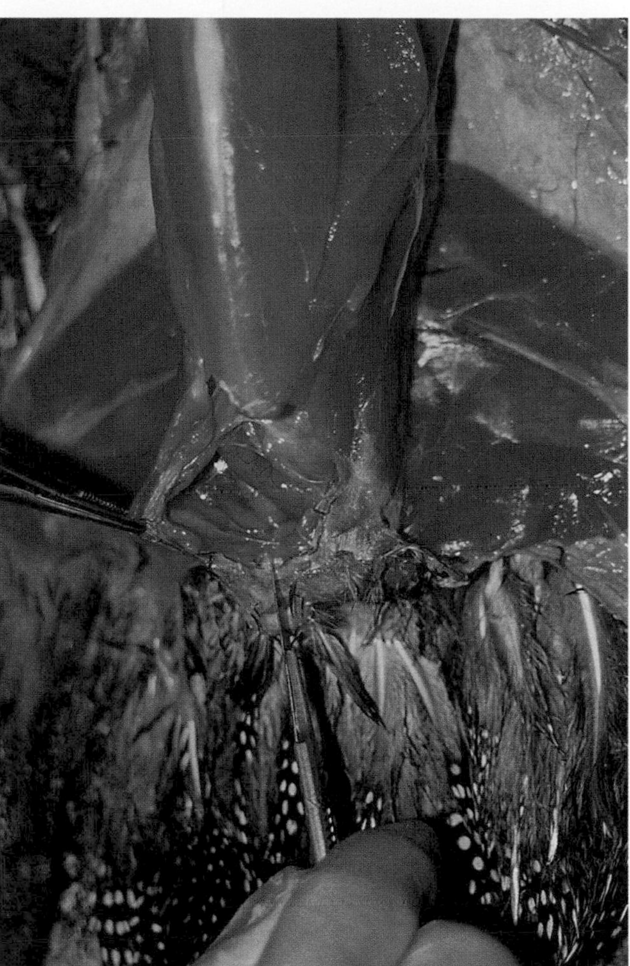

• **Fig. 18.6** Make a small incision in the abdominal wall near the cloaca using fine scissors to expose the abdominal viscera. Enlarge it forward to the sternum and open the abdomen. (From Samour J: Avian medicine, London, 2000, Mosby.)

9. Expose the thoracic cavity by cutting the rib cage, coracoid, and clavicles from both sides (Fig. 18.7). It is then reflected, along with the pectoral muscles, to expose the underlying organs. Identify the **heart**, **liver**, and **gizzard** (Fig. 18.8).

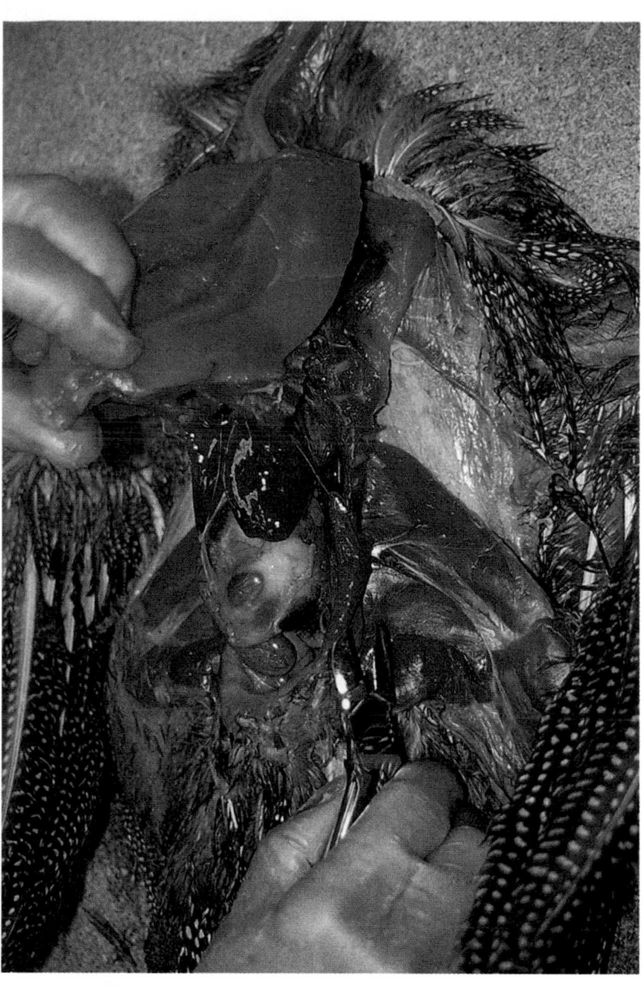

• Fig. 18.7 The abdominal cavity has been exposed and the sternum partly deflected anteriorly to expose part of the lung on one side, the liver overlapping part of the gizzard, the duodenal loop surrounding the pancreas, and a small part of the lower intestinal tract. (From Samour J: Avian medicine, London, 2000, Mosby.)

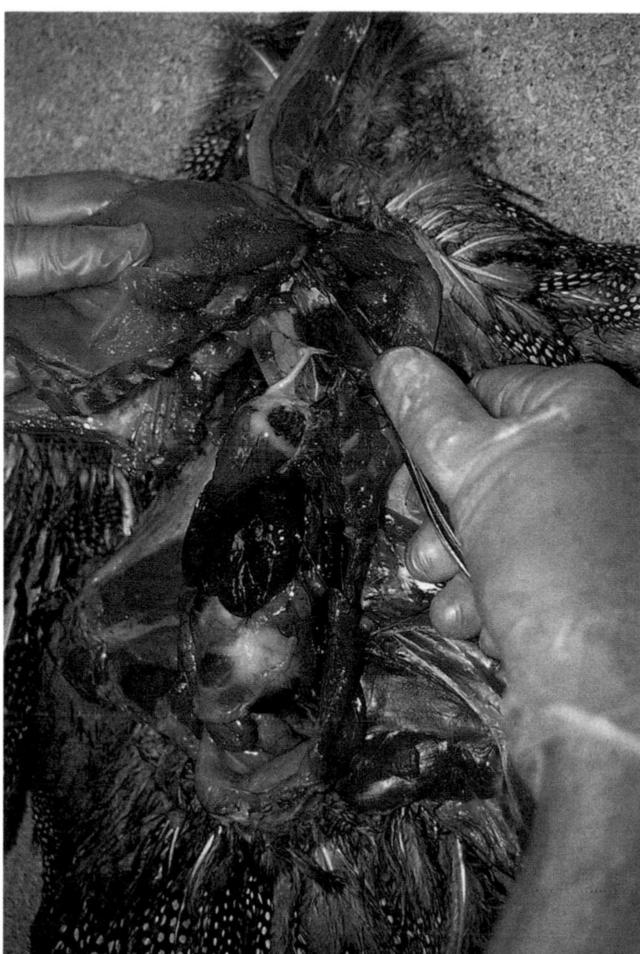

• Fig. 18.8 Deflect the sternum to the right side of the bird to expose the left lung, heart, liver, left kidney, gizzard, and part of the gut. (From Samour J: Avian medicine, London, 2000, Mosby.)

10. To better visualize other internal structures, partially remove the liver (Fig. 18.9). Identify the heart, **spleen**, **proventriculus**, and gizzard (Fig. 18.10).
11. Examination of the internal structures of the thoracic and abdominal cavity requires a systematic approach to ensure that all structures are examined. One method of accomplishing this objective is to examine structures according to body systems. This would follow a format similar to the one listed below:
    a. Cardiovascular and respiratory systems: heart, cardiac vessels, trachea, syrinx, lungs, and air sacs
    b. Endocrine system: thyroid glands and adrenal glands
    c. Digestive system: liver, esophagus, crop, proventriculus, gizzard, small intestines, and large intestines
    d. Lymphoreticular system: spleen
    e. Urinary system: kidneys
    f. Reproductive system: left ovary and left oviduct (female); testes (male)

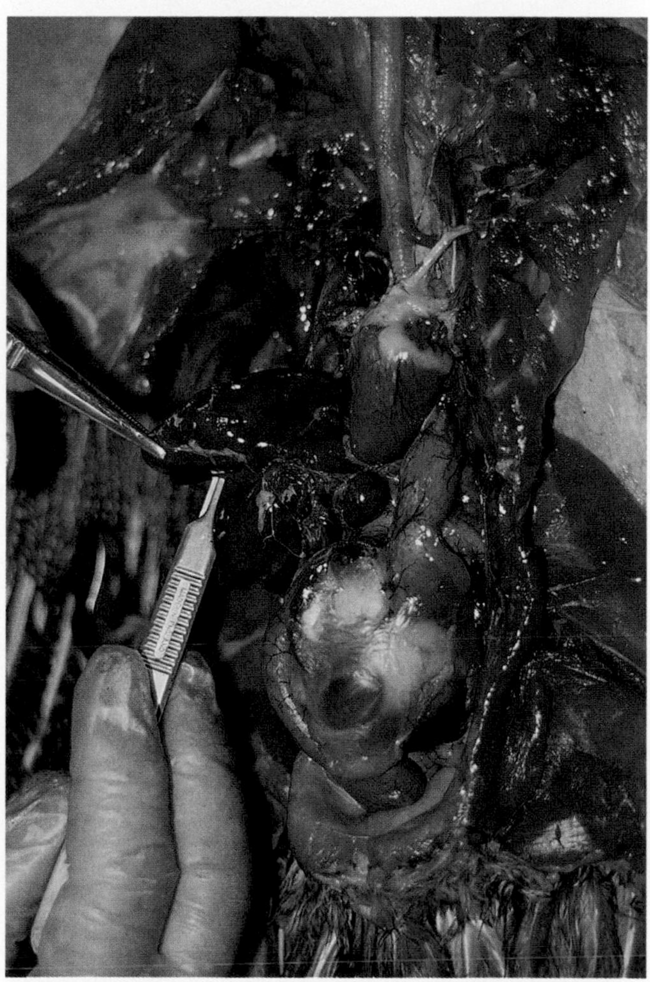

• **Fig. 18.9** The liver has been carefully removed and deflected to one side, exposing the oval-shaped spleen, which is situated between the proventriculus and the liver and gallbladder. The heart is anterior and the gizzard posterior to the spleen. (From Samour J: Avian medicine, London, 2000, Mosby.)

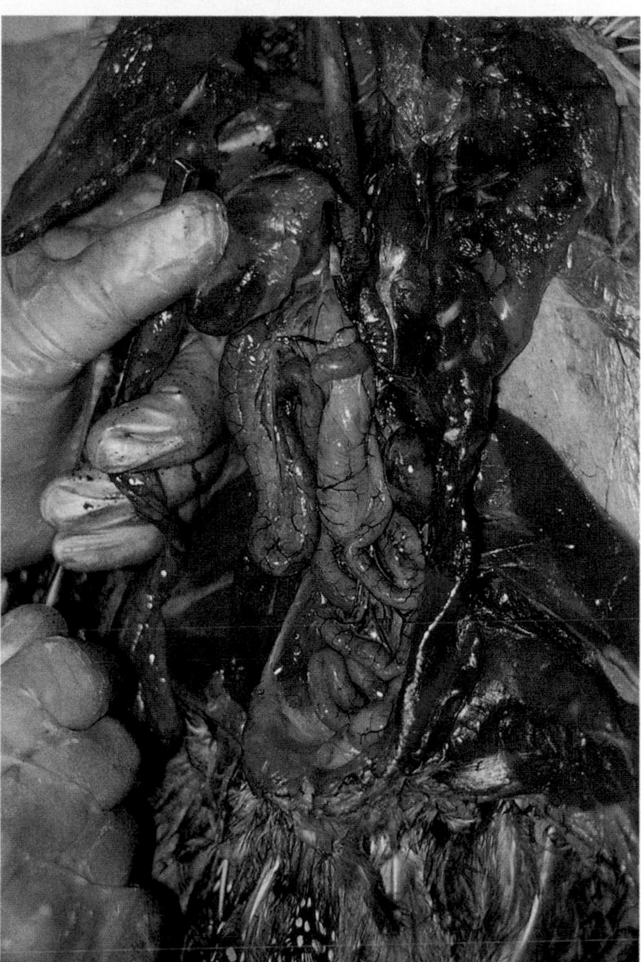

• **Fig. 18.10** The gizzard is deflected to show where the left bronchus has been cut immediately posterior to the syrinx. The left testis is visible immediately posterior to the left lung. (From Samour J: Avian medicine, London, 2000, Mosby.)

EXERCISES

Feather Types and Structure

Exercise 1

Label and Describe Feather Structure

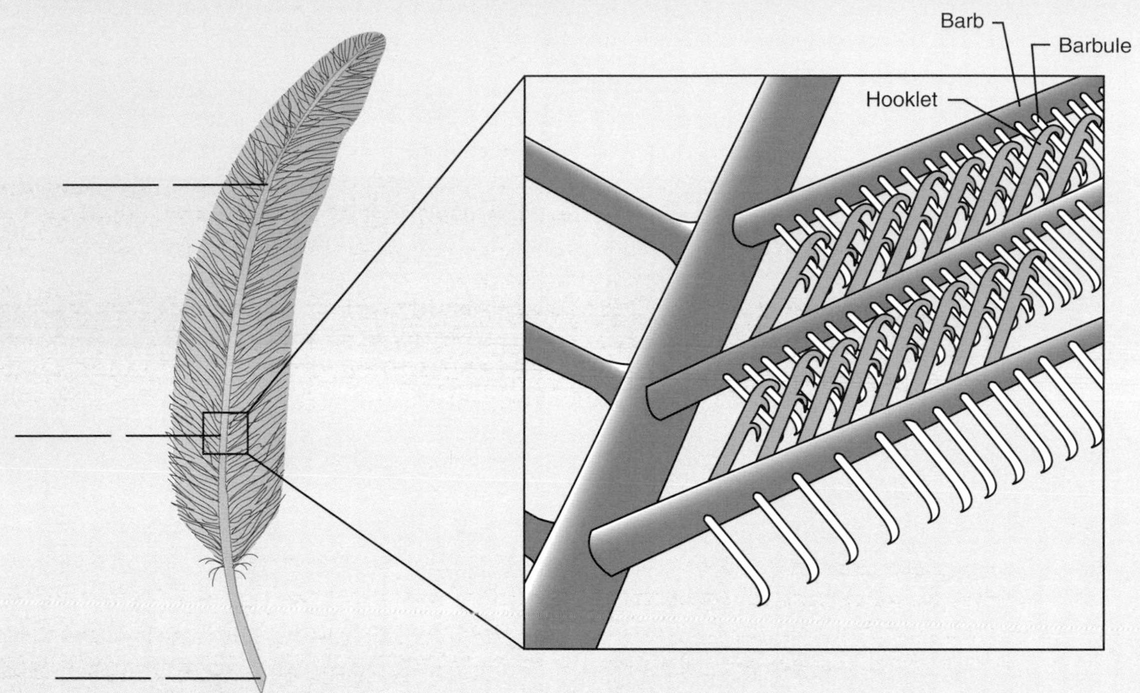

1. Label the inferior umbilicus on the drawing.
2. What is the function of the inferior umbilicus?

   ____

3. Label the rachis on the drawing.
4. Provide a definition for rachis:

   ____

   ____

5. Label the vane on the drawing. The three components of the vane include the barbs, barbules, and hooklets.
6. What is the function of these components? ______________________________

   ____

   ____

Exercise 2

Draw Feather Types

Draw the following feather types in the boxes provided below: contour feather, semiplume feather, down feather, filoplume feather, and bristle feather.

Contour

Filoplume

Semiplume

Bristle

Down

Exercise 3

Feather Identification

Identify the type of feather in each of the four examples.

1: ____________________

a. Contour
b. Filoplume
c. Bristle
d. Semiplume
e. None of the above

Question 1

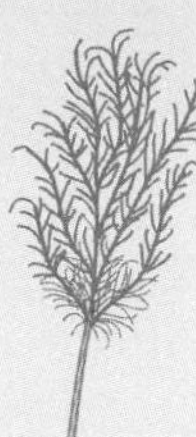

3: ____________________

a. Contour
b. Filoplume
c. Bristle
d. Semiplume
e. None of the above

Question 3

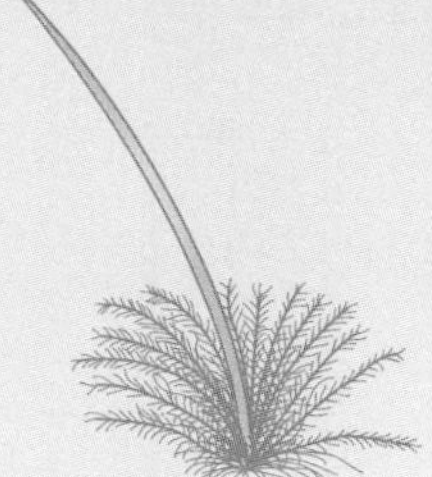

2: ____________________

a. Down
b. Filoplume
c. Bristle
d. Semiplume
e. None of the above

Question 2

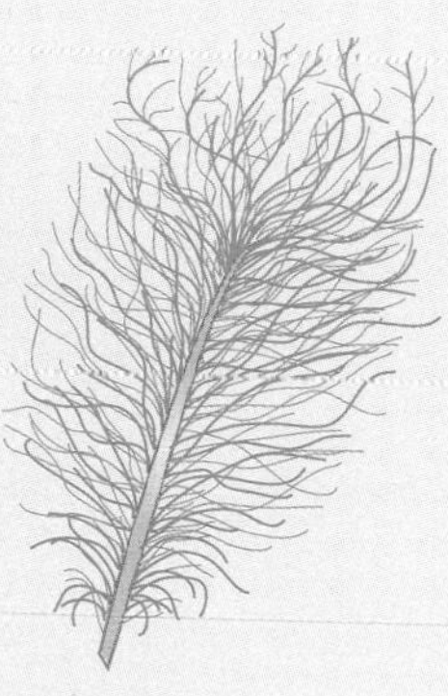

4: ____________________

a. Down
b. Filoplume
c. Bristle
d. Semiplume
e. None of the above

Question 4

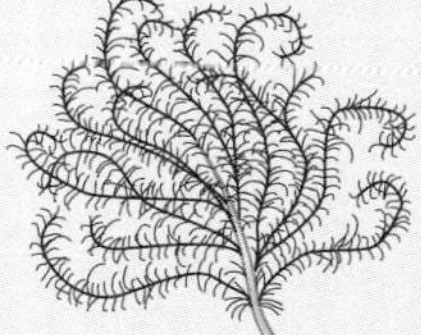

Skeletal Anatomy

Exercise 4

Explore the Avian Lightweight Skeletal Structure

What four evolutionary modifications of the avian skeleton account for its lightweight nature?

1. ______________________________

2. ______________________________

3. ______________________________

4. ______________________________

Exercise 5

Label an Avian Skeleton

Label the structures listed below on the diagram:

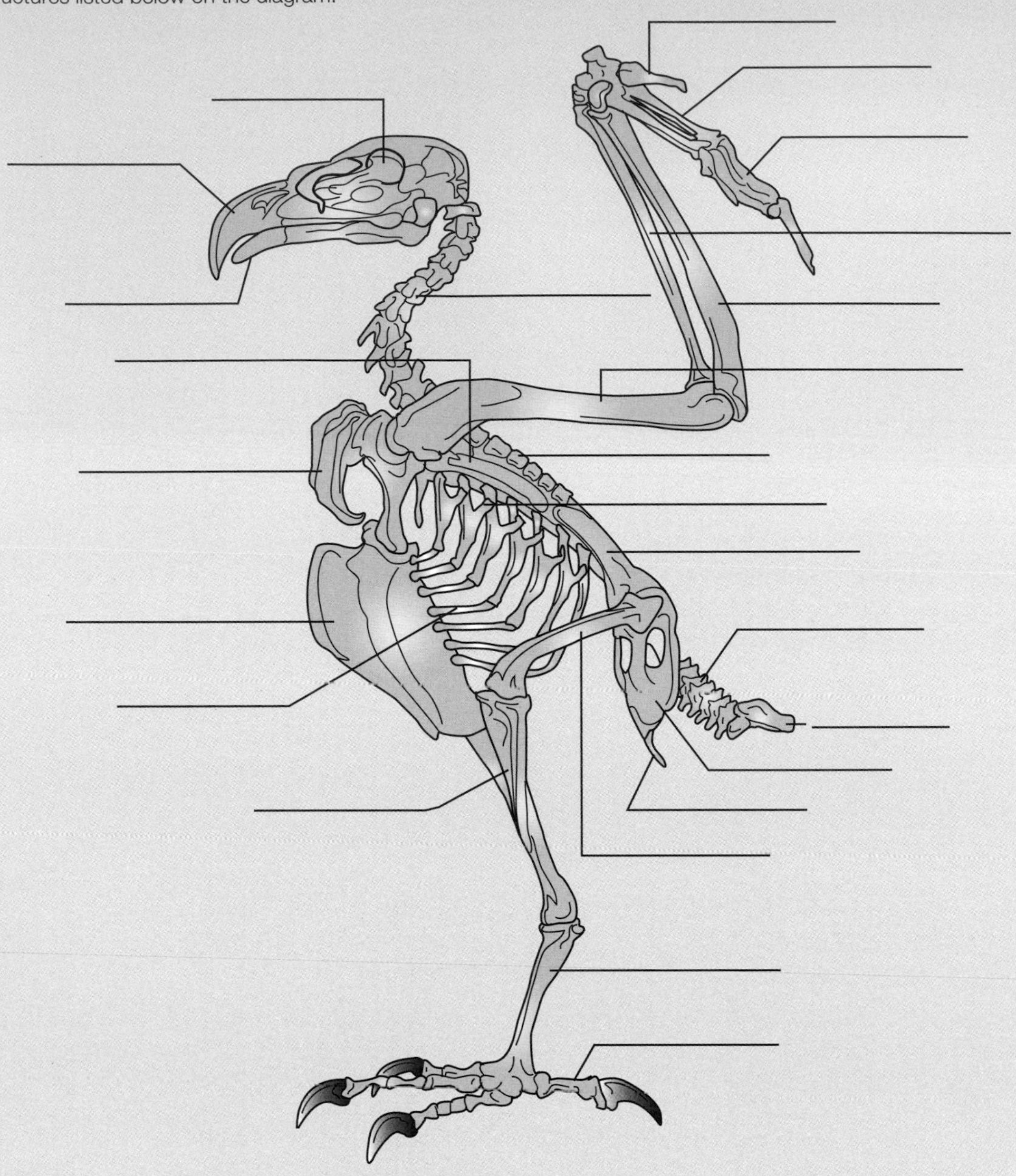

Orbit	Coccygeal vertebrae	Humerus
Cervical vertebrae	Sternum	Radius
Thoracic vertebrae	Coracoid	Ulna
Synsacrum	Scapula	Femur
Upper mandible	Lower mandible	Hallux
Complete rib	Tibiotarsus	Ischium
Tarsometatarsus	Pubis	Second digit
Pygostyle	Uncinate process	
Major metacarpal	Alula (first digit)	

Wing Anatomy

Exercise 6

Explore an Avian Pectoralis Muscle

Where does the pectoralis muscle originate and where is its insertion?

1. Origin ______________________________

2. Insertion ______________________________

Exercise 7

Clinical Application: Label an Avian Leg Skeleton

In clinical practice, you will be responsible for radiographing various structures in avian patients. It is essential to understand avian anatomy to ensure all appropriate structures are included in your radiographic view. The two figures below represent a radiograph of an avian leg from a cockatoo and a corresponding schematic diagram. Identify the following structures on the radiograph and the schematic: femur, tibiotarsus, tarsometatarsus, and phalanges.

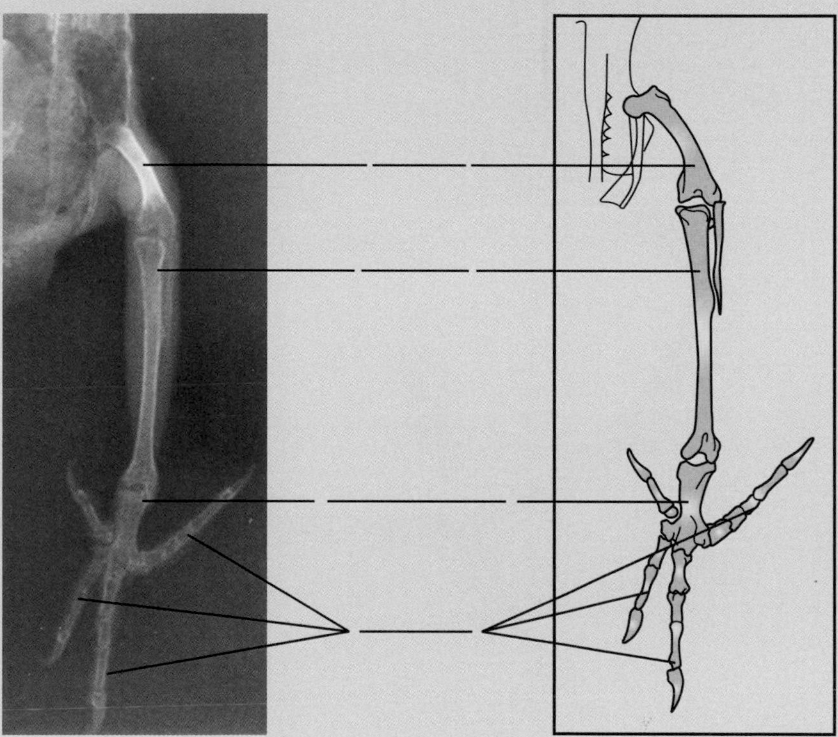

Exercise 8

Clinical Application: Identify Avian Foot Type

Based on the radiograph and schematic of the cockatoo in the previous question, is this bird considered *anisodactyl* or *zygodactyl?*

Why? ____

____

____

Ocular Anatomy

Exercise 9

Label an Avian Eye

Label the structures listed below on the figure:

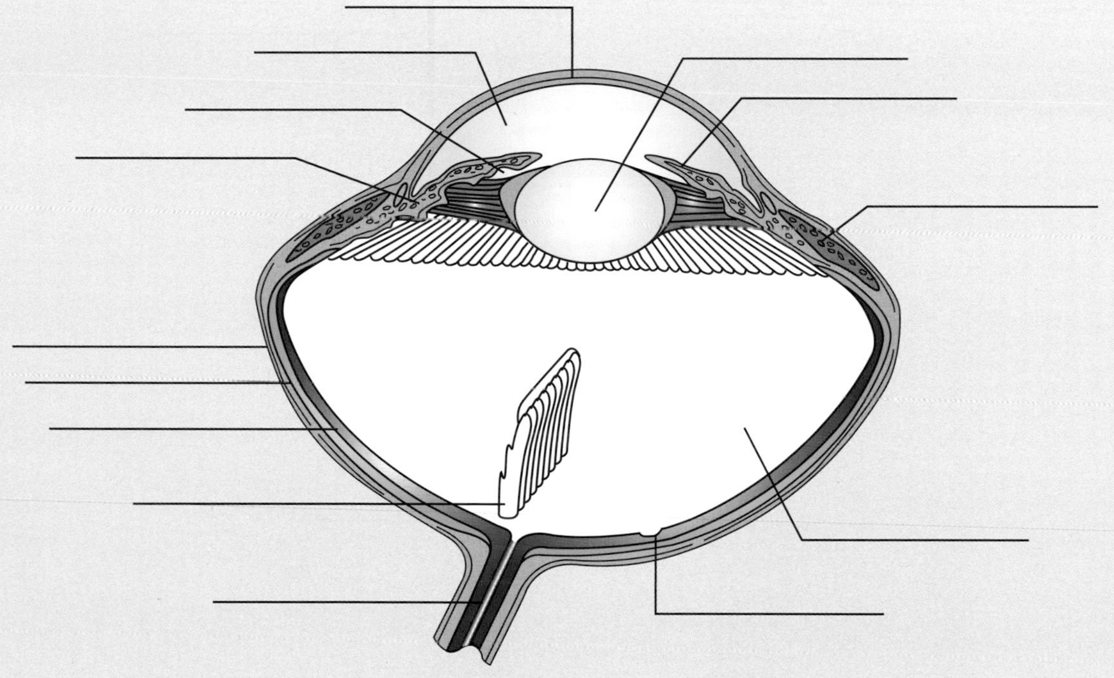

Sclera	Choroid	Lens
Cornea	Iris	Anterior chamber
Sclerotic ring	Retina	Posterior chamber
Optic nerve	Pecten	Ciliary body
Vitreous	Central fovea	

Exercise 10

Explore an Avian Eye

There are three tissue layers within the avian eye: the fibrous tunic, uveal tunic, and neural tunic. Name the structures that compose each of these layers.

Fibrous tunic ______________________________

____

Uveal tunic ______________________________

____

Neural tunic ______________________________

____

Beak Anatomy

Exercise 11

Explore an Avian Beak

Based on your readings from the textbook and your knowledge of the variation in beak structure, describe the type of beak for each of the birds that follow and indicate how the beak aids in consumption and foraging.

1. Seed eaters ______________________________

   ____

2. Woodpeckers ______________________________

   ____

3. Raptors ______________________________

   ____

4. Shorebirds ______________________________

   ____

Digestive Anatomy

Exercise 12

Label and Describe an Avian Digestive System

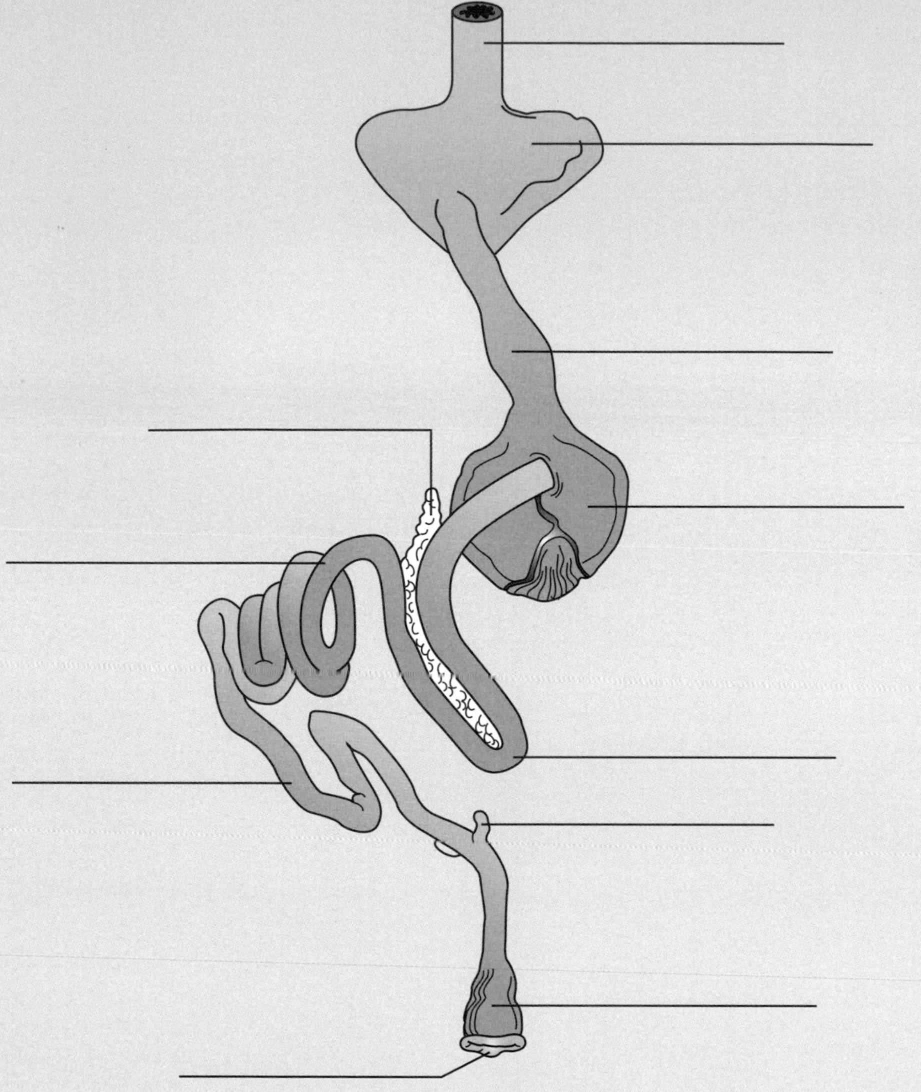

1. Label the crop on the drawing, and then define the function of the crop. ______________________________

____

2. Label the proventriculus, and then define the function of the proventriculus. ______________________________

____

3. Label the gizzard, and then define the function of the gizzard. ______________________________

____

4. Label the cloaca, and then define the function of the cloaca. ______________________________

____

5. Label the esophagus, vent, pancreas, ileum, jejunum, rudimentary ceca, and duodenum.

Cardiac Anatomy

Exercise 13

Label an Avian Heart

Label the following structures on the diagram: right atrium, left atrium, right ventricle, left ventricle, right coronary artery, pulmonary trunk, right and left pulmonary arteries, right and left brachiocephalic trunk, and aorta.

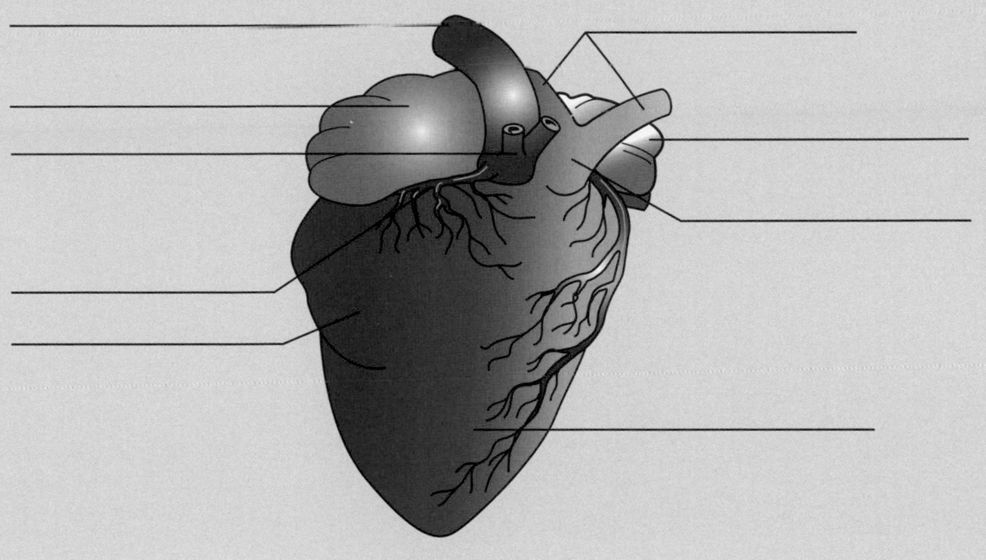

Respiratory Anatomy

Exercise 14

Label, Color, and Describe an Avian Respiratory System

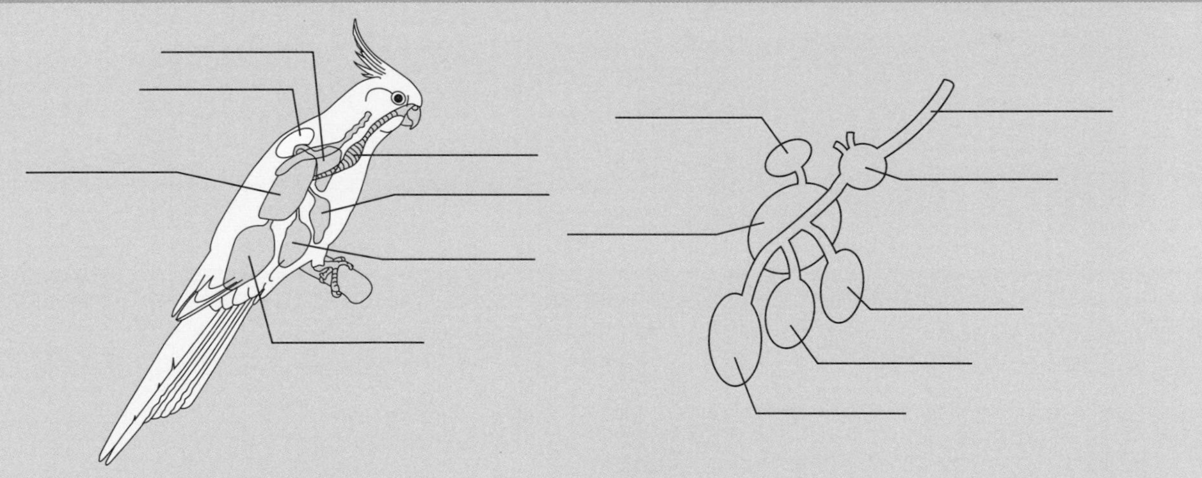

1. How does a bird create sound using the syrinx? ____
____
____
2. Label and shade in the following air sacs: cranial thoracic, caudal thoracic, cervical, abdominal, and interclavicular, as well as the lung and trachea.
3. What are the three functions of the air sacs?
   a. ____
   b. ____
   c. ____

Reproductive Anatomy

Exercise 15

Label, Color, and Discuss an Avian Reproduction System

Using colored pencils, label and shade in the following structures: ovary, infundibulum, magnum, isthmus, uterus, and vagina.

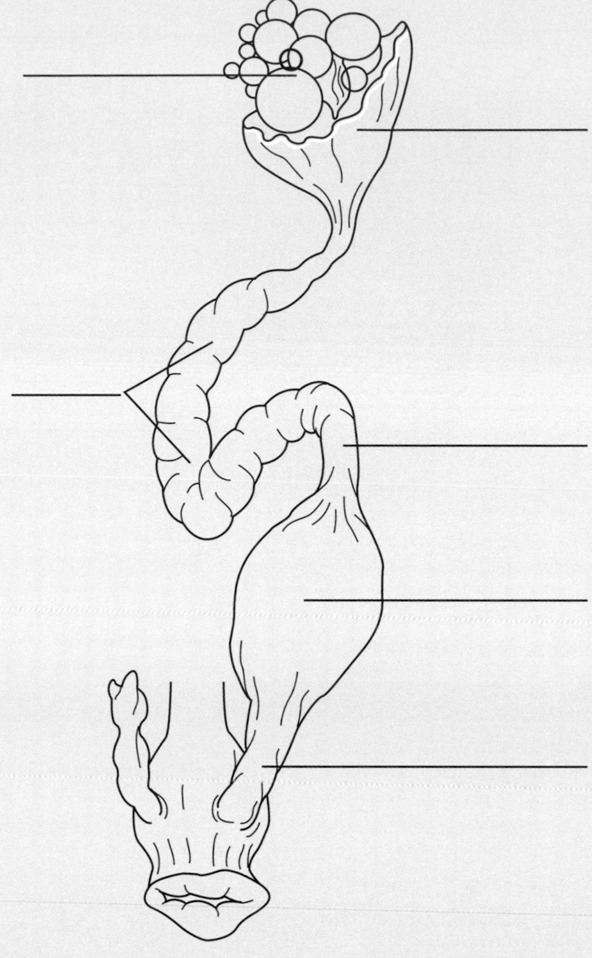

Exercise 16

Describe Avian Ovulation

Describe the process of ovulation and the function of each anatomic structure of the oviduct: ______________________________

____

____

____

____

____

____

Critical and Clinical Thinking

Exercise 17

Define the Term Necropsy

Exercise 18

Explore the Anatomic Structure of the Avian Species

1. Name the three chambers of the ear:
2. Name the three pairs of bones that compose the pectoral girdle:
3. Name the bony structure that acts as a "shock absorber" when a bird lands from flight:
4. Name the arteries that supply blood to the flight muscles:
5. Name the three parts of the cloaca:
6. Name the bronchi that are connected to air capillaries and function in gas exchange:
7. Name the air sac that extends into the humerus, sternum, syrinx, and pectoral girdle:
8. Name the avian cell that is equivalent to the mammalian neutrophil:
9. Name which ovary in female birds is nonfunctional:
10. Name the avian third eyelid:
11. Name the web of skin (extending from the shoulder to the wrist) that aids in aerodynamics:
12. Name the major skin gland of birds, located at the upper base of the tail:

Exercise 19

Clinical Thinking Challenge

Support each of the following correct statements with appropriate rationale, stating why or in what way each statement is correct.

1. Depressor muscles are important to thermal fluctuation. Unlike mammals, birds do not possess sweat glands.
2. Beaks vary in their hardness and flexibility, and function in many ways.

Continued

Exercise 19—cont'd

Clinical Thinking Challenge

3. For birds in captivity, beak and claw maintenance is critical to a bird's health.

4. Feathers serve several important functions.

5. The configuration of owl feathers allows silent flight.

6. In some species, such as Mallard ducks *(Anas platyrhynchos)* and European starlings *(Sturnus vulgaris),* the males of the species appear more colorful before the breeding season.

7. During feather development, a growing feather is called a blood feather.

8. The lightweight nature of the skeleton is due to several factors.

9. In most species of birds, the sternum is large and concave for two main reasons.

10. When handling birds, and especially when restraining them, it is important not to apply excessive pressure over the keel.

11. The two most prominent muscle pairs controlling the wings are those responsible for depressing and elevating the wing. Both pairs originate on the sternum but differ in where they insert.

12. In birds, the position of the eyes on the head differs among species and appears to depend on their feeding habits.

13. Birds are sensitive when just the tips of their feathers are touched.

14. Egestion of pellets can be used as a clinical indicator of normal gastrointestinal mobility in some species.

15. The cloaca is located at the end of the digestive tract and is divided into three sections.

16. Evaluation of a bird's mutes is an important diagnostic tool in assessing overall health.

Exercise 19—cont'd

Clinical Thinking Challenge

17. The delivery of oxygen and removal of carbon dioxide from the body tissues must be quick and efficient.

18. Air sacs are connected to the primary bronchi (abdominal sacs) or ventrobronchi (cervical, cranial thoracic, caudal thoracic, and interclavicular sacs) and serve several functions.

19. In the avian species, each breath of air reaches the lung capillaries with the maximum amount of oxygen possible—close to the 21% present in atmospheric air.

20. In chickens, the nitrogenous waste eliminated by the kidneys consists of 75% uric acid and this is significant for several reasons.

21. Lengthwise, the avian oviduct can be divided into five sections.

Glossary

A

abomasum: Animals not containing a single stomach have, instead, a multichambered system comprised of a reticulum, rumen, omasum, and abomasum.

accessory carpal bone: The accessory carpal bone protrudes backward on the lateral side of the carpus (useful landmark for radiography).

acetabulum: The socket portion of the ball-and-socket hip joint. It is formed at the junction of the ilium, ischium, and pubis bones of the pelvis.

action: The body movement that a contraction of the muscle will produce.

adipose tissue: Adipose connective tissue is fat.

afferent glomerular arterioles: Arterioles that carry blood into the glomerulus for filtration.

air sacs: The respiratory system is composed of the oral cavity, trachea, syrinx, bronchi, parabronchi, air sacs, and lungs. There are a total of nine air sacs in the bird.

anconeal process: A "beak shaped" process at the proximal end of the trochlear notch of the ulna. If it fails to unite with the ulna, an ununited anconeal process can cause the elbow joint to become unstable, leading to lameness.

anterior chamber: The portion of the aqueous compartment of the eye in front of the iris.

antrum: One of the components that make up the monogastric stomach.

aorta: The major artery of the systemic circulation that receives blood from the left ventricle.

aortic arch: After leaving the heart in a cranial direction, the point at which the aorta turns caudally to go to the abdominal cavity.

aortic valve: The valve between the left ventricle of the heart and the aorta.

apex: The pointed tip of the heart. It faces in a generally caudal direction in the living animal, tipped ventrally and to the left.

apical: Toward the tip of the root of a tooth.

aponeurosis: Dense fibrous connective tissue much like a tendon but organized into a thin sheet of tissue.

aqueous compartment: The compartment of the eye in front of the lens and ciliary body. It is divided by the iris into the anterior chamber and the posterior chamber.

aqueous humor: The watery fluid that fills the aqueous compartment of the eye.

arachnoid: The middle layer of the meninges.

arch: The long flexible tunnel formed by the adjacent arches of the vertebrae. Contains and protects the spinal cord.

arm: Part of a microscope. The arm connects the eyepieces to the objectives.

artery: A blood vessel that carries blood away from the heart.

articular cartilage: The thin layer of hyaline cartilage that covers the articular (joint) surfaces of bones in synovial joints. It forms a smooth layer over the joint surfaces of the bones that decreases friction and allows free joint movement.

articular process: The process of a vertebra that forms a synovial joint with an adjacent vertebra.

articular surface: The smooth joint surface of a bone that contacts another bone in a synovial joint.

arytenoid cartilage: Cartilage in the larynx to which the vocal folds attach.

atlas: The first cervical vertebra. It forms the atlanto-occipital joint with the occipital bone of the skull and the atlanto-axial joint with the axis, the second cervical vertebra.

atrium: The heart chamber that receives blood from the large veins. The right atrium receives blood from the vena cava and the left atrium receives blood from the pulmonary vein.

auricle: The externally visible part of an atrium.

axial skeleton: The bones along the central axis of the body. Made up of the skull, hyoid bone, spinal column, ribs, and sternum.

axis: The second cervical vertebra. It forms the atlanto-axial joint with the first cervical vertebra—the atlas.

B

barrel: Trunk of the body—formed by the ribcage and the abdomen.

base (heart): The base of the heart is where all the blood vessels enter and leave. It faces in a generally cranial direction in the living animal, tipped dorsally and to the right.

base (microscope): Bottom support of microscope.

bifurcation of the trachea: The point at which the trachea subdivides into two primary bronchi.

blastocyst: An early stage of an embryonic development where the cells undergoing change form a hollow sphere of these cells.

body of the uterus: The most caudal part of the uterus where the two horns meet.

body tube: Part of a microscope holding the lenses, connected to the base and stage by the arm.

bones of the cranium: The bones of the skull that surround the brain. The externally visible bones of the cranium are the occipital bone, the interparietal bones, parietal bones, temporal bones, and frontal bones. The internal (hidden) bones of the cranium are the sphenoid and ethmoid bones.

bones of the face: The skull bones that do not surround the brain. The externally visible bones of the face are the incisive bones, nasal bones, maxillary bones, lacrimal bones, zygomatic bones, and mandible. The internal (hidden) bones of the face are the palatine bones, pterygoid bones, vomer bone, and turbinates.

Bowman's capsule: Part of the renal corpuscle that surrounds the glomerulus. It consists of two layers, an inner (visceral) layer that lies directly on the glomerular capillaries and an outer (parietal) layer. The space between the two layers, the capsular space, is continuous with the proximal convoluted tubule.

brachiocephalic trunk: The first artery that branches off the aortic arch.

brain stem: The most primitive section of the brain responsible for subconscious functions, such as cardiac and respiratory functions, swallowing, and blood pressure.

brisket: Area at the base of the neck between the front legs that covers the cranial end of the sternum.

bristle: There are six types of feathers: contour, semiplume, down, filoplume, bristle, and powder down.

broad ligament: The largest ligament that supports the female reproductive organs in the abdominal cavity.

bronchus: At its caudal end, the trachea bifurcates (divides) into two branches called primary bronchi, which enter the lungs.

buccal: Surface of a tooth facing the cheeks.

bulb of the glans: The bulbus glandis; it is erectile tissue in the dog penis that swells after ejaculation. It allows the bitch and dog to tie.

bulbar conjunctiva: The transparent membrane that covers the front portion of the eyeball.

bulbourethral glands: The most caudal male accessory reproductive gland that secretes a mucuslike liquid that lubricates and clears the urethra.

C

calcaneal tuberosity: Large process of the fibular tarsal bone that projects upwards and backwards. Commonly referred to as the point of the hock. Site of attachment of the gastrocnemius (calf) muscle. Equivalent to the human heel.

cancellous bone: "Spongy" bone. A form of bone composed of seemingly randomly arranged "spicules" of bone separated by spaces filled with bone marrow. Appears spongelike to the naked eye. Found in the ends (epiphyses) of long bones and the interiors of short bones, flat bones, and irregular bones.
canine teeth: The teeth located just lateral to the incisor teeth.
cannon bone: Large metacarpal or metatarsal bone of hoofed animals.
capsule: Outer fibrous covering of the kidney.
cardia (cardiac sphincter): A thickening where the esophagus joins the stomach. It is important in preventing the reflux of ingesta into the esophagus, which could cause discomfort and esophageal ulceration.
carpal bones: The bones of the carpus. Consist of two parallel rows of short bones located between the distal ends of the radius and ulna and the proximal ends of the metacarpal bones.
caudal: Toward the tail, also the "back" surface of a limb proximal to the carpus or tarsus.
caudal vena cava: Large vein that returns blood to the heart from the caudal part of the body.
cecum: The cecum is a blind-ended pouch from which the ascending colon arises. It is located in the caudal right quadrant of the abdomen, and in humans and rabbits it has an added extension attached to it called the appendix.
cellular component: The cellular component of whole blood is made up of erythrocytes (RBCs, red blood cells), leukocytes (WBCs, white blood cells), and thrombocytes (platelets).
central nervous system: The brain and spinal cord. Abbreviated CNS.
cephalic vein: The vein on the cranial aspect of the forearm in most domestic mammals; much favored for intravenous injection in dogs.
cerebellum: The section of the brain responsible for coordinated movement, balance, posture, and complex reflexes.
cerebrum: The section of the brain responsible for learning, intelligence, and awareness.
cervical vertebrae: The bones of the neck portion of the spinal column.
cervix: The smooth muscle valve between the uterine body and the vagina.
chordae tendineae: Fine, threadlike cords that connect the free edges of the atrioventricular valves to the papillary muscles in the ventricles.
choroid: A portion of the middle vascular layer of the eye. It consists mainly of pigment and blood vessels and is located between the sclera and the retina.
ciliary body: The portion of the middle vascular layer of the eye located immediately behind the iris. It contains ciliary muscles that adjust the shape of the lens.
clavicular intersection: A small tendinous band embedded in the brachiocephalic muscle near the point of the shoulder in animals, such as the horse and dog.
clitoris: Part of the female vulva, it contains erectile tissue and is covered by many sensory nerve endings. Homologous to the penis of the male.
cloaca: Cavity located at the end of the digestive tract of birds that receives waste products from the intestinal, urinary, and genital tracts. It is divided into three sections: the coprodeum, the urodeum, and the proctodeum.
clotting factors: Clotting factors are proteins and other chemicals normally dissolved in the plasma portion of whole blood.
coarse adjustment: Part of a microscope. Large focusing knob used for low power only.
coccygeal vertebrae: The bones of the tail portion of the spinal column.
cochlea: The snail shell–shaped cavity in the temporal bone of the skull that contains the hearing portion of the inner ear.
collecting ducts: The tubes in the kidney that collect fluid from the distal convoluted tubules and carry it to the renal pelvis.
common bile duct: Delivers bile acids from the liver and gall bladder to the small intestine.
common pancreatic duct and Vater's ampulla: The main port though which bile and pancreatic enzymes are delivered to the duodenum.
compact bone: Heavy, dense bone made up of tiny, tightly compacted laminated cylinders of bone called Haversian systems. Makes up the shafts (diaphyses) of long bones and the outer surfaces of all bones.
condenser: Part of a microscope. The condenser is located above the light source and focuses light into the objective.
condenser knob: Raises or lowers the condenser on a microscope.
condyle: A large rounded articular (joint) surface. Examples are found on the distal ends of the humerus and femur.
cones: Photoreceptors in the retina of the eye that perceive color and detail.
conical papillae: Projections of the epidermis on the surface of a dog's foot pad.
conjunctival sac: The space between the bulbar and palpebral portions of the conjunctiva. The space between the eyelid and the eyeball.
connective tissue: Connective tissue is responsible for supporting and connecting other tissues.
contour feather: There are six types of feathers: contour, semiplume, down, filoplume, bristle, and powder down.
control knob of mechanical stage clips: Knobs, located below and to the right side of the stage on a microscope, used to direct the brackets to move the slide to the right and left, and forward and backward.
cornea: The clear "window" on the front of the eye that admits light to the interior of the eye. It is part of the outer fibrous layer of the eyeball.
cornual process: The "horn core" of horned animals. A process of the frontal bone. The hollow cavity within the cornual process is continuous with the frontal sinus—the paranasal sinus of the frontal bone.
coronal: Toward the crown of a tooth.
coronoid processes: Medial and lateral coronoid processes on distal end of trochlear notch are located on the ends of the horizontal, concave radial notch where the proximal end of the radius articulates with the ulna.
corpus callosum: Structure in the brain composed of nerve fibers that connect the right and left cerebral hemispheres.
corpus cavernosum penis: The larger of the two penile erectile tissues. It is located dorsal to the urethra.
corpus cavernosum urethrae: The smaller of the two penile erectile tissues that forms a sleeve around the penile urethra.
corpus luteum: The corpus luteum (Latin for yellow body) develops after ovulation and will secrete progestin hormone to maintain the pregnancy.
cortex: The outer portion of the kidney where renal corpuscles and the convoluted tubules of the nephrons are located.
costal arch: Caudal ventral border of the rib cage formed by the costal cartilages of the 10th, 11th, and 12th ribs in dogs and cats.
costal cartilage: The cartilaginous ventral portion of a rib.
costochondral junction: The junction between the bony and cartilaginous portions of a rib.
cotyledonary attachment: Cotyledonary attachment is seen in ruminants, and contains multiple smaller, round, raised attachment sites that resemble inverted mushroom caps.
cranial: Toward the head. Also the "front" surface of a limb proximal to the carpus or tarsus.
cranial vena cava: Large vein that returns blood to the heart from the head and forelimbs.
cremaster muscle: The muscle attached to the scrotum that allows the testes to be brought closer to or further away from the body to control their temperature.
crop: Dilation of the esophagus in some species of birds that acts as a storage pouch for food.
crown: The exposed part of a tooth above the gum line. The part of the tooth covered by enamel.

D

deep: Toward the center of the body or a body part.
dental arch: The complete arched arrangement of upper or lower teeth. Also known as the dental arcade.
dentin: The connective tissue layer surrounding the tooth pulp; is more dense than bone but not as dense as overlying enamel.
diaphragm: The thin, dome-shaped muscular structure that forms the boundary between the thoracic and abdominal cavities.
diencephalon: The section of the brain that is a passageway between the brain stem and cerebrum.
diffuse attachment: One of four types of placental attachment.
distal (direction): Away from the body (used for appendages).
distal (surface): For canine, premolar, and molar teeth, the surface or edge facing toward the caudal end of the mouth. For the incisor teeth, the surface or edge farthest from the center (midline).
distal convoluted tubule: The last tubular part of the nephron before it enters the collecting duct.
distal sesamoid bone: The "navicular bone" of horses. It is located in the digital flexor tendon deep in the hoof behind the joint between the middle and distal phalanges.
dorsal: Toward the top (backbone) surface of the body. Also the top/"front" surface of a limb distal to the carpus or tarsus.
dorsal plane: Divides the body into dorsal and ventral parts.
dorsal recumbency: Lying on the back (dorsal body surface) with the ventral surface facing up.
down: There are six types of feathers: contour, semiplume, down, filoplume, bristle, and powder down.
duodenum: The first segment of the small intestine after the stomach. Chyme enters the duodenum from the stomach.
dura mater: The outer fibrous layer of the meninges.

E

ectoderm: An embryonic tissue that develops into the integumentary and nervous systems.
efferent duct: Spermatozoa enter the epididymis from the efferent ducts of the testis and exit into the vas deferens.
efferent glomerular arterioles: Arterioles that carry blood away from the glomerulus after it has been filtered in the renal corpuscle.
enamel: Outer coating layer of the tooth; toughest substance in the body.
endoderm: An embryonic tissue that develops into mucous membranes, respiratory system, and digestive system.
endometrium: This inner layer contains mucous membranes and blood vessels that enlarge during pregnancy to nutritionally support the embryo until it implants. This layer is also important in placental development.
epicondyles: Knoblike projections.
epididymis (head, body, tail): The head of the epididymis is where spermatozoa enter from the efferent ducts; the body of the epididymis is the main portion of the epididymis that lies along the side of the testis; the tail of the epididymis continues on as the vas deferens.
epiglottis: The cartilage of the larynx that projects forward from the ventral portion of the larynx. It is the "trapdoor" of the larynx.
esophagus: Carries food from the oral cavity to the stomach.
Eustachian tube: The tube that connects the middle ear cavity with the pharynx.
external acoustic meatus: The bony canal in the temporal bone that leads into the middle ear cavity. In the living animal it contains the external ear canal.
external auditory canal: The tube that carries sound waves from the pinna to the tympanic membrane.
external ear: The externally visible part of the ear made up of the pinna and external auditory canal.
extraocular muscles: Muscles that move the eyeball.
eyepiece or ocular (10× or 5× each): Part of a microscope that contains a magnifying lens.

F

fabella: One of two small sesamoid bones located in the proximal gastrocnemius (calf) muscle tendon just above and behind the femoral condyles of dogs and cats.
facet: A flat articular surface, such as between carpal bones and between the radius and ulna.
facial nerve: Cranial nerve VII. Mixed nerve that is sensory and motor to areas of the face.
femoral artery and vein: Blood vessels located on the medial surface of the "thigh" region of the hind leg.
femoral nerve: The nerve found on medial surface of thigh near the femoral artery and vein.
femur: The long bone of the "thigh" region. It forms the hip joint with the pelvis at its proximal end and the stifle joint with the tibia at its distal end.
fetlock: Joint between cannon bone (large metacarpal/metatarsal) and the proximal phalanx of hoofed animals.
fibrous joint: An immovable joint also known as a synarthrosis. The bones of a fibrous joint are firmly united by fibrous tissue. The sutures that unite most of the skull bones are fibrous joints.
fibula: A thin bone located beside the tibia in the lower leg region of the pelvic limb. It is a complete bone in the dog and cat, but only the proximal and distal ends are present in horses and cattle. The fibula does not support any appreciable weight. It mainly acts as a muscle attachment site.
filiform papilla: Best known for their sharp spicules, which enable the cat to groom itself.
filoplume: There are six types of feathers: contour, semiplume, down, filoplume, bristle, and powder down.
fimbriae: Fingerlike projections from the edge of the infundibulum on the oviduct that surround a follicle. They guide the released ovum into the infundibulum at ovulation.
fine adjustment: Part of a microscope. Small focusing knob used to give a sharper image after object has been focused using the coarse adjustment knob.
flank: Lateral surface of the abdomen between the last rib and the hind legs.
flat bone: Bones that are relatively thin and flat. They consist of two thin plates of compact bone separated by a thin layer of cancellous bone. Many of the skull bones are flat bones.
Flehmen response: An animal behavior in which the animal curls back the upper lip.
fleshy: An apparent direct attachment of muscle to the bone; in reality, the muscle attaches to the periosteum of the bone by very short tendons.
foliate: Receptors on the tongue that detect salty tastes.
foliate papilla: One of the four types of papillae in the cat.
foramen: A hole in a bone.
foramen magnum: The large hole in the occipital bone through which the spinal cord exits the skull.
fossa: A depressed or sunken area on the surface of a bone. Fossas are usually occupied by muscles or tendons in living animals.
frontal bones: Skull bones. External bones of the cranium. The two frontal bones make up the "forehead" region of the skull. They contain the large frontal sinuses. The cornual process (horn core) in horned animals is an extension of the frontal bone.
fundus: The fundus is referred to as a "blind pouch" and is located dorsal to the cardia. The body is considered the "middle" portion of the stomach. Both the fundus and the body contain gastric glands with parietal cells, chief cells, and mucous cells.
fungiform: Receptors on the tongue that detect sweet, salty, and sour tastes.
furcation: The area where the roots of a multirooted tooth join the crown.

G

gingiva: The epithelial tissue that composes the "gums."
gizzard: Muscular stomach in birds that grinds food into a digestible form.
glenoid cavity: The concave articular surface of the scapula. The socket portion of the ball-and-socket shoulder joint.
glomerular capillaries: The "tuft" of capillaries at the center of the renal corpuscle. Urine production begins when plasma is filtered out of the capillaries and into Bowman's capsular space.
gray matter: Area of the central nervous system made up primarily of neuron cell bodies and unmyelinated nerve fibers. Appears brownish-gray grossly.
greater trochanter: Greater trochanter on proximal end of the femur is large process to which gluteal muscles attach.
greater tubercle: Greater tubercle on proximal end of the humerus is large process to which shoulder muscles attach.
gustatory cells: Structures found mainly on certain papillae of the tongue that contain the receptor cells for taste.
gyri: Folds in the cerebrum and cerebellum.

H

head: A spheroidal articular surface on the proximal end of a long bone. Present on the proximal ends of the humerus, femur, and rib. The head of a bone is joined to the shaft by an area that is often narrowed, called the neck.
high-power or high dry objective (40×, 43×, or 45×): The high power (HP) objective or the high dry lens offers high magnification without the use of oil and may magnify 40×, 43×, or 45×, depending upon the objective.
hilus: The indented area on the medial sides of the kidneys where blood and lymph vessels, nerves, and the ureters enter and leave the kidney.
hock: Tarsus.
humerus: The long bone of the brachium or "upper arm."
hypothalamus: A portion of the brain stem that has extensive links to the brain and to the pituitary gland. It functions as an important bridge between the nervous and the endocrine systems.

I

ileum: The ileum is the shortest portion of the small intestine and forms a transitory link between the lengthy jejunum and the beginning of the large intestine.
iliac artery and vein: Main blood vessels to and from the hind legs. The terminal branches of the abdominal aorta and caudal vena cava.
ilium: The cranial-most area of the pelvis. It forms the sacroiliac joint with the sacrum.
illuminator or light source: Source of light in a microscope that is directed through the slide and into the objective and ocular lenses.
incisal edge: The cutting edge of a sharp tooth's crown.
incisive bones: Skull bones that are part of the external bones of the face. The two incisive bones are the most rostral of the skull bones. In all common domestic animals, except ruminants, the incisive bones house the upper incisor teeth.
incisor teeth: The most rostral group of teeth.
incus: One of three ossicles that help transmit sound waves across the middle ear. It is also known as the anvil. It is the middle of the three ossicles.

infundibulum: A funnel-like enlargement at the ovarian end of the oviduct. It catches the released ovum.
insensitive lamina: Inner surface of the horny wall of a hoof. Interdigitates with the sensitive lamina.
insertion: The attachment at the more movable end of the muscle; in the limbs this is usually the most distal end.
integral proteins: The proteins located within the lipid bilayer of the cell membrane that create channels, which aid in selective permeability.
interatrial septum: The "wall" of myocardium that separates the left and right atria of the heart.
intermediate filaments: Thin filaments that provide the structural support for certain membrane junctions. They are especially important in tissue that needs to flex. Also called tonofilaments.
interparietal bones: Skull bones that are part of the external bones of the cranium. The two interparietal bones are located on the dorsal midline just rostral to the occipital bone. The interparietal bones are usually distinct in young animals, but in older animals they may fuse together into one bone and may even fuse to the parietal bones and become indistinguishable.
interproximal space: Space between adjacent teeth.
interproximal surface: Surface of a tooth that faces an adjacent tooth.
interventricular groove: The fat-filled groove on the outside of the heart that corresponds to the location of the interventricular septum. Also known as the interventricular sulcus.
interventricular septum: The "wall" of myocardium that separates the left and right ventricles of the heart.
iris: The colored portion of the eye. It is a pigmented, muscular diaphragm that controls the amount of light that enters the posterior part of the eyeball.
iris diaphragm: Part of a microscope. A device that controls the diameter of the light beam coming up through the condenser, so that when the diaphragm is stopped down (nearly closed) the light comes straight up through the center of the condenser lens and contrast is high. When the diaphragm is wide open, the image is brighter and contrast is low.
irregular bone: A bone whose shape does not fit into the long bone, short bone, or flat bone categories. Irregular bones either have characteristics of more than one of the other three shape categories, or a truly irregular shape. Examples include vertebrae and some strangely shaped skull bones such as the sphenoid bone and sesamoid bones.
ischium: The caudal-most area of the pelvis.
isthmus: Section of the avian oviduct that deposits the keratin shell membrane.

J

jejunum: The jejunum is the longest portion of the small intestine and, not surprisingly, absorbs the bulk of the nutrients derived from food.
jugular groove: The groove on each side of the neck in which the jugular vein is located. It is formed by the sternocephalicus muscle and the brachiocephalicus muscle.
jugular vein: Large vein in the neck region. The left and right jugular veins are located in a groove on either side of the trachea.

K

knee: Carpus of hoofed animals.

L

labia: Lips of the vulva.
labial: Surface of a tooth facing the lips.
labial frenulum: The labial frenulum is the mucosal attachment to each lip along the upper and lower midlines.
lacrimal bones: Skull bones. External bones of the face. The two small lacrimal bones form part of the medial portion of the orbit of the eye. In the living animal the lacrimal bones house the lacrimal sacs—part of the tear drainage system of the eye.
lacrimal puncta: The openings into the nasolacrimal drainage system that carries tears away from the surface of each eye. They are located near the medial canthus on both the upper and lower eyelid margins.
large intestine: In companion animals, the large intestine is composed of the cecum, and the ascending, transverse, and descending colon.
larynx: The voice box. A short irregular tube of cartilage and muscle that connects the pharynx with the trachea.
lateral: Away from the median plane.
lateral canthus: The lateral corner of the eye where the upper and lower eyelids come together.
lateral malleolus: Lateral malleolus is the laterally facing rounded process on the distal end of the fibula (the lateral "knob" on our ankle is our lateral malleolus).
lateral recumbency: Lying on the side; left lateral recumbency means left side down and right lateral recumbency means right side down.
latissimus dorsi muscle: This large triangular muscle lies caudal to the scapula and covers much of the thoracic wall. It draws the limb caudally and flexes the shoulder joint.
left: The animal's left.
left atrium: The heart chamber that receives blood from the large veins. The right atrium receives blood from the vena cava and the left atrium receives blood from the pulmonary vein.
left ventricle: The left ventricle pumps blood out through the aorta and the right ventricle pumps blood out through the pulmonary artery.
lens: The soft, transparent structure in the eye made up of layers of microscopic fibers that are arranged like layers of an onion. Its main function is to help focus a clear image on the retina.
limbus: The junction of the cornea and sclera of the eye.
lingual: Surface of a lower tooth facing the tongue.
lingual frenulum: The mucosal attachment located along the midline under the tongue.
long bone: Bones that are longer than they are wide. Most of the limb bones, such as the humerus, femur, and radius, are long bones.
long digital extensor muscle: This spindle-shaped muscle lies lateral to the cranial tibial muscle and is partly covered by it. It extends digital joints, flexes the tarsal joint, and extends the stifle joint.
longitudinal fissure: The longitudinal fissure separates the cerebrum into right and left cerebral hemispheres.
loop of Henle: The narrowest part of the tubular portion of the nephron. It dips into the medulla of the kidney and makes a U-turn to return to the cortex.
low-power objective (10×): The low-power (LP) objective is a 10× magnification, and one power higher than a scanning objective lens.
lumbar vertebrae: The group of vertebrae located dorsal to the abdominal region.
lungs: Two spongy, respiratory organs in the thoracic cavity. They remove carbon dioxide from the blood and replace it with oxygen.
lysosome: A cytoplasmic organelle that fights pathogens, repairs damaged tissues, and aids in intracellular digestion by engulfing materials with its membrane-bound vesicle bodies. It contains the digestive enzymes that help destroy microorganisms that have been phagocytized by the neutrophil.

M

magnum: Section of the avian oviduct that secretes albumin (the egg white) of the egg.
malleus: One of the three ossicles of the middle ear. Also known as the hammer, it helps transmit sound waves across the middle ear from the tympanic membrane. It is attached to the tympanic membrane.
mammary papilla (or teats): Projections from mammary glands through which milk exits the glands.
mandible: A skull bone. One of the external bones of the face. The mandible is the lower jaw. The only movable skull bone. The mandible houses all of the lower teeth. It is usually referred to as a single bone, but in dogs, cats, and cattle the two halves of the mandible are separate bones joined by a cartilaginous mandibular symphysis at the rostral end.
manubrium: The first, most cranial sternebra. Its full name is manubrium sterni.
maxillary bones: Skull bones. External bones of the face. The two maxillary bones make up most of the upper jaw and house the upper canine teeth, if present, and all of the upper cheek teeth (premolars and molars).
medial: Toward the median plane.
medial canthus: The medial corner of the eye where the upper and lower eyelids come together.
medial malleolus: Medial malleolus is medially facing rounded process on the distal end of the tibia (the "knob" on the medial side of our ankle is our medial malleolus).
median nerve: The middle of the three major branches of the brachial plexus.
median plane: Divides the body into equal left and right halves.
medulla: The renal medulla is the inner layer that is darker in color and has a smooth striated appearance.
medulla oblongata: The medulla oblongata is the area of the brain stem that connects with the spinal cord.
Meissner's corpuscles: Nerve endings in the dermal papilla, which are receptors for touch.
meninges: Connective tissue layers that cover the brain and spinal cord.

mesial: For canine, premolar, and molar teeth, the surface or edge facing toward the rostral end of the mouth. For the incisor teeth, the surface or edge facing toward the center (midline).
mesoderm: An embryonic tissue that develops into connective tissue, muscle, and the urinary, circulatory, and reproductive systems.
mesometrium: This outer layer attaches the uterus to the dorsal abdominal wall.
metacarpal bones: The bones of the thoracic limbs located between the carpus and the phalanges.
metatarsal bones: The bones of the pelvic limbs located between the tarsus and the phalanges.
microfilaments: Closely associated with microtubules, these submicroscopic structures are found in most cells and are composed mostly of actin.
microtubules: Tiny, hollow, tubelike structures that aid certain cells with rigidity and transportation. They also form the spindle fibers in the process of mitosis.
midbrain: The midbrain is located between the pons and the cerebrum.
mitochondria: The primary source of ATP formation for aerobic cell respiration. This cytoplasmic organelle also contains DNA and RNA, making the mitochondria capable of its own protein synthesis and replication.
mitral valve: The valve between the left atrium and the left ventricle of the heart.
modulation (pain): Modification (amplification or suppression) of pain impulses that occur in the spinal cord.
molar teeth: The caudal cheek teeth.
monogastric stomach: Made up of five compartments.
multiparous: A multiparous species typically has multiple corpora lutea (one per released follicle).
muzzle: Rostral part of the face formed mainly by the maxillary and nasal bones.
myocardium: The thick muscular layer of the heart wall.
myometrium: This layer consists of smooth muscles that will contract at the time of parturition to deliver the fetus. It is sensitive to the hormone oxytocin.

N

nasal bones: Skull bones that are part of the external bones of the face. The nasal bones form the "bridge" of the nose—the dorsal part of the nasal cavity.
nasal cavity and turbinates: Skull bones that are part of the internal bones of the face. Also known as the nasal conchae. The turbinates are four thin, scroll-like bones that fill most of the space in the nasal cavity. In the living animal the turbinates are covered by the moist, vascular lining of the nasal passages. Their scroll-like shape helps the nasal lining warm and humidify the inhaled air and trap tiny particles of inhaled foreign material.
nasal septum: The wall dividing the nasal cavity into left and right passages, composed of a central area of bone covered by a mucous membrane.
nasolacrimal duct: The tube that carries tears from the lacrimal sac to the nasal cavity.
nasopalatine duct (incisive duct): A small nodule located directly behind the incisors, forming a connection between the oral cavity and the nasal passage above it.
neck: The area of a bone that joins the head with the main portion of the bone.
necropsy: Postmortem examination of an animal cadaver.
nephron: The basic functional unit of the kidney.
nervous tissue: Nervous tissue is responsible for controlling work through electrical and chemical signals.
nociception: The process of experiencing pain.
nonpolar tails (hydrophobic): The water-fearing and nonpolar head of a phospholipid.
nosepiece: The part of a microscope that holds the objective lenses. It is able to rotate so that lenses can be interchanged.
nostrils (nares): The nostrils open into the nasal cavity.
nuclear pores: Pores that traverse through both layers of the nuclear envelope, allowing the passage of protein molecules in and RNA molecules out of the nucleus of a cell.
nucleoli: One or more small round nonmembranous structures located within the nucleus.
nucleus: The nucleus is often described as the control center of the cell and is necessary for protein synthesis and reproduction because it contains the vital genetic instruction, DNA. A mature red blood cell, for example, lacks a nucleus and therefore cannot survive for long without the ability or instructions needed to make protein.
nutrient foramen: A large channel through the cortex of a large bone through which large blood vessels pass carrying blood to and from the bone marrow.

O

objectives lenses: Part of a microscope. Interchangeable magnifying lenses attached to a revolving nosepiece.
oblique recumbency: The body is tilted between dorsal or sternal recumbency and lateral recumbency. Referred to by a combination of the other position terms.
obturator foramen: One of a pair of large holes in the pelvis located on either side of the pelvic symphysis. The role of the obturator foramina seems to be to lighten the pelvis, because no large nerves or vessels pass through them.
occipital bone: A skull bone that is one of the external bones of the cranium. The occipital bone is the caudal-most bone of the skull. It forms the atlanto-occipital joint with the first cervical vertebra—the atlas—through the occipital condyles. The large foramen magnum in the occipital bone is where the spinal cord exits the skull.
occipital condyle: One of two articular surfaces on the occipital bone. The occipital condyles are located on either side of the foramen magnum and form the atlanto-occipital joint with the first cervical vertebra—the atlas.
occlusal surface: The flat grinding surface of molar teeth.
oculars: Part of a microscope. Eyepieces that contain a magnifying lens.
oil immersion (97× or 100×): The highest power lens is in the oil immersion objective with a magnification of 97× or 100×, used with oil to improve resolution.
olecranon process: The large process on the proximal end of the ulna that forms the point of the elbow. The olecranon process is the site where the tendon of the powerful triceps brachii muscle attaches.
olfactory bulb: The olfactory bulbs receive information from the olfactory (sense of smell) nerves, then send the impulses to the cerebrum via the olfactory tracts.
olfactory cells: Receptors (olfactory cells) that detect chemical substances are located in two patches of olfactory epithelium in the upper part of the nasal passages.
olfactory epithelium: Two patches in the upper part of the nasal passages that detect chemical substances dissolved in the nasal mucus layer.
olfactory sense: The sense of smell.
omasum: Animals not containing a single stomach but instead a multichambered organ comprised of a reticulum, rumen, omasum, and abomasum.
omnivore: An animal whose diet is a mixture of plants and meat.
omotransversarius muscle: This straplike muscle is partially covered by the brachiocephalicus muscle. It advances the limb and/or pulls the head and neck to the side.
opening of the stage: A hole in the stage of a microscope through which the light from the condenser passes.
optic chiasm: The area where half the fibers of each optic nerve cross to the other side of the brain.
optic disc: The area of the retina where nerve fibers on its surface converge to form the beginning of the optic nerve. The blind spot of the eye.
optic nerve: Formed from retinal nerve fibers. It carries visual nerve impulses to the optic chiasm and on to the brain.
origin: The attachment at the less movable end of the muscle or usually the more proximal end.
os penis: A bone that partially surrounds the penile urethra of a dog.
ossicles: Skull bones that are the bones of the ear. They are located in the middle ear and transmit sound wave vibrations from the tympanic membrane to the inner ear.
otoliths: Tiny crystals in the gelatinous mass of the vestibule that help it sense the position and linear motion of the head.
ovary: The female gonad.
oviducts: Short convoluted tubes that attach to the tips of the horns of the uterus and conduct the fertilized ovum to the uterus. The usual site of fertilization of an ovum by a spermatozoon.
oxyphil cell: Parathyroid cell found in humans and horses. Thought to be retired parafollicular cells.
oxytocin: One of the posterior pituitary hormones. It is produced in the hypothalamus and then stored and released from the posterior pituitary gland. It stimulates contraction of the myometrium of the uterus at breeding and parturition and contraction of the myoepithelial cells of the lactating mammary gland.

P

palatal: Surface of an upper tooth facing the hard palate.
palmar: Ground/"back" surface of front limb distal to the carpus.
palpebral conjunctiva: The transparent membrane that lines the inner portion of the eyelid.

pancreas: Endocrine and exocrine gland that produces and secretes digestive enzymes into the intestines and produces hormones, such as insulin and glucagon.
papilla (plural—papillae): Receptors (gustatory cells) that detect these substances are organized into taste buds.
papillary layer: The uppermost layer of the dermis composed of loose irregular connective tissue. It is called the papillary layer because there are various dermal papillae that project into the epidermis.
paranasal sinuses: Air-filled cavities in some bones of the skull that are outpouchings of the nasal passage.
parathyroid glands: Endocrine glands consisting of several small nodules located in, on, or near the thyroid gland. They produce parathyroid hormone.
parietal bones: Skull bones that are among the external bones of the cranium. The two parietal bones form the dorsolateral walls of the cranium. They are large and well developed in the dog and cat, but relatively small in horses and cattle.
parietal vaginal tunic: The outer, thick connective tissue sac around each testis.
pastern: Area of the proximal phalanx of hoofed animals.
patella: The "kneecap." The largest sesamoid bone in the body. The patella is located on the front surface of the stifle joint in the tendon of the large quadriceps femoris muscle. It rides in the trochlea of the femur.
pectineus muscle: A medial muscle of the thigh, this small spindle-shaped muscle adducts the limb.
pectoralis muscle: The pectoralis muscle and the supracoracoideus muscle are two essential muscular components that generate wing motion.
pelvic limb: The hind limb.
pelvic urethra: The portion of the urethra located in the pelvic canal.
pelvis: The most proximal bone of the pelvic limb. Also known as the os coxae. The pelvis attaches to the sacrum dorsally at the sacroiliac joints and forms the hip joints with the heads of the femurs. It has three parts, the ilium, ischium, and pubis.
penile urethra: The portion of the urethra located in the penis.
penis: The male breeding organ.
perception (pain): The part of the pain sensation that involves the brain consciously recognizing pain.
pericardial sac: The outermost layer of the pericardium that surrounds the heart.
periople: Soft, light-colored horn produced by a germinal layer (perioplic corium). It covers the coronary band of the hoof.
peripheral nervous system: Portion of the nervous system made up of cordlike nerves that are bundles of nerve fibers that link the CNS with the rest of the body.
peristalsis: A rhythmic, wavelike motion that progressively moves through a tube organ, such as the small intestine. Peristalsis assists with the movement of food through the alimentary canal.
peritubular capillaries: Capillaries in the network that surrounds the tubular part of the nephron of the kidney that eventually converge to form the renal vein. They are involved in the processes of tubular secretion and reabsorption.
peroxisome: Found in high numbers in kidney and liver cells of most vertebrate animals, this single-membraned vesicle detoxifies the body by releasing catalase and other enzymes.
phalanx: A bone of a digit (toe or finger). Plural, phalanges.
pharynx: The "throat." A common passageway for the respiratory and digestive systems located between the mouth and nasal passages, and the esophagus and trachea.
Pheromones: Small, chemical molecules that, when released by one organism, act as chemical signals to induce a certain behavior in another organism.
phospholipids: A molecule composed of three parts: phosphorus, fatty acids, and a nitrogenous base. Any lipid that contains phosphorus. Phospholipids are the main components of the cell membrane.
photoreceptors: The sensory receptors of the eye that convert photons of light energy to nerve impulses that are interpreted by the brain as vision. The rods and cones of the retina.
pia mater: The inner layer of the meninges that is closely adhered to the brain and spinal cord.
pineal body: A structure in the brain located at the caudal end of the deep cleft that separates the two hemispheres of the cerebrum, just rostral to the cerebellum. It produces the hormonelike substance melatonin that appears to influence the body's biological clock.
pinna: The externally visible part of the ear that collects sound waves and funnels them down into the external ear canal. The ear flap.
pituitary gland: The "master endocrine gland." A pea-sized endocrine gland located at the base of the brain; made up of the anterior pituitary gland, which produces seven known hormones, and the posterior pituitary gland, which stores and releases two hormones from the hypothalamus. The pituitary gland is also called the hypophysis.
placenta: The multilayered, fluid-filled sac around the developing fetus that attaches to the uterine lining. It provides nutrients for the fetus as well as gas exchange and waste removal.
plantar: Ground/"back" surface of hind limb distal to the tarsus.
planum nasale: Touch receptors found in the hypodermis.
planum nasolabial: The nose of the horse and cow, commonly called the muzzle.
plasma: Plasma is the liquid portion of whole blood after the blood cells have been removed.
plasma membrane: The plasma membrane surrounds the internal structures of the cell, forming a flexible barrier between the intracellular and extracellular environments.
polar head (hydrophilic): The water-loving polar head of a phospholipid.
poll: Top of the head between the bases of the ears.
polygonal plates in the canine planum nasale: Plaques packed together on the skin of the nose. This pattern is caused by the presence of deep grooves in the epidermis.
pons: The pons is located just rostral to the medulla oblongata. It is separated from the medulla oblongata by a horizontal groove. Nerve fibers running transversely across the pons give it a rounded, plump look.
posterior chamber: The portion of the aqueous compartment of the eye behind the iris.
posterior pituitary gland: The neurohypophysis; the caudal portion of the pituitary gland that stores and releases two hormones (antidiuretic hormone and oxytocin) that are produced in the hypothalamus.
powder down: There are six types of feathers: contour, semiplume, down, filoplume, bristle, and powder down.
premolar teeth: The rostral cheek teeth.
prepuce: The sheath of skin that encloses the penis when it is not erect.
process: A general name for a lump, bump, or other projection on a bone. Processes can be either articular processes, which contribute to joint formation, or nonarticular processes, which are usually sites where tendons attach.
progesterone: The principal progestin hormone produced by the corpus luteum of the ovary. It helps prepare the uterus for implantation of the fertilized ovum and helps maintain pregnancy once it begins.
prolactin: The anterior pituitary hormone that helps trigger and maintain lactation.
prostate: The single male accessory reproductive gland that surrounds the pelvic urethra and sends many ducts into the urethra. The only accessory reproductive gland in the dog.
proventriculus: Anterior glandular stomach of birds in which chemical digestion of proteins begins.
proximal: Toward or closest to the body (used for appendages).
proximal convoluted tubule: The first tubular part of the nephron of the kidney nephron. Continuous with Bowman's capsular space.
proximal sesamoid bones: Paired sesamoid bones in the legs of horses. They are located in the large digital flexor tendons behind the "fetlock" joints—the joints between the large metacarpal and metatarsal bones and the proximal phalanges.
pubis: The smallest and most medial area of the pelvis. The pubis forms the cranial portion of the floor of the pelvis.
pulmonary artery: The large blood vessel that leaves the right ventricle is the pulmonary artery.
pulmonary valve: The valve between the right ventricle and the pulmonary artery. Also known as the pulmonic valve.
pulmonary vein: The large blood vessel that enters the left atrium is the pulmonary vein.
pulp: The latticelike material in the center of the tooth; contains the nerve and blood supply for the tooth.
pupil: The opening in the center of the iris.
pylorus (pyloric sphincter): The "end" portion of the stomach is the pylorus, a muscular sphincter. The pylorus allows digested material to enter the small intestines at the duodenum while preventing any retrograde movement of these contents back into the stomach.

Q

quadrant: The left or right half of each dental arch.
quarters: The hoof is divided roughly into the toe or cranial portion, the medial and lateral quarters on the sides, and the medial and lateral heels or rear portion of the hoof.

R

radial nerve: The largest and most cranial of the three major branches of the brachial plexus. It is found running between the triceps muscle and the humerus.

radial notch: Medial and lateral coronoid processes on distal end of trochlear notch are located on the ends of the horizontal, concave radial notch where the proximal end of the radius articulates with the ulna.
radius: One of the two bones (the ulna is the other) that form the antebrachium (forearm). The radius is usually the main weight-bearing bone.
ramus of the mandible: The vertical portion of the mandible located at its caudal end. The ramus is where the powerful jaw muscles attach to the mandible.
raphae: Seams; lines of union of the halves of various symmetrical anatomic parts.
receptor proteins: Receptor proteins contain specific receptor sites that bond only to specific molecules such as hormones.
rectum: The end of the intestinal tract.
relaxin hormone: In sows and cows, the ovaries secrete relaxin hormone to assist in relaxation of the cervix in preparation for parturition.
reticular layer: The lower layer of the dermis composed of dense irregular connective tissue.
reticulum: Animals not containing a single stomach, but instead a multichambered system comprised of a reticulum, rumen, omasum, and abomasum.
retina: The inner nervous layer of the eye where the photoreceptors are located.
retractor penis muscle: The muscle that pulls the penis of bulls, rams, and boars back into its nonerect S-shape.
rheostat: Part of a microscope. Regulates the intensity of the light.
ribosome: A cytoplasmic organelle composed of ribonucleic acid located on the rough endoplasmic reticulum or suspended in the cytoplasm, where protein synthesis takes place.
ribs: Long bones of the axial skeleton that form the lateral walls of the thorax. Their dorsal portions are made of bone and form synovial joints with the thoracic vertebrae. Their ventral portions are made of cartilage—the costal cartilages.
right: The animal's right.
right atrium: The heart chamber that receives blood from the large veins. The right atrium receives blood from the vena cava and the left atrium receives blood from the pulmonary vein.
rods: Photoreceptors in the retina of the eye that perceive dim light images in shades of gray.
root: The hidden part of a tooth below the gum line.
rostral: Toward the tip of the nose (used only on the head).
round ligament: The round ligament of the uterus is a lateral fold of the broad ligament made up of fibrous tissue and blood vessels.
rugae: Covering of the hard palate.
rumen: The rumen is the largest compartment of the forestomach and acts as a fermentation vat. It is lined with papillae and is separated into compartments by internal muscular walls called pillars, which allow selective regions of the rumen to mix and stir its contents as needed.
ruminant "stomach": Ruminants, such as cows, sheep, and goats, do not have a single stomach like dogs, cats, horses, and humans, but instead have a four-chambered organ composed of a "forestomach," containing the reticulum, rumen, and omasum, and the "true stomach," which is called the abomasum.

S

sacral vertebrae: The vertebrae of the pelvic region. The sacral vertebrae fuse into a solid structure called the sacrum. The sacrum forms a joint with the pelvis on each side called the sacroiliac joint.
sacrum: The solid structure formed by the fusion of the sacral vertebrae.
salivary glands: Glands that assist in the mastication of food in the mouth.
saphenous vein: Vein of the lower portion of the hind leg. Found between the hock and the stifle joints.
scanning objective (3.29, 3.59, or 49): Lowest power objective lenses on a microscope.
scapula: The shoulder blade. The most proximal bone of the thoracic limb. In domestic animals there is no bony connection between the scapula and the axial skeleton.
sciatic nerve: Runs along the caudal aspect of the femur beneath the biceps femoris muscle. It is important to avoid this nerve when giving intramuscular injections.
sclera: The white portion of the eye. It is part of the outer fibrous layer of the eyeball.
scrotum: The sac of skin that houses the testes.
sebaceous glands: Associated with hair follicles, cells within the glands rupture and release the white oily sebum that they contain. Sebum is important in lubricating the hair shaft.
semicircular canals: The portion of the inner ear that senses rotary motion of the head.
seminal vesicles: The most cranial of the male accessory reproductive glands. They are not found in the dog and cat.
seminiferous tubules: Testes produce spermatazoa in microscopic seminiferous tubules.
semiplume: There are six types of feathers: contour, semiplume, down, filoplume, bristle, and powder down.
semitendinosus muscle: This strap-like muscle lies medial to the biceps femoris muscle and lateral to the semimembranosus muscle. It extends the hip, flexes the stifle, and extends the tarsal joints.
serum: The liquid portion of whole blood if no anticoagulant is added to a blood sample.
sesamoid bone: A bone present in some tendons. They act as bearings over the joint surfaces, allowing powerful muscles to move the joints without the tendon wearing out as they move over the joints.
shaft of the mandible: The horizontal portion of the mandible that houses all the lower teeth.
short bone: A small bone shaped like a small cube or marshmallow. The bones of the carpus are examples of short bones.
sigmoid flexure: An S-shaped bend in the nonerect penis of the bull, ram, and boar.
sole: The thick, horny tissue between the wall, the frog, and the bars.
sole corium: Sensitive connective tissue layer that lies underneath the soft horn of the sole. Contains the germinal cells that create the horn of the sole.
spermatic cord: A structure that links the testes with the rest of the body. It consists of blood and lymphatic vessels, nerves, and the vas deferens.
spinal cord: The caudal continuation of the brain stem outside the skull that continues down the spinal canal formed by the vertebrae of the spine. It conducts sensory information and motor instructions between the brain and the periphery of the body.
spine: Spine is a ridge that projects laterally.
spinous process: The single dorsally projecting process of a vertebra.
splint bones: The vestigial metacarpal and metatarsal bones of a horse's leg. There are two splint bones in each leg: one on either side of the "cannon bone"—the large metacarpal or metatarsal bone.
stage: Part of a microscope. Platform upon which a specimen slide is mounted.
stage clips: Part of a microscope, found on older styles without mechanical stages, used to hold and move the slide.
stapes: The ossicle in the middle ear shaped like a stirrup.
sternal recumbency: Lying on the sternum (ventral body surface) with the dorsal surface facing up.
sternum: The breastbone. The series of rodlike bones called sternebrae that form the floor of the thorax.
stifle joint: Femorotibial/femoropatellar joint. The joint between the femur and the tibia. In humans it is called the knee joint.
stratum basale: The lowest layer of keratinocytes is called the stratum germinativum or stratum basale (basal layer) and consists of a single layer of cells along the basement membrane of the epidermis.
stratum corneum: The topmost layer of the epidermis is the stratum corneum (horny layer). This is a layer of dead remnants of squamous epithelial cells.
stratum granulosum: The cells of the epidermis begin to become diamond-shaped or elongated. The nuclei and cellular organelles in these cells are starting to degenerate. Keratin is being created and is starting to fill the cytoplasm of the cells.
stratum lucidum: A layer of the epidermis composed of elongated dead cells, which are mostly filled with keratin and have lost their nuclei. The cells appear to be clear when they are stained.
stratum spinosum: A layer of the epidermis consisting of about three layers of squamous epithelial cells. There is some evidence of cell division in this layer and the cells still contain their nuclei.
styloid process: On the distal end of the radius and articulates with the carpus.
subclavian arteries: Blood vessels that supply blood to the front legs.
sublingual gland: A salivary gland.
superficial: Toward the surface of the body or a body part.
superficial cervical lymph node: One of the lymph nodes in the neck region that are routinely palpated during physical examinations.
suspensory ligament of the ovary: A ligament that comes off the cranial end of the broad ligament and attaches to the body wall near the last rib.
synovial fluid: Viscous fluid formed by the lining layer of the joint capsule of a synovial joint. Serves to lubricate the joint surfaces.
syrinx: Enlargement of the trachea above the sternum in birds. Contains muscles, air sacs, and vibrating membranes that collectively form the voice box.

T

tactile elevation: A type of hair seen in animals connected to specialized nerves, allowing an animal to "touch" objects in its environment.
tailhead: Dorsal part of the base of a tail.
tapetum (a.k.a. tapetum lucidum): The highly reflective area of the choroid in the back of the eye of most domestic animals.
tarsal bones: The bones of the tarsus. Consists of two rows of short bones located between the distal ends of the tibia and fibula and the proximal ends of the metatarsal bones.
tarsal glands (a.k.a. meibomian glands): Glands on the eyelid margins that produce a waxy substance that helps prevent tears from overflowing onto the animal's face.
tarsus: The joint composed of the tarsal bones. Referred to as the "hock" of most animals and the "ankle" of humans.
taste buds: Structures found mainly on certain papillae of the tongue that contain the receptor cells for taste.
temporal bones: Skull bones that are part of the external bones of the cranium. The two temporal bones form the lateral walls of the cranium, contain the middle and inner ear structures, and are the skull bones that form the temporomandibular joints with the mandible (lower jaw).
tendon: An extension of the epimysium that consists of dense cordlike connective tissue.
testes: The male gonads. They produce the male reproductive cells, spermatozoa, as well as androgen hormones.
testicular capsule (tunica albuginea): The capsule of the testis.
testis: A male gonad.
testosterone: The principal male sex hormone.
thalamus: Part of diencephalon that acts as a relay station for regulating sensory impulses to the cerebrum.
third eyelid (a.k.a. nictitating membrane): A T-shaped plate of cartilage covered by conjunctiva located medially between the eyelids and the eyeball. It also contains lymph nodules and a gland that contributes to the tear film on its back (ocular) surface.
thoracic cavity: The chest. The body cavity occupied by the heart and lungs, along with many blood vessels, nerves, and lymphatic vessels.
thoracic limb: The front limb.
thoracic vertebrae: The group of vertebrae located dorsal to the thoracic region.
thyroid gland: An endocrine gland made up of two parts located on either side of the larynx in the neck region. It produces thyroid hormone and calcitonin.
tibia: The main weight-bearing bone of the lower leg. It forms the stifle joint with the femur proximal to it and the hock with the tarsus distal to it.
tibial crest: A longitudinal ridge on the front of the proximal end of the tibia.
toe: The cranial portion of the equine hoof.
trachea: The windpipe. A thin-walled tube descending from the larynx to the bronchi that carries air to the lungs.
transduction (pain): The part of the pain sensation that involves conversion of the painful stimulus to a nerve impulse.
transmission (pain): The part of a pain sensation that involves sending the impulse up nerve fibers to the spinal cord.
transverse plane: Divides the body into cranial and caudal parts.
transverse process: A lateral-projecting process of a vertebra.
tricuspid valve: The valve between the right atrium and the right ventricle of the heart.
trochlea: Trochlea is a smooth articular surface on the cranial surface of the distal end in which the patella (kneecap) rides.
trochlear notch: Trochlear notch is half-moon–shaped, concave articular surface that wraps around the trochlea of the humeral condyle to help make the elbow joint a very tight, secure joint.
turbinates: Skull bones that are part of the internal bones of the face. Also known as the nasal conchae. The turbinates are four thin, scroll-like bones that fill most of the space in the nasal cavity. In the living animal the turbinates are covered by the moist, vascular lining of the nasal passages. Their scroll-like shape helps the nasal lining warm and humidify the inhaled air and trap tiny particles of inhaled foreign material.
tympanic membrane: The eardrum. The paper-thin connective tissue membrane that is tightly stretched across the opening of the external ear canal into the middle ear.

U

ulna: One of the two bones (the radius is the other) that form the antebrachium (forearm). The ulna forms a major portion of the elbow joint with the distal end of the humerus.
ulnar nerve: The most caudal of the three major branches of the brachial plexus. It is easily found near the olecranon.
umbilical cord: The umbilical cord is the only direct point of placental attachment to the fetus, and contains multiple vessels in addition to the urachus.
umbilicus: A small scar that will either be flat or slightly raised on the ventral midline of the abdomen about one third the distance from the xiphoid cartilage to the penis or vulva. It is where the umbilical cord was attached to the fetus.
uniparous: A uniparous species typically only has a single corpus luteum.
ureters: Muscular tubes that carry urine from the kidneys to the urinary bladder.
urethra: Tubular structure that carries urine from the urinary bladder out of the body.
urinary bladder: Saclike organ that stores urine until it is ready to be released out of the body.
uterine body: The portion of the uterus of common domestic animals that connects the horns with the cervix.
uterine horns: The most cranial parts of the uterus. They are paired structures that attach to the body of the uterus.
uterus: The hollow, muscular organ where pregnancy is maintained.
uvea: The middle vascular layer of the eye.

V

vagina: The birth canal and the tube that receives the penis during breeding.
vallate: Receptors on the tongue that detect sour.
vallate papilla: One of the four types of papillae in the cat.
vas deferens: The tube that connects the tail of the epididymis with the urethra.
vena cava: Large vein that returns blood from the systemic circulation to the heart.
ventral: Toward the bottom (belly) surface of the body.
ventricle: The heart chamber that pumps blood out through the large arteries. The left ventricle pumps blood out through the aorta and the right ventricle pumps blood out through the pulmonary artery.
Vermonasal organ: The paired auxiliary olfactory sense organ located in the soft tissue of the nasal septum.
vertebra: One of the bones of the spinal column.
vertebral body: A typical vertebra consists of a ventral body, a dorsal arch, and a group of processes.
vestibule (ear): The entrance into the vagina. It is part of the vulva located between the labia and the entrance into the vagina.
vestibule (oral): The space between the teeth and the lips.
vestibule (vagina): The portion of the inner ear that senses position and linear motion of the head.
visceral vaginal tunic: The inner, thin connective tissue sac that is tightly adhered to the surface of the testis.
vitreous compartment: The compartment of the eye behind the lens and ciliary body.
vitreous humor: The soft, gelatinous fluid that fills the vitreous compartment of the eye.
vocal cords: Two fibrous connective tissue bands attached to the arytenoid cartilages of the larynx that vibrate as air passes over them.
vulva: The only externally visible part of the female reproductive tract. It is composed of the labia, clitoris, and vestibule.

W

wall: The portion of the equine hoof visible while the horse is standing.
white line: The innermost layer of the hoof wall; central to it are deeper, sensitive tissues.
white matter: Collection of nerve fibers in the CNS that are surrounded by myelin, making them appear white grossly.
withers: Area dorsal to scapulas.

X

xiphoid: The last, most caudal sternebra. Its full name is the xiphoid process.

Z

zonary attachment: One of four types of placental attachment.
zygomatic bones: Skull bones that are part of the external bones of the face. The zygomatic bones form a portion of the orbit of the eye and the rostral portion of the zygomatic arch.

Index

Note: Page numbers followed by *f* indicate figures, *t* indicate tables, and *b* indicate boxes.

A

Abdomen, muscles of
  origin, insertion, action, 175*t*
  superficial, 176*f*
Abdominal aorta, 309*f*
Abdominal cavity, important blood vessels in, 315
  canine, 311*f*
  feline, 309–310*f*
  nonpregnant, 311*f*
  pregnant, 312*f*
    identification exercises for, 326–327, 326–327*f*
Abdominal oblique
  external, 190
  internal, 190–191
Abdominal wall, muscles of, 175, 189–191, 189–192*f*
  exercises for, 199–203, 199*b*, 199–201*f*, 202*b*, 202*t*
Abductor pollicis longus muscle, 165–166*f*, 167
Abomasum, 370, 371–373*f*
Accessory carpal, 122
Acetabulum, 126
Acromion, 161
Adductor magnus et brevis muscle, 180*f*
Adductor muscle, 178*f*, 181*f*, 182, 187–188*f*
Adipose tissue, 77–78*f*
  photomicrograph of, 64*f*
Adrenal gland, 270, 279–281
  anatomy and histology of, 270
  clinical applications of, 270
  exercises for, 279–280*b*, 279*t*, 281*f*
  hormone physiology of, 270
  identification exercises for, 279*b*
  in-class activity, 270
Adrenocorticotropic hormone (ACTH), 265
Air sacs, avian, 461
Aldosterone, 270
Allantoic sac, 451
Alopecia, 270, 271*f*
Alpha cells, 272*f*, 273
Amniotic sac, 451
Amphiarthroses, 130
Anaphase, 44
Anatomic terms, 2–15
  anatomic planes, 2–3, 2*f*
  basic, 2–3
  dental, 4–9, 6*b*
  directional, 3–4
  exercises for, 9–19
  for general body position, 4, 5*b*
  regional, 4
Anconeal process, 122
Anconeus muscle, 164*f*
Androgens, 422
Anestrus period, 432*f*
Anorectic, 61
Antebrachial muscles
  caudomedial, 172*f*
  craniolateral, 171*f*
Anterior chamber, 244
Antidiuretic hormone (ADH), 265
Antigen-antibody complexes, 293*f*
Antrum, of stomach, 370
Aorta, 302, 309
  abdominal, 312, 312*f*
    feline, 310*f*
  avian, 461
  feline, 305*f*, 309*f*
  of sheep, 303*f*
Aortic arch, feline, 308*f*
Aortic valve, 302
Aperture diaphragm, 24–25
Apex of the frog, 82
Apical, defined, 6*b*, 8, 8*f*
Aponeurosis, defined, 149
Appendicular skeleton, 120–130, 121*b*, 122*f*
Aqueous compartment, 244
Aqueous humor, 244
Arachnoid, 216*f*, 217
Arm, of microscope, 24
Arrector pili muscle, 76, 77*f*
Arrhythmogenic right ventricular cardiomyopathy, 69*b*
Arteries, 299
Atlas, wings of, 110*f*
Atria, 302, 303*f*
Atrophy, 61
Attachment, definition of, 149
Auricles, 300, 308*f*, 315
Auricular cartilage, 158*f*
Auscultation, of breath sounds and lungs, 347–348
  clinical significance of, 348
Automated hematology instruments, 287
Avian anatomy, 458–479
  beak, 460
  cardiac, 461
  clinical significance of, 458–459
  critical and clinical thinking exercises for, 477–479, 477*b*
  digestive, 460–461
  exercises for, 466–479
  feather types and structure, 466–469
  in-class necropsy exercise for, 461–465, 462–465*f*
  introduction to, 459
  ocular, 460
  reproductive, 461
  respiratory, 461
  skeletal, 460
  wing, 460
Axillary artery, 305*f*
Axillary vein, 305*f*
Axillobrachialis vein, 160*f*
Axon, 60, 204
Azygous vein, 305*f*

B

Bacterial skin infection, 77, 77*f*
Bacteria, stained, 20, 21*f*
Ball and socket joint, 130, 132*f*
Barbs, 459–460
Barbules, 459–460
Bars, 82
Base, of microscope, 24
Basophil, 289*f*
Beak, anatomy of, 460
  exercise for, 473*b*
Beta cells, 272*f*, 273
Biceps brachii muscle, 162, 163–164*f*, 171*f*
Biceps femoris muscle, 176–177*f*, 178–179, 187*f*
Big Head, 268–270
Bile duct, common, 373
Bitter tastes, 233*b*

Blastocyst, 452
Blood, 285–298
exercises for, 293–298
film, 288*f*
hematology stains, 287–288, 295–296
exercises for, 295*b*
immunoassays, 291–292, 297–298
exercises for, 297*b*
introduction, 286
smear, 287, 294–295
exercises for, 294*b*
regions of, 288*f*
transfusions, 288–291
exercises for, 296*b*
types or groups, 290, 291*f*
crossmatch testing, 291, 297
veterinary technician's responsibilities, 286–287
exercises for, 293–294*b*
Blood flow, 303
to and from kidneys, 400, 400*f*, 409–410
tracing through heart, 318, 322*f*, 323
Blood groups, 290
Blood smear, 20, 22*f*
Blood vessels
of abdominal cavity, 309–312*f*, 315
of neck and thoracic cavity, 304–308*f*, 312, 312*f*
of pelvic limb, 312–315*f*, 315
of thoracic limb, 308–309*f*, 315–319
Body, of stomach, 370, 370*f*
Body position
anatomic terms for, 4, 4*f*
oblique, 4
terms for, 4, 5*b*
Body tissues, hormone production and action, 273*t*
Bone, decalcified compact, photomicrograph of, 65*f*
Bones, 98. *See also* specific bones
cancellous, 99
in horse, 100*f*
compact, 99
in horse, 100*f*
features, 101–105, 132
articular surfaces, 101, 104*f*
holes and depressed areas, 105, 111–112*f*
processes, 105, 108–110*f*
flat, 99
bovine, 102*f*
canine, 102–103*f*
head of, 105, 106–107*f*
irregular, 101, 103*f*
bovine, 104*f*
canine, 103*f*
in equine, 103*f*
as levers, 98
long, 99
shapes, 99–101, 101–103*f*, 132
short, 99
in equine, 101–102*f*
Bones *(Continued)*
skull, 112–113
types, 99
Bone spavin, 182*b*
Bovine horn, 82–84, 83*f*
Bowman's capsule, 401
Brachial artery, 305*f*
Brachial fascia, feline, 151*f*
Brachialis muscle, 160–161*f*, 162, 164*f*, 171*f*
Brachial plexus, 219, 219*f*
Brachial vein, 305*f*
Brachiocephalic trunk, 302*f*, 303, 305–308*f*
Brachiocephalicus muscle, feline, 153–154
Brachioradialis muscle, 164*f*, 166*f*
Brain, 205–214
divisions of, 205, 205–207*f*
gray matter and white matter in, 214, 214–215*f*
Brain stem, 205, 205–207*f*, 207
external structures of, 213, 213*f*
gray and white matter in, 214, 214–215*f*
Bran Disease, 268–270
Breath sounds, auscultation of, 347–348
clinical significance of, 348
Bristle feathers, 459
Broad ligament, of uterus, 434
Bronchi, 340, 344*f*
avian, 461
Bronchial tree, 343*f*
Brush border, 61
Buccal surface, 6*b*, 8
Bulbar conjunctiva, 244, 245*f*
Bulb of glans, 429, 430*f*
Bulbourethral glands, 427, 427*f*
Bulbs of the heel, 82
Bumps, 101–105

C

Cadaver, retractable nails of, 80
Calcanean tendon, common, 178–179*f*, 181*f*, 182–185, 186–188*f*, 189
Calcaneus, 128–129
Calcitonin, 268
Calcitriol, 268
Calcium, regulation of, 268
Canine
structure of, 80
thorax, radiograph of, 304*f*
Canine skin, 78*f*
Canine teeth, 6
defined, 6*b*
Capillaries, 299
Capillary refill time, 69*b*
Capsular space, 401
Carbohydrates, digestion of, 373–374
Cardiac muscle, photomicrograph of, 65*f*
Cardia, of stomach, 370
Cardiovascular system, 299–333
basic blood flow through, 300–312, 322*f*
exercises for, 321, 323*f*
identification exercises for, 320–328, 320*f*
Cardiovascular system *(Continued)*
clinical significance of, 299
critical and clinical thinking exercises for, 328–333
exercises for, 322*f*, 327*f*
heart
external, 301–302*f*, 308
identification exercises for, 320–328, 320–321*f*, 324–327*f*, 332–333
in-class activities in, 315–319
internal, 303*f*, 309
Carotid arteries, 303, 305–307*f*
Carpal bones, 99, 122, 124–126*f*
accessory, 170*f*, 173*f*
equine, 102*f*
Carpal pad, 174*f*
Carpus, 4, 4*f*
equine, 124*f*
Carrier proteins, of plasma membrane, 35
Cartilage
elastic, photomicrograph of, 63*f*
hyaline, 101, 104*f*
Cartilaginous joints, 130
Cat declaw nerves, 220, 220*f*
Cats lack receptors, 233*b*
Caudal artery, 309*f*
mesenteric, 309*f*
Caudal, defined, 3, 3*b*
Caudal surface, 4, 4*f*
Caudal vein, 310*f*
Cecum, 375–377, 376–377*f*
Celiac artery, feline, 309*f*
Cell anatomy, 34–53
cytoplasm in, 38–40, 39–42*f*
exercises for, 44–46, 44–45*b*, 45*f*
nucleus in, 37–38, 38*f*
plasma membrane in, 35–37, 37*f*
preparing and examining wet mount slide in, 49*b*
Cell body, 60
Cell division
exercises for, 49–52, 49–51*b*, 50*f*
stages of, 42–44, 43*f*
mitosis, 43–44
in sex cells (meiosis), 44, 44*f*
Cell membrane. *See* Plasma membrane
Cellular component, 286
Cellular microscopy, exercise for, 46–49, 46*b*, 47*f*, 48–49*b*
Central nervous system (CNS), 204
Centrioles, 38
Centromere, 43
Centrosome, 38
Cephalic vein, 308
canine, 309*f*
feline, 151*f*, 154*f*, 160*f*, 308*f*
Cerebellum
external structures of, 207, 208*f*
gray matter and white matter in, in brain, 215*f*
internal structures of, 210, 210*f*

Cerebrum, 205, 205–207*f*
external structures of, 207, 208*f*
gray matter and white matter of, 214*f*
internal structures of, 210, 210*f*
Cervix, 434–436, 435*f*, 451
Channel proteins, of plasma membrane, 35
Chestnuts, 74–76, 76*f*
location of, 87*b*, 87*f*
Cholesterol molecules, of plasma membrane, 35
Chordae tendineae, 302, 303*f*, 316
Choroid, 238–241, 240*f*
Chromatids, 43
Chromatin, 37, 43
Chromosomes, 37
Ciliary body, 238, 239*f*
Clavicle, 152*f*, 160*f*
Claws, 80, 174*f*
Cleidocephalicus muscle, feline, 152*f*, 158*f*
Cleidomastoideus muscle, feline, 152*f*, 160*f*
Clitoris, 436
Cloaca, 460
Clotting factors, 286
Coffin bone, 82
Collateral cartilages, 82
Colon, 376–378*f*, 377
Commercial immunoassay kits, 291
Compact bone, decalcified, photomicrograph of, 65*f*
Complete blood count (CBC), 286
Compound light microscope
care of, 25
coarse and fine adjustment of, 25
critical and clinical thinking, 32–33
estimating size of objects with prepared blood film in, 30*b*
labeling parts of, 26*b*
measurements and calculations for magnifications of, 28*t*
parts of, 21–25, 23*f*
putting away of, 25
stage and stage brackets or clips of, 25
use of, 20, 27–32
Condenser, 24
Condyles, 101, 104–105*f*
canine, 104*f*
Cones, 241
Conical papillae, 73, 74*f*
Conjunctiva, 244–246, 245*f*
Conjunctival sac, 244
Connective tissue, 58–59, 58*b*, 78*f*
function of, 55
Connective tissue papilla, 79
Connective tissue root sheath, 79
Contour feathers, 459–460
Cookie cutter lesions, 77
Coracobrachialis muscle, 163*f*
Coracoids, 460
Corium, 80, 82
Corium layers, function and location of, 90*b*, 90*t*
Cornea, 248*f*
Cornual process, 82, 113
Coronal, defined, 6*b*, 8, 8*f*
Coronary band, 82
Coronary corium, 82
Coronet, 82
Coronoid processes, 122
Corpora lutea, 432*f*
Corpus cavernosum penis, 429
Corpus cavernosum urethrae, 429
Corpus luteum, 451
Corpus spongiosum, 429
Cortex, 78–79
Corticotropin-releasing hormone (CRH), 265
Cortisol, 270
Costal arch, feline, 150
Costal (rib) cartilage, 120
Costochondral junction, 120
Cotyledonary attachment, of placenta, 451
Cowper's glands, 427–428
Cow skull and horn, 83*f*
Cranial, defined, 3*b*
Cranial mesenteric artery, feline, 309*f*
Cranial nerves, 209, 209*f*, 209*t*
Cranial surface, 4, 4*f*
Cranial tibial muscle, 177–179*f*, 181*f*, 182, 183–184*f*, 187–188*f*
Cranium
bones of, 113
protective roles of, 98
Cremaster muscle, 422
Crop, 461
Crossmatch testing, 291, 297
exercises for, 297*b*
Crown, 6–7
defined, 6*b*
Crusts, 77*b*
Cushing disease, 79*b*
Cushing's syndrome, 281*f*
Cutaneous trunci muscle, feline, 151*f*
Cuticle, 78–79
Cytokinesis, 43–44
Cytoskeletal elements, 38
Cytosol, 38

D

DCT. *See* Distal convoluted tubule (DCT)
Decalcified compact bone, photomicrograph of, 65*f*
Deep, defined, 4
Dehorning, 83*b*
Delta cells, 273
Deltoideus muscle, 160*f*, 161, 171*f*
Deltoid muscle, feline, 153–154*f*, 160*f*
Dendrites, 60
Dental arcade, 6
Dental arch, 6
defined, 6*b*
Dental charting, 381*b*, 381*f*
Dental formulas, 380–382
Dental terms, 4–9
Dentition
canine, 380*f*
of cat, 369*f*
equine, 380*f*
Dermal papillae, 76
Dermis, 71, 76–78, 77–78*f*
Diabetes mellitus, feline, 282*b*
Diaphragm, 304–306*f*, 308–310*f*, 342
Diaphysis, 99
Diarthroses, 130
Diencephalon, 205–207, 206–207*f*
external structures of, 211, 211*f*
gray matter and white matter of, 214
internal structures of, 212, 212*f*
Diffuse attachment, of placenta, 451
Digastricus muscle, 157–158
Digestive system, 364–398
avian
labeling exercise for, 474–475, 474*f*
clinical significance of, 365
critical and clinical thinking for, 396–398
digestion-related organs in, 379
esophagus in, 367, 368*f*, 369–373
dissection of, 369–373
exercises, 379–398
intestinal tract in, 373–378
introduction of, 365
labeling exercises for, 384*f*, 387*f*, 389*f*, 394–396*f*
oral cavity in, 367–369
review of, 390–394, 391–393*f*
salivary glands in, 366–367, 366*f*
stomach in
dissection of, 369
exercise for, 382–385, 382*f*
monogastric, 370, 370*f*
ruminant, 370–373, 371–373*f*, 384*f*
Digital annular ligaments, 173*f*
Digital cushion, 82
Digital extensor muscle
common, 164–166*f*, 174*f*
lateral, 164–166*f*, 167, 171–172*f*, 178*f*, 184*f*
long, 177–178*f*, 182, 183–184*f*, 186–187*f*
tendon of, 183–184*f*
Digital extensor tendon
division of, 165*f*
lateral, 174*f*
Digital flexor muscle
deep, 167–173, 169–173*f*, 179*f*, 181*f*, 187*f*, 188–189
branches of, 169*f*
superficial, 170*f*
tendons of, 168*f*, 170*f*, 174*f*, 182–185, 186*f*
superficial, 167, 168–171*f*, 178–181*f*, 183*f*, 185–187*f*, 187–188
tendon, 170*f*
tendons of, 169*f*, 173–174*f*
tendons of, 173*f*

Digital flexor tendon, deep, 185*f*
Digital pad, 174*f*
Digit pad, 166*f*, 170*f*
Discoid attachment, of placenta, 451
Distal, 7–8
  defined, 3*f*, 4, 6*b*
Distal convoluted tubule (DCT), 401
Distal hind leg
  caudal muscles of, 174
  craniolateral muscles of, 174, 174*f*
Distal phalanx, 80
Distal sesamoid bone, 130
Dog, nose and paw pads of, 86*b*, 86*f*
Dorsal, defined, 3, 3*b*
Dorsal plane, 3*b*
Dorsal recumbency, 5*b*
Dorsal surface, 4, 4*f*
Down feathers, 459
Duodenum, 373

E

Ear, 235*f*
Ear canal, depths of, 249
Eccrine sweat glands, 76–77, 77*f*
Ectoderm, 452
Efferent ducts, 424
Elastic cartilage, photomicrograph of, 63*f*
Elastic ligaments, 174*f*
Endocrine pancreas, 270–273
  exercises for, 281–282*b*
Endocrine system, 262–265, 270–284
  adrenal gland, 270
  and control of hormone secretion, 262, 263*f*
  endocrine pancreas, 270–273
  exercises for, 273–284, 273–278*b*, 274*f*, 280*b*, 282*b*, 284*b*
  gonads, 273
  hypothalamus and pituitary gland, 262–265
    exercises for, 274–275*b*, 274*f*
  identification exercises for, 281–282*b*
  introduction, 262
  parathyroid gland, 268–270
    exercises for, 278*b*, 278*t*
  thyroid gland, 265, 266*f*
    exercises for, 275–277*b*
  tissues, 282–284
    exercises for, 282–284*b*
  word search, 284*b*
Endoderm, 452
Endometrium, 451
Endoplasmic reticulum (ER), 39
Endotracheal tube, placement of, 338
Energy, 38
Enzyme-linked immunosorbent assay (ELISA), 291–292
  membrane, 293*f*
Eosinophil, 289*f*
Epicondyles, 122
Epidermis, 71, 77*f*
  layers of, 71–72
  of nose and paw pads, 72–73, 74*f*
Epididymis, 424, 426*f*
Epiglottis, 338, 338*f*, 367–368*f*, 368
Epinephrine, 270
  identification exercises for, 280*b*
Epiphyseal plates, 99
Epiphyses, 99
Epithelial tissue, 55–58
  function of, 55
  identification of, 55
Equilibrium, 236–237
  semicircular canals, 237
  vestibule, 236
Equine foot, 80–82, 81*f*
Equine intestinal mucosa, photomicrograph of, 63*f*
Ergots, 74–76, 76*f*
  location of, 87*b*, 87*f*
Esophagus, 367, 368*f*, 369–373
  avian, 461
  dissection of, 369
Exocrine gland, classification, 57*b*
Extensor carpi radialis muscle, 161*f*, 164–165*f*, 170–171*f*
Extensor carpi ulnaris muscle, 165–167, 165–166*f*, 171*f*
  attachment of, 165*f*
Extensor retinaculum, 166*f*, 174*f*, 183*f*
  proximal, 177–179*f*, 181*f*
External acoustic meatus, 113
External auditory canal, 235
External ear, 235
External eye-related landmarks, 246, 247*f*
External root sheath, 78–79*f*, 79
Extraocular muscles, 246
Eye
  avian, 460
    exercise for, 473*b*
    labeling exercise for, 472*f*, 473*b*
  compartments of, 244, 244*f*
  dissection of, 247–249
  identification exercises for, 252–255*b*, 252–255*f*
  outer fibrous layer of, 237–238, 237–238*f*
Eyelids, 244–246, 245*f*
  third, 460

F

Fabellae, 126, 128*f*
Face, bones of, 113–118, 113*b*
Facet, 105, 107–108*f*
  bovine, 107*f*
  equine, 108*f*
Facial muscles, paralysis of, 217
Facial nerve, 158*f*, 217, 217*f*
Fat, digestion of, 373–374
Feather, types and structure of, 459–460
  drawing exercises for, 467*b*
  identification exercises for, 468*b*, 468*f*
  labeling exercises for, 466*b*, 466*f*
Feces, microscopy of, 20
Feet
  canine, 130*f*
  feline, 130*f*
Feline claws
  color structures in, 91*b*, 91*f*
  structure of, 80
Feline immunodeficiency virus (FIV), 291
Feline skin, observation of, 86*b*
Femoral artery, 179*f*, 309*f*, 312, 319
Femoral fascia, feline, 151*f*
  lateral, 176–177*f*
Femoral nerve, 220–221, 220*f*
Femoral triangle, 179*f*
Femoral vein, 179*f*, 310*f*, 312, 312–313*f*
Femur, 126
  avian, 460
  bovine, 127*f*
  canine, 105*f*
    greater trochanter of, 108*f*
  equine, nutrient foramen of, 111*f*
  greater trochanter of, 180*f*
Fibrous joints, 130
Fibula, 128, 128*f*
  avian, 460
Fight or flight response, 262
Filiform papillae, 233, 234*f*, 367*f*, 368
Filoplume feathers, 459
Fimbriae, 433
Fixation, 62
Fleshy, definition of, 149
Flexor carpi radialis muscle, 167
  cut stump of, 173*f*
  tendon of, 170*f*
Flexor carpi ulnaris muscle, 167, 168–171*f*
  humeral head of, 169*f*
  tendon of, 169*f*
  ulnar head of, 169*f*
Flexor muscle, deep, 185*f*
Flexor retinaculum, 170*f*
Flexures, in equine hindgut, 378
Fluid mosaic, 35
Fluid therapy, exercises for, 52–53, 52*b*
Foliate papillae, 233*b*, 234*f*
Follicle-stimulating hormone (FSH), 264*f*, 431
Foot
  avian, exercise for, 472*b*
  equine, structures of
    exercises for, 90–91*b*, 92*f*
  rear, muscles of, 189
Foramen, 105
Foramen magnum, 113
Forefoot, muscles of, 173*f*
  lateral aspect, 174*f*
  palmar aspect, 173*f*
Foreleg
  caudal muscles of, 160–161*f*, 162–163, 163*f*, 169–170*f*
  caudomedial muscles of, 167–173
  cranial muscles of, 162, 163–164*f*, 166*f*
  craniolateral muscles of, 163–167
  intrinsic muscles of, origin, insertion, action, 159*t*

Foreleg *(Continued)*
lateral aspect of, 161*f*, 171*f*, 174*f*
palmar aspect of, 173*f*
upper, medial muscles of, 163*f*
Fossa(e), 105, 112*f*
of canine scapula, 112*f*
of feline mandible, 112*f*
Frog, 82
Frog corium, 82
Frontal bones, 113
Frontal sinus, 340*f*
Fundus, of stomach, 370
Fungiform papillae, 233*b*, 234*f*
Furcation, 9
defined, 6*b*

G

Gastrocnemius muscle, 178–179*f*, 181*f*, 182–185, 184*f*, 187*f*
lateral head of, 180*f*, 183*f*, 186*f*
medial head of, 186*f*
Gastrointestinal tract, of rabbit, 389*f*
Gingival, defined, 6*b*, 8, 8*f*
Gingivitis, 381
Gizzard, 461
Glenoid cavity, 122
Gliding joint, 130, 132*f*
Glomerulus, 401
Glottis, 338, 368
Glucocorticosteroid, identification exercises for, 280*b*
Gluteal fascia, feline, 151*f*, 176*f*
Gluteal muscle
deep, 178*f*, 187*f*
middle, 177–178, 177*f*
superficial, 176*f*, 177
middle, 180*f*, 187*f*
superficial, 176*f*, 180*f*, 187*f*
Gluteofemoralis muscle, 176*f*
Goiter, 268*f*
Golgi apparatus, 39
Gonads, 273
avian, 461
Gracilis muscle, 179*f*, 181, 187*f*
Granulation tissue, 75
Gray matter
in brain, 214, 214–215*f*
of cerebellum, 210*f*
in spinal cord, 215
Greater tubercle, canine, 108*f*, 122
Grooves, 101–105
Growth hormone (GH), 264*f*
Gustatory cells, 233
Gyri, 207, 214

H

Hair
structure of, 78–80
types of, 88*b*
Hair bulb, 76
Hair follicle, 76, 79*f*
color structures of, 89*b*
microscopic exam of, 90*b*, 90*f*
Hair loss, 270
Hair root, 79
Hair shafts, 78, 78*f*
Hair, structure of, exercises for, 88–90, 88–90*b*, 88*f*
Hard palates, 367, 367–368*f*
Head
of bones, 105
muscles of, 155–156
origin, insertion, and action, 150*t*
Healing process, in tissue, 67*b*
Hearing, 235–236, 250–251
exercises for, 250–251*b*, 250*f*
external ear, 235
inner ear, 236
middle ear, 235–236
Heart, 299
auscultate to, 318–319, 318*f*
clinical significance of, 319
avian, 461
labeling exercises for, 475*b*, 475*f*
canine in thoracic cavity, 304*f*
diagram of, 321*f*
external structures of, 301–302*f*, 308*f*
internal structures of, 303*f*, 309*f*
of sheep, 301–303*f*, 320–321*f*
dissection of, 316–317*f*, 317–318
tracing flow of blood in, 318*f*
tracing flow of blood in, 318, 322–323*f*
Heart sounds, 318
Heels, 82
Hematology stains, 287–288, 295–296
exercises for, 295*b*
Hepatic vein, 310*f*
Hilum, 342
Hilus, 402
Hind leg
caudal muscles of, 182–189
craniolateral muscles of, 182
Hind limb, blood vessels of, 312*f*
Hinge joint, 131*f*
Hip
lateral muscles of, 174*f*, 176–178, 176*f*
muscles of, 177*f*
Hirsutism, 270
Holes, 101–105
Hoof, 82
injuries of, 70
Hoof wall, 82
Hooklets, 459–460
Hormones, 263*f*, 452
identification exercises for, 278*b*, 456*b*
male, 422
secretion of, control in, 262, 273–274, 273–274*b*
exercises for, 273*b*
Humerus, 120, 122, 163*f*
avian, 460
bovine, 123*f*
canine, 105*f*
greater tubercle of, 108*f*
distal, 163*f*
Hyaline cartilage, 101, 104*f*
rings, 340
Hydrolase, 39
Hyoid bone, 118
Hyperadrenocorticism, 270
exercises for, 280*b*
in horse, 270*f*
Hypercalcemia, 268
identification exercises, 281*b*
Hyperparathyroidism, 268–270
in iguana, 278*b*
Hyperthyroidism, 265, 278*b*
exercises for, 277*b*
Hypocalcemia, 268
Hypodermis, 71
Hypoglycemia, 273
Hypothalamus, 212, 262–265, 264*f*
exercises for, 274–275*b*
Hypothyroidism, 79*b*

I

Ileocecal junction, 375–377
Ileum, 373
Iliac arteries, 309*f*, 312*f*
Iliac veins, 310*f*, 312*f*
Ilium, 126, 176*f*
Immunoassays, 291–292, 297–298
exercises for, 297*b*
Incisal edge, 6*b*, 9, 9*f*
Incisive bones, 113
Incisive duct, 367
Incisor teeth, 6
defined, 6*b*
Inclusion bodies, 40
Incus, 236
Indirect ELISA technique, 292*f*
Infection, microscopy of, 20
Inferior umbilicus, 459–460
Infraspinatus muscle, 160–161*f*, 161–162, 164*f*, 171*f*
Infundibulum, 433
avian, 461
Injuries, to hooves, 70
Inner ear, 236
Inner nervous layer, 241–242, 241*f*
Insensitive lamina, 82
Insulin, 273
Insulinoma, 273
identification exercises for, 281*b*
Integral proteins, 35
Integumentary
layers of, 71–76, 84–86
exercises for, 84*b*, 84*f*, 85*t*
special features of, 76–80
exercises for, 86–88, 86–87*b*, 86–87*f*
Integumentary system, 70–84, 90–93
associated structures, 80–84
bovine horn, 82–84, 83*f*
canine and feline claws, structure of, 80
equine foot, 80–82, 81*f*
retractable nails, of cadaver, 80
critical and clinical thinking, exercises for, 93, 93–96*b*

Integumentary system *(Continued)*
features of, 76–80
dermis, 76–78, 77–78*f*
hair, structure of, 78–80
layers of, 71–76, 84–86
Intermediate filaments, 38
Internal root sheath, 78*f*, 79
Interosseous muscles, 187–188*f*
branches of, 165*f*
tendons of, 184*f*
Interparietal bones, 113
Interphase, 42–43
Interproximal space, 6*b*, 9
Interproximal surfaces, 6*b*, 9
Interstitial cells, 422
Interventricular groove, 300
Interventricular septum, 303*f*
Intestinal mucosa, equine, photomicrograph of, 63*f*
Intestinal tract, 373–378
exercise for, 385–387, 386*f*
Iris, 238, 239*f*, 241*f*
Iris diaphragm, 23*f*, 24–25
Ischiadicus nerve, 176*f*
Ischiatic tuberosity, 176*f*
Ischium, 126
Islets of Langerhans, 272*f*, 273
Isthmus, avian, 461

J

Jejunum, 373, 377*f*
Joints, 130, 131*f*. *See also* specific joints
cartilaginous, 130
fibrous, 130
identification exercises of, 143–144, 143*b*, 143*f*
synovial, 130
Jugular vein, 151–152*f*, 164*f*, 303, 305–307*f*

K

Keratinocytes, 71–72
Kidney, 402–403
external features of, 402, 402–403*f*, 414*b*, 414*f*
hormone production and action, 273*t*
internal features of, 403, 403–404*f*, 415–416, 415*b*, 415*f*

L

Labia, 436
Labial frenulum, 367, 367*f*
Labial surface, 6*b*, 8
Lacrimal bones, 113
Lacrimal puncta, 246
Lactation, 452
definition exercise for, 455*b*
Laminar corium, 82
Langerhans cells, 71–72
Large intestine, 375–378
Laryngopharynx, 367, 368*f*
Larynx, 338, 350–351, 368*f*
of calf, 338*f*
Larynx *(Continued)*
labeling exercises for, 350*b*, 350*f*
openings of, 338
Lateral canthus, 244, 246
Lateral malleolus, 128
Lateral recumbency, 5*b*
Latissimus dorsi muscle, 152*f*, 155, 164*f*
Left atrium, avian, 461
Left, defined, 3*b*, 4, 5*b*
Left ventricle, avian, 461
Leg
avian, 460
caudal muscles of, 185*f*
craniolateral, 184*f*
deep muscles, 178*f*, 180*f*
equine, 126*f*
lateral aspect of, muscles of, 176*f*, 183*f*, 186*f*
origins and insertions of, 187*f*
medial aspect of, muscles of, 181
muscles of, 177*f*
Lens, 238, 240*f*, 248*f*
Light microscopy. *See also* Compound light microscope
clinical significance of, 20
Light source, 24
Limbs, terms for, 3, 3*f*
Lingual frenulum, 367, 368*f*
Lingual surface, 6*b*, 8
Liver, 377–378*f*, 379
Lobe, 342
Longitudinal fissure, 207
Loop of Henle, 401
Lower respiratory tract, structures of, 351–356
labeling exercises for, 351–355*b*, 351–355*f*
Lumps, 101–105
Lungs, 304*f*, 342
auscultation of, 347–348
clinical significance of, 348
avian, 461
capillaries of, 300
labeling exercises for, 356*b*, 356*f*
of pig, 345*f*
Luteinizing hormone (LH), 264*f*, 422, 431
Lymph, 285–298
Lymph nodes, 285–298
axillary, 156*f*
cervical, 156*f*
deep, 164*f*
feline, 155
mandibular, 158*f*
parotid, 158*f*
popliteal, 176*f*
Lysosome, 39

M

Magnification
degree of, 24
measurements and calculations for, 28*t*
Magnum, avian, 461
Major crossmatch test, 291
Major slide crossmatch, 291
Malleolus, medial, 184*f*
Malleus, 235, 236*f*
Mammal, pregnant, dissection questions for, 453
Mammary gland
gross anatomy of, 452, 452*t*
location of, 452
microscopic anatomy of, 452
Mammary papillae, feline, 150
Mandible, 113–118
cow, 336*f*
defined, 6*b*
of equine, 9*f*
feline, fossa on, 112*f*
Mandibular salivary gland, 366, 366*f*
Manubrium, 120
Masseter muscle, 152*f*, 154*f*, 157
Mastication, muscles of, 157–158
Masticatory myositis, 159*b*
Matrix, 78*f*, 79
Maxilla, defined, 6*b*
Maxillary bones, 113
Medial canthus, 244, 246
Medial, defined, 3, 3*b*, 3*f*
Medial saphenous vein, feline, 310*f*
Median nerve, 173*f*, 219, 219*f*
Median plane, 3, 3*b*
Mediastinum, 342
Medulla, 78–79
Medulla oblongata, 213
Meiosis, 42, 44, 44*f*
Meissner's corpuscles, 76–77
Melanin, 71–72
Melanocytes, 71–72
Melanocyte-stimulating hormone (MSH), 265
Meninges, 216–217, 216*f*
Merkel cells, 71–72
Mesial, 7–8
defined, 6*b*
Mesoderm, 452
Mesometrium, 451
Metacarpal bones, 124
Metacarpal pad, 174*f*
Metacarpophalangeal joint, 174*f*
Metaphase, 43
Metatarsal bones, 129
second, 184*f*
Microfilaments, 38
Microscope, parts of, 21–25
Microscopy, 20–33
Microtubules, 38
Microvilli, 61, 61*f*
Midbrain, 213, 213*f*
Middle ear, 235–236
Minor crossmatch test, 291
Minor slide crossmatch test, 291
Mitochondria, 38
Mitosis, 42
stages of, 42–44
Mitral valve, 302, 303*f*, 318

Modulation, 233
Molar teeth, 6
  defined, 6*b*
  of dire wolf, 16*f*
Monogastric stomach, 370, 370*f*
Motor fibers, 205
Mucous membranes, 69*b*
Multiparous, 451
Muscles
  action of, 150
  attachment of, 149
  dissection of, 151, 176*f*
  extrinsic, 149–151
    of thoracic limb and related areas, 149–151
  of head and neck, 149, 155–156
  insertion of, 150
  of mastication, 149
  and neck, origin, insertion, and action of, 150*t*
  origin of, 150
  subcutaneous, 149
  superficial, feline, 151*f*
Muscle tissue, 59–60, 59*b*
  function of, 55
Muscular system, 148–203
  critical and clinical thinking for, 203
  exercises for, 192–203, 192*b*, 192*f*, 194*b*, 194*t*, 196*b*, 198–199*b*, 199*f*, 202*b*, 202*t*
  introduction of, 148–149
Mylohyoideus muscle, 152*f*, 158
Myometrium, 451
Myositis, masticatory, 159*b*

N

Nail, 80
Nasal bones, 113
Nasal cavity, 335
Nasal passage, 335
Nasal septum, 335
  in deer, 337*f*
  ovine, 337*f*
Nasal turbinates, 337*f*
Nasolacrimal ducts, 249
Nasolacrimal system, 246
Nasopalatine duct, 367
Nasopharynx, 367, 368*f*
Navicular bone, 82
Neck, 122, 349–350
  blood vessels of, 312
    canine, 304*f*
    feline, 305–308*f*
  muscles of, 155–156
    origin, insertion, and action, 150*t*
  palpation of, 347
Necropsy exercise, for avian anatomy, 461–465
Negative feedback system, 263*f*, 265
  exercises for, 276*b*
Neonatal isoerythrolysis (NI), 290
Nephron notables, 401
  exercise for, 410–411, 410*b*, 410*f*
Nerve fibers, myelinated, 214
Nervous system, 204–231
  brachial plexus, radial nerve, median nerve, and ulnar nerve, 219, 219*f*
  brain, 205–214, 205–207*f*
  brain stem, 205, 205–207*f*
  cat declaw nerves, 220, 220*f*
  cerebral and cerebellar internal structures, 210, 210*f*
  clinical significance of, 204
  comparison of endocrine and, 274*t*
  cranial nerves and, 209, 209*f*, 209*t*
  diencephalon
    external structures of, 211, 211*f*
    internal structures of, 212, 212*f*
  exercises for, 222–231, 222–228*b*, 222–224*f*, 225*t*
  facial nerve, 217, 217*f*
  femoral nerve and, 220–221, 220*f*
  gray matter and white matter in, in brain, 214, 214–215*f*
  introduction of, 204–205
  meninges, 216–217, 216*f*
  sciatic nerve and, 221, 221*f*
  spinal cord and, 215, 215*f*
  vagus nerve and, 218, 218*f*
Nervous tissue, 60, 60*b*, 60*f*
  function of, 55
Neurons, 60
Neutrophil, 289*f*
Nictitating membrane, 246, 460
Nociception, 233
Nonpolar tails, of phospholipids, 35
Norepinephrine, 270
  identification exercises for, 280*b*
Nose
  of common animals, 356*b*
  of dog, 86*b*, 86*f*
  epidermis of, 72–73, 74*f*
  of exotic animals, 358*b*, 358–359*f*
Nostrils, 335, 336*f*
  ovine, 336*f*
Nuclear pores, 38
Nucleoli, 38
Nucleus, 37–38, 38*f*
Nutrient foramen, of equine femur, 111*f*

O

Objective lenses, 23–24
Oblique positions, 4
Oblique recumbency, 5*b*
Obturator foramen, of canine pelvic bone, 111*f*
Obturator foramina, 126
Occipital bone, 113
Occipital condyles, 113
Occlusal surface, 6*b*, 9, 9*f*
Oculars, 21–23
Offspring, naming of, 456*b*
Olecranon, 161*f*
  of ulna, 163*f*, 166*f*, 170*f*
Olecranon fossa, 122
Olecranon process, 122
  of canine ulna, 110*f*
Olfactory bulbs, 207
Olfactory cells, 235
Olfactory epithelium, 235
Omasum, 370, 371–373*f*
Omotransversarius muscle, 153–154*f*, 155, 157*f*, 160*f*
Ophthalmoscope, using of, 249
Optic chiasm, 242–244, 243*f*
Optic disc, 242, 242*f*
Optic nerve, 242, 243*f*
Oral cavity, 367–369, 367–368*f*
  cow, 336*f*
  exercises for, 379–398, 379*f*
  in-class activity for, 369
Organelles, 38
Organs, digestion-related, 379
  exercise for, 387–390, 387–388*f*
Oropharynx, 367, 368*f*
Os penis, 429, 429*f*
Otoscope, using, 249
Ovarian arteries, 309*f*, 311*f*
Ovarian cycle, exercises for, 453*b*, 453*f*
Ovarian vein, 310*f*
Ovaries, 431, 432*f*, 451
  avian, 461
Oviducts, 433, 433*f*
Ovulation, 431
  avian, description of, 476*b*
  development of, 431
Ovum, fertilized, 433
Oxyphil cells, 268, 269*f*
Oxytocin, 265, 452
  exercises for, 275*b*

P

Pacinian corpuscles, 76–77, 78*f*
Pain, 250, 250*b*
  exercises for, 250*b*
Palatal surface, 6*b*, 8
Palatine tonsils, 367, 367–368*f*
Palmar surface, 3*b*, 4, 4*f*
Palpebral conjunctiva, 245*f*, 246
Palpebral reflex, 217
Pancreas, 377–378*f*, 379
  anatomy and histology of, 270–273, 272*f*
Papilla, 78*f*, 233
Papillary layer, 76, 77*f*
Papules, 77*b*
Paralysis of facial muscles, 217
Paranasal sinuses, 335
Parathyroid gland, 268–270, 269*f*
  anatomy and histology of, 268, 269*f*, 278*b*
  clinical applications, 268–270
  comparative anatomy of thyroid and, 267*b*, 267*f*
  exercises for, 278*b*
  hormone physiology of, 268
  identification exercises for, 278*b*
  in-class activity, 268

Parathyroid hormone, 268
overproduction, 268–270
Parfocal, defined, 24
Parietal bones, 113
Parietal vaginal tunic, 424
Parotid duct, 158*f*, 367
Parotid salivary gland, 158*f*, 366
Parturition, 433–434, 451
Patella, 126
Patellar ligament, 187–188*f*
Paw pads
of dog, 86*b*, 86*f*
epidermis of, 72–73, 74*f*
PCT. *See* Proximal convoluted tubule (PCT)
Pectineus muscle, 179*f*, 181*f*, 182, 187–188*f*
Pectoralis muscle, avian, 460
exercise of, 471*b*
Pectoral muscle
deep, 152*f*, 153, 156*f*, 160*f*
superficial, 152–153, 152*f*, 160*f*
Pelvic bone, canine, obturator foramen in, 111*f*
Pelvic limb
important blood vessels of, 312, 312–315*f*
muscles of, 173*f*
exercises for, 199–203, 199*b*, 199–201*f*, 202*b*, 202*t*
origin, insertion, action, 175*t*
superficial, 176*f*
Pelvic urethra, 427
Pelvis
bovine, 131*f*
tuber ischium of, 109*f*
canine, 127*f*
Penile urethra, 427
Penis, 427–428*f*, 428–429
Perception, 233
Pericardial sac, 301*f*, 306*f*
Periodontal fibers, 6–7
defined, 6*b*
Perioplic corium, 82
Peripheral nerves, 217–221. *See also* specific nerves
Peripheral nervous system (PNS), 204
Peroneal nerve, 186*f*
Peroneus brevis, 178*f*
Peroneus longus muscle, 177–178*f*, 180*f*, 182, 184*f*, 186–187*f*
tendon of, 186*f*
Peroneus longus tendon, 185*f*
Peroxisomes, 40
Phalanges, 124–125, 129–130, 129–130*f*
Pharynx, 338, 338*f*
cow, 336*f*
Phospholipids, 35
Photoreceptor cells, avian, 460
Photoreceptors, 241
Pia mater, 216*f*, 217
Pineal body, 212, 212*f*
hormone production and action, 273*t*
Pinna, 235, 236*f*
Piriformis muscle, 178*f*
Pituitary gland, 211, 211*f*, 262–265
anterior, 265
exercises for, 275*b*
exercises for, 274*b*, 274*f*
posterior, 265
Pituitary hormones, exercises for, 274*b*, 274*f*
Placenta, 437–440, 437–438*f*, 451–452
hormone production and action, 273*t*
retained, 437*b*
Placental attachment
identification exercise for, 455*b*, 455*f*
matching exercise for, 454*b*
Placentome, 437*b*
Plantar surface, 4, 4*f*
Planum nasale, 72
Planum nasolabiale, 72
Plasma, 286
difference between blood serum, 287*f*
Plasma membrane, 35–37, 37*f*
Platelets, 289
Platysma muscle, 151*f*, 156
Polar heads, of phospholipids, 35
Polydactyl, 80
Polydactyl dog, 80, 80*f*
Polygonal plates, 72, 73*f*
Pons, 213, 213*f*
Popliteus muscle, 185*f*, 187–188*f*
Positional terminology, dental, 7*f*
Positive feedback system, 263*f*
Posterior chamber, 244
Power down feathers, 459
Pregnancy, 451–452
clinical thinking challenge for, 455*b*
Premolar teeth, 6
defined, 6*b*
Prepuce, 427*f*, 429
Processes, 105, 108–110*f*
Progesterone, 452
Prolactin, 264*f*, 265, 452
Pronator teres muscle, 165*f*
Prophase, 43
Prostate gland, 427, 427*f*
Proteasomes, 39–40
Protein, digestion of, 373–374
Proud flesh, 75
of horse, 75*b*, 75*f*
Proventriculus, 461
Proximal convoluted tubule (PCT), 401
Proximal, defined, 3*b*, 3*f*, 4
Proximal interphalangeal joint, 174*f*
Proximal sesamoid bones, 130
Pubis, 126
Pulmonary artery, 300, 302
feline, 305*f*
Pulmonary valve, 318
Pulmonary vein, 302, 316
Pulse points, palpation of, 319
clinical significance of, 319
Pustules, 77*b*
Pygostyle, 460

Q

Quadrant, defined, 6, 6*b*
Quadriceps femoris muscle, 182, 186–188*f*
Quarters, 82

R

Rachis, 459–460
Radial nerve, 156*f*, 219, 219*f*
avoiding damage to, 163*b*
deep, 164*f*
superficial, 164*f*, 166*f*
Radial notch, 122
Radiographs, urinary system on, 408, 408*f*
Radius, 122
canine, 124*f*
Ramus, 118
Receptor proteins, of plasma membrane, 35
Rectus abdominis, 191
Rectus femoris muscle, 178*f*, 181*f*, 187*f*
Recumbency
dorsal, 4, 5*f*
lateral, 4, 5*f*
sternal, 4, 5*f*
Regional terms, 4, 5*f*
Relaxin hormone, 451
Renal artery, 309, 309*f*
feline, 310*f*
Renal corpuscle, 401
Renal cortex, 403
Renal medulla, 403
Renal pelvis, 403
Renal vein, 310*f*
Reproductive cycle, exercise for, 456*b*
Reproductive glands, accessory, 427–428, 428*t*
Reproductive system, 421–449
avian, 461
labeling exercise for, 476*b*, 476*f*
clinical significance of, 421
critical and clinical thinking, exercises for, 445–449, 445*b*, 447–448*b*
exercises for, 440–449
female, 431–440, 434–435*f*
cervix, 434–436, 435*f*
comparison of, 435*f*
identification, exercise for, 445, 445*f*
labeling, exercise for, 444, 444*f*
ovaries, 431, 432*f*
oviducts, 433, 433*f*
placenta, 437–440, 437–438*f*
suspensory ligaments, 434, 435*f*
uterus, 433–434, 434*f*
vagina, 436
vulva, 436, 436*f*
introduction to, 421
male, 422–431, 430–431*f*
accessory reproductive glands, 427–428, 428*t*
bulb of glans, 429, 430*f*
epididymis, 424, 426*f*
identification, exercise for, 442–443, 442–443*f*

Reproductive system *(Continued)*
labeling, exercise for, 440, 440*f*
os penis, 429, 429*f*
penis, 428–429, 428*f*
prepuce, 429
scrotum, 422, 423*f*
sigmoid flexure, 431, 431*f*
spermatic cord, 425–427, 426*f*
testes, 422, 424*f*
urethra, 427, 427*f*
vaginal tunics and testis capsule, 424, 425–426*f*
vas deferens, 425, 426*f*
Resolving power, 24
Respiratory rate, 348
Respiratory system, 334–335, 349–363
avian, 461
labeling, exercise for, 475–476, 475*f*
clinical significance, 334
critical and clinical thinking, exercises for, 356–363, 356*b*, 356–358*f*, 358*b*, 362*b*
exercises for, 349–363, 349–351*b*, 349*f*, 351*f*, 353–356*b*, 358–359*b*, 362*b*
in-class activities, 347–348
introduction to, 334
labeling exercises for, 350*b*, 350*f*
larynx, 338, 338–339*f*
trachea, 340
upper ovine, 336*f*
Respiratory tract
lower, 342, 342*t*, 343–346*f*
upper, 335
in cow, 336*f*
in deer, 337*f*
in dog, 335*f*
in sheep, 336*f*
Reticular layer, 76, 77*f*
Reticulitis, traumatic, 373, 373*f*
Reticulorumen, 370
Reticuloruminal contractions, 370
Reticulum, 370, 371–373*f*
Retina, 241–242
avian, 460
Retractable nails, of cadaver, 80
Retractor penis muscle, 431
Rhabdomyolysis, 177*b*
Rheostat, 24
Rhomboideus muscle, 155
Rib cage, rabbit, 120*f*
Ribosomes, 38
Ribs, 107*f*, 120
roles of, 98
Right atrium, avian, 461
Right, defined, 3*b*, 4, 5*b*
Rods, 241
Romanowsky stain, 287–288
Root, 6–7
defined, 6*b*
Rostral, defined, 3, 3*b*
Rotator cuff injuries, 162*b*
Rough endoplasmic reticulum, 39, 40*f*
Round ligament, of uterus, 434
Rugae, 367, 367*f*
Rumen, 370
Ruminants
horn of, 93*b*
stomach, 370–373, 371–373*f*

S

Sagittal plane, 3*b*
Salivary gland, 366–367, 366*f*
mandibular, 152*f*, 154*f*
parotid, 154*f*, 158*f*
Saphenous vein, 151*f*
canine, 314–315*f*
lateral, 312*f*, 314*f*
medial, 313*f*
Sartorius muscle, 176–177*f*, 179–180*f*, 187–188*f*
Scapula, 120, 122, 156*f*, 163–164*f*
canine, 102*f*
spine of, 110*f*
dorsal border of, 161*f*
lateral muscles of, 161–162
spine, 161*f*
Sciatic nerve, 221, 221*f*
Scrotum, 422, 423*f*
Sebaceous glands, 76–77, 77–78*f*
Sebum, 76–77
Semicircular canals, 237
Semimembranosus muscle, 178–180*f*, 187–188*f*
Seminal vesicles, 427
Seminiferous tubules, 422
Semiplume feathers, 459–460
Semitendinosus muscle, 177–180*f*, 179, 187–188*f*
Sense organs, 232–256
exercises for, 250–256
matching exercises for, 256*b*
suggested in-class activities, 247–249
vision, 237–246, 237*f*
compartments of eye, 244, 244*f*
external eye-related landmarks, 246, 247*f*
extraocular muscles, 246
eyelids and conjunctiva, 244–246
identification exercises for, 251
inner nervous layer, 241–242, 241*f*
middle vascular layer, 238–241
optic chiasm, 242–244, 243*f*
optic disc, 242, 242*f*
optic nerve, 242, 243*f*
outer fibrous layer of eye, 237–238, 237–238*f*
third eyelid, 246, 246*f*
Sensitive lamina, 82
Sensory fibers, 205
Serratus ventralis muscle, 155, 157*f*, 189*f*
Serum, 286
difference between plasma, 287*f*
Sesamoid bones, 125
bovine, 104*f*
Sex cells, cell division in, 44, 44*f*
Shaft, 113
Sheath of hair follicle, 78*f*
Sheep, heart of, tracing flow of blood in, 318
Shoulder
lateral muscles of, 161–162, 164*f*
medial muscles of, 162, 163*f*
superficial muscles of, 154*f*
Shoulder slip, 162*b*
Sigmoid flexure, 431, 431*f*
Sinus, 82
Sinuses, paranasal, 335
Skeletal muscle, photomicrograph of, 64*f*
Skeletal system, 97–105, 112–130, 132–144
bone features, 101–105, 132
articular surfaces, 101, 104*f*
holes and depressed areas, 105, 111–112*f*
processes, 105, 108–110*f*
bone shapes, 99–101, 101–103*f*, 132
bone types, 99, 100*f*
clinical significance, 97–98
critical and clinical thinking, exercises of, 144*b*
identification exercises of, 134–137, 134*b*, 134*f*
in-class activities, 132–133
introduction, 98
joints, 130, 131*f*
medical word parts, 99–130
skeleton, 112–130
axial, 112–120, 112–113*b*, 113*f*, 132–133
Skeleton, 82, 112–130
appendicular, 112, 120–130, 121*b*, 122*f*, 133
bones of, 121*b*
avian, 460
labeling exercises for, 470–471*b*, 470–471*f*
lightweight structure of, exercise for, 469*b*
axial, 112–120, 112–113*b*, 113*f*, 132–133
feline, 122*f*
identification exercises of, 137–143, 137–142*b*, 137–142*f*
labeling exercises of, 142*b*, 142*f*
Skin. *See also* Integumentary system
role of, 70
and signal of internal disease, 79*b*
thin, of pig, 88*b*
Skin scrapings, microscopy of, 20, 21*f*
Skull, 112–113, 113*b*, 349–350
bones of, 112–113
bovine, 115*f*
canine, 116–117*f*, 132*f*
equine, 117*f*
feline, 116*f*
Small intestine, 373–375, 376*f*
dissection of, 374–375, 374–375*f*
hormone production and action, 273*t*
Smell, 235
Smooth ER, 39

Soft palate, 367
Sole, 82
Sole corium, 82
Somatostatin, 273
Spermatic cord, 425–427, 426*f*
Spermatozoa, 421–422
Spinal column
  bones of, 118–120
  feline, 119*f*
Spinal cord, 204–205, 213*f*, 215, 215*f*
  gray and white matter of, 215
Spine, 122
Stapes, 236
Sternal recumbency, 5*b*
Sternoccipitalis muscle, 154*f*
Sternocephalicus muscle, 155–156, 158*f*
Sternum, 120
  avian, 460
  rabbit, 120
Stethoscope, esophageal, placement of, 340*f*
Stifle joint, canine, 104*f*
Stomach, 369–373
  avian, 461
  dissection of, 369
  exercise for, 382–385, 382*f*
  hormone production and action, 273*t*
  monogastric, 370, 370*f*
  ruminant, 370–373, 371–373*f*, 384*f*
Stratum basale, 72, 73*f*
Stratum corneum, 72, 73*f*
Stratum germinativum, 72, 73*f*
Stratum granulosum, 72, 73*f*
Stratum lucidum, 72, 73*f*
Stratum spinosum, 72, 73*f*
Styloid process, 122
Subclavian artery, 303, 305–308*f*
Subcutaneous adipose tissue, 78*f*
Subcutaneous artery Subcutaneous vein, 78*f*
Subcutaneous layer, 71
Subcuticular layer, 77*f*
Sublingual salivary gland, 366, 366*f*
Subscapularis muscle, 156*f*, 162
Suicide sacs, 39
Sulci, 207, 214
Superficial, defined, 3*b*, 4
Superficial veins, 300
Supracoracoideus muscle, 460
Supraspinatus muscle, 161*f*, 162, 164*f*, 171*f*
Suspensory ligaments, 238, 434, 435*f*
Sweat gland, 79*f*
Synarthroses, 130
Synovial joints, 130
Synsacrum, 460
Syrinx, 461

T

Tactile (Meissner) corpuscle, 78*f*
Tactile elevation, 78
Tactile hair, 78
Tapetum, 238, 240–241*f*
Target cells, 263*f*
Tarsal, 99
Tarsal bones, 128–129
Tarsal glands, 246
Tarsometatarsus, avian, 460
Tarsus, 4, 4*f*
Taste, 233–235
Taste buds, 233
Tears, 246
Teats, feline, 150
Teeth
  structure of, 368, 379*f*
  types of, 6, 6*f*, 368
Telophase, 44
Temporal bones, 113
Temporalis muscle, 154*f*, 157
  feline, 154*f*
Temporal muscle, 158*f*
Temporomandibular joint (TMJ), 112
Tendon
  of abductor pollicis longus muscle, 168*f*
  bowed, 167*b*
  common calcanean, 178–179*f*, 181*f*, 186–188*f*, 189
  of deep digital flexor muscle, 185*f*
  definition of, 149
  of flexor carpi radialis muscle, 170*f*
  of flexor carpi ulnaris muscle, 169*f*
  of interosseous muscles, 184*f*
  of long digital extensor muscle, 183–184*f*
  patellar, 176*f*
  peroneus longus, 185*f*
Tensor fasciae antebrachii muscle, 163*f*
Tensor fasciae latae muscle, 176–177*f*, 180*f*
Teres major muscle, 161*f*, 162, 163–165*f*, 171*f*, 187*f*
Teres minor muscle, 164*f*
Testes, 422, 424*f*
Testicular arteries, 309, 309*f*
Testicular vein
  canine, 311*f*
  feline, 310*f*
Testis capsule, 424, 426*f*
Tetraiodothyronine, 265
Thalamus, 212
Thick skin, 71–72, 73*f*
Thigh
  caudal muscles of, 174, 178–181
  cranial muscles of, 174, 182
  medial muscles of, 174, 181–182
Thin skin, 72, 73*f*
Third digit, 82
Third eyelid, 246, 246*f*
Thoracic cavity, 342
  blood vessels of, 304*f*, 307–308*f*, 312
    feline, 305–307*f*
    identification exercises for, 321, 324, 324–325*f*
  canine organs, 348*f*
Thoracic limb, 120–125
  blood vessels of, 315–319
    canine, 309*f*
    feline, 308*f*
Thoracic limb *(Continued)*
  extrinsic muscles of, 152–155
    exercises for, 192–194, 192*b*, 193*f*, 194*b*, 194*t*
  intrinsic muscles of, 159–173
    exercises for, 194–199, 194*b*, 194–195*f*, 196*b*, 198*b*, 198*t*
  muscles of, 149–151
Thoracolumbar fascia, 189*f*
Thorax
  canine, radiographs of, 304*f*
  feline, 306–308*f*
  organs of, 371–373*f*
  radiographs of, 304*f*
  superficial muscles of, 153 154*f*
Thymus, hormone production and action, 273*t*
Thyroglobulin, 265
Thyroid gland, 265, 275–278
  anatomy and histology of, 265, 266*f*
  clinical applications of, 265
  exercises for, 275–277*b*
  hormone physiology of, 265
  identification exercises for, 276*b*
  in-class activity, 265
Thyroid hormone, systemic effects of, 268*f*
Thyroid-stimulating hormone (TSH), 264*f*, 265
Thyrotropin-releasing hormone (TRH), 265
Thyroxine, 265
Tibia, 126–128, 179*f*
  canine, 128*f*
  equine, tibial crest of, 109*f*
Tibial nerve, 186*f*
Tibiotarsus, avian, 460
Tissues, 55, 60
  arrhythmogenic right ventricular cardiomyopathy, 69*b*
  capillary refill time, 69*b*
  clinical thinking challenge, 66*b*
  connective, 58–59, 58*b*
  epithelial, 55–58
  healing process of, 67*b*
  histologic preparation of, 62*b*, 62*f*
  identification of, 55
  microscope exercise for, 63*b*
  mucous membranes and clues, 69*b*
  muscle, 59–60, 59*b*
  nervous, 60, 60*b*, 60*f*
  types of, 54
Toe, 82
Tongue, cow, 336*f*
Trachea, 304*f*, 306–307*f*, 338, 350–351, 367, 368*f*
  avian, 461
  bifurcation of, 346*f*
  labeling exercises for, 350*b*, 350*f*
Transduction, 233
Transmission, 233
Transverse plane, 3*b*
Transversus abdominis muscle, 191
Trapezius muscle, 153*f*, 155

Traumatic reticulitis, 373, 373*f*
Triceps brachii muscle, 153–154*f*, 161*f*, 162–163, 163–164*f*, 171*f*
Tricuspid valve, 302, 303*f*, 318
Trigone of bladder, 405
Triiodothyronine, 265
Tripe, 370
Trochlear notch, 122
Tuber calcanei, 185*f*
Tuber ischium, of bovine pelvis, 109*f*
Tuber olecrani, 168–169*f*
Tuber sacrale, 176*f*
Turbinates, 118, 335, 337*f*
Tympanic bullae, 113
Tympanic membrane, 235

U

Ubiquitin protein, linear, 39–40
Ulna, 122
  canine, 123*f*
    olecranon process of, 110*f*
Ulnaris lateralis, 167
Ulnar nerve, 170*f*, 219, 219*f*
Umbilical cord, 437, 438–439*f*, 451–452
Umbilicus
  feline, 150
  inferior, 459–460
Ungual process, 80
Uniparous, 451
Urachus, 406
Ureters, 405, 405*f*
Urethra, 407, 407–408*f*
  male, 427, 427*f*
Urinary bladder, 406, 406*f*
  palpation of, 409
Urinary system, 399–420
  blood flow in, 400, 400*f*
  clinical and critical thinking for, 416, 416*b*, 416*f*
  clinical significance of, 399
  exercises for, 409–416, 409*b*, 416–420*b*
  in-class activities for, 409
  introduction of, 399–400
  kidney in, 402–403
    external features of, 402, 402–403*f*, 414–415
    internal features of, 403, 403–404*f*, 415–416
Urinary system *(Continued)*
  labeling exercises for, 410–415*f*, 420*f*
  location, 401–402, 401–402*f*, 411–414, 411–414*b*, 411–414*f*
  nephron notables in, 401
  on radiographs, 408
  ureters in, 405, 405*f*
  urethra in, 407, 407–408*f*
  urinary bladder in, 406, 406*f*
Uterine blood vessels, 311*f*, 435*f*
Uterine horn, 432*f*
Uterine layer, identification exercise for, 454*b*
Uterus, 433–434, 434*f*, 451
  avian, 461

V

Vagina, 436
  avian, 461
Vaginal smear, 20, 22*f*
Vaginal tunics, 424, 426*f*
  formation of, 425*f*
  identification exercise for, 441, 441*f*
Vagus nerve, 218, 218*f*
Vallate papillae, 233*b*, 234*f*
Vane, feather, 459–460
Vas deferens, 425, 426*f*
Vastus lateralis muscle, 178–181, 180*f*, 187*f*
Vastus medialis muscle, 181*f*
Vater's ampulla, 375
Vaults, 40
Veins, 299–300
Vena cava, 302
  caudal, 303, 308*f*, 309, 310*f*, 312, 312*f*
  cranial, 303, 305–306*f*, 308*f*
  in sheep heart, 315
Venipuncture sites, palpation of, 318
  clinical significance of, 318
Ventral, defined, 3, 3*b*
Ventricles, 300, 316–317*f*
Vertebra(e)
  anatomy of, 118*f*
  avian, 460
  canine cervical, 119*f*
  rabbit, 120–121*f*
  regions of, 118–119, 119*b*
  roles of, 98
  wings of atlas of, 110*f*
Vestibule, 236, 367, 367*f*, 436
Visceral vaginal tunic, 424
Vision, 237–246, 237*f*
  compartments of eye, 244, 244*f*
  external eye-related landmarks, 246, 247*f*
  extraocular muscles, 246
  eyelids and conjunctiva, 244–246
  inner nervous layer, 241–242, 241*f*
  middle vascular layer, 238–241
    choroid, 238–241, 240*f*
    ciliary body, 238, 239*f*
    iris, 238, 239*f*
    lens, 238, 240*f*
  optic chiasm, 242–244, 243*f*
  optic disc, 242, 242*f*
  optic nerve, 242, 243*f*
  outer fibrous layer of eye, 237–238, 237–238*f*
  third eyelid, 246, 246*f*
Vitamin D, 268
Vitreous compartment, 244
Vitreous humor, 244
Volatile fatty acids (VFA), 370
Vulva, 436, 436*f*

W

Wet mount slide, preparing and examining, 49*b*
Whiskers, 78
White line, 82
White matter, 210
  in brain, 214, 214*f*
  of cerebellum, 210*f*
  in spinal cord, 215
Whole blood, 286
Wings, anatomy of, 460
Working distance, 24
Wounds, microscopy of, 20

X

Xiphoid process, 120

Y

Yeast, photomicrograph of, 20, 21*f*

Z

Zonary attachment, of placenta, 451
Zygomatic bones, 113
Zygote, 452